Brudvik's Advanced Removable Partial Dentures
Second Edition

Dedication

To my wife, Deanne, and our children, Alice and Elliot,
for tolerating all those nights I would come home after a 10-hour workday
only to type away in my office all night.

One book, one tree: In support of reforestation worldwide and to address the climate crisis, for every book sold Quintessence Publishing will plant a tree (https://onetreeplanted.org/).

Library of Congress Cataloging-in-Publication Data

Names: Waliszewski, Michael P., author. | Brudvik, James S. Advanced removable partial dentures.
Title: Brudvik's advanced removable partial dentures / Michael P. Waliszewski.
Other titles: Advanced removable partial dentures
Description: Second edition. | Batavia, IL : Quintessence Publishing Co, Inc, [2022] | Preceded by Advanced removable partial dentures / James S. Brudvik. c1999. | Includes bibliographical references and index. | Summary: "Technical manual describing the function of each element of removable partial dentures, clinical and laboratory steps of RPD design and fabrication, and discussions of various types of prostheses and when/how to use them"-- Provided by publisher.
Identifiers: LCCN 2022014309 (print) | LCCN 2022014310 (ebook) | ISBN 9781647241025 (hardcover) | ISBN 9781647241445 (ebook)
Subjects: MESH: Denture, Partial, Removable
Classification: LCC RK667.I45 (print) | LCC RK667.I45 (ebook) | NLM WU 515 | DDC 617.6/93--dc23/eng/20220408
LC record available at https://lccn.loc.gov/2022014309
LC ebook record available at https://lccn.loc.gov/2022014310

A CIP record for this book is available from the British Library.
ISBN: 978-1-64724-102-5

QUINTESSENCE PUBLISHING USA

Quintessence Publishing Co, Inc
411 N Raddant Road
Batavia, IL 60510
www.quintpub.com

5 4 3 2 1

Editors: Marieke Z. Swerski and Leah Huffman
Design: Sue Zubek
Production: Angelina Schmelter

Printed in Croatia

BRUDVIK'S

ADVANCED REMOVABLE PARTIAL DENTURES

SECOND EDITION

Michael P. Waliszewski, DDS, MsD
Private Practice Limited to Prosthodontics
Brookfield, Wisconsin

Visiting Lecturer
University of Washington School of
Dentistry - Graduate Prosthodontics
Seattle, Washington

with contributions from

Hai Zhang, DMD, PhD
Professor
University of Washington School of Dentistry
Seattle, Washington

QUINTESSENCE PUBLISHING

Berlin | Chicago | Tokyo
Barcelona | London | Milan | Mexico City | Paris | Prague | Seoul | Warsaw
Beijing | Istanbul | Sao Paulo | Zagreb

CONTENTS

PREFACE

It was the Wednesday before Thanksgiving 2016. The day prior, I had lectured to the current graduate prosthodontic residents at my alma mater, the University of Washington Graduate Prosthodontics (UWGP) Program. Dr James Brudvik, affectionately referred to as "The Colonel" by UWGP alumni, had attended. He of course wouldn't miss the opportunity to listen to anything related to removable partial dentures. The phone call was out of the ordinary; email usually sufficed in the interim between my Seattle visits:

> "I have a favor to ask you, Mike."
> "Yes, Colonel."
> "I think it's time to update 'Das Book' [as he called it], and I think you're the only one who might have any interest in doing it."

As usual, he was correct on both counts. Originally published in 1999, *Advanced Removable Partial Dentures* was Dr Brudvik's effort to share "a more sophisticated look at this treatment modality." It was legendary among the residents. Most of us would wait until graduation was assured, and then we would ask him to sign the inside cover as evidence of prosthodontic knowledge well earned. While it was never meant to be more than a monograph, the information it contained was the rare resource that helped us manage actual (rather than theoretical) technical problems. Throughout the course of this update and really ever since I met the Colonel in 2002, the energy and enthusiasm he has for this topic never waned. The lack of this level of RPD energy within dentistry is palpable.

Now, nearly 6 years since the Colonel's phone call, it's clear that this project was always going to be more than a simple update. I am honored to present this topic in greater depth and intensity than in the first edition. All of the original diagrams, drawn by Dr Brudvik himself, remain. These have been supplemented with images of relevant clinical cases where highlighting was necessary. These images come from one of three sources: *(1)* my own clinical cases and work, *(2)* images from Dr Brudvik's University of Washington archive, or, where I was able to identify specific UWGP alumni, *(3)* images from past students of Dr Brudvik's.

References to specific RPD and related research has also been added. This reference list is a biased one, as it includes the entirety of Dr Brudvik's peer-reviewed RPD literature. Beyond these additions, there is a 40% increase in subject matter and four additional chapters. Despite this updating, the intention was to maintain the original feel and purpose of the first edition. The introduction to the first edition, included for context, explains how this is a text for experienced RPD providers and graduate students looking to provide care at a higher level.

The volume of information included reflects how influential Dr Brudvik has been in keeping the RPD a relevant, successful, and advanced means of tooth replacement. The philosophy and ideas presented here come from Dr Brudvik and the many colleagues, residents, and technicians with whom he interacted and shared RPD enthusiasm. As I see it, my most worthwhile contribution beyond organizer was selecting the title of this work. When informing the Colonel that the plan was to title it *Brudvik's Advanced Removable Partial Dentures*, he was hesitant. In what is the only time I ever superseded the Colonel's authority, my reply was that this is the way it has to be. No more was said on the issue. This reflects the humble nature and goodwill that so many at the University of Washington, and I gather during his military days as well, came to know. He was more interested in what the student could do with the knowledge given than the accolades the teacher would receive. Now 89 and recently entered into memory care, Dr Brudvik will unfortunately no longer be encouraging students and clinicians to do better RPDs. It is therefore left to the rest of us to not let the RPD remain neglected and ill-considered. While his name will live on with his many students and this title, his legacy can only continue if more read this book and put its lessons into practice.

Acknowledgments

Beyond Dr Brudvik himself, there are many who have at various points contributed to the information and philosophy within this textbook. This is one of the reasons why all of Dr Brudvik's peer-reviewed and published articles are included. In them the reader will find numerous worthy coauthors, all sharing and contributing to Dr Brudvik's philosophy and energy. It must be noted that there was an unofficial edit of *Advanced Removable Partial Dentures* that Dr Brudvik completed with Dr Sami Dogan in January 2014. This was a digital copy, with some updating and editing, that was shared among many after the 1999 version went out of print in 2008.

Dr Hai Zhang, now full professor at the University of Washington, was a most valuable contributor to this project. Chapters 5, 6, 7, and 13 were all first handled by Dr Zhang prior to further editing. His greater contribution, however, was being the on-site contact at the University of Washington. Between finding old slides, contacting the company 3DRPD, and detailing many of the digital fabrication concepts, Dr Zhang was a key man throughout this project.

Acknowledgments for certain specific images can be found in the margin here. As previously mentioned, all but a single drawing comes from the first edition, with Dr Brudvik as the original artist. The vast majority of images, listed without any acknowledgment, are my own. There are a fair number of images that come from the "Dr James Brudvik archive." This is the collection of material that Dr Brudvik used to lecture with extensively. These are images of his own cases, images taken by or for the University of Washington School of Dentistry, as well as images from cases treated by various University of Washington residents while in the Graduate Prosthodontics Program. Where I was able, I acknowledged the name of the resident who treated the case in the photograph. There are, however, a handful that went unidentified and are therefore listed simply under "Dr James Brudvik archive." For not being able to match 100% of these images to a specific resident, I apologize. For all those who were able to share images for this book, I thank you once again. These include Dr Hongseok An, Ruth Bourke (BSc), Dr Jacopo Castelnuovo, Dr Kinsey Chitswe, Dr Daniel Domagala, Dr Yoshihiro Goto, Dr Yu-Bin (Crystal) Hsu, Dr Jack Keesler, Dr Seungbum Lee, Dr Marie (Val) Lim, Dr Shwey-Chun (Polly) Ma, Dr Tal Morr, Dr Ricardo Mitrani, Dr Rosario Palacios, Dr Alexander Shor, Dr Kavita Shor, Dr Kenneth Waliszewski, Dr Keng Mun Wong, Dr Hai Zhang, and the company 3DRPD.

In this list above, one should notice a Dr Kenneth Waliszewski. This is my father. By accounts more unbiased than my own, he is the most honest, well-respected, and selfless retired prosthodontist in Wisconsin. Without his (and my mother's) loving encouragement for our entire family, things would not have turned out so well for all. His lessons of hard work, honesty, and giving were more valuable than anything I learned in school (including his crown and bridge course at Marquette).

IMAGE CREDITS

Dr James Brudvik archive
1-15, 1-16, 1-17, 1-19, 1-20(a,b), 3-21(a–c), 4-2(a,b), 4-5(a–d), 5-2(a,b), 5-4(a,b), 5-5, 5-11(a–d), 5-12, 5-13, 5-15, 5-16(a,c), 6-37d, 7-1b, 8-3, 8-4, 8-7, 8-9, 9-9, 9-20, 9-22, 9-23, 9-24, 10-26(a–d), 12-2a, 12-7, 12-8, 13-5, 13-7, 13-17, 13-18, 13-19, 13-37, 13-41

Dr Jack Keesler
2-8(a,b)

Dr Kinsey Chitswe
2-12a

Dr Yoshihiro Goto
2-12b, 3-18, 11-5, 11-6, 11-26(a–c)

Dr Rosario Palacios
2-23, 3-12b

Dr Kenneth Waliszewski
3-4

Dr Shwey-Chun (Polly) Ma
4-6, 4-16, 12-2b, 12-3(a,b), 13-34

Dr Hongseok An
5-1(a,b), 6-37(a–c), 6-38(a–e)

Dr Seungbum Lee
6-31(a,b)

Dr Daniel Domagala
6-35

Dr Hai Zhang
6-39

3DRPD
6-40, 6-41, 6-42

Dr Val Lim and Ruth Bourke, BSc
8-13, 8-19

Dr Jacopo Castelnuovo
12-5(a–f), 13-38

Dr Tal Morr
13-3(a,b), 13-16

Dr Yu-Bin Hsu
13-4, 13-6(a,b), 13-8

Dr Ricardo Mitrani
13-10, 13-11, 13-12, 13-13, 13-14(a,b), 13-32, 13-40, 13-42b

Dr Kavita Shor
14-14, 14-15, 14-16

Dr Keng Mun Wong
14-17(a–e)

INTRODUCTION TO THE SECOND EDITION

Michael P. Waliszewski, DDS, MSD

The Philosophy of Care outlined by Dr Brudvik in the Introduction to the First Edition remains a modern, logical, and successful approach to successful RPDs. There have, however, been significant changes to how this approach is applied. These changes are most obvious in the new or most extensively expanded chapters 1, 3, 10, 13, 14, and 15.

Dentistry in general is more attuned to risk assessment than in the past. If dentists can control why dental disease occurs, logically they should be able to prevent it. Focusing on prevention rather than replacement, as recommended and highlighted in the first edition, has finally become the standard-of-care approach. For patients who are good at losing teeth, like partially edentulous patients, there can be no other way to treatment plan. The caries management by risk assessment (CAMBRA) protocols are tools that were not available to traditional RPD clinicians. These types of modern disease management protocols are highlighted in chapter 1. Chapter 3 reflects in great detail the need to separate tooth and tissue support when planning and designing. This is noted as even more necessary when "extreme" Kennedy classifications are considered.

Chapter 10 advances the disease management mentality of chapter 1, through a discussion of interim protheses. Often mentioned but previously little detailed, nonmetal RPDs now have a full chapter dedicated to their use. Advances in material technology and their influence on real-world, everyday clinical care are highlighted within this chapter.

A greatly expanded and better organized chapter 13 deals with dental implants and partial dentures. The early adoption of implants into RPD therapy at the University of Washington has given graduates the advantage of long-term outcome analysis. Multiple methods and philosophies for incorporating implants, even preexisting ones, into RPD treatment is detailed. Chapter 14 is more or less an extension of chapter 13, as metal frameworks are so integral to implant prostheses. An earlier version of this chapter on frameworks for implant overdentures was created for the unpublished edit of *Advanced Removable Partial Dentures* when it became obvious that the volume and detail of information on this neglected topic warranted dedicated space.

Having graduated from Marquette University School of Dentistry in 2002 and then from the University of Washington Graduate Prosthodontics Program in 2005, I had access to direct mentorship from exceptionally experienced prosthodontists who still remembered a time "before dental implants." Their respect for and appreciation of osseointegration offered a level-headed and unbiased comparison with conventional means of tooth replacement. With their retirement and the overall thinning of the dental educator ranks (I now list myself as a former faculty member), one wonders where current students might receive unbiased mentorship in regard to conventional prosthodontics. It does not appear Dr Brudvik's assessment that "dental schools make a serious effort to teach the subject" is still the case in the year 2022.

Where does this leave the RPD if the quality seen in most commercial laboratories and updated cross-sectional studies indicate further deterioration? Chapter 15 has been added to highlight key historical reasons for how and why the RPD has evolved. The turning point in RPD philosophy, predicted when the parent article to this chapter was written, no longer appears accessible for the average dental patient at the corner dental service organization chain location. In today's environment of large group or managed practices providing ever faster, cheaper, and more efficient care, one wonders if most dentists will do anything other than "install" partial dentures made from digital scans that the assistants made and sent immediately to a lab. The counter to this pessimistic outlook, confirmed by the experience of nearly all prosthodontists interested in RPDs, is that the volume of partially edentulous patients who could benefit from the philosophy of this textbook is ever-increasing. Patients frustrated by poor results overseen by uneducated or disinterested providers will seek out those who can help in an unbiased, conventional, and economical way. Herein lies the path to continued relevance for the RPD.

INTRODUCTION TO THE FIRST EDITION

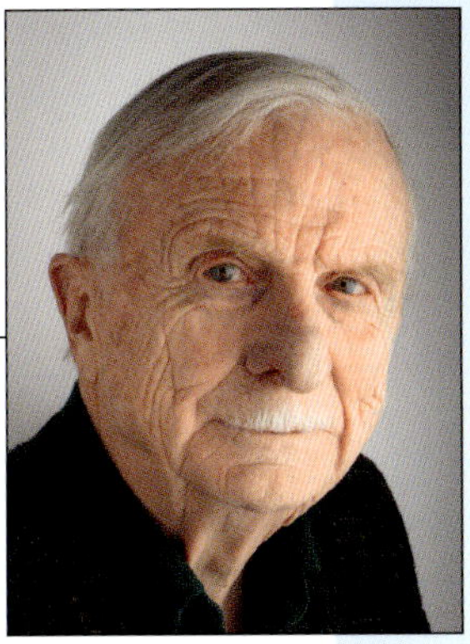

(1933–2022)

James S. Brudvik, DDS, FACP
Professor Emeritus of Prosthodontics
University of Washington School of Dentistry
Seattle, Washington

The removable partial denture has long been considered an inferior means of replacing missing teeth and associated structures when compared with the fixed partial denture. Some have even spoken of it as a stepping stone to a complete denture. The old rhyme, "Little RPD, don't you cry, you'll be a CD by and by," may best express past feelings toward this treatment modality. Many surveys, published over the years in our journals, indicate that dentistry does a rather poor job with the RPD. These reports testify to the fact that most RPDs are created entirely by the technician with a minimum of input from the clinician in the form of mouth preparation or design.

Dental schools make a serious effort to teach the subject, and excellent texts are available for the undergraduate. Nonetheless, the state of RPDs seen in the commercial laboratories and in the cross-sectional studies available to us indicates that, in general, RPDs are poorly designed and constructed and poorly maintained.

Therefore, it is no wonder that patients dislike their RPDs to the point of not wearing them and, if they can afford alternative treatment, request it routinely. It has been our experience that the patient who states, "I had a partial once and couldn't wear it!" most likely had a substandard prosthesis and, when treated with a partial denture that is made to the state of the art, finds it tolerable and easily accepts the limitations of this form of tooth and tissue replacement.

Plainly stated, there is a dramatic difference between the standard RPD and the one that approaches the state of the art as we know it today. It was in the attempt to create that quality RPD that this manuscript was written. It is intended to serve as a guide to both graduate students in prosthodontics and concerned general practitioners; to challenge them to think of the removable appliance as they would the fixed partial denture, with all the same considerations of soft tissue management, caries control, periodontal support, orthodontic therapy, and implant involvement. In almost every clinical situation, the patient who requires a removable partial denture will have a need for some form of fixed prosthodontics as well, from a simple bonded rest to the most complex precision attachments extending from fixed units.

This work is not intended to be a textbook in the classical sense. It will not have a bibliography or extensive illustrations. It is, rather, a monograph on the removable partial denture, written with the expectation that the reader will already have covered the basics of the partial denture and is now ready to take a more sophisticated look at this treatment modality. Here, then, are our thoughts as they have evolved in over 50 years of practice and teaching in this fascinating area.

Philosophy of Care

What makes a successful RPD? At the risk of oversimplification, one could say that the successful removable appliance need be only six things:

1. **Strong:** It does not wear, break, distort, or come apart when worn.
2. **Stable:** It will have maximum lateral contact with abutment teeth through parallel guide planes, which will limit the path of removal to as close to 0 degrees as possible.
3. **Retentive:** It remains in position in the patient's mouth during use and gives the patient confidence that it will continue to do so over its life.
4. **Esthetic:** It will satisfy the patient's expectations without undue evidence of its presence.
5. **Comfortable:** It will have the minimal amount of metal and resin necessary to support abutments and replace missing tissue.
6. **Pain-free:** It does not cause discomfort when in the mouth for the short term and causes no long-term damage to either hard or soft tissue over its life.

If these six requirements can be met, the RPD stands a good chance of long-term success. Unfortunately, the success of the RPD in and of itself does not guarantee the long-term health of the remaining teeth and soft tissues. Maintenance therefore becomes the primary factor in the long-term success of the treatment. The profession has usually substituted concern over the type of clasp to be used for the more fundamental requirements of regularly scheduled recall and appropriate maintenance. Preparing the mouth to its very best state of health before starting prosthodontic procedures and then keeping the tissues in that state of health over the life of the RPD is far more important than any design considerations. It has become obvious to us that a partial denture in a healthy mouth—assuming that it meets our six requirements—will be successful regardless of its design. Rest placement and clasp design, interesting as they may be to argue over from a theoretical point of view, are simply not germane to the real question of what makes a successful RPD. Suppositions derived from bench studies do not necessarily transfer to the clinical realities of long-term care. We can think of the factors that compose successful RPD treatment in these percentages:

- Maintenance: 50%
- Mouth preparation: 23%
- Construction: 23%
- Design: 4%

How long should a properly designed, constructed, and maintained RPD last? Good evidence exists that this state-of-the-art partial could be expected to last a minimum of 10 years, assuming that the patient was seen at regular intervals and that both the mouth and the RPD received the indicated maintenance. RPDs providing good service for 20 years are not unheard of, although the long-term maintenance requirements increase dramatically after 10 years.

The construction of the RPD, more than any other form of dental therapy, is almost always delegated to the dental laboratory because the equipment required to produce an acceptable cast framework is not going to be found in the dental office. In many cases, the clinician may have never even met the technicians creating the prostheses. This fact requires that the clinicians maintain control by inserting themselves into the process at the critical steps in construction. These steps will be covered in depth in this manuscript. Because the actual construction is relegated, the average clinician is apt to have very little confidence or experience in these matters and is likely to take the technician's view of the design and construction process—a view that will be more mechanical than biologic. The wise clinician will make a point of remaining in close contact with the technician and bringing these auxiliaries into the clinical aspects of care whenever possible.

The modern removable partial denture combines fixed and removable prosthodontics with implant support when key abutments are missing and requires a thorough understanding of both aspects of care by the clinician and by the technician. Unfortunately, the evolution of the dental laboratory industry has separated technicians into often isolated specialties: complete dentures, removable partial dentures, and fixed partial dentures and implant prostheses. The technician who is knowledgeable in all areas is a vanishing breed. In order to direct the construction of the most sophisticated restorations, the clinician must assume the responsibility of coordinating the laboratory phases. This text is intended to set standards of care for the comprehensive management of the partially edentulous patient who will require some form of a removable restoration.

Patient satisfaction with their RPD has been studied and several factors identified. Age, general health, previous experience with a partial denture, and the opposing dentition all have been shown to play a role in how the patient views their new partial denture. Older patients are more apt to accept the limitations of the partial. The better the patient's overall health, the greater their satisfaction with the same effect based on the amount of experience they have had. As could be expected, what they have in the opposing arch will be a factor as well. Having a removable appliance in both arches increases their dissatisfaction with their partials. These factors must be discussed with the patient as a part of their informed consent to treatment with RPDs and may well influence their decision to consider other forms of treatment, especially now when implant options have become a clinical reality.

TREATMENT PLANNING

1

These patients have demonstrated the ability to lose teeth.

The Challenges of Partial Edentulism

Patients with RPDs, having demonstrated the ability to lose teeth, are high risk and will remain that way as long as they have remaining natural teeth. To forget this fundamental fact is to disregard the dental history of the average RPD patient. Why have these teeth been lost? What has been or will be done to keep more teeth from being lost? Dentists are all too quick to consider the patient "cured" after several fillings and a visit for root planing. What is the value of this treatment if the etiologic factors remain unresolved, as is typically the case? The traditional focus of RPD therapy has been on the technical expertise required to make a quality partial denture. Unfortunately, the technical outcome is far less influential than disease management in maintaining the remaining dentition. In other words, maintenance of dental health is the primary determinant of long-term success with RPDs. Maintenance, as a separate and distinct part of the patient's ongoing treatment plan, is the core requirement for good outcomes.

RPDs are typically unfairly blamed for contributing to tooth loss. This association often overlooks an error in judgment when the treatment was originally planned. Patients with multiple recent extractions are typically rushed through the process of RPD fabrication without regard to continued disease risk. The patient, now with tooth replacements, often goes on their way with the etiologic factors still present. It should not be a surprise then when caries or periodontitis returns a short time later and the process of treatment begins all over again.

Modern RPD therapy must address the dental disease process rather than continue to be overwhelmingly focused on technical issues. As with any definitive prosthodontic therapy, initial therapy must first manage the reasons why disease occurred in the first place. Only after successful initial therapy can definitive (long-term) therapy be considered. This requires patience on the part of the patient and the provider. It may also mean that an interim prosthesis will be necessary while time is given for the patient to demonstrate whether the disease is truly under control.

Caries

Caries is currently the most prevalent dental disease by a wide margin. Since the 1990s, the caries experience within the adolescent and adult population appears to have leveled off with little recent change.[1,2] Among US adults aged 50 to 64 years evaluated in 2011 and 2012, 97% had dental caries experience (either active caries or a dental restoration). Some data show that the dental caries experience for older adults may even be increasing.[3] It appears that the influence of fluoride in general has

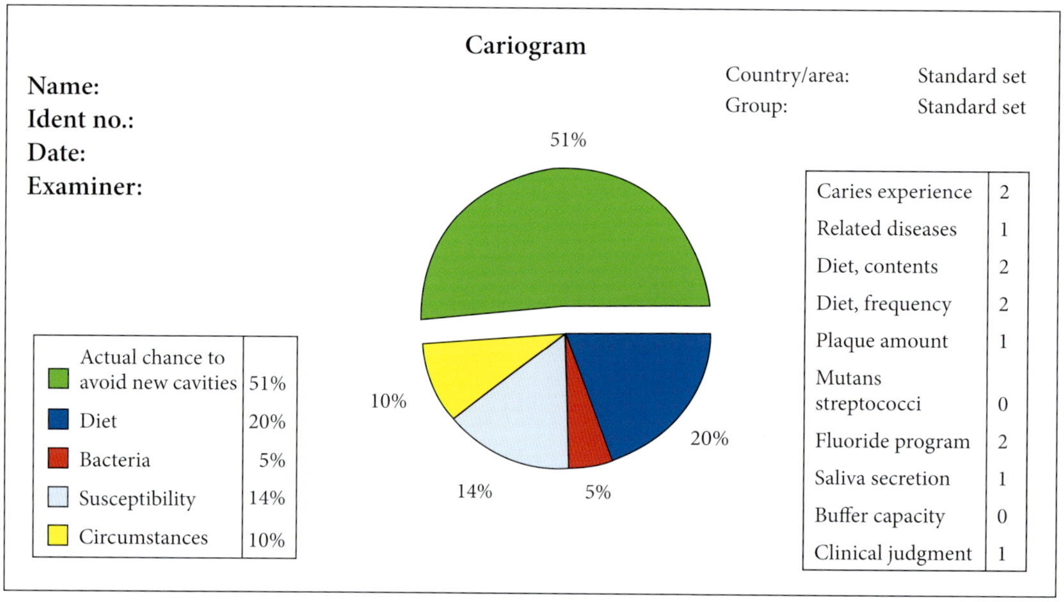

FIG 1-1 An example Cariogram from the open-access software. A "preliminary interpretation and proposed measures" are also created after data input is complete. It therefore provides risk assessment as well as guidelines for preventive treatment.

been maximized. Further gains may be difficult considering the current cariogenic diets of developed countries. Much of the lack of improvement is due to high rates of caries and tooth loss within lower socioeconomic populations. This is also the population of patients least likely to be able to afford more expensive fixed prosthodontic treatment options.

Using diagnostic aids to determine future risk prior to treatment decision-making is an absolute requirement. This is a major philosophical shift away from dentistry's "drill and fill" approach that does nothing more than manage the consequences of caries. Articles such as those by Anderson et al[4] are classic summaries about changing the mindset of the profession to one focused on disease prevention rather than treatment. Once caries experience has been confirmed, determining future risk by use of a caries risk assessment tool is now considered the standard of care. Traditionally, the Venn diagram was a good starting point for this risk assessment. However, this limited analysis has been expanded to include the many significant challenges imposed by socioeconomic and medical realities. The American Dental Association has a more appropriate yet still efficient standardized caries risk assessment form available free online.[5] It assists with evidence-based classification of low-, medium-, or high-risk individuals. A third method to determine risk is the Cariogram. This is an open-access computer program that graphically illustrates caries risk and the etiologic factors behind it (Fig 1-1). It was designed as an educational tool for both dentists and patients and is also easily available online.[6]

Several systems exist that incorporate caries risk analysis with caries risk prevention recommendations. One such system utilized frequently in the United States is the CAMBRA protocol. CAMBRA stands for Caries Management By Risk Assessment. It was developed as an evidence-based approach to preventing and managing cavities at the earliest stages. Internationally, the ICCMS (International Caries Classification and Management System) is another. The ICCMS is a comprehensive way of using and following the modern noninvasive caries management philosophy. Its purpose is to deliver effective risk-based caries therapy that prevents new lesions, controls initial caries nonoperatively, and preserves tooth tissue at all times. These systems are most effective when used before patients lose teeth or—better still—before patients experience carious lesions.

Unfortunately, for the patients we wish to treat with RPDs, the consequences of disease have already been severe, and reversal of the risk factors may not be possible (Figs 1-2 and 1-3). This makes the philosophical shift to disease prevention more challenging within prosthodontics. The preventive strategies employed must therefore be more aggressive and thoroughly applied if further tooth loss is to be prevented.[7] While not always successful, caries experience can be reduced when preventive strategies are

FIG 1–2 A Cariogram with the data input as shown.

Cariogram

Name: Mrs Lotsa Caries
Ident no.: 4321
Date: April 1, 2020
Examiner: Dr James Brudvik

Country/area: Standard set
Group: Standard set

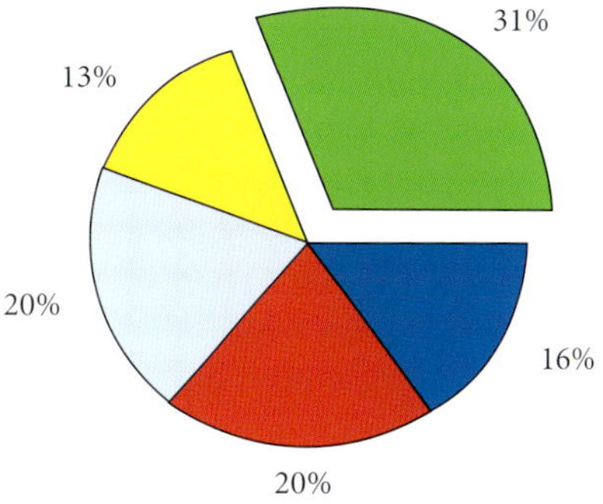

Actual chance to avoid new cavities	31%
Diet	16%
Bacteria	20%
Susceptibility	20%
Circumstances	13%

Caries experience	2	Worse than normal for age
Related diseases	1	A diabetic with mild hypertension, taking medication
Diet, contents	2	Moderate content of fermentable carbohydrates
Diet, frequency	1	4 to 5 intakes per day, including snacks
Plaque amount	2	Plaque Index of 2
Mutans streptococci	_	Not tested, no number is input
Fluoride program	2	Fluoride toothpaste, no supplements
Saliva secretion	2	Tested rate was 0.5–0.9 mL stimulated saliva/min
Buffer capacity	0	Adequate, Dentobuff test result is blue
Clinical judgment	1	Normal setting, risk in line with evidence

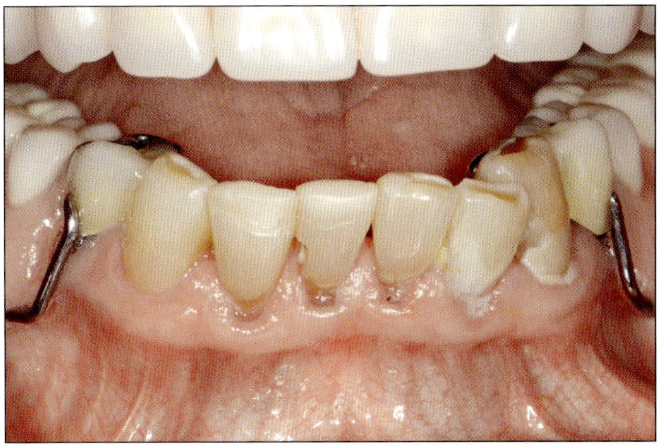

FIG 1–3 In the Cariogram in Fig 1-2, the "chance" to avoid caries was 31%. This is quite low. The severity of these risk factors predicts new caries lesions in this environment. Unsurprisingly, caries returned 2 years after this patient was treated. The patient factors listed are typical of the average RPD patient.

applied as designed. Due to the desire to reduce recurrent disease, dental benefit plans are beginning to require caries risk assessments prior to restorative intervention. This trend is likely to continue.

Periodontal disease

Periodontal disease is commonly a more generalized disease process, resulting in the loss of multiple teeth rather than on an individual basis as with caries. When severe periodontal disease is considered on its own, the prevalence was found to be 9%.[8] It is currently accepted that periodontitis largely stems from various biologic, systemic, and pro-inflammatory mediators.[9] Due to the complexity of the disease, the etiologic factors can be many and varied. On a population level, sex, age, smoking, diabetes, and ethnicity are just a few of the factors that may predict an individual's risk.[10]

Management of periodontal disease is admittedly noncurative. Patients at risk due to systemic or genetic predispositions will remain at risk for attachment loss after treatment. The necessity to continually address the etiologic factors for the disease was identified much earlier within the periodontal community than the same philosophy was for caries management. The need for posttreatment periodontal maintenance is clear. The standard of care established for all high-risk periodontal disease patients is more frequent professional cleanings with dedicated oral hygiene instruction and reinforcement. That being said, even after disease is established and without any further treatment, the rate of progression at specific teeth may be slow and infrequent.[11]

The idea that the RPD complicates the oral environment by its presence has been extensively researched. Certain results indicate that this is the case. Plaque retention, bacterial levels, and gingival inflammation have been shown to increase after an RPD is placed. However, when this research is more closely evaluated, the RPDs in use by the research population often fail to meet the standard of care for long-term prostheses.[12–16] The presence of acrylic resin, gingival coverage, and tissue impingement all contribute to negative tissue response and can be managed by prosthesis design. That makes the negative periodontal conclusions made by these articles pertinent only to RPDs that fall below the standard of care.

Often, the result of the research is speculative in nature rather than proof of causation. If we know the risk remains after losing teeth due to periodontitis, is it fair to blame the RPD that follows for the periodontitis? Taken as a whole, when controlled studies on patients wearing definitive RPDs are conducted, the results show that the RPDs are not contributing to disease progression if the patients consistently follow standard disease management protocols. This means that if these high-risk patients receive RPDs that adhere to certain standards of care, and if these patients follow the disease management protocols dentistry has developed, then the RPD will not be the cause of further destruction.[17–21] The idea of poorly maintained and designed RPDs contributing to inflammation and bacterial colonization in the mouth will continue to be highlighted throughout this textbook.

Malocclusion

On the most basic level, all occlusal concepts begin with the goal of having even and simultaneous bilateral contact. Due to lost, migrated, restored, or fractured teeth, this type of contact is often missing in debilitated partially edentulous situations. Assuming that there are opposing occlusal contacts in each arch, these contacts must occur evenly, simultaneously, and bilaterally. From a treatment perspective, this allows accurate and reliable articulation of casts or digital scans. It also gives the clinician a defined point from which to assess whether the prosthesis itself creates any interferences that need adjustment. Easy-to-miss, subtle interferences can contribute to further migration, more rapid attrition, framework displacement, and fractures (Fig 1-4a). This means an equilibration is almost always indicated before prosthesis fabrication (Fig 1-4b). If it is not done, the dentist will be relying on the prosthetic teeth to restore a comfortable and stable articulation. This is exceedingly difficult and infrequently maintained when there are limited opposing natural tooth contacts. For these reasons, the goal of having centric occlusion coincident with maximal intercuspal position needs to be met more stringently in RPD patients than in completely dentate patients.

On an arch relationship level, there is a belief that Class II malocclusions have significant biologic cost in the form of attrition, fracture, and reduced longevity of restorations.[22–27] Perhaps this is why prosthodontists believe that a larger percentage of their patient-practice base is Class II, when compared with that of the average general dentist. This in turn implies that patients with these malocclusions, and with malocclusions in general, have significant dental consequences.

Research into the effects of malocclusion on masticatory efficiency has been inconclusive.[28–30] This is partly due to the lack of correlation between the subjective experience of masticatory performance and the objective masticatory efficiency.[28] If muscle forces and mandibular movement patterns are not in harmony with the hard tissue determinants of occlusion (namely the teeth), excessive and more frequent contact of the opposing teeth may result.[31] This type of dysfunction may have symptoms of increased rates of attrition, periodontal concerns, or fracture. In some examples, this type of dysfunction has been described as *traumatic occlusion*.[32–34] In essence, a biologic problem like caries weakens the restorative condition of the teeth, creating an environment where malocclusions are now much more influential. The implication is that significant malocclusions are tolerated without biologic complications until the physiology is disrupted. Once this occurs, these malocclusions often need more aggressive correction to prevent damage to oral structures. This is clearly the situation for

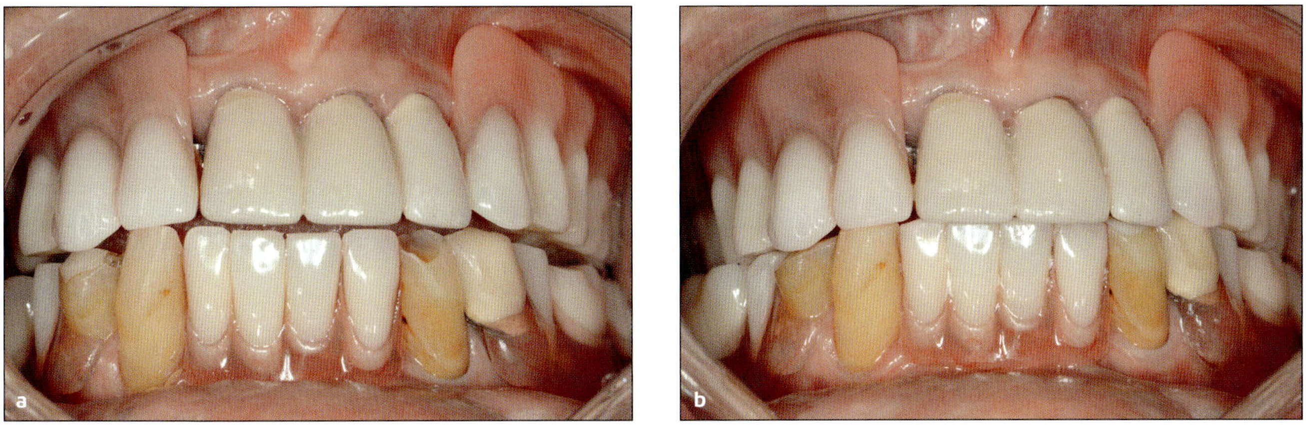

FIG 1-4 *(a)* An obvious interference between prosthetic and natural teeth. This particular interference is contributing to instability, wear, and tooth fracture of both prostheses. *(b)* The same patient, now after an occlusal equilibration done as part of initial therapy. This allows the clinician to confirm the diagnoses and helps predict the outcome with the new prostheses.

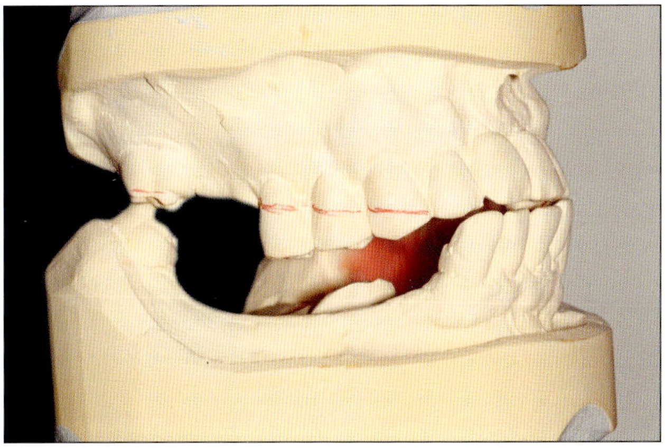

FIG 1-5 Properly articulated diagnostic casts are necessary to determine the extent of a malocclusion. These casts demonstrate the significant problem this skeletal Class III patient has with his occlusal plane.

partially edentulous patients. Normal physiology has been disrupted, typically by the loss of several teeth, which allows the negative influence of a previously tolerated malocclusion to become significant.

Diagnosis of a malocclusion is not always possible with simple examination. More often than not, articulated diagnostic casts are required to accurately and thoroughly diagnose occlusal relationships (Fig 1-5). While experienced operators can find more occlusal interferences than can novices, even they must rely on diagnostic casts for the complex situations that often present. Beyond defining interferences, diagnostic casts help demonstrate the extent of occlusal plane and interocclusal space issues. Casts, when properly articulated, will demonstrate these issues and the clinician's options to address them. Most common among these is the lack of space for prosthetic teeth or components of the RPD. It is also the author's opinion that with the current state and cost of the technology, this procedure is more efficient and accurate when done on an analog rather than digital basis.

Disease Management

In practice, the sequence of treatment for potential RPD patients can take three basic routes. The particular sequence is based on the patient's risk profile determined at the initial examination. While all RPD patients are high risk when compared with the average dental patient, we must further subdivide them into low-, high-, and extreme-risk categories. A low-risk profile is one where we would expect to be successful in managing the risk factors and disease. Commonly, these are long-time RPD or fixed partial denture patients who require a new removable prosthesis due to a technical rather than biologic failure. These patients can typically proceed rapidly into definitive prosthodontic therapy.

A high-risk profile is one where the patient presents with active generalized disease. These patients commonly have existing or recently failed prostheses (Fig 1-6). The challenge with these patients is determining whether their disease can be controlled long-term. This determination cannot be made

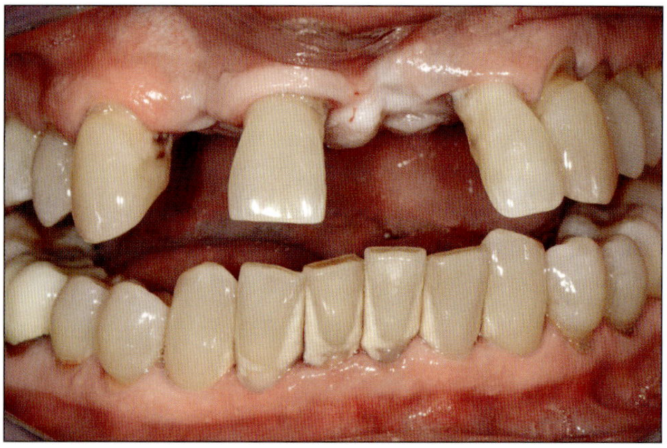

FIG 1-6 Pretreatment photograph of a patient with severe generalized periodontal disease. It will take time to reestablish oral health. It is not advisable to proceed with definitive prosthodontics until this has occurred.

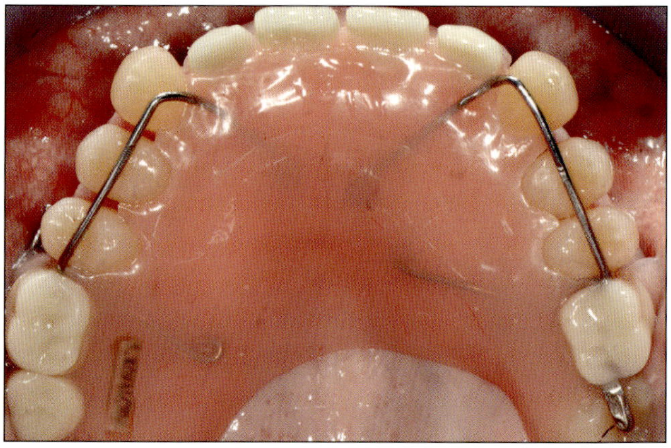

FIG 1-7 After beginning initial therapy. An interim resin-based RPD was used during the disease-control phase for this patient.

quickly. It often requires a period of initial therapy to first manage and then prevent disease. The only way to determine whether disease has been controlled is to recall and evaluate the patient over time. This presents many challenges for those in everyday clinical practice. The idea of delaying definitive prosthodontic care is given little more than cursory lip service in dental school. Once in practice, the day-to-day demands of production-oriented care pushes providers to "complete care." Likewise, the patient frequently demands that their functional and esthetic condition be improved. Most certainly, these are the main reasons that brought them to the dentist in the first place. This means the definitive RPD is made as soon after active disease removal as the dentist's schedule allows. Unfortunately, this eliminates the time period for actual risk reduction and leaves the new RPD in an oral environment just as at-risk for disease as when the patient first entered the dental office. Herein lies the main reason for so many of the biologic RPD failures.

These high-risk patients must have their dental health reestablished. This means the patient is free from active caries, periodontitis, and other dental disease processes. When RPD patients are managed this way, definitive crowns and other complex restorative dentistry is avoided at all costs. This may require long-term provisional crowns or large core build-ups that are not prepared for full-coverage crowns. If the patient is missing anterior teeth or long spans of posterior teeth, an interim RPD will likely be required as well (Fig 1-7). This common and important treatment modality allows the dentist to address immediate need without committing to more expensive and extensive therapy. These prostheses are discussed in detail in chapter 10. Once the patient is "under control," they are placed in a personalized maintenance program. Examples of typical disease-control and maintenance procedures are listed in Table 1-1. The frequency and type of treatment is dependent on the patient's risk level. The higher the risk, the more intense and frequent the recall and procedures.

When RPD patients are maintained by regularly attending a professional prophylaxis appointment with dedicated oral hygiene instruction, the recurrence of disease is low and the continued successful use of the RPD is high.[16–20] Recent research into risk-based caries and periodontal disease-control supports the risk-based management philosophy.[35,36]

Many of the commonly cited references for RPDs being a risk factor for disease actually indicate that the RPD itself has no significant detrimental effect when oral hygiene protocols are followed.[37–41] In fact, many of the plaque or bacteriologic tests were completed after the test subjects were told to not brush their teeth or during the time period between regular prophylaxis appointments. Regardless, all the research noted reinforces the critical need of increasing the frequency of regular prophylaxis with oral hygiene instruction for RPD patients.

The key point to be repeatedly stressed is that definitive therapy is not conducted until a demonstrated reduction in risk has occurred. Evidence of risk reduction is only found when patients present disease-free at reevaluations. The dentist must then determine the length of time needed before proceeding to definitive therapy. In general, the higher the risk, the longer the period required to determine successful disease control. A major advantage of this protocol is that the posttreatment maintenance program has already been established and proven successful prior to the definitive RPD being fabricated. This tends to greatly increase the odds of long-term RPD survival. It does so by weeding out those

Table 1-1 The most popular and effective preventive procedures for RPD patients

RISK FACTOR	PREVENTIVE MEASURE	PROVIDER	SUGGESTED PROTOCOL
All RPD patients	Increased recall frequency	In office	Minimum two times per year with frequency determined by risk assessment. Extreme risk cases may require recall as frequently as every 2 months.
	Oral hygiene instruction	Dental hygienist	Repeated at every recall. A dedicated time period of personal interaction to review and critique previous effectiveness. Time must be given to practice proper technique and demonstrate results. Plaque-disclosing agents facilitate patient understanding. This time includes instruction on cleaning of the RPD itself.
	Dental prophylaxis	Dental hygienist	A prophylaxis appointment duration should be at least 1 hour. This includes time for operatory setup and cleaning. Effectiveness of the necessary preventive measures listed here is questionable if less time is available. As fewer teeth are present, the time shifts from cleaning of the natural teeth to cleaning of the prosthesis and oral hygiene instruction.
Caries (low risk)	Diet counseling and modification	Dental team and at home	A discussion and review of risk factors found in a patient interview. Review of a 5-day diet history completed by the patient tends to be more effective and can be analyzed by a nutritionist or online at https://www.esha.com/products/food-processor/. Follow-up is required for assessment of modification and can be completed efficiently with front-office phone calls.
	Xylitol lozenges	At home	Frequent dosing required for effectiveness. Must ensure product provides effective concentration. Some risk of gastrointestinal disturbance. Chewing-gum versions not appropriate for RPD patients.
	Prescription-strength fluoride toothpaste	At home	Generally for the average-risk RPD patient. Typically used after regular hygiene procedures prior to bed and/or before leaving the house in the morning. The patient brushes on teeth, spits out excess, and does not rinse.
Caries (medium risk)	Topical fluoride varnish	In office or at home	Generally for the moderate-risk RPD patient. Applied to all teeth after completion of prophylaxis appointment. Frequency determined by risk. Patient is not to eat or drink for at least 2 hours after application. A protocol of three applications within a 10-day period is often suggested for initial caries control regimens.
Caries (high risk)	Fluoride gel tray	At home	Generally for high/extreme caries risk. A flexible pull-down shell with drops of 1.1% fluoride gel in the areas of the teeth. Used after regular oral hygiene daily for 30 minutes.
	Silver diamine fluoride	Dental hygienist or dentist	Applied to early or active carious lesions to arrest progression. Little current evidence for the adult population but may be an effective means to control root surface caries in the high-risk elderly population where the black discoloration is not an issue.
	Chlorhexidine varnish	Dental hygienist or dentist	Currently not available in the United States. Some early evidence of benefit in root caries prevention.
Caries/ periodontitis	Chlorhexidine rinse	At home	Nonalcoholic version recommended. Used to reduce bacterial load on recurring rather than continuous basis. Use 0.12% rinse (or stronger if available) for 2 minutes prior to bed for 2 weeks prior to upcoming recall appointment. This minimizes stain formation and times its removal efficiently. Must use at least 60 minutes after any product that contains sodium lauryl sulfate (most toothpastes) to avoid possible inhibitory interaction.
Xerostomia	Salivary substitutes	At home	Several versions now available on mainstream pharmacy shelves. Must ensure they do not reduce PH of oral environment.

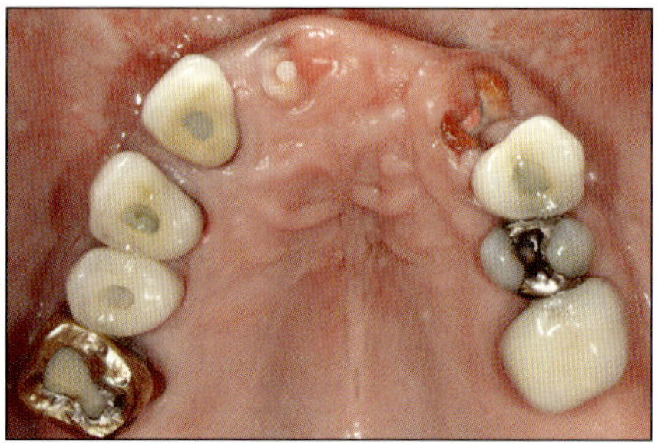

FIG 1-8 A complex tooth-supported fixed-removable reconstruction would not be advised in this patient, considering the poor restorative condition of the remaining teeth, the cost to manage that condition, and the continued disease risk.

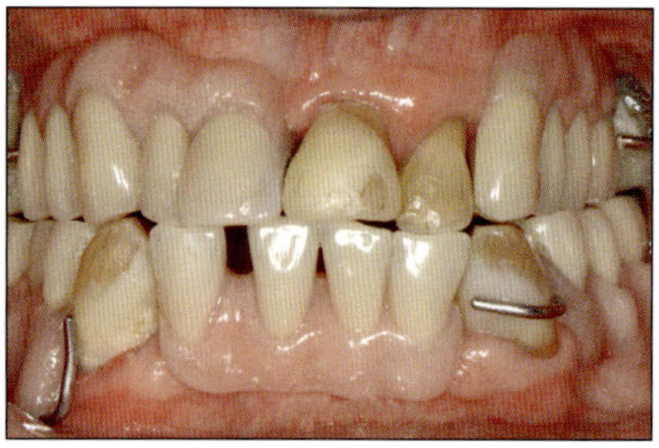

FIG 1-9 Example of interim RPDs being used in a high-risk elderly patient.

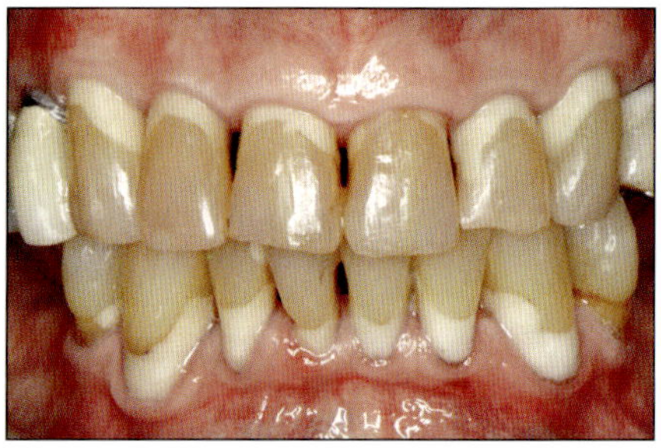

FIG 1-10 Example of a shortened dental arch. This patient, a cancer survivor, functions on two occluding units.

patients who are either not motivated or unable to reduce their risk of disease. In these instances, disease will return despite the management steps taken. When this occurs, there is less at stake because the more expensive and extensive therapies have been avoided. These saved resources can then be invested in alternative therapies.

When we look ahead to the complex fixed-removable reconstructions later in this textbook, the comment on saving resources for a more predictable alternative therapy must be remembered. The more complex the tooth-tissue-supported reconstruction, the higher the risk of failure.[42] This likely indicates the poor condition of the preoperative condition as well as the higher disease risk profiles that required the more extensive reconstruction in the first place (Fig 1-8). The clinician must decide if the extensive rehabilitation efforts needed for these more complex situations are worthwhile in terms of function, cost, and time. If not, alternatives must be strongly considered.

Alternatives

It must not be assumed that preventive strategies will always work. If the evidence collected by the risk assessment points to disease recurrence, then treatments not involving the natural teeth must be recommended. This brings us to the third category, an extreme-risk patient. If RPDs are made within an uncontrollable extreme-risk environment (which, in spite of the evidence, they often are), they will fail. The sequence of treatment in these scenarios is typically direct, with edentulation and implant therapy being the basis of the reconstruction choices.

Interim RPD

When an RPD is not indicated, there are six basic alternatives. One option is the interim acrylic RPD. For the extreme-risk patient, the word *interim* is in reference to both the teeth and the RPD. These patients will generally never have a definitive RPD. Instead, this type of plan is used to delay the undesired use of complete dentures. This is often a very appropriate choice for very elderly or terminally ill patients in whom quality of life for the remaining months is the most important goal (Fig 1-9).

Shortened arch

In certain situations, a second alternative to RPDs can be the shortened-arch concept.[43–45] Popularized in Europe by Dr Kayser and others, this concept utilizes the fact that a significant percentage of partially edentulous patients function well enough with a limited number of occluding posterior units (Fig 1-10). This can be as extreme as the patient having only one or two opposing premolar teeth in their entire mouth.

Dentists have a tendency to want to replace missing teeth. However, this should be a patient-driven choice. The patient should have a comfort or function complaint directly related to the lack of posterior occluding units before an RPD is considered. Research has shown no significant detrimental effects long-term from lacking posterior occluding units.[46,47] This concept is particularly appropriate for elderly patients or patients who have never worn removable devices. Part of the reason for the high rate of patients not using Kennedy Class I RPDs is the fact that patients can often function acceptably well with the limited numbers of natural teeth that they have. Two common contraindications to the shortened arch are esthetics in broad smile situations and the need for additional occluding units opposing a conventional complete denture.

Conventional complete denture

Conventional complete dentures are another obvious alternative. A simple analysis of the patient's edentulous anatomy often demonstrates a favorable prognosis (Fig 1-11).

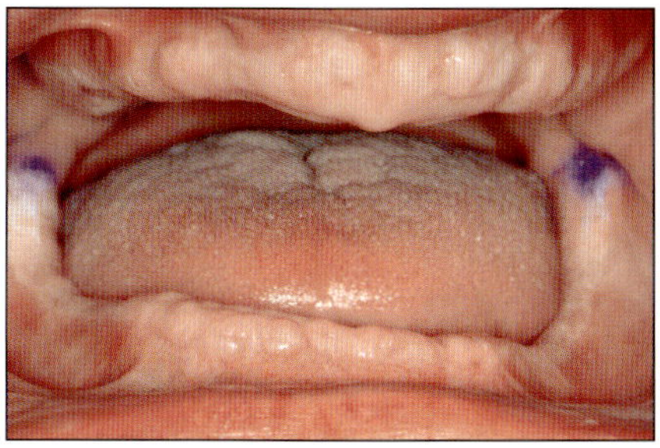

FIG 1-11 Favorable denture anatomy.

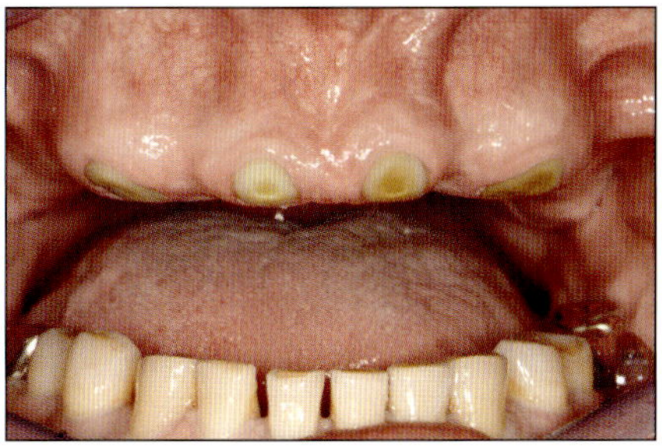

FIG 1-12 These maxillary roots have been maintained as overdenture abutments. They are critical to maintain favorable denture anatomy that resists the force of the dentate mandible.

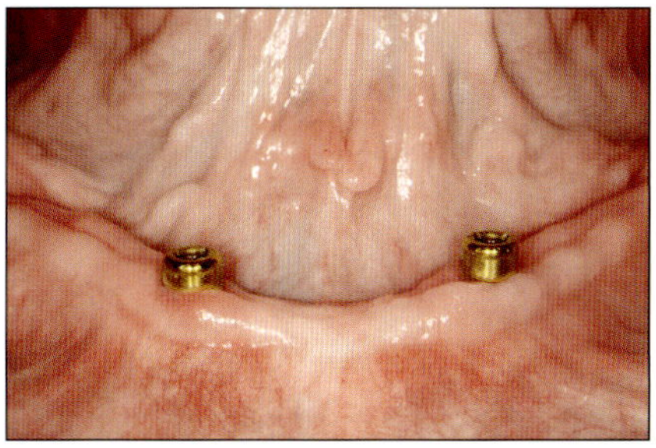

FIG 1-13 Two stud attachments for an implant overdenture.

Experience has also shown that a favorable maxillary arch form has the potential to support a maxillary complete denture at least as well as a Kennedy Class I RPD supported by only anterior teeth. This is due to common challenges with gravity and retention faced by the maxillary RPD. The esthetic improvement in this scenario is also often dramatic. There is frequently no better way to improve the cosmetic result when heavily restored, discolored, and malpositioned maxillary incisors are present. Replacement by a well-designed complete denture also has the potential to compensate for age, lip support, and disease management issues where an RPD cannot. This choice is also often economical, as investment in the anatomically inferior mandibular arch is preferred. This is to more predictably avoid the use of a mandibular conventional complete denture, which often results when first-round treatment fails and the patient no longer has resources for retreatment. It has been the author's experience that maxillary conventional complete dentures have a high success and satisfaction rate. While not as common, there are scenarios where a mandibular conventional complete denture can be made predictable and successful. Therefore, they too should be a consideration when the anatomy is favorable and the disease burden/risk too high.

Overdenture

Some anatomical situations are predictive of poor denture function. If edentulation is indicated and conventional dentures are economically and/or cosmetically preferred, then an overdenture should be considered (Fig 1-12). It is common to find teeth that have previous root canal therapy in partially edentulous patients. These can be fairly easily and economically utilized to maintain the residual ridge and lend support where the edentulous anatomy is otherwise lacking. A significant volume of research from the 1980s shows good results and offers suggestions to manage the high rate of caries found on the root abutments. These roots can be used with various types of attachments as well, further increasing their benefit and effect on retention.

Implant overdenture

The fifth alternative to RPDs has been the most influential in treatment planning. The implant overdenture has been so successful biologically and functionally that much of the prosthodontic profession considers it the standard of care for edentulous patients. Here we are speaking specifically about the mandible and the tissue-supported implant-retained overdenture concept. By placing two mandibular anterior dental implants—or even a single implant—most issues with retention and stability in mandibular complete dentures are vastly improved (Fig 1-13). When this therapy is compared to the typical Kennedy Class I RPD, it is often the implant overdenture that comes out ahead. Consider this in terms of future disease risk, function, esthetics, comfort, and long-term management. The two most positive factors are the elimination of caries risk and near-total control over tooth position/occlusion. While maintenance is a continual challenge and cost is somewhat greater than an RPD, this is among the most successful and gratifying treatments in prosthetic dentistry. It must be noted that there is concern with long-term implant health when the same concept is used on the maxillary arch.

Full-arch implant-supported prosthesis

The sixth and final alternative to RPDs is also the most expensive. The mainstream use of full-arch implant-supported fixed complete dentures is a reality. The transition into this fixed prosthetic solution commonly also occurs in a single visit (Fig 1-14). The success rates in the long term continue to be very high. The fact that this is a fixed solution that eliminates the caries risk and reduces

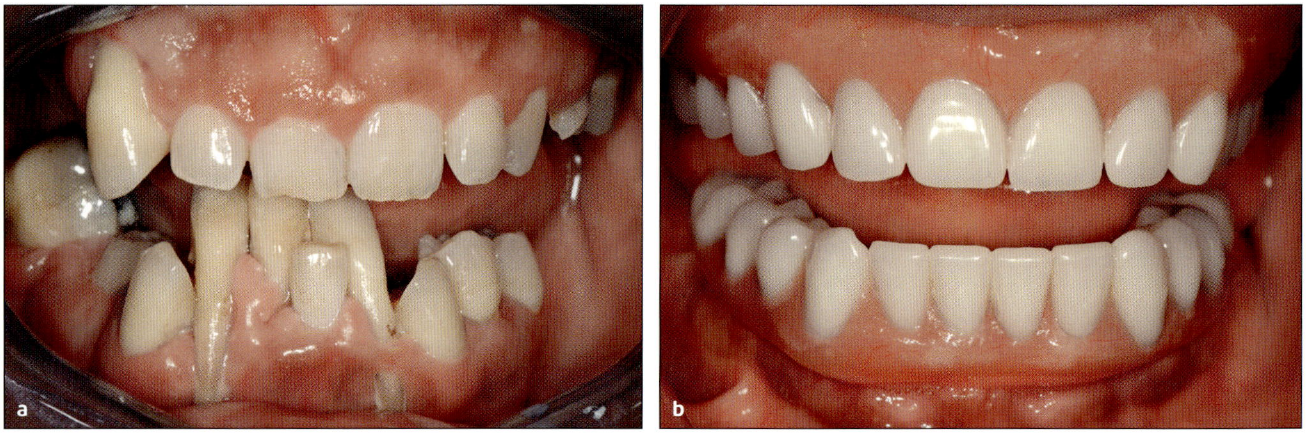

FIG 1-14 *(a)* Pretreatment view. *(b)* Immediately placed maxillary denture and mandibular implant-supported fixed complete denture (hybrid).

maintenance issues makes the economic cost worthwhile for many patients. Traditionally, Kennedy Class I patients have been left with RPDs as the primary recommendation because they lack adequate bone volume to safely accept dental implants in the posterior region. This alternative uses the favorable anterior anatomy to provide a fixed prothesis. This widens the patient base for which it is appropriate and beneficial. The experienced reader will no doubt remember Kelly syndrome and its relation to mandibular Kennedy Class I situations. This treatment modality restores rigid posterior support and therefore theoretically eliminates the proposed etiology for combination syndrome.

Diagnostics

The challenges of partial edentulism, risk factor analysis, disease management, and alternatives all highlight the complex planning required for RPD patients. As discussed, in many situations it will take weeks or months to make final decisions and finalize an RPD treatment plan. The obvious first step in treatment for the partially edentulous patient is the phase that includes the gathering of diagnostic data and those diagnostic procedures commonly grouped under the heading of treatment planning. The preceding discussion about treatment planning focused on mouth-level issues. Tooth-level and arch-level prognoses must also be gathered. Intimate detail of every aspect of the patient's remaining teeth is required to assess prognosis at an individual tooth level. Tooth-level prognosis is almost exclusively an assessment of the structural integrity and durability of the tooth. Simply put, the more remaining healthy tooth structure and periodontal support an individual tooth has, the better the prognosis.

Arch-level prognosis is the viability of the total amount of teeth within a specific arch to support and resist the function placed on it by the opposing arch. Arch-level prognosis typically cannot be determined until articulated diagnostic casts have been evaluated. Better still, a diagnostic wax-up and tooth arrangement that includes a tentative RPD design will fully illustrate the arch-level challenges. It may well be that the diagnostic phase is second only to maintenance as an indicator of long-term success. This is because the more accurate the thought process during the diagnostic phase, the more likely it is that complicating factors are avoided or eliminated.

An experienced clinician can make many early determinations at the initial examination appointment. This requires a skilled interviewer and focused questions. At a minimum, the following questions (in no particular order) must be addressed as part of the evaluation of the gathered data:

- Are the patient's expectations achievable?
- Can the patient's dental disease be adequately managed?
- What further analysis of disease risk factors is necessary to predict the patient risk profile?
- Is an RPD indicated/necessary for this patient at this time?
- What prosthodontic/restorative needs are apparent in the opposing arch, and how will their treatment affect the RPD?
- Are the hard and soft tissues that would relate to a removable appliance acceptable (ie, in an ideal state of health) at this time, or will they require preprosthetic therapy? This could include everything from orthognathic surgery to a bonded rest. Will the abutment teeth provide all the required support, or will additional support be required from the soft tissues of the edentulous areas (stress relief)?

- Would the patient be better served with implant-supported/implant-retained prostheses, and can the increase in cost of care be justified?
- Should ideal treatment be modified because of age, chronic systemic disease, or psychologic factors?
- Will the patient be able to provide the required level of home care that will be necessary for long-term success?

Some of these answers will require direct questioning of the patient. Others may only need to be a part of the clinician's thought process but should be considered while the patient is still present. Some questions will result in referrals to other specialists and/or additional diagnostic tests. The following basic information must be obtained before definitive treatment planning can occur:

- Identification of the chief complaint
- Evaluation of existing prostheses (if available)
- Head and neck examination
- Evaluation of mandibular movement and temporomandibular disease screening to include sounds and mouth opening
- Intraoral examination of both soft and hard tissues with emphasis on cancer screening

Accurate and complete charting of the following is required:

- Caries and caries risk assessment
- Existing restorations
- Periodontal tissues to include probing, gingival location/volume, mobilities, and general bone levels
- Pulp testing for vitality, especially on potential abutment teeth
- Radiographic evaluation of both a full-mouth series and a panoramic film are a minimum (in cases where jaw discrepancies and malocclusions are severe, radiographic or other imaging of the TMJ areas should be considered)
- Occlusal contacts, centric and eccentric, presence and location of interferences
- Diet analysis
- Impressions for diagnostic casts
- Interocclusal jaw relation record (if indicated)
- Shade and mold selection

The need for these diagnostic data should be obvious to any clinician; unfortunately, the planning for the average RPD seldom includes all this information, and as a result, the treatment is compromised from the very beginning. There is no point even considering the "design" portion of the treatment plan until this information is available and has received some consideration and reflection.

The wise clinician will not give the patient any definitive plan or fee at the time of the initial examination. The more complex the situation, the more likely this is to be the case. It is far better to tell the patient that no intelligent response can be made until all of the diagnostic data have been evaluated and any required consultations obtained. However, postexamination discussion is very valuable to explain the initial findings and the basics of the possible treatment options. This serves to narrow the discussion on which options the patient is willing to entertain. Effort can then be focused on assimilating the data and creating the final list of necessary procedures.

Preliminary impressions

The quality of the initial impressions and the casts that result from them, although diagnostic only, need to be of far higher quality than that normally seen. Most every specialist in removable prosthodontics has had the experience of attending a meeting or seminar when someone asks for help in treatment planning a case: A plaster cast, pulled from a pocket, usually without a decent base, full of blebs and voids and with no evidence of ever having been on a dental surveyor and then, "I apologize for this cast, but can you help me with a design?"

The preliminary impression and resultant cast should be of the same quality as the final impression as far as extensions, hard and soft tissue details, and integrity of the occlusal surface are concerned. This impression should be considered as a trial impression for the final. Tray size is evaluated, patient compliance with instructions noted, ease of placement discovered, and the patient's ability to sit still during the set of the alginate evaluated. Everything that can be learned from this impression will aid the clinician in making an accurate final impression.

Sometimes no stock tray will adequately fit the mouth, indicating that a custom tray will have to be included in preparation for the final impression. Modification of the stock tray with wax or compound may be necessary to allow the impression of border tissues or high palatal vault. All these issues must be evaluated at the preliminary impression so that in the final impression, the clinician can concentrate on those factors related to accuracy of the impression of the hard tissues.

Alginate can be expected to give overextended borders due to its consistency when properly mixed. Under no circumstances should the powder/water ratio be changed to reduce the viscosity of the mix. Rather, the amount of alginate required to make a quality impression should be carefully estimated and only that amount placed in the tray.

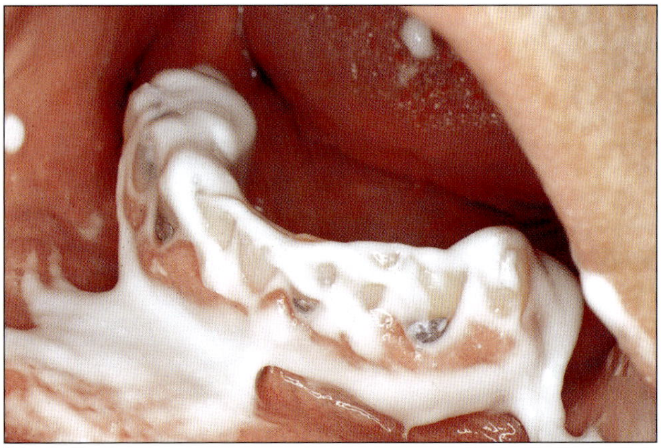

FIG 1-15 Alginate applied to critical areas to reduce bubbles and voids.

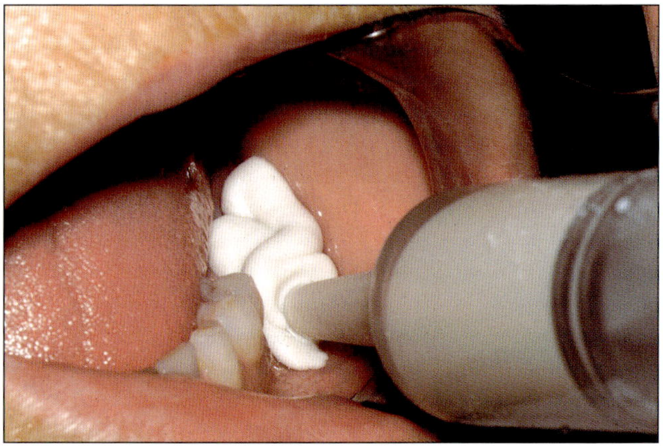

FIG 1-16 Large-diameter syringes can be used to fill difficult-to-reach anatomical areas.

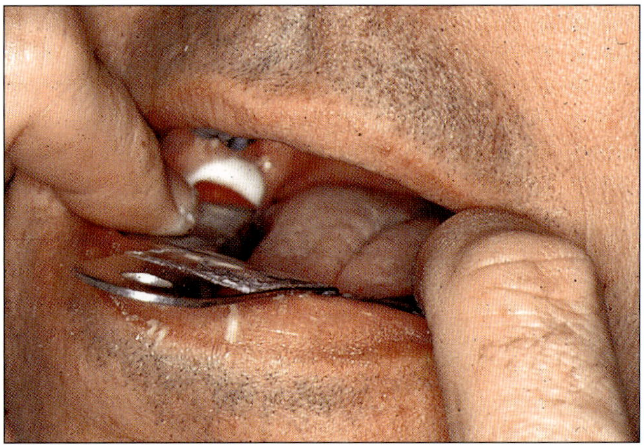

FIG 1-17 Stock tray seated and stabilized throughout the complete setting of the alginate.

Alginate must be placed into the critical areas: occlusal surfaces, marginal gingival crevices, soft tissue undercuts, etc (Fig 1-15). One cannot count on the material flowing to these areas of its own accord. The material can be placed with the finger or injected using a syringe, but in no instance should the tray be placed in the mouth until all critical areas are wiped with alginate. Borders should be filled using a syringe (Fig 1-16). The critical areas are buccal to the tuberosities and the retromylohyoid space, places where voids are often found in the completed impression. Another advantage of placing alginate in the mouth before seating the tray is that less material needs to be placed in the tray, resulting in increased visibility for tray placement.

Whenever possible, the stock tray is modified by adding wax or compound to allow a minimum of 0.25 inch of alginate around all critical structures. A common problem with alginate is overseating of the tray, resulting in less than the required 0.25 inch of material over the occlusal surfaces. Stops can be placed in the tray using hard wax or dental compound to restrict the overseating. Unfortunately, the area of the stop will often be distorted due to the minimal alginate present. The required occlusal spacing may be obtained by placing the empty tray in the mouth, seating it to contact with the occlusal surfaces, and evaluating the relative position of the handle to the lips when the tray is lifted the 0.25 inch. In making the impression, the tray is seated to that lifted position and held in place until the impression is set (Fig 1-17).

When the impression is removed from the mouth, it must be rinsed and lightly dried and then inspected for tears because alginate will usually tear before it distorts. Visual inspection will also show any evidence of the material breaking free from the Rim-Lock or retentive holes. When using a Rim-Lock tray, excess alginate should be cut from the borders with a sharp knife so that the edge of the tray can be seen and the retention of the alginate verified.

Alginate is clearly an imperfect impression material—often due to user error—but it is the material of choice for both preliminary and often final impressions for the RPD. Seldom is the alginate mixed for the manufacturer's recommended time. Likewise, it is often not allowed time for a complete set before removal from the mouth. Many inaccurate impressions can be traced to the patient's inability to remain motionless during the setting phase. When the time in the mouth has been altered by using very cold water or not mixing for the usual 60 seconds, the patient is forced to remain motionless for longer than necessary. Because alginate sets not all at once but in scattered "islands" of setting material, any movement by the clinician or patient during the setting period runs the risk of reorienting the partially set material, producing a distorted impression. Ideally, the set should begin promptly after the tray is in its proper position and any border molding has occurred. Alginate mixed with the proper measure of room-temperature (65°F

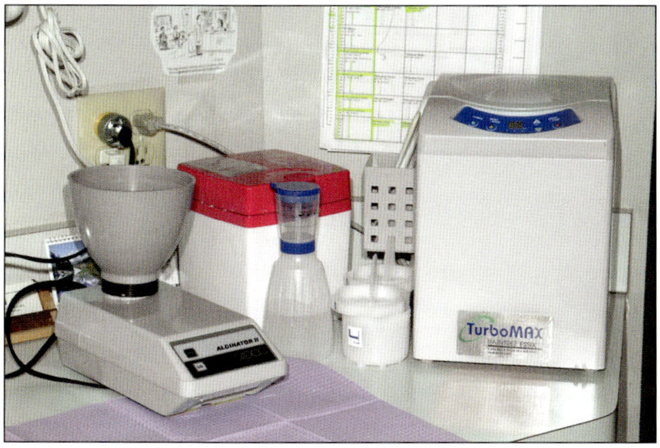

FIG 1-18 Mechanical alginate mixing bowl *(left)* and centrifugal-style alginate mixer *(right)*. Both result in improved consistency. Note also the measuring device for room-temperature water in the center.

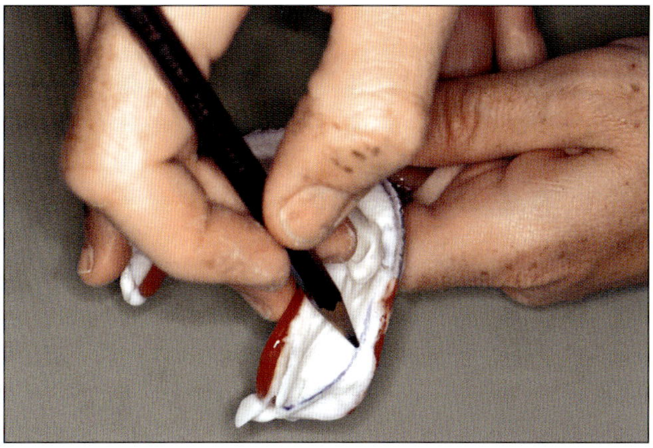

FIG 1-19 After verification and prior to patient departure, key anatomical extensions, such as the buccal shelf, are outlined with an indelible marker.

to 70°F) water will allow roughly 1 minute for loading the tray and placing it in the mouth before the set begins. Optimal gelation time should be between 3 and 4 minutes using 68°F water. The patient is instructed to remain motionless during this time. The initial impression gives the clinician the opportunity to test the patient's ability in this regard. This should increase the probability that the final impression will be accurate. Should the patient move during the final impression, it must be remade and the patient informed again of their part in this procedure. Following the manufacturer's instructions for handling properties is obviously necessary.

If the mixing of the alginate is incomplete, a reduction of up to 50% in the strength of the gel can be expected. On the other hand, alginate mixed beyond the manufacturer's stated time will have reduced gel strength because the forming gels will be broken. Mechanical mixing devices, including vacuum mixing, are more apt to give consistency and thereby accuracy and should be considered as essential instrumentation (Fig 1-18). The cost of centrifugal alginate mixing machines has become much more reasonable over the last decade. These machines accurately, efficiently, and reliably create a nearly bubble-free, completely integrated mix. A typical mixing time is 6 to 8 seconds. For clinicians who regularly use alginate, this machine becomes almost a necessity to create reliable and predictable mixes every time. The hand-mixing method should only be used when no other options are available because it is impossible to accurately, efficiently, and reliably mix alginate by hand.

Alginate adhesives must be considered essential for all final impressions, but because they are not easy to remove from the tray, they are not required for the diagnostic impression. When a stock Rim-Lock tray is used, however, care must be taken to force the alginate into the Rim-Lock with the spatula when loading the tray. Once this has been done, the alginate is not likely to pop free of the lock. As more offices move to disposable plastic trays, the location and extent of perforations become more important, and the use of adhesive is required. Another advantage to plastic trays is that they can be easily modified. Regardless, the impression should be carefully inspected before pouring so that if a separation has occurred, the set alginate can be replaced in the lock of the tray. While this maneuver would be unacceptable for a final impression, it will normally produce a cast that is accurate enough for diagnostic procedures.

Once the impression has been removed from the mouth, the following series of steps will maximize chances for an accurate diagnostic cast:

1. Rinse the impression under running water.
2. Using a cotton tip, gently clean the tooth impressions. (Plaque and other oral debris, if left in the impression, will reduce the surface hardness of the resultant cast because the surface-hardening agents in the alginate must come into contact with the dental stone to gain the maximum quality of cast).
3. Blow excess fluid from the impression and evaluate the impression under good light for tears and defects.
4. With an indelible pencil or other marker, trace the outline of the proposed denture on the alginate (Fig 1-19). Because the patient is still in the chair, extensions can be quickly verified. Should contours seen in the mouth and essential to the construction not be present in the impression, the decision to remake the impression will not require an additional appointment. Attempts to identify denture base extensions from a stone cast days after the impression was made often lead to problems with extensions and will never be as accurate as

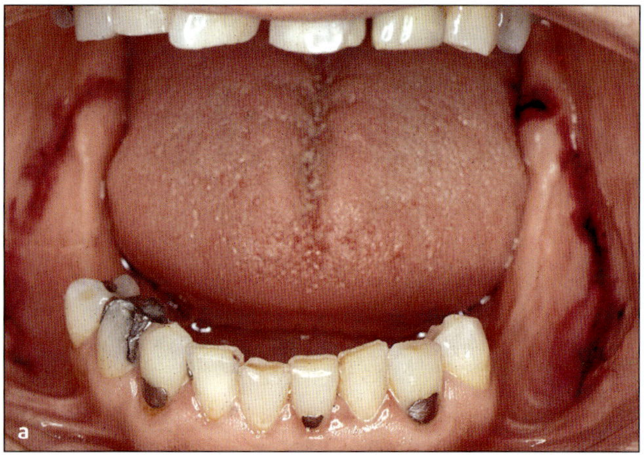
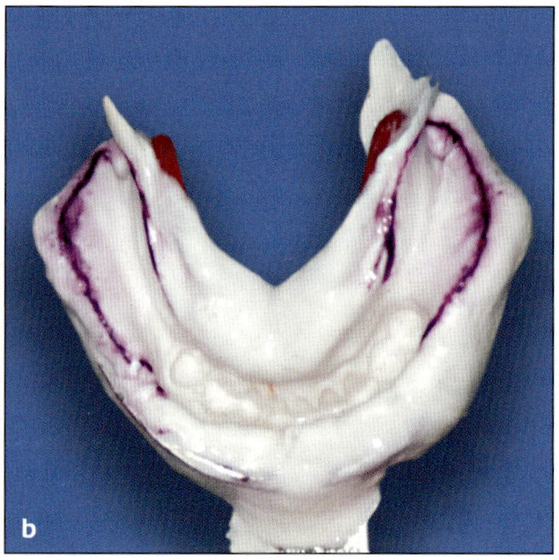

FIG 1-20 *(a)* If moisture can be controlled, markings can be made prior to the impression. *(b)* An adequately extended impression, now marked, is poured as soon as possible.

those determined via this method of drawing on the alginate impression. Anatomical landmarks can also be outlined prior to the impression (Fig 1-20a), with the highlighted areas transferring into the alginate and eventually to the cast (Fig 1-20b).

5. The technique used to pour the preliminary impression is immaterial, and any approach that results in a dense cast with no voids and a base suitable for mounting in the dental surveyor will suffice for diagnostic purposes. As a general rule, boxing the alginate impression is discouraged because any pressures on unsupported alginate will cause distortion. The double-pour approach will be more dependable. As a minimum, the cast should be trimmed so that a land area of 3 mm is established, and any and all blebs are removed because this cast may be seen by the patient as well as by the technician. The author's experience has been that a neat diagnostic cast with a careful design, properly drawn, goes a long way to indicating that the clinician really knows what the standards are, and technicians are impressed when they see a quality diagnostic cast.

Preprosthodontic therapy

One of the essentials of the state-of-the-art RPD is the level of mouth preparation that is required before the actual partial denture is constructed. Mouth preparation is, regrettably, usually interpreted to mean only the creation of rest preparations on some of the remaining teeth. Unfortunately, reviews of cases submitted to the dental laboratories show that many mouths do not have even this level of mouth preparation.

For the modern RPD, mouth preparation will cover any and all therapy required to bring the mouth to optimum health and to modify tissue in such a manner as to make the final prosthesis ideal. Obviously, a removable appliance can still be made accepting the mouth as it presents. In fact, most of the RPDs seen in any review of prosthetic treatment will fall into this category, with little or no recontouring of teeth, occlusal plane discrepancies, malocclusions, and the like. A discussion of the basic therapies for mouth preparation at this point in the treatment planning process is necessary to fully develop the concept of ideal mouth preparation.

While the sequencing of the actual care is a critical issue, the sequencing of consultations is not. The prosthodontist almost always manages the restorative dental examination and caries risk assessment. The periodontal examination is a different matter because most prosthodontists work with a circle of periodontists with an exchange of referrals. No matter how the data are gathered, a baseline of pocket depth, furcation involvement, plaque scores, mobilities, and general periodontal soft tissue conditions must be made. Baseline data of this magnitude provide the clinician with a starting point for referrals as well as protection for medicolegal matters. When determined, periodontal therapy referrals are best made as soon as a preliminary treatment plan has been confirmed. This allows initial therapy and the long-term process of disease management to begin.

Endodontic referrals are apt to be more common, especially those regarding existing endodontic restorations. Retreatment decisions can greatly affect the treatment plan, both in regard to abutment selection and to total cost of care. Root canal filling material exposed for any reason may need to be retreated before definitive care is undertaken as a protection against failure after crowns have been cemented. In addition, as debilitated individual teeth are disassembled and reconstructed, the need for endodontic intervention often becomes clearer as treatment proceeds.

Orthodontic and oral and maxillofacial surgical consultations are almost always case specific and may not always be necessary, although to plan treatment without them, the clinician must be assured that they cannot contribute to the care of the patient. A large number of cases will require minor tooth movement to align the arch and to establish the ideal occlusal plane. In practice, it may be difficult to find an orthodontist willing and able to manage the unique challenges of individual tooth movements in older partially edentulous patients. Direct consultation in these instances is in order rather than simple letters or phone calls. Often, these consultations can best be done after a preliminary treatment plan and design has been established. This is particularly true when one is considering tori removal or adjunctive dental implant therapy.

Along with the periodontal examination, the evaluation of existing restorations and tooth contours is critical to our treatment. In far too many instances, restorations of marginal quality are left in the mouth and the partial denture built around them.

A critical component of treatment planning involves the use of dental implants. Obviously, patients with unlimited funds can avoid an RPD entirely. However, there will be situations where implants cannot be placed, usually in very complex treatments. Implants and considerations for their use are discussed later in this book.

Once the aforementioned information has been gathered, the clinical findings can be summarized as a part of the patient's record and included in the treatment plan letter. This document establishes a diagnosis and prognosis of the mouth with and without treatment. At this point, the diagnostic casts, radiographs, and periodontal charting are reviewed together and the cast "surveyed" to determine the RPD options. The treatment plan and the patient's informed consent letter can only be completed after the tentative design of the final appliance has been established.

Is all this really necessary? Must a written treatment plan and consent letter be given to the patient? Should we make an orthodontic consult as part of our chain of diagnostic procedures? The answer to these and similar questions is, of course, most certainly yes! The type of treatment described in this book, the partial denture at the most advanced level, does require more work, both in planning and execution. The results are, very obviously, worth our time and our best efforts.

References

1. Dye BA, Li X, Beltran-Aguilar ED. Selected oral health indicators in the United States, 2005–2008. NCHS Data Brief, no. 96. Hyattsville, MD: National Center for Health Statistics, 2012.
2. Dye BA, Thornton-Evans G, Li X, Iafolla TJ. Dental caries and tooth loss in adults in the United States, 2011–2012. NCHS Data Brief, no. 197. Hyattsville, MD: National Center for Health Statistics, 2015.
3. Centers for Disease Control and Prevention. Oral Health Surveillance Report: Trends in Dental Caries and Sealants, Tooth Retention, and Edentulism, United States, 1999–2004 to 2011–2016. https://www.cdc.gov/oralhealth/publications/OHSR-2019-index.html. Accessed 24 March 2022.
4. Anderson MH, Bales DJ, Omnell KA. Modern management of dental caries: The cutting edge is not the dental bur. J Am Dent Assoc 1993;124:37–44.
5. American Dental Association. Caries Risk Assessment Form (Age > 6). https://www.ada.org/resources/research/science-and-research-institute/oral-health-topics/caries-risk-assessment-and-management. Accessed 21 March 2022.
6. Bratthall D, Petersson, GH. Cariogram—A multifactorial risk assessment model for a multifactorial disease. Community Dent Oral Epidemiol 2005;33:256–264.
7. Featherstone JDB, Singh S, Curtis DA. Caries risk assessment and management for the prosthodontic patient. J Prosthodont 2011;20:2–9.
8. Eke PI, Dye BA, Wei L, et. al. Update on prevalence of periodontitis in adults in the United States: NHANES 2009 to 2012. J Periodontol 2015;86:611–622.
9. The pathogenesis of periodontal disease. J Periodontol 1999;70:457–470.
10. Eke PI, Wei L, Thornton-Evans GO, et al. Risk indicators for periodontitis in US adults: NHANES 2009-2012. J Periodontol 2016;87:1174–1185.
11. Lindhe J, Haffjee AD, Socransky SS. Progression of periodontal disease in adult subjects in the absence of periodontal thereapy. J Clin Periodont 1983;10:433–442.
12. Carlsson GE, Hedegard B, Koivumaa K. Studies in partial denture prosthesis, III. A longitudinal study of mandibular partial dentures with double extension saddles. Acta Odontol Scand 1962;20:95–119.
13. Mine K, Fueki K, Igarashi Y. Microbiological risk for periodontitis of abutment teeth in patients with removable partial dentures. J Oral Rehabil 2009:36;696–702.
14. Markkanen H, Lappalainen R, Honkala E, Tuominen R. Periodontal conditions with removable complete and partial dentures in the adult population aged 30 years and over. J Oral Rehabil 1987:14:355–360.
15. Zlatarić DK, Celebic A, Valentic-Peruzovic M. The effect of removable partial dentures on periodontal health of abutment and non-abutment teeth. J Periodontol 2002;73:137–144.
16. Tuominen R, Ranta K, Paunino I. Wearing of removable partial dentures in relation to periodontal pockets. J Oral Rehabil 1989;16:119–126.
17. Bergman B, Hugoson A, Olsson CO. Caries, periodontal, and prosthetic findings in patients with removable partial dentures: A 10-year longitudinal study. J Prosthet Dent 1982;48:506–510.
18. Chandler JA, Brudvik JS. Clinical evaluation of patients eight to nine years after placement of removable partial dentures. J Prosthet Dent 1984;51:736–743.
19. Wilding RJ, Reddy J. Periodontal disease in partial denture wearers—A biological index. J Oral Rehabil 1987;14:111–124.
20. Vanzeveren C, D'Hoore W, Bercy P, Leloup G. Treatment with removable partial dentures: A longitudinal study. Part I. J Oral Rehabil 2003;30:447–458.
21. Kapur KK. Veterans Administration cooperative dental implant study—Comparisons between fixed partial dentures supported by blade-vent implants and removable partial dentures. Part II: Comparisons of success rates and periodontal health between two treatment modalities. J Prosthet Dent 1989;62:685–703.
22. Akerly WB. Prosthodontic treatment of traumatic overlap of the anterior teeth. J Prosthet Dent 1977;38:26–34.
23. Curtis TA, Langer Y, Curtis DA, Carpenter R. Occlusal considerations for partially or completely edentulous skeletal Class II patients. Part I: Background information. J Prosthet Dent 1988;60:202–211.

24. Curtis TA, Langer Y, Curtis DA, Carpenter R. Occlusal considerations for partially or completely edentulous skeletal Class II patients. Part II: Treatment concepts. J Prosthet Dent 1988;60:334–342.
25. Drago CJ, Caswell CW. Prosthodontic rehabilitation of patients with Class II malocclusions. J Prosthet Dent 1990;64:435–445.
26. Capp NJ, Warren K. Restorative treatment for patients with excessive vertical overlap. Int J Prosthodont 1991;4:353–360.
27. Ambard A, Mueninghoff L. Planning restorative treatment for patients with severe Class II malocclusions. J Prosthet Dent 2002;88:200–207.
28. Omar SM, McEwen JD, Ogston SA. A test for occlusal function. Br J Orthod 1987;14:85–90.
29. Akeel R, Nilner M, Nilner K. Masticatory efficiency in individuals with natural dentition. Swed Dent J 1992;16:191–198.
30. Luke DA, Lucas PW. Chewing efficiency in relation to occlusal and other variations in the natural human dentition. Br Dent J 1985;159:401–403.
31. Schuyler CH. Factors contributing to traumatic occlusion. J Prosthet Dent 1961;11:708–715.
32. Glickman I, Smulow JB. Further observations on the effects of trauma from occlusion. J Periodontol 1967;38:280–293.
33. Branschofsky M, Beikler T, Schäfer R, Flemming TF, Lang H. Secondary trauma from occlusion and periodontitis. Quintessence Int 2011;42:515–522.
34. Panek H, Matthews-Brzozowska T, Nowakowska D, et al. Dynamic occlusions in natural permanent dentition. Quintessence Int 2008;39:337–342.
35. Evans, RW, Clark P, Jia N. The caries management system: Are preventive effects sustained postclinical trial? Community Dent Oral Epidemiol 2016;44:188–197.
36. Tada S, Allen PF, Ikebe K, Matsuda K, Maeda Y. Impact of periodontal maintenance on tooth survival in patients with removable partial dentures. J Clin Periodontol 2015;42:46–53.
37. Ghamrawy E. Quantitative changes in dental plaque formation related to removable partial dentures. J Oral Rehabil 1976;3:115–120.
38. Brill N, Tryde G, Stoltze K, El Ghamrawy E. Ecological changes in the oral cavity caused by removable partial dentures. J Prosthet Dent 1977;38:138–148.
39. Bates JF, Addy M. Partial dentures and plaque accumulation. J Dent 1978;6:285–293.
40. Costa L, do Nascimento C, Pagnano de Souza VO, Pedrazzi V. Microbiological and clinical assessment of the abutment and non-abutment teeth of partial removable denture wearers. Arch Oral Biol 2017;75:74–80.
41. Mihalow DM, Tinanoff N. The influence of removable partial dentures on the level of *Streptococcus mutans* in saliva. J Prosthet Dent 1988;59:49–51.
42. Studer SP, Mader C, Stahel W, Scharer P. A retrospective study of combined fixed-removable reconstructions with their analysis of failures. J Oral Rehabil 1998;25:513–526.
43. Jepson N, Allen F, Moynihan P, Kelly P, Thomason M. Patient satisfaction following restoration of shortened mandibular dental arches in a randomized controlled trial. Int J Prosthodont 2003;16:409–414.
44. Kayser AF, Witter DJ, Spanuaf AJ. Overtreatment with removable partial dentures in shortened dental arches. Aust Dent J 1987;32:178–182.
45. Kayser AF. The shortened dental arch: A therapeutic concept in reduced dentitions and certain high-risk groups. Int J Periodontics Restorative Dent 1989;9:427–449.
46. Witter DJ, de Haan AF, Käyser AF, van Rossum GM. A 6-year follow-up study of oral function in shortened dental arches. Part I: Occlusal stability. J Oral Rehabil 1994;21:113–125.
47. Witter DJ, De Haan AF, Käyser AF, Van Rossum GM. A 6-year follow-up study of oral function in shortened dental arches. Part II: Craniomandibular dysfunction and oral comfort. J Oral Rehabil 1994;21:353–366.

ELEMENTS OF DESIGN

2

Ever since the publication of Dr W. Frantz's study of the variations in partial denture design, I have been troubled by the seemingly total lack of consensus on the design of a conventional partial denture.[1] I can understand that there would be some different approaches to any partial design, but to find that there is apparently no commonly held approach to the design that would result in a minimum of variations is troubling. It may well be that the average clinician simply does not have sufficient repetitions of similar partially edentulous situations to develop a consistent philosophy for designing a partial denture.

For any situation where there are inadequate repetitions or where the consequences of overlooking a particular step are unacceptable, the development of a checklist, not unlike that used by the pilot of an airplane, is in order. The checklist that I have used and taught for these many years is based on what I believe to be the most logical approach to determining the design of any removable partial situation. It focuses on clinical rather than laboratory decision-making and is broken down into the following categories, always in this order since it ranks the components by clinical importance:

1. Abutments (rests and guiding planes)
2. Connectors (major and minor)
3. Resin retention (metal, bead, or pontics)
4. Retention (clasp or attachment)

—James S. Brudvik, 1999

Abutments

As described under "Philosophy of Care" (page viii), an RPD must possess only six characteristics to be successful: strong, stable, retentive, esthetic, comfortable, and pain-free. The relationship between the abutment tooth and the framework is the most important of all design and construction considerations. In keeping with this thought, the selection of the remaining teeth to be used as abutments becomes critical. The *Glossary of Prosthodontic Terms*[2] defines an *abutment* as:

> **Abutment:** 1. that part of a structure that directly receives thrust or pressure; an anchorage; 2. a tooth, a portion of a tooth, or that portion of a dental implant that serves to support and/or retain a prosthesis.

An individual tooth must possess the anatomy, position, and strength to effectively serve as an abutment. A tooth that is deficient in any of these factors becomes either expendable or an ancillary abutment. Deficient teeth may best be considered "not present" during the design and are often removed to achieve a more predictable result. Let us briefly consider these three factors.

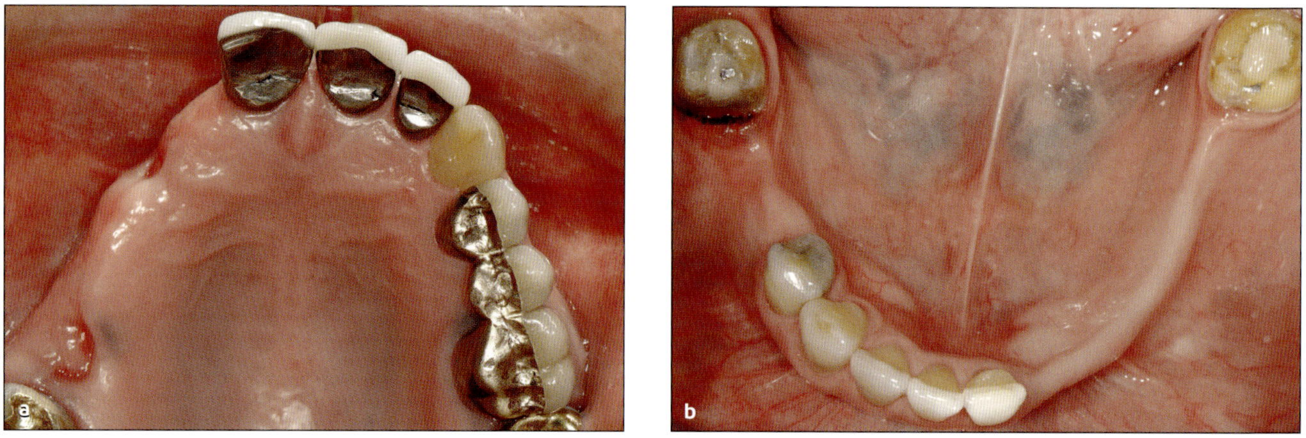

FIG 2-1 *(a and b)* These patients have been left with anatomically inferior anterior abutments.

Anatomical value

The anatomical differences between teeth are a focal point in prosthodontics. Ante's so-called "law" is just one example. The support offered by a molar is dramatically different from that of a premolar. Likewise, canines have significantly greater support and stability value than lateral incisors. Anatomically inferior teeth should not be utilized as primary abutments if long-term results are a goal (Fig 2-1). These include mandibular premolars with their typically short, singular, and conical root form.

Proper evaluation of root form anatomy requires current radiographs. Situations where these weaker teeth must be used as abutments require special management with design modifications and/or splinting. These situations are discussed throughout this text. Nonetheless, it is best to find alternatives to using anatomically inferior teeth.

Positional relationship

The positional relationship of potential abutments is determined by articulated diagnostic casts as discussed in chapter 1. These casts will demonstrate malpositioned teeth far better than clinical evaluation alone. An anatomically superior abutment is often rendered useless or potentially destructive when it is malpositioned (Fig 2-2). Classic examples include overerupted maxillary first molars or mesially tipped mandibular third molars. While minor discrepancies can be managed with judicious enameloplasty, major displacement issues will be chronic occlusal interferences. These interferences are common causes of breakage, instability, and chronic soreness in ill-managed RPDs. Likewise, arch form distortions such as lingually tipped premolars can both interfere with major connector placement and leave a buccal contour devoid of any undercut. A potential abutment that is outside the dental arch or plane of occlusion must be managed or removed. Treatment options may include minor orthodontics, root canal therapy to allow appropriate occlusal reduction, or removal and replacement with a repositioned dental implant.

Structural integrity

The third factor to consider is the structural integrity of the potential abutment tooth as measured by remaining tooth structure and periodontal support. Teeth that would not be able to structurally or periodontally support an individual crown in a dentate arch should not be expected to do so in a partially edentulous one. A pervasive challenge in RPD patients is that the majority of remaining teeth have been previously restored, which adds to risk. In an ideal world, previous restorations and crowns would be replaced to allow thorough evaluation and reconstruction (Fig 2-3). Only in this scenario can the structural integrity of a tooth be evaluated. This must be done for critical abutment teeth such as canines and lone-standing molars. For this reason, the surveyed crown is a common design necessity in the advanced RPD, not due to the desire to change tooth contour, but to address the structural deficiencies of teeth with extensive operative dentistry. In the treatment flow for the common RPD patient, these evaluations are completed as part of disease management.

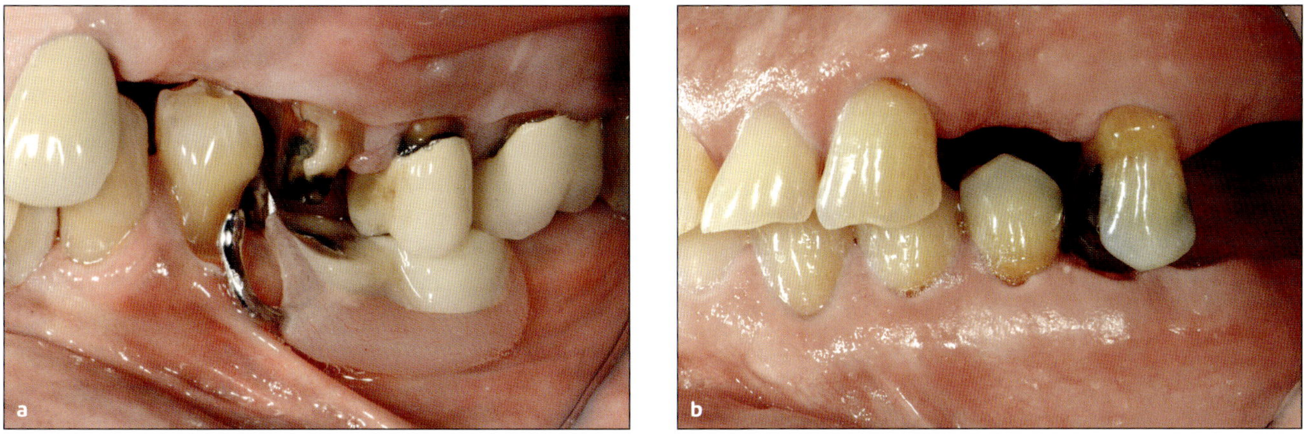

FIG 2-2 *(a and b)* Positional issues can be so severe as to require tooth removal.

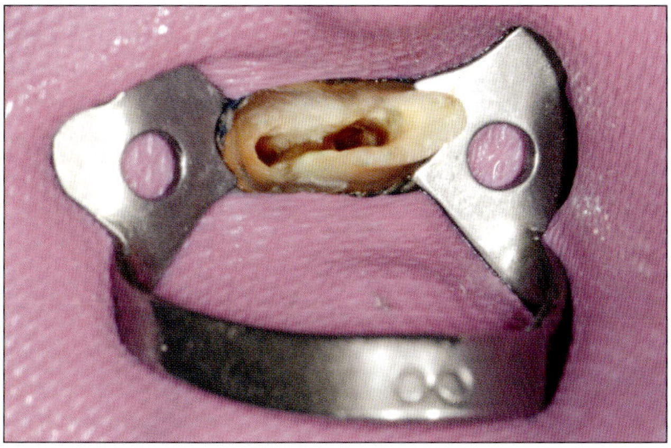

FIG 2-3 Disassembly to evaluate a potential abutment.

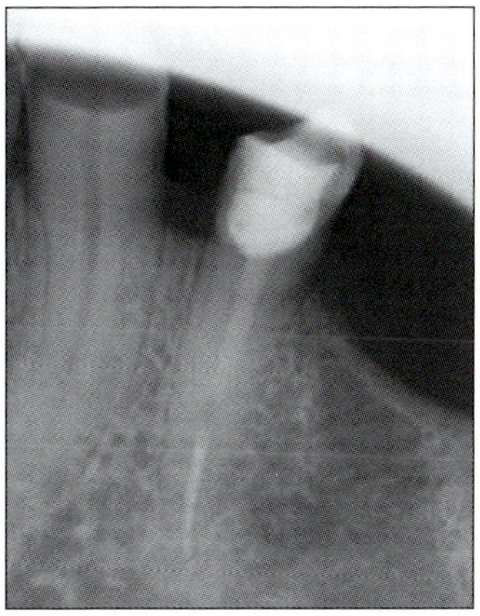

FIG 2-4 An endodontically treated terminal abutment is at high risk for failure under these loading conditions.

Endodontically treated teeth are four times more likely to fail when used as an RPD abutment than teeth that have not been endodontically treated.[3] When a terminal abutment is compromised to the point of requiring or having received root canal therapy, it should no longer be considered a viable abutment. An otherwise strong canine may be a possible exception. However, premolars and incisors are universally weakened beyond reliability once they are heavily restored and endodontically treated. These teeth have typically been restored several times and are often already crowned. To invest in root canal therapy, core restoration, possible clinical crown lengthening, and a new crown is unwise, and in the cost-conscious RPD patient, one might say foolhardy. This cost must also be considered in terms of more reliable alternatives or strategic use of resources. One example discussed in detail later is the use of a single dental implant to eliminate a distal extension. Moreover, we are commonly debating costly rehabilitation of anatomically inferior mandibular premolars when a strong mandibular canine is typically available one tooth space anterior.

When endodontically treated teeth are being considered as abutments, they should not be critical to the design of the partial denture. Their future loss should be assumed, and the partial denture should be able to function with as minimal modification as possible if they are lost (Fig 2-4). It must be noted that the philosophy of advanced RPDs is not to crown everything, because this in and of itself does not improve the prognosis. Rather, the strategic use of coronal reinforcement for structurally compromised yet otherwise strong teeth has proven to do so over time.

On an individual tooth level, periodontal support is evaluated much the same as tooth structure. Unfortunately, periodontally compromised patients commonly present with significant bone loss on all remaining teeth. In these situations, there is often a lack of satisfactory individual abutment teeth. This is a good example of evaluating prognosis at the arch level. If disease has been controlled, the total value of all remaining periodontal support is considered, and it becomes an all-or-none situation. As discussed later in this book, either all remaining teeth will be utilized as abutments, or an alternative treatment plan should be considered.

Teeth that are healthy but mobile are major clinical challenges. If not managed, the mobility will prevent accurate impressions, cause restoration dislodgement, and tend to prevent ideal tooth-frame interfacing.[4] If initial therapy has not improved mobility, these teeth may need to be splinted. If adjacent teeth require crowns for structural reasons, they are typically best splinted. If the teeth do not require crowns, alternative methods such as metal or (in rare instances) ceramic splints can be considered. The need for splinting increases for terminal abutments.

Number of abutments

With the remaining teeth now assessed, we must make our determinations. As a general rule, we must consider the strongest remaining teeth first and then progress to weaker teeth as we decide on the number of teeth necessary to support the partial denture. Whether or not a tooth is ultimately selected to be clasped is immaterial at this time. However, a tooth selected as an abutment will receive some sort of rest. It is always preferable to include more abutments rather than fewer because the only downside is a more complicated casting with the attendant risk of a poor fit. Obviously, the number of teeth to be replaced is related to the number of abutments needed for support. The evidence suggests that long-term health is directly related to the number of abutments.

Teeth that are unlikely to remain for the expected life of a partial denture, ie, 10 years, must either be extracted, or the framework must be designed with their replacement in mind. In general, if a tooth is in a satisfactory positional relationship and is easy to replace when lost, it should be kept. The most common example of this is a debilitated mandibular second or third molar that is the last remaining posterior tooth on that side of the arch. When such a tooth is preventing a distal extension, it is providing an invaluable improvement in prognosis and should be maintained. In distal extension situations, terminal premolars in poor condition are difficult to replace and if kept are often better utilized as overlays (see chapter 12).

As we now consider specific design components, we must clarify each in terms of its function during force transmission. Rests serve to *support* the prosthesis by resisting the vertical forces toward the tissue. Guiding planes and similarly designed minor connector surfaces serve to *stabilize* the prosthesis by resisting lateral forces. Clasps typically serve to retain the RPD by resisting vertical displacement in a coronal direction. Advanced RPD design achieves consistency, simplicity, and effectiveness by using each component to resist its designated force. The tradition-based idea that clasps are the means by which the RPD achieves support, stability, and retention all together is fraught with complexity and negative biologic consequences. The philosophical design difference with advanced RPDs begins here.

Rests

Rests are the primary means by which an RPD will resist vertical forces toward the tissue. They are exponentially more important than soft tissue support derived from a distal extension base. A tooth that is contacted by the partial denture but not through a positive rest cannot be considered an abutment. A good example of what might happen in this situation can be illustrated by a Class I mandibular partial denture where a lingual plate is used as the major connector and, after a period of time, a clinical evaluation shows that the incisors have moved out of contact with the plate.

Positive rests are defined as rests that form acute angles with the minor connectors that join them to the major connector. With a rest-connector angle of less than 90 degrees, the partial denture framework, if it really contacts the abutments, cannot move away from the tooth, and the tooth cannot move away from the partial denture without vertical movement (Fig 2-5). Of these rest designs, the proximal rest form is typically used for the foundation of the lingual ledge rest on a fixed restoration.

The choice of rest preparation that is placed on the selected abutment tooth is generally obvious: occlusal rests for posterior teeth and cingulum rests for incisors. For either of these primary rest designs, you will find that laboratories and dentists alike chronically undersize them. Mainstream textbooks cite one-half to one-third as a target size for both the buccolingual width or mesiodistal length. Even a cursory evaluation of everyday RPDs will find the dimensions much closer to one-fourth or even one-fifth of those measures on molars. This undersizing has several negative effects. First, it complicates the ability to fit the casting. The smaller dimensions are more difficult to evaluate and adjust while also requiring more precision when casting. Second, it becomes technically very challenging to achieve a positive rest form with rounded angles. A larger rest is more easily made round, which will aid fitting procedures. Likewise, the larger rests will be stronger and more resistant to fracture.

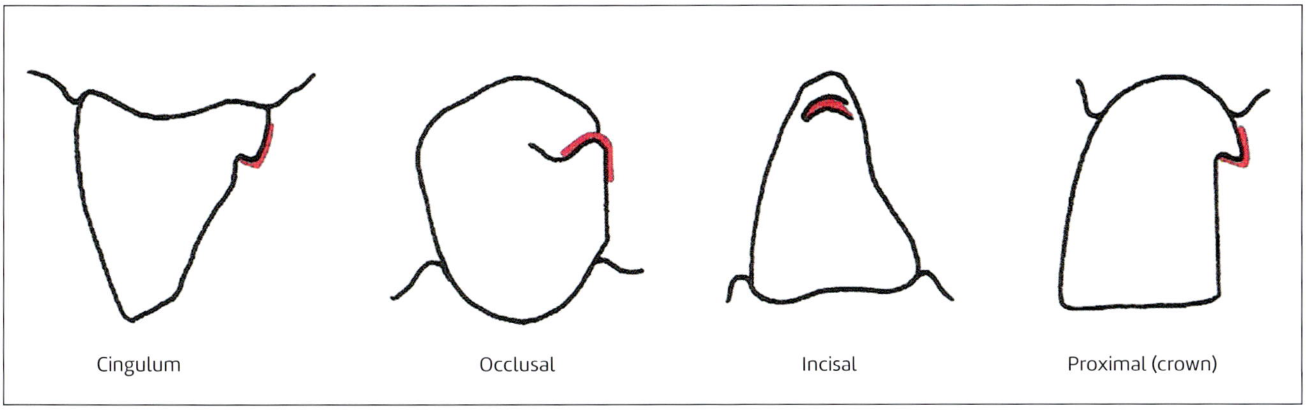

FIG 2-5 Illustration of "positive" rest form on the four primary types of rests.

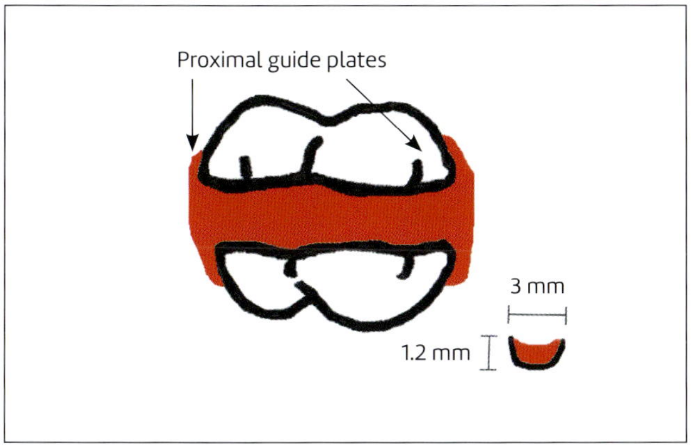

FIG 2-6 Strut rest.

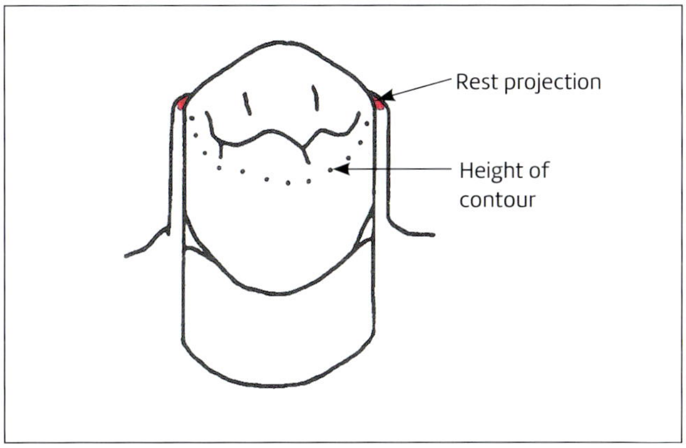

FIG 2-7 Rest projections.

The supposed contraindication to these rest dimensions is the belief that the smaller preparation is more conservative. This ignores the fact that the vast majority of abutment teeth in clinical practice have previous restorations. The larger the restoration, the larger the rest preparation can safely be while still conserving tooth structure. The larger size of the rest also serves as a means to judiciously "shoe" smaller or weakened cusps. This concept is discussed further later in this textbook with the concept of overlays. In the world of RPDs, an overlay is really nothing more than a large and very effective occlusal rest.

Another reason for undersized rests is the inadequate enamel thickness present for cingulum rests, especially on mandibular canines and incisors. Even well-undersized cingulum preparations will perforate through to dentin. Dentists therefore underprepare these areas. Incisal rests make for a good alternative but are often objectionable esthetically. To facilitate positive cingulum rest form of an adequate size, these rest seats are most likely to be made with either bonded etched metal, composite, or ceramic.

There are several uncommon types of rests that will be discussed throughout this textbook. Really, any design feature that can serve to support the prosthesis can be considered a rest. Embrasure clasp assemblies, when properly designed, include adjacent occlusal rests as the assembly passes through the embrasure. Overlays are a second rest example. Strut rests are another. Strut rests are commonly used to support and help splint periodontally compromised teeth (Fig 2-6). Rest projections can also be used. The effect of a positive rest is obtained with minor connectors (guide plates) only if they touch the tooth on opposing sides and above the height of contour. This tooth is not able to move away from the partial denture. This situation is rare and usually limited to the management of existing crowns with porcelain occlusal surfaces where preparing an adequate rest may damage a crown that need not otherwise be replaced (Fig 2-7).

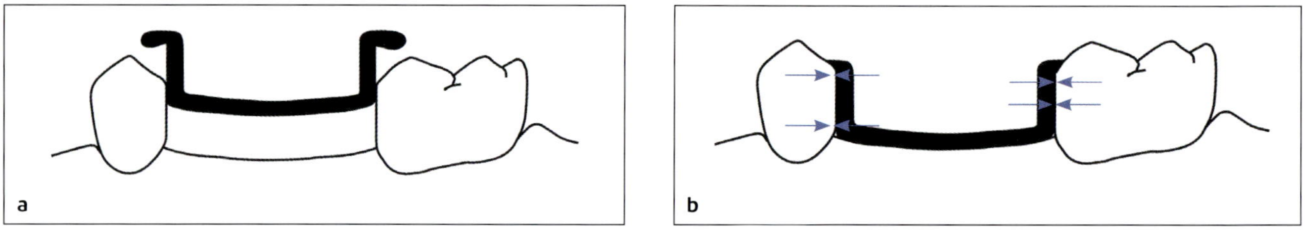

FIG 2-8 *(a)* Vertical seating along a precise path of placement/removal. *(b)* The fully seated guiding planes prevent lateral movement of any sort. No tipping, bending, or rotating can occur until the guiding plane contact is lifted beyond its effective length.

Guiding planes

With the quantity and quality of abutments determined and rest seats placed, we move on to establishing the stability of the partial denture. Resistance to lateral forces is best established with guiding planes. Traditionally, guiding planes were only considered to control the path of placement and removal of an RPD. This reflects the extent of "textbook" understanding. A quick review of the bibliography of traditional RPD textbooks shows how seldom guiding planes are considered. This is unfortunate because the guiding plane has replaced the clasp in terms of importance in modern RPD design. Guiding planes can achieve three very important goals: *(1)* controlling the path of placement and removal, *(2)* maximizing stability, and *(3)* improving the retention of an RPD if properly utilized in tooth-bound situations.[5–9] Achieving contact between the guide plates of a framework and accurately prepared guiding planes on abutment teeth will greatly increase the stability and frictional retention of the RPD.

With these featured goals in mind, the author prefers the following definition of *guiding planes*, based on the definition from the *Glossary of Prosthodontic Terms*[2]:

> **Guiding planes:** Two or more vertically parallel surfaces on abutment teeth and/or fixed dental prostheses oriented so as to control the path of placement and resistance to displacement of a tooth-borne removable dental prosthesis.

As highlighted in chapter 15, the modern concept of guiding planes developed as clinicians recognized the clinical benefits of maximizing stability. The frictional contact of the stabilizing surfaces has the added effect of increasing retention. By precisely controlling the path of placement and increasing the amount of friction, retention is achieved. Once a tooth-bound guiding plane–stabilized partial denture is fully seated, the partial denture cannot be dislodged without first rising vertically beyond the effective length of the guiding planes (Fig 2-8).

There are five basic requirements to utilize guiding planes in this fashion. First, a rigid major connector is required for cross-arch force distribution. A flexible vinyl major connector, for example, allows the frame to bend away from tooth-contacting surfaces. Second, there must be opposing surfaces. This eliminates Kennedy Class I situations where there are no posterior abutments of any kind. Without opposing surfaces, frictional retention cannot occur. Third, adequate abutment surface area is needed. The amount of frictional retention is mathematically related to the amount of surface area available. More surface area allows for more friction. This means the unmodified distal surface of short mandibular canines tends to be a poor choice. The triangular shape and narrow buccal lingual dimension leaves limited total surface area for friction to occur. Fourth, optimum parallelism between the abutments must be achieved. This can be challenging and is discussed in detail in chapter 4. Fifth, optimum framework fit must be achieved. A poorly fit framework, with space between the guiding planes and guide plates, will not achieve the desired frictional fit. The issue of fit is a major point of focus throughout this textbook and is where the majority of effort and clinical ingenuity are currently focused.

If these five factors are achieved, one can expect improvements in longevity, design simplification, function, periodontal response, and esthetics. It has been the author's experience that as guiding plane surfaces are achieved, clasps can be eliminated.[10] In certain Kennedy Class III situations where guiding planes are maximized, clasps can in fact be entirely eliminated. While this should not be taken as a goal, it demonstrates a hierarchy that values rests and guiding planes above clasps.

While guiding plane surfaces are generally the proximal surfaces of teeth adjacent to edentulous spaces, other lateral surfaces can and should be utilized for this purpose as well. Minor connectors rising through embrasures can also be designed as guiding surfaces. In fact, guiding planes are typically considered minor connectors because they often connect rests to the major connector. The coping prosthesis philosophy, popular in Germany, applies the guiding plane principles to all four tooth surfaces. This is the primary reason these designs are also able to eliminate the use of conventional clasps.

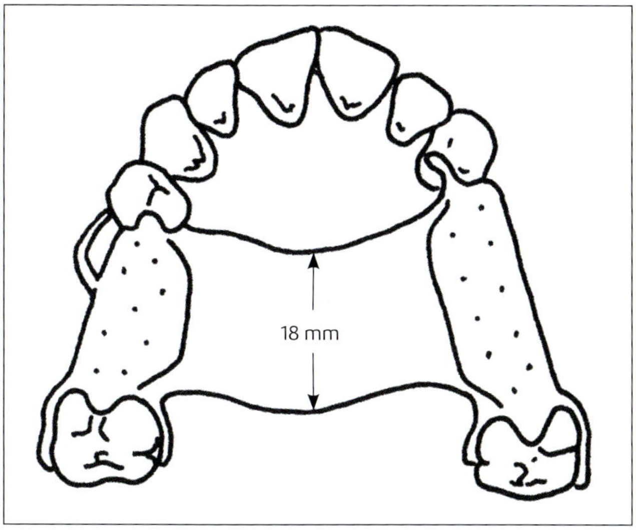

FIG 2–9 Palatal strap.

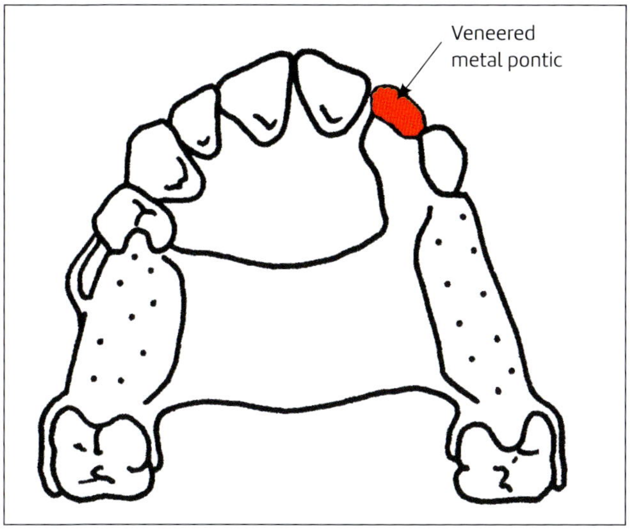

FIG 2–10 Cantilever from palatal strap.

Connectors

Once the abutments have been selected and the need for restorations (if any) verified, we move on to the second design consideration, that of choosing the connectors, both major and minor. The three primary factors for major connector selection are patient comfort, rigidity, and hygiene. If we expect patients to wear RPDs, they must cover as little surface area, in as subtle a way, as possible.[11] Rigidity is necessary to evenly distribute forces to the remaining teeth.[12] The often overlooked need to maintain periodontal health requires the RPD to cover as little soft tissue as possible.[13] The clinical reality for the average RPD is that the major connector is uncomfortable, is too large, and covers excess gingival tissue.[14]

The tendency to use large major connectors with extensive plating stems from the belief that size is required to achieve adequate rigidity. While this may have been true when the majority of frames were made from type IV gold alloys, today's cobalt-chromium or nickel-chromium alloys achieve clinically acceptable levels of strength and rigidity in much smaller dimensions. This makes plating to increase strength unnecessary and also facilitates the use of smaller, more hygienic frames like the dental lingual bar. Obviously, one issue with the recent popularity of nonmetallic frameworks is their lack of rigidity or strength in comfortable hygienic dimensions. Because the options for the major connectors are arch specific, it is best to consider them independently.

Maxillary major connectors

The major connector of choice is one that will, whenever possible, cover neither the anterior nor the posterior palate. Studies have shown that the connector commonly called the *palatal strap* is the one most acceptable to the patient.[11] This connector crosses the palate in the area of the mesial of the second premolar to the distal of the first molar and should be in the range of 15 mm to ensure sufficient rigidity without being too thick (Fig 2-9). There are instances, in smaller mouths, where this dimension can be significantly less. A palatal strap measuring, for example, 15 mm in width and having a cross-sectional thickness of 0.5 mm will, for all practical purposes, be rigid in normal function.

Unless anterior teeth are being replaced by the partial denture, this design is compatible with all posterior replacement situations. In situations where an isolated lateral incisor is being replaced, the casting can be extended as a cantilever from the canine to keep the anterior palate (speaking area) uncovered (Fig 2-10). It is essential that the canine have a very positive cingulum rest to support the cantilever against lateral forces.

In distal extension situations, the lateral extensions of the major connector are brought posteriorly to flow into the pterygomaxillary notch, thus assuring maximum coverage of the edentulous ridge. An alternative design often used for the maxilla is the anteroposterior strap, which seems to place metal in the least acceptable portions of the palate. These are the areas where the tongue, when in function, primarily contacts. The anterior strap will be in the speaking area, and the posterior strap will often be too far posterior for comfort. The resulting open central palate will have an extended border that can lead to excessive food collection under the partial denture.

Potential for further tooth loss within the life of the partial denture must always be considered in the major

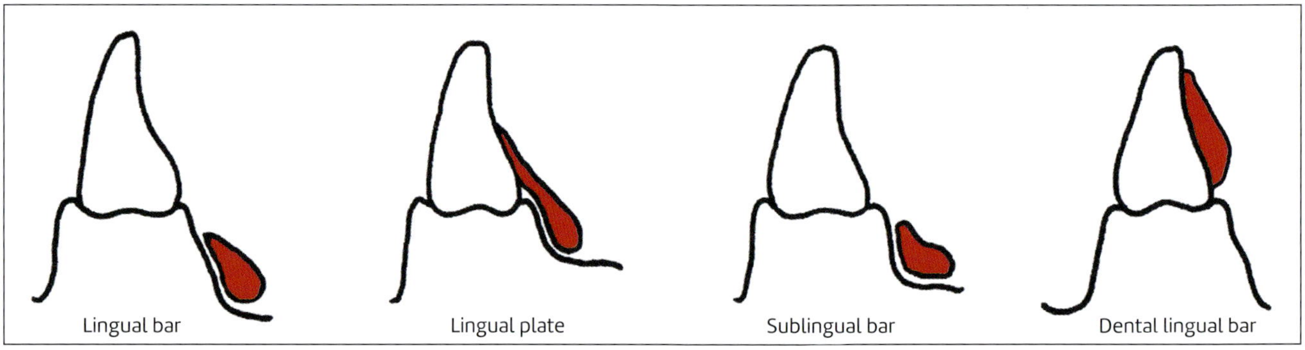

FIG 2-11 The four most common mandibular major connector designs.

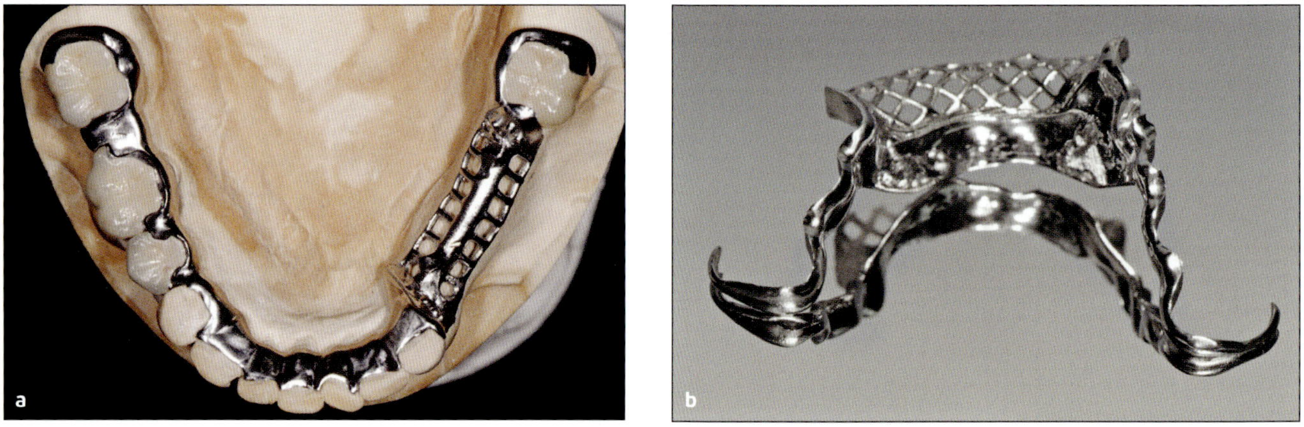

FIG 2-12 Dental lingual bar used for a Class III *(a)* and a Class IV *(b)* major connector.

connector design because the teeth in question need to have a lingual plate contact with the casting if they are to be easily added to the partial denture without affecting the quality of the prosthesis. A laser-welded component can always be added, but this will require a sizeable additional cost.

Mandibular major connectors

Designing a major connector for the mandible should be far easier than for the maxilla. Choices are limited to lingual bars, lingual plates, sublingual bars, dental lingual bars, some combination of these four, and—in very isolated instances—labial bars. The connector of choice will be the one that covers the minimum amount of soft tissue. The standard lingual bar does have space considerations that must be observed. The superior border of the bar must be 3 mm from the gingival margin of the remaining teeth to minimize soft tissue irritation. There must be 4 mm of space for the casting below this point in order to have a rigid major connector with minimum bulk. The commercial clasp patterns used by laboratories are very close to 4 mm in width. Therefore, 7 mm of space between the gingival marginal tissue of the remaining teeth and the functional depth of the floor of the mouth is essential if a lingual bar is desired.

When less space than this is available, the clinician must choose either a lingual plate, dental lingual bar, or sublingual bar. This connector has the same relationship with the gingival tissues of the remaining teeth but with some portion of the inferior extension of the bar rotated 90 degrees and placed on the anterior floor of the mouth (Fig 2-11). The dental lingual bar has almost the same dimensions as the conventional lingual bar, with the only difference being the simulation of lingual anatomy. The superior border is above the level of the cingulum and contacts the remaining anterior teeth above the gingival margin. Herein lies the periodontal benefit to this design.

The dimensions for a dental lingual bar are suggested by the size of the abutment teeth (Fig 2-12). It is therefore indicated when the clinical height of the teeth is great and the available major connector space is limited. With these connectors, the soft tissues can be left uncovered when

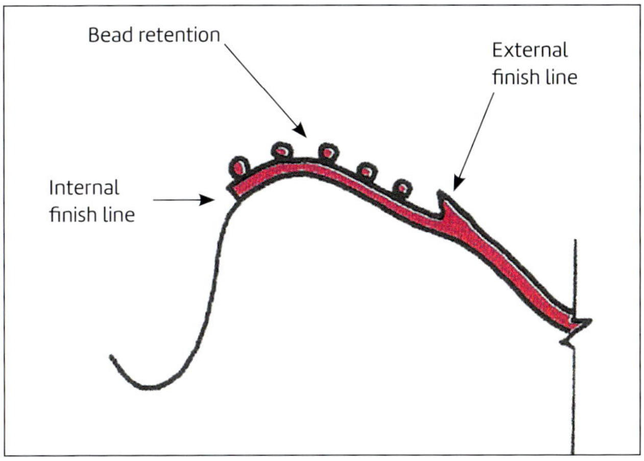

FIG 2-13 Diagram of the preferred resin retention method: bead retention. Note the design and position of the internal and external finish lines.

4 to 5 mm of space remains in the coverage area. The dental lingual bar may appear to be too narrow to have sufficient rigidity, but because it is supported by multiple abutments, there has been no evidence of problems that can be related to flexibility.[12] It certainly has been appreciated by the patients for whom it has been used.

In the very few situations where the remaining mandibular teeth are severely lingually inclined, the entire major connector can be brought out into the labial vestibule. The dimensions of the bar must be increased for rigidity because the arc will be longer. The soft tissues are given the same 3-mm clearance as in the lingual bar.

Minor connectors

As the name implies, minor connectors are the intervening metal between the major connector and the other RPD components. Traditionally, this has been the extent of minor connector use. They will most likely be found on the proximal surfaces of abutment teeth adjacent to edentulous areas. In special situations, they are added to lingual surfaces of teeth to isolate the path of insertion/removal. This will most often be done when teeth remain on only one side of the arch, as in extreme Kennedy Class II situations or maxillary obturators for hemi-maxillary resections.

As noted previously, we have found that minor connectors used as guiding planes have extensive value in stabilizing and even retaining the RPD. With that in mind, the minor connectors are to be placed onto prepared tooth surfaces whenever possible in order to restrict the path of removal. These prepared surfaces ultimately take the form of guide plates and rest extensions and, where necessary, lingual plates. How intently the tooth surfaces are paralleled and contacted will be determined by how much resistance to lateral forces (stability) the dentist wishes to design into the RPD and whether movement of the framework in function is required.

Whenever possible, minor connectors should contact preparations in enamel, augmented with bonded metal or composites. The use of contoured surveyed crowns is an excellent opportunity to maximize minor connector or guiding plane form and effectiveness.

The ideal minor connector relationship will be one where the marginal soft tissues will be uncovered. Six millimeters of clearance from the marginal tissues in the maxilla and 3 mm in the mandible are considered adequate. Numerous studies have shown that soft tissues that are not covered by the partial denture will be healthier than those that are covered, regardless of the patient's oral hygiene.[13] Metal dimensions for minor connectors that end in occlusal rests are based primarily upon having enough metal present (ie, > 1.5 mm) so that the rests will not fracture with time at the marginal ridge. The guide plates can be quite thin (eg, 0.5 mm) because they take little or no flexing stress and are not apt to be in occlusal contact. The approach arm of the minor connector must have a minimum of 1.5 mm of metal, both mesiodistally and buccolingually, to ensure adequate strength.

Resin Retention

The third element of RPD design is one that is almost always left to the laboratory technician to select, even though it is a decision that is clinically based. For the most part, the choice of retention for the denture teeth and associated base resin is simple. When it is certain that the edentulous area will need to be relined during the life of the partial denture, then the standard raised mesh is selected. These situations will be limited to those involving distal extension bases and areas of recent extraction. In every other instance, a metal base with appropriate retentive lugs or loops is indicated. The internal finishing line for these metal bases will be a butt joint slightly to the buccal of the ridge crest with the external as shown in Fig 2-13.

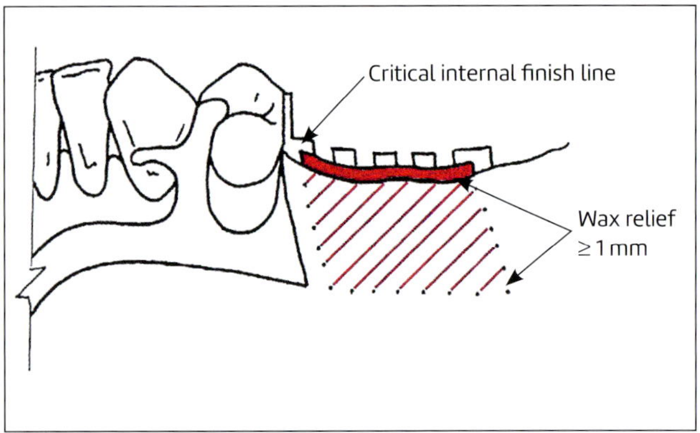

FIG 2-14 For the raised mesh, the internal line is formed by the shape of the wax relief pad.

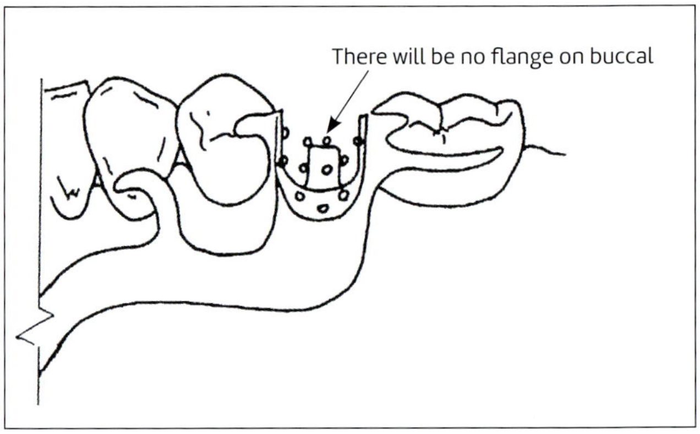

FIG 2-15 Example of a single posterior tooth replacement.

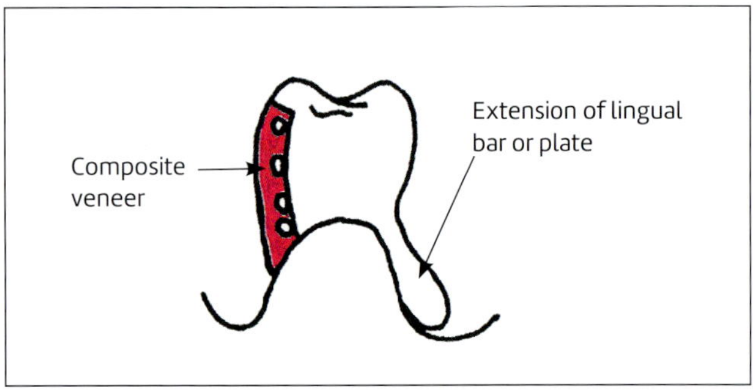

FIG 2-16 A solid metal prosthetic tooth veneered with composite is often the ideal choice for situations with limited space.

The reason why metal coverage is preferred is that it places highly polished metal over the gingival marginal tissue rather than the thin flash of resin that is commonly found with the standard raised retentive mesh. When mesh must be used, the laboratory must be instructed to use a minimum of one thickness of baseplate wax as the relief pad rather than the usual 24- to 28-gauge wax. The thin 24- to 28-gauge wax sheets leave inadequate acrylic below the mesh. This leads to leakage because the limited thickness of acrylic is porous, and the metal is often exposed during adjustments or relines.[14]

The angle of the internal finishing line is a critical component of the retentive mechanism. For an ideal internal finishing line, the angle formed in the wax must be acute so that the resultant contour in the casting will trap the resin in place and reduce the percolation that occurs with thermal changes (Fig 2-14). Resin bonding agents, properly placed, will overcome the potential for resin-metal separation, but their use is not currently a part of the normal processing protocol in most dental laboratories. The external finishing line must also provide an acute angle so as to lock in the resin and reduce leakage. The finishing line must extend from the appropriate line angle to the occlusal surface so that the denture tooth can be placed in a normal position with a small amount of resin between it and the finish line.

Whenever possible, missing anterior teeth are to be replaced with fixed partial dentures (FPDs), leaving the RPD to replace posterior teeth. Attempting to replace both anterior and posterior teeth on the same casting is a compromise that may affect both esthetics and abutment stability. As an additional benefit of anterior fixed replacements, the FPD will be given ideal contours to support the posterior partial denture and to allow the elimination of buccal clasp arms. A variety of precision attachments can be added to these abutment crowns to eliminate anterior clasping as well.

For the single-tooth edentulous space, there are various options available to the clinician and the technician. Most commonly, some form of reinforced acrylic pontic is chosen. These can be best described as metal ridge coverage with a post extending into the denture tooth. Additional metal beads will enhance the retention (Fig 2-15).

Only in the rarest of circumstances should raised mesh retention be selected for the single tooth, because the amount of retention created in the constricted mesh space is inadequate to retain the denture tooth. When space is lacking, a metal backing, waxed as part of the casting but having the attributes of the lingual aspects of a fixed pontic, is indicated because additional support is required against the forces of incision. This "pontic" is then veneered with a composite resin (Fig 2-16).

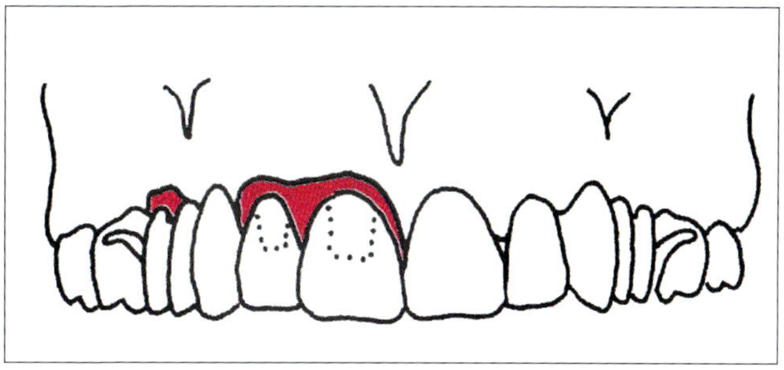

FIG 2-17 A short flange, often tinted, is indicated to restore the esthetics of interdental papillae.

When the occlusal surface of the pontic is an integral part of the casting, the opposing cast, if there is any, must accompany the definitive cast to the laboratory. When the opposing occlusion is a denture tooth, the anatomy of the occlusal surface of the metal pontic should mimic the selected denture tooth.

The most efficient way to manage the single-tooth replacement is to select the denture tooth before the master cast is sent to the laboratory for the framework. The tooth is ground in to fit the edentulous area, an esthetic try-in is arranged (if appropriate), and a matrix, made of either firm putty or plaster, is formed to positively position the denture tooth on the master cast. The technician will utilize the matrix and the denture tooth when waxing the framework, and the result will be a retentive form keyed to the ideal tooth position. Obviously, this technique is most often needed for the replacement of anterior teeth and is essential when two or more adjacent anterior teeth are being replaced on the partial denture. On some occasions when a denture tooth cannot be found that matches the shade of the adjacent natural teeth, a composite veneer made from an indirect hybrid composite like Sinfony (3M ESPE) can be placed on a properly designed metal pontic. These materials can be blended and stained to match almost any tooth. They are, however, quite brittle in shear and, as a result, should have metal at the incisal to protect the veneer. The partial denture casting can be 0.3 mm thick at the incisal or occlusal and still be rigid enough to withstand direct functional forces. Whenever possible, the single-tooth replacement should be planned to exit from the tissue as a fixed pontic, without any resin flange. When two adjacent teeth are replaced, a very short flange may be required to provide for the interdental papilla (Fig 2-17).

Often, this short flange can be kept very thin and made to closely match the surrounding attached gingiva with a minimum of tinting of the base with colored resin (Earl Pound technique). For heavily pigmented gingiva, the flange can be packed in clear resin with appropriate tinting so that the patient's gingiva can be seen through the very thin flange. The red fibers normally found in standard denture resins must be removed by sifting the polymer through a 2 × 2 gauze because the presence of the fibers in the area of the attached gingiva can never be anatomically correct and will spoil the esthetic effect of even the most carefully tinted resin.

The purpose of a flange on an RPD is quite a bit different than a flange on a complete denture. While the flanges of distal extensions in Class I situations will be very much like denture flanges, tooth-bound flanges serve only to prevent food impaction and restore lost contour for comfort and esthetics. Because tooth-bound segments are entirely supported by the adjacent abutments, there is no soft tissue support. This means that the extension and dimension of an RPD flange is determined by the volume and location of the residual ridge resorption in that specific edentulous segment. The flange should only restore the contour necessary to restore the lost anatomy. This is best tested at a trial placement with a finalized wax-up.

Clasp Retention

The fourth and final consideration in the design of the RPD is that of "spring" retention, usually a retentive clasp arm. Clinicians continue to feel that clasp selection is the most important consideration in design. Clasp types, be they I-bar, circumferential, reverse back action, or any other of the many clasps that have found a place in prosthodontics, do not appear to have any clearly defined effect on the clinical success of the partial denture. What is more important is that the clasp be properly made to be strong, retentive, and esthetic and to do no harm. We will base our selection on these factors alone and will consider the type of clasp the least important component of our advanced partial denture.

Because the laboratory plays such a large role in the design of the standard RPD, it is not strange that they may emphasize clasp construction. Our technicians are often forced to create castings with little or no evidence of preparation of the remaining teeth. The undesirable undercuts that may exist force technicians to devise ways to work around them, resulting in clasps that are

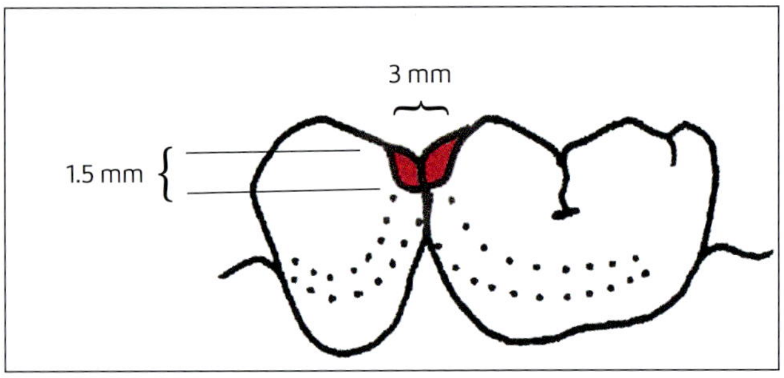

FIG 2-18 Minimum preparation dimensions for a typical two-armed embrasure clasp assembly.

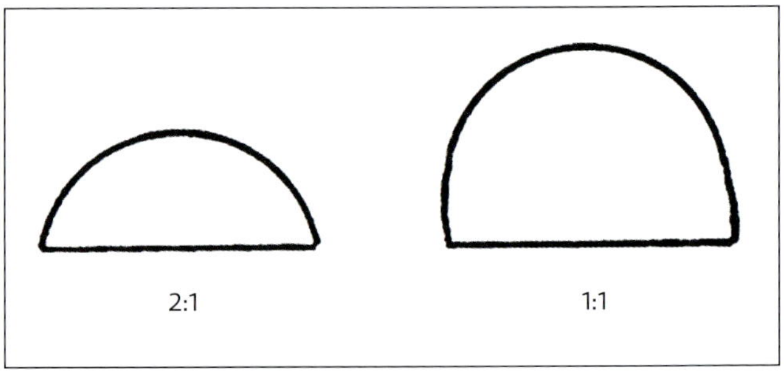

FIG 2-19 Width-to-thickness ratios for two cast clasp patterns.

excessive in number and generally unesthetic. A laboratory-designed RPD will usually have more retentive clasps than one designed by a prosthodontist, because careful mouth preparation can be expected to maximize stability, which will in turn reduce the overall retentive requirements. The number of clasps, especially those that are unesthetic, can also be reduced by the way the casting is managed when fitting, finishing, and polishing. These techniques are fully discussed later in this text.

When retentive clasps are contemplated, their length, taper, and cross-sectional width-to-thickness ratio must be taken into account. The alloy from which they are made and the degree of retentive undercut in which they are placed also affects their flexibility and resistance. All these factors will describe a retentive clasp arm of any configuration that can be expected to function below its proportional limit. Factors that result in a distortion of the clasp arm from any cause must be altered so that the clasp will perform as desired for the life of the partial denture.

Given a mouth that has had ideal mouth preparation, either subtractive or additive, there are only four forms of retentive clasp arms that need be used: circumferential clasp, circumferential wire, I-bar, and L-bar.

Circumferential cast clasp

This clasp is the most commonly used of all the clasp forms and is easily constructed by the laboratory and adjusted by the clinician. While it is strong, it is also rigid and potentially unesthetic. It is therefore indicated for the posterior part of the mouth and, because of its rigidity, best used in tooth-borne situations. A modification of the circumferential clasp is the embrasure clasp, which is nothing but two circumferential clasps back to back. This clasp, used primarily in fully dentate sextants, is rarely necessary in conventional RPDs but does have a place in some maxillofacial prostheses. The amount of retention gained from the anterior projecting arms of the embrasure clasp is usually excessive, and when that anterior component is on a premolar, it will become quite rigid due to its reduced length. The buccal clasp arm is apt to be unesthetic as well. In the well-prepared mouth, the posterior component on the molar provides adequate retention for the conventional partial denture. The embrasure clasp passing through a contact area is a clasp that often breaks in service. The reason for this is that there is seldom enough space created through the contact areas of the two teeth at the embrasure. As a result, the clasp is often found to be in hyperocclusion. The adjusting of the metal to allow tooth contact with the opposing arch weakens the clasp by making it thinner at the buccal extension of the marginal ridge than it is further along the clasp arm. This thin area sets up a flexure point in the clasp, and after repeated movement of the clasp arm in function, a stress fracture develops. Repair of this broken embrasure clasp is difficult, if not impossible, to accomplish with any hope of long-term success. To create adequate space for the most commonly used clasp pattern, the clinician must prepare a channel measuring 1.5×1.5 mm for one clasp coming through the embrasure and 1.5×3.0 mm if two clasps are run through that same embrasure (Fig 2-18).

The cast circumferential clasp pattern that should be requested when maximum flexibility is required is one with a width/thickness ratio of near 2:1; the 3MA40 pattern is one example. Unfortunately, this pattern ratio is somewhat difficult to find, and some pattern manufacturers do not even provide width/thickness ratios on their products. The 1:1 ratio clasp is a 1BA55 pattern and is about three times as stiff as the 2:1 clasp[15] (Fig 2-19).

The conventional approach to the cast circumferential clasp requires that a bracing arm, theoretically placed more gingivally on the tooth, be used to provide reciprocation.

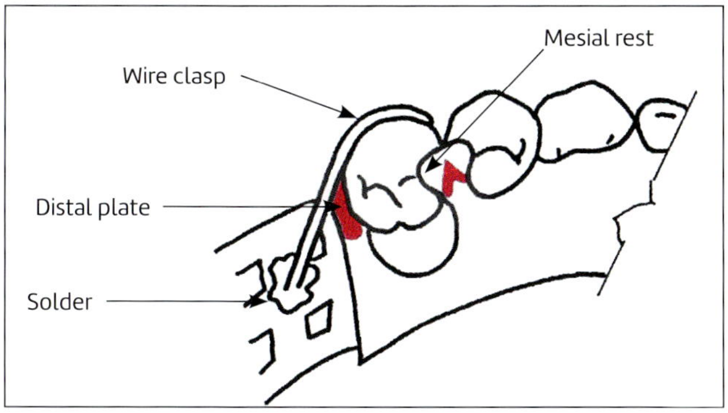

FIG 2-20 Elimination of lingual bracing arm (reciprocation) with guiding planes *(red)*.

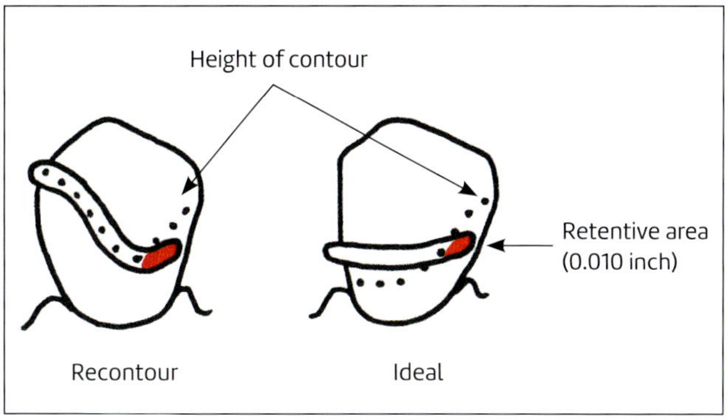

FIG 2-21 Tooth contour for retentive clasps (wire or cast). The contour on the *left* requires recontouring to increase clasp flexibility and avoid occlusal interference.

The need for this bracing arm, customary since the end of the band clasp era (see chapter 15), has never been clearly demonstrated. If a bracing arm is placed to reciprocate, it should be made from a pattern having a width-to-thickness ratio that approaches 1:1 in order to resist the more appropriately flexible 2:1 ratio retentive clasp.

There are other ways to achieve reciprocation that are not clasp dependent. These would include precise guiding planes on the minor connectors to the rests as well as the natural contact of the tooth to the adjacent tooth. In order for the so-called "bracing arm" to function as it has been proposed it should, it must contact the abutment on a surface parallel to the path of insertion in such a way as to hold the abutment tooth in position as the retentive clasp arm passes over the height of contour and the rest seats fully. This situation normally only occurs when a milled surface has been prepared on a casting for the abutment since the natural tooth is unlikely to have parallel walls opposite the retentive clasp arm. Once the partial denture is fully seated, the prepared guiding planes provide lateral bracing for the partial denture in a way that clasp arms cannot (Fig 2-20).

Circumferential wire clasp

The wrought wire clasp, as it is universally known, has long been considered the clasp of choice for Class I and II partial dentures, especially for the mandible. It is obvious that a structure that is cold rolled, as all wires are, is going to be more flexible than a cast clasp of similar dimensions.[16] In addition, because it is round, this clasp will be roughly three times more flexible than a half-round cast clasp when loaded in a direction other than horizontally, as it would be as the prime retentive element on a mandibular bilateral distal extension partial denture. The retentive properties of wire are dependent on alloy, length of the active clasp arm, and gauge.[17]

The means of attachment of the wire to the framework also has an effect on the flexibility of the clasp, with the most ideal situation being one where the wire is attached some distance from where it is expected to flex. This would normally be on the resin retention area 0.33 inch back from the tooth. Both precious and nonprecious wires can and have been used for retentive clasp arms. There is generally one gauge difference between a precious wire and one that is an alloy of nickel-chromium or similar material, with the nonprecious wire being stiffer.[18] The Jelenko Standard wire was for a long time the clasp wire of choice (Au 63%, Ag 11%, Pt 10%, Pd 2%, and Cu 13%). However, because it is no longer made, other wires like Argenco 12 (Argen) have been used instead with similar clinical results.

In order to get maximum flexibility from the circumferential wire clasp, every effort must be made to keep the bend placed in the wire in two planes. Historically (and before mouth preparation), wires took the place of plate gold clasps. They were bent to conform to the unmodified tooth contours and, as a result, were bent in the three planes of space as the clasp made an abrupt bend from the marginal ridge toward the gingival and was then contoured around to the mesial of the tooth to enter the undercut. As each successive bend was made, the wire flexibility was reduced.

Accurate tooth modification to reduce the undercuts on the proximal two-thirds of the buccal surface allow the clasp to exit from the flange area close to the gingiva and enter the retentive area in the terminal one-third to a depth of 0.01 inch to 0.15 inch (Fig 2-21). Another advantage of most wires is that if one is bent beyond its proportional limit, for example when a patient mishandles a clasp, there appears to be no clinically significant effect on flexibility or displacement.[19] The wire is simply readapted to the tooth contour.

The selection of gold wires is based primarily on active length according to this simple rule, which allows each wire to perform below its proportional limit: clasps with

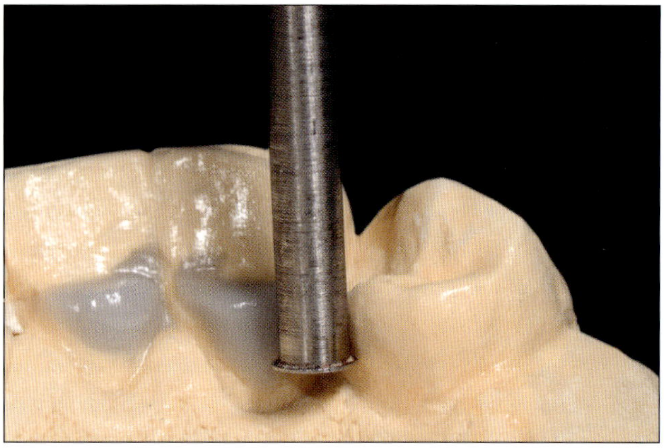

FIG 2-22 Typical mesiolingual undercut on a mandibular premolar.

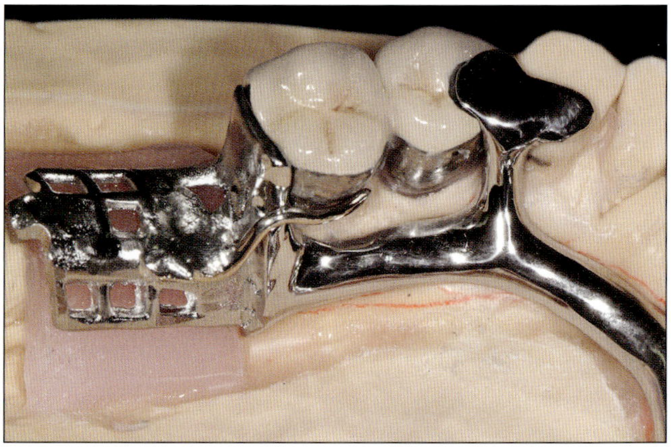

FIG 2-23 Lingual retentive clasp arm on a splinted mandibular premolar.

an active length of < 7 mm should be of 20 gauge, those with a length of 8 to 10 mm will be of 19 gauge, and those > 10 mm will be of 18 gauge.[17] At these distances and these gauges, the wires will give approximately the same amount of retention and remain below their proportional limit. While it may be possible to place some wires into undercuts of > 0.15 inch and still have them function without distortion, there is no clinical evidence that this increase in undercut depth is of any value.

The wire clasp can be used successfully on the lingual surface of most mandibular premolars, in conjunction with a distal guide plate that extends slightly beyond the distal facial line angle and a mesial rest or positive contact with the adjacent tooth, to provide retention without any display of buccal metal[20] (Fig 2-22). In these situations, the clasp arm will be very short and must therefore be of 20 gauge or finer (Fig 2-23). The major connector is normally a lingual or sublingual bar, at least in the area of this clasp, to allow the required 3 mm space at the bar's superior margin.

In the maxilla, the major connector is opened to the lingual as a matter of course whenever possible. This ensures that finding a lingual surface for the wire retentive clasp arm will not normally be a problem if the tooth contours provide any retentive areas of 0.01 inch or greater. There is no need for a buccal bracing arm in these situations. When the major connector cannot be opened for any reason in either arch, it is still possible to utilize only a lingual circumferential retentive clasp arm if sufficient tooth height exists to permit the wire to sit on the occlusal border of the lingual plate at the level of the height of contour and then enter the undercut at the terminal third where the lingual plate dips below the 0.01-inch undercut. The only disadvantage to this design is the very slight opening of the major connector beneath the clasp tip (Fig 2-24).

Unlike cast clasp arms that can be expected to break if they are deformed and then recontoured more than a few times, wire clasps (especially those of high gold alloys) will withstand repeated readaptation without any change in their retentive properties. Because these clasps are more flexible, they have the disadvantage of being far easier for the patient to deform if they are used as handles to remove the partial denture from the mouth. Patients must be warned that deformation of a properly placed wire clasp can only occur if the wire is loaded beyond its proportional limit, and that will not happen if the clasp is not distorted by the patient. Some patients insist on biting their partial dentures into place rather than placing them with the fingers of both hands. Patients must be shown that they should use the flanges of the denture base as a purchase point for removing the denture. Sometimes the placement of a simulated Class V cavity on a denture tooth will give the patient a purchase point to apply a dislodging force. When the clasp has been placed on the lingual surface, the patient is unable to use it as a lever and the clasp is less likely to be overstressed or bent.

Infrabulge clasps: I-bar and L-bar

Infrabulge clasps have long been advocated as an alternative to the circumferential wire clasp for Class I and II situations. They have been proposed as a more esthetic alternative to the circumferential cast clasp as well. These clasps can come in a number of forms and can be either cast or wrought. The most commonly used infrabulge clasp has been the I-bar, which was to be placed at the greatest convexity of the tooth mesiodistally as seen from the horizontal (there is no clinical evidence that this precise placement makes any difference). When combined with a proximal

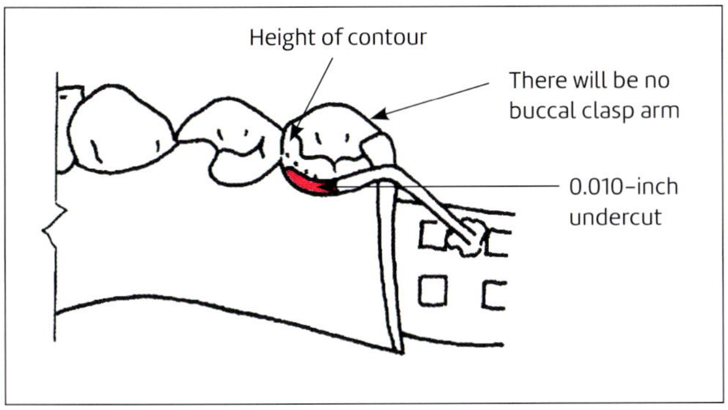

FIG 2-24 Lingual retentive wire clasp above lingual plate.

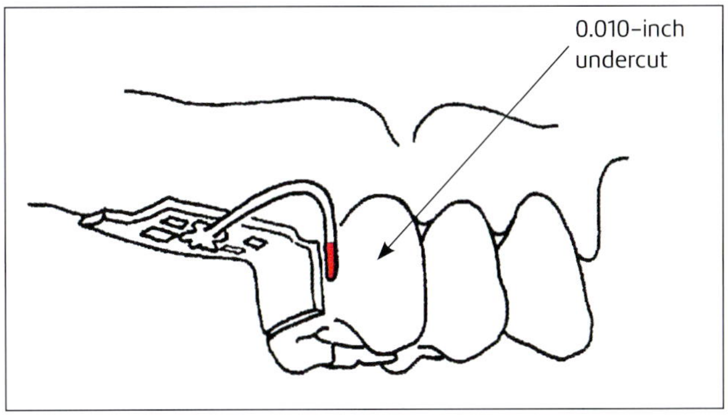

FIG 2-25 Short-wire I-bar to distobuccal retentive area.

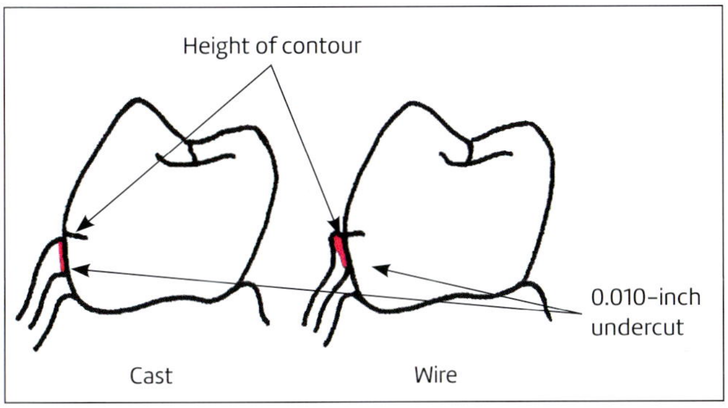

FIG 2-26 Tooth-bar clasp relationship.

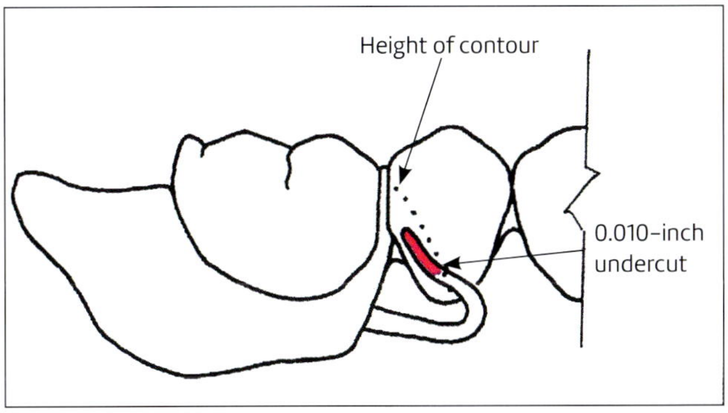

FIG 2-27 Contour indicating the L-bar clasp.

guide plane at the edentulous side of the prime abutment and a rest at the other end of the occlusal surface, no bracing arm is required because the tooth cannot be displaced by the action of the retentive clasp arm. Depending on the contact of the guide plane, stress relief can be created with this system for the Class I situation. When the I-bar clasp is made of a suitable length and gauge of wire, additional advantages are possible. Because the wire is added to the casting by soldering after the frame has been finished and polished, it is possible to place the clasp arm very close to the buccal extension of the guide plate (Fig 2-25).

With this distal positioning, the clasp arm becomes shorter and must therefore be of a higher gauge to retain flexibility (normally a 20-gauge wire will be chosen). The guiding plane and plate must extend fully to the line angle, and a positive rest on the opposite side of the abutment must be used to provide reciprocation if the distally placed I-bar is on a terminal abutment. If this type of clasping is used on the anterior abutment of a Class III partial denture, the need for precise reciprocation is not as great because the posterior abutment will restrict distal movement of the partial denture.

The contact between the I-bar and the retentive area must not be a point contact. Instead, the wire is contoured in such a way as to present a line contact or a surface contact. When a cast I-bar is used, the surface contact is created in the blockout and waxing of the framework (Fig 2-26). These expanded contact areas provide a margin of error for the technician because placing a clasp tip at point contact on a repeated basis is an unreasonable request.

While the I-bar clasp is by far the most common of the infrabulge clasps, there is an occasional need for an L-bar when the only available usable undercut is immediately adjacent to the edentulous area and where even a light-wire I-bar will be too short and therefore too rigid. By bringing the approach arm up to the mid buccal of the tooth and then bringing the base of the L-bar distally to the retentive area, sufficient clasp length can be developed in most situations (Fig 2-27). This clasp form can be created in either cast metal or with wire, again remembering to choose the appropriate gauge based upon the active length of the clasp.

Other forms of bar clasps have been advocated over the years, primarily the T-bar and occasionally a U-bar. These forms have no place in the modern RPD and are generally unesthetic and difficult (if not impossible) to adjust, especially if they are made in cast metal.

There is one major contraindication for the infrabulge clasp. The height of contour of the soft tissue in the area of the proximal approach arm and the degree of soft tissue undercut can make the bar clasps unacceptable. If the height of contour is very close to the buccal marginal tissue, the approach arm will have to stand out from the tissue because it cannot be in an undercut relative to the path of insertion as determined by the guiding planes. If that soft tissue undercut is severe, the clasp may abrade the buccal mucosa in normal function.

Even the most casual glance at any text about RPDs will identify many other clasp forms, such as ring clasps, back-action clasps, "C" or fishhook clasps, and more. These clasp forms have all been created to work around contours that have not been adequately modified with appropriate mouth preparation or, in some cases, teeth that need minor orthodontia to return them to a normal position in the arch. If there is no useable mesial undercut for a circumferential wire clasp, undercuts on the lingual surface will have to be used or the tooth modified with some form of additive preparation. Given quality mouth preparation, no other forms beyond the cast and wrought circumferential clasps and the I-bar and L-bar clasps, either wrought or cast, are indicated.

There are two other general categories of cast retentive elements that will be considered later in this textbook: the rotational path of insertion partial and the hinged connector (commonly referred to as a *swinglock*). These two special types of frameworks may include conventional clasping in addition to their special retentive devices.

Attachments, whether precision, semiprecision, or resilient, obviously take the place of the retentive clasp and are described in detail later as well. The use of attachments for the retentive elements have little effect on the principles of design. They serve only as substitutes for the retentive clasp and are placed on proximal surfaces adjacent to the edentulous area or in a pontic, should one exist, in posterior fixed restorations.

References

1. Frantz WR. Variability in dentists' designs of a removable maxillary partial denture. J Prosthet Dent 1973;29:172–182.
2. The Glossary of Prosthodontic Terms: Ninth Edition. J Prosthet Dent 2017;117(5S):e1–e105.
3. Sorensen J, Martinoff J. Endodontically treated teeth as abutments. J Prosthet Dent 1985;53:631–636.
4. Jasim FA, Brudvik JS, Nicholls JI. Impression distortion from abutment tooth inclination in removable partial dentures. J Prosthet Dent 1985;54:532–538.
5. Stewart KL, Rudd KD. Stabilizing periodontally weakened teeth with removable partial dentures. J Prosthet Dent 1968;19:475–482.
6. Kratochvil FJ. Maintaining supporting structures with a removable partial prosthesis. J Prosthet Dent 1971;25:167–174.
7. Brudvik JS, Shor A. The milled surface as a precision attachment. Dent Clin North Am 2004;48:685–708.
8. Ahmad I, Waters NE. Value of guide planes in partial denture retention. J Dent 1992;20:59–64.
9. Ali M, Waters NE, Nairn RI, West F, Sheriff M. A lab investigation of the role of guide planes in the retention of cast cobalt-chromium alloy partial denture frameworks. J Dent 2001;29:291–299.
10. Ahmad I, Sherriff M, Waters NE. The effect of reducing the number of clasps on removable denture retention. J Prosthet Dent 1992;68:928–933.
11. Campbell LD. Subjective reactions to major connector designs for removable partial dentures. J Prosthet Dent 1977;37:507.
12. Walter RD, Brudvik JS, Raigrodski AJ, Mancl LA, Chung KH. A comparison of the rigidity of five mandibular major connectors for partial removable dental prostheses via load deflection. J Prosthet Dent 2010;104:182–190.
13. Bissada NF, Ibrahim SI, Barsoum WM. Gingival response to various types of removable partial dentures. J Periodont 1974;45:651–659.
14. Pun DK, Waliszewski MP, Waliszewski KJ, Berzins D. Survey of partial removable dental prosthesis types in a distinct patient population. J Prosthet Dent 2011;106:48–56.
15. Morris HF, Asgar K, Brudvik JS, Winkler S, Roberts EP. Stress-relaxation testing. Part IV: Clasp pattern dimensions and their influence on clasp behavior. J Prosthet Dent 1983;50:319–326.
16. Frank RP, Brudvik JS, Nicholls JI. A comparison of the flexibility of wrought wire and cast circumferential clasps. J Prosthet Dent 1983;49:471–476.
17. Brudvik JS, Morris HF. Stress-relaxation testing. Part III: Influence of wire alloys, gauges, and lengths on clasp behavior. J Prosthet Dent 1981;46:374–379.
18. Morris HF, Asgar K, Roberts EP, Brudvik JS. Stress-relaxation testing. Part II: Comparison of bending profiles, microstructures, microhardnesses, and surface characteristics of several wrought wires. J Prosthet Dent 1981;46:256–262.
19. Matheson GR, Brudvik JS, Nicholls JI. Behavior of wrought wire clasps after repeated permanent deformation. J Prosthet Dent 1986;55:226–231.
20. Brudvik JS, Palacios R. Lingual retention and the elimination of the visible clasp arm. J Esthet Restor Dent 2007;19:247–254.

CLASSIFICATION-BASED DESIGN

3

Different support requires different design.

With an understanding of the components of the partial denture, we can now look to specific design considerations for each of the four basic classifications of RPD. Each classification must be considered independently. The differences in tooth versus tissue support dictate how the prosthesis will behave and therefore require variable design strategies. This is the value of the Kennedy classification.[1] So, while there will be many similarities in design, the intent of this chapter is to identify basic principles for each class independently. Despite these differences, the priority and sequence of the four components of partial denture therapy remain the same.

Much frustration with RPD design and teaching comes from the fact that the discipline covers such a wide variety of clinical scenarios. It is impossible to discuss any design feature regarding an RPD without first mentioning the Kennedy classification. When compared with other classification systems, the main differentiation of the Kennedy classification system is its ability to quickly and clearly demonstrate the location of tooth support in relation to edentulous spaces. Applegate's rules for use of the Kennedy classification are required for proper application[2] (Box 3-1 and Fig 3-1).

With dental implants available to replace strategic abutments, one must consider how this alters the Kennedy classification. An implant, when present, can be used in a multitude of ways. But what is always present with a healthy and integrated dental implant is support. For this reason, it seems logical to simply consider the dental implant a potential abutment. For the purpose of the Kennedy classification, it would therefore be considered the same as a natural tooth. This preserves the system's simplicity in defining the relationship between hard and soft tissue support. With that in mind, a ninth rule for application of the Kennedy classification is added[2] (Fig 3-2; see Box 3-1).

The classifications were originally ordered based on their prevalence, with Class I being the most commonly encountered situation and Class IV being the least.[3] However, with time and changing epidemiologic factors, this may no longer be the case.[4] Preventive dentistry, improved endodontic therapy, and the strategic use of dental implants all contribute to an increased percentage of Class II and III cases.

Applegate proposed two further classifications, Class V and Class VI.[5] His suggested Class V is a Class III with a very weak anterior abutment tooth (see Fig 2-1); for example, a lateral incisor with small root form. This class highlights the need for design modifications with anatomically weak abutments. His suggested Class VI situation is a single missing molar. This is commonly referred to as a *Nesbett partial* after Dr Norman Nesbett. This single-tooth RPD is regaining popularity with the use of flexible polyamide materials. It is considered compromised care due to the risk of aspiration, lack of stability, and periodontal challenges. Moreover, the superior predictability and long-term success of fixed options gives little reason to consider this design.

Box 3-1 Applegate's rules for Kennedy classification[2]

1	The classification should follow rather than precede extractions of teeth that might alter the original classification.
2	If a third molar is missing and not to be replaced, it is not considered in the classification.
3	If a third molar is present and is to be used as an abutment, it is considered in the classification.
4	If a second molar is missing and is not to be replaced, it is not considered in the classification.
5	The most posterior edentulous area (or areas) always determines the classification.
6	Edentulous areas other than those determining the classification are referred to as *modifications* and are designated by their number.
7	The extent of the modification is not considered, only the number of additional areas.
8	There can be no modification areas in Class IV arches. Any edentulous area lying posterior to the single bilateral area determines the classification; see Rule 5.
9*	If an osseointegrated dental implant is present and exposed to the oral cavity (ie, not buried subgingivally), it is considered the same as a natural tooth when determining the classification.

*Added by the authors.

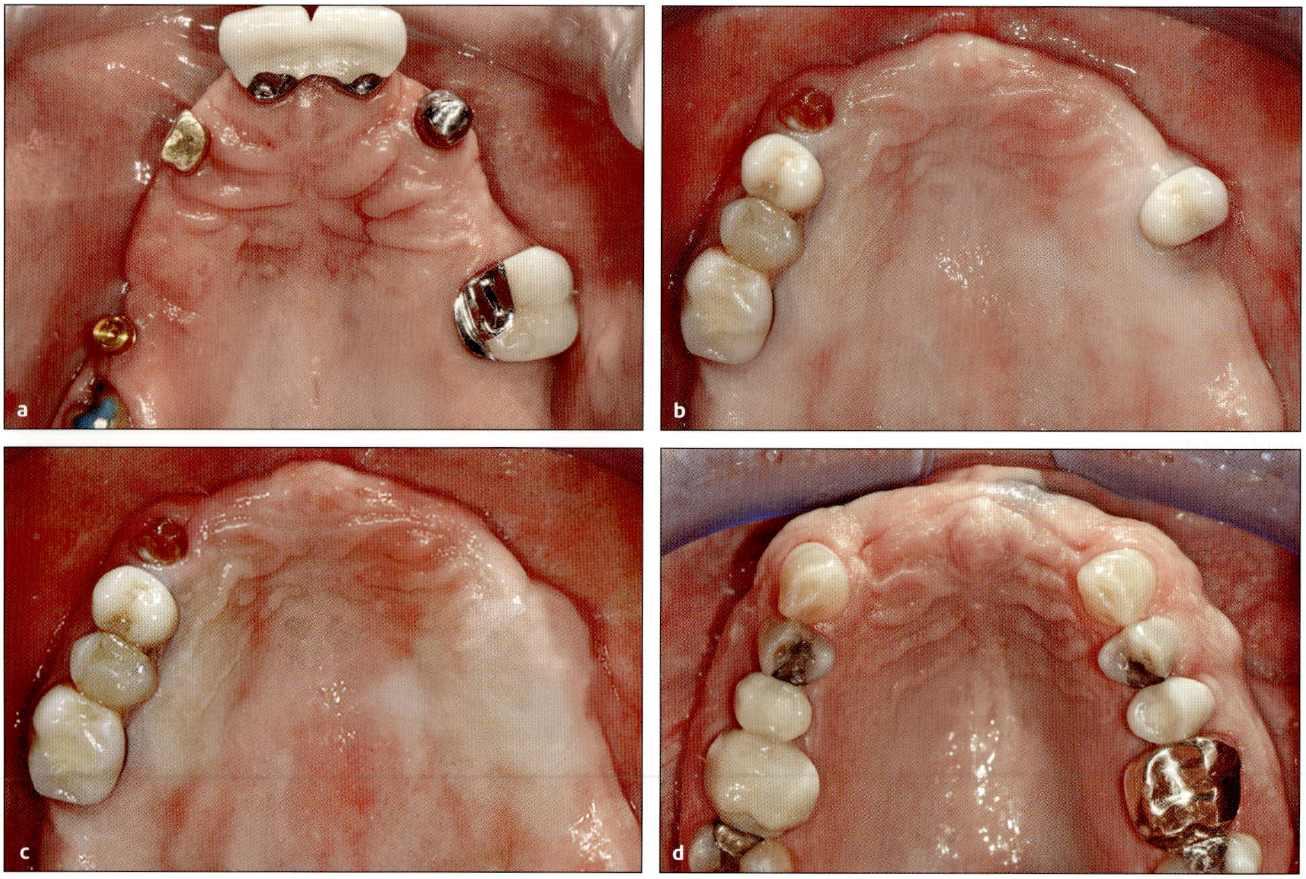

FIG 3-1 *(a)* Tooth no. 15 will not be replaced. Teeth nos. 2, 3, 6, and 11 are overlays. This is a Class III Mod 3. Rules 4, 6, 7. *(b)* Tooth no. 2 will not be replaced. This is a Class II Mod 1. Rules 4, 5, 6. *(c)* Tooth no. 2 will not be replaced. This is a Class II arch. Rules 4, 5. *(d)* A Class IV arch. Rule 8.

NOTE: The Universal numbering system is used in this book.

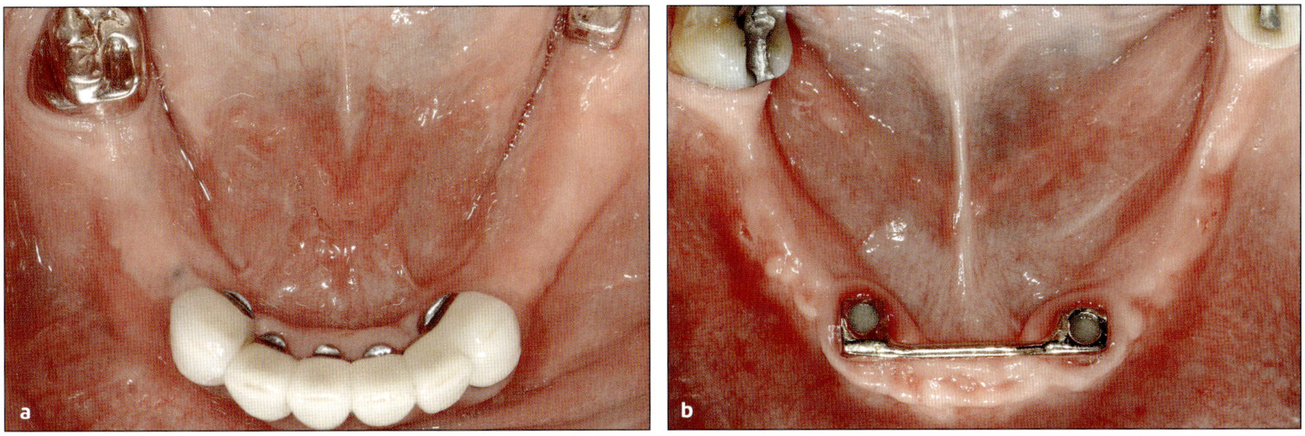

FIG 3-2 *(a)* An implant at site no. 18 creates a Class III Mod 1 arch from the previous Class II Mod 1. Rule 9. *(b)* Two splinted anterior implants create a Class III Mod 1 arch from the previous extreme Class IV. Rule 9.

Finding the Path of Insertion

Before any specific designs can be established, a quality diagnostic cast must be available for surveying. The cast must accurately represent all remaining teeth as well as those soft tissue areas that will be within the denture space. This includes retromolar pads, frenum extensions, and vestibules when bar clasps are being considered.

The first step will always be to determine the path of insertion and removal. Here the emphasis is on the path of removal because the goal will be to limit the possible directions that the partial denture can exit from the mouth through preparation of hard tissues. The path of insertion is, of course, the reciprocal of the more important path of removal and is most often presented as being of some importance. In all but one instance, the path of removal should be parallel to the long axis of the prime abutment(s). There will be occasions, usually in Class IV situations and especially in those where a rotational path of insertion is planned, when the path of removal is primarily determined by the soft tissue contour height.

The path of insertion/removal is frozen in space by the prepared guiding planes and the cast guide plates (minor connectors) that touch them. Undercuts on hard or soft tissue exist only relative to that path, so tilting the cast on the surveyor in order to alter the relative heights of contour to obtain retention will not produce real undercuts unless the path is controlled by the planes. Given the frictional retention that parallel guide plates can provide, there is seldom any need to be concerned about retention. If there are no usable retentive areas anywhere on the desired abutment teeth, then they must be created by either subtractive or additive mouth preparation.

Class I RPD

The Class I RPD is both tooth and tissue supported. Maximum support of and on the remaining abutment teeth is therefore essential. Provision must be made to allow or create stress relief in the casting, especially on the mandibular arch, so that some support can be placed on the edentulous ridges to dissipate the load of heavy mastication. This can only occur if the casting allows some degree of rotation around the terminal axis when loaded.

Abutment selection and rests

Only when canines are the prime abutments (ie, the abutments adjacent to the distal extension base) should a single abutment be chosen per side for the Class I partial denture. When the first premolar is the prime abutment, then that side will have two abutments. The lone premolar must have an occlusal rest and the adjacent canine either a distal incisal or a cingulum rest. A first premolar used by itself does not provide sufficient support to replace the missing molars and the second premolar. If the second premolar is the prime abutment, then there will be either two or three abutments, based on the level of bone support. If they have excellent bone support and the opposing arch is a complete denture, the canine or first premolar rest can be eliminated, leaving only two abutments (Fig 3-3). For the mandible, this rest cannot be made deep enough and kept in enamel, so either bonded metal, composite, or ceramic must be used to create the rest seat. Because it is rare to replace only a second molar on a Class I RPD, the only options we need concern ourselves with are those mentioned in this section.

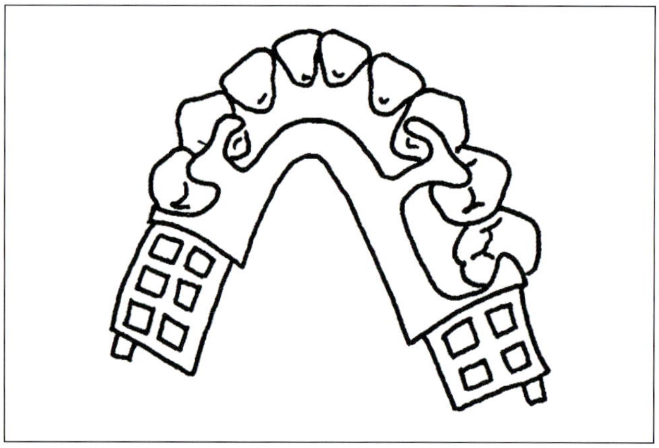

FIG 3-3 Multiple abutments are used when possible. Note that the lingual of tooth no. 21 is plated, while the larger area lingual to teeth nos. 28 and 29 is able to be left open when the rest is placed on the distal of the prime abutment.

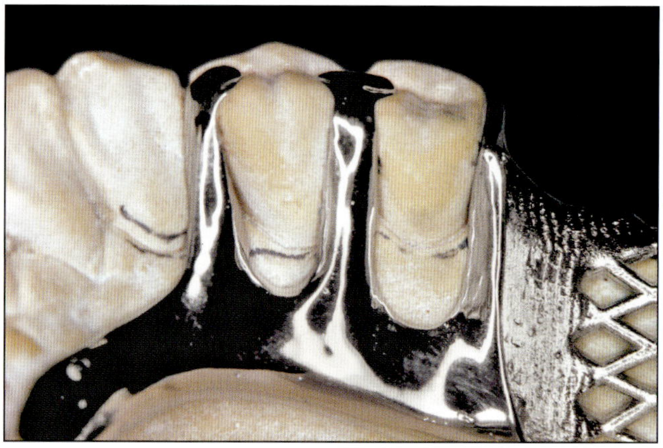

FIG 3-4 Even if shortened or relieved, this distal guide plate is the point of rotation (first contact with teeth). Placing the rest to the mesial creates negative periodontal consequences and increases the complexity of the casting due to the additional minor connector required to support the rest.

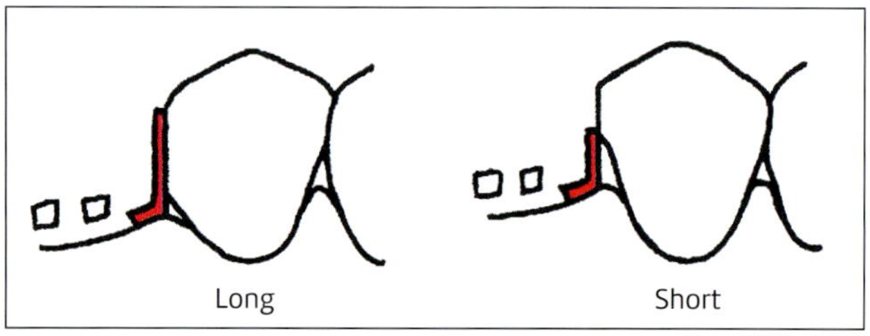

FIG 3-5 Guiding plane options for Class I partial dentures.

From a functional standpoint, the position of the occlusal rests on the premolars is immaterial, although some would say that a mesial rest on the prime abutment is more beneficial than a distal. While there may well be theoretical differences here, there appears to be no difference clinically in the well-made and well-maintained RPD. The theoretical difference comes from the historical belief that the occlusal rest is the point of rotation for the RPD framework. This long-held notion comes from 1930s RPD design that has persisted in RPD textbooks.[6] These historical designs had a gap or space between the lateral surface of the abutment tooth and the RPD. This allowed the rest to be the first point of contact with the tooth. The difference in the vast majority of modern RPDs is that the rest is not the first point of contact between the partial denture and the abutment tooth. It is the first point of contact with the tooth that is the point of rotation (Fig 3-4). This is more commonly the distal guide plate or minor connector. It can also be a clasp approach arm, prosthetic tooth, or lingual plating.

The path of insertion/removal will be chosen to allow parallelism of the distal surfaces of the prime abutments with minimal subtractive mouth preparation. The guiding planes created on the prime abutments require a basic decision. In order to allow some stress relief (rotation), two techniques have been proposed over the years. Kratochvil suggested that the guiding plane be prepared to be as long as possible with the stress relief coming from a functional relief of the casting before the altered cast impression was made.[7] Krol, on the other hand, described a shorter guiding plane extending from the marginal ridge roughly one-third the way down the tooth with the occlusal limit of the guide plate being the gingival extension of this shorter guiding plane[8] (Fig 3-5).

In the short option, often called *proximal plate design*, the stress relief is created in the blockout of the undercut gingival to the guiding plane. The guide plate is effective in reciprocation but can also rotate into the undercut rather than bind on the guiding plane during loading of the posterior denture bases. There is no clinical evidence that would favor one of these approaches over the other. The decision may well rest on the quality of the laboratory support because the reduced-length guiding plane/plate requires a greater attention to detail in both blockout and finishing of the casting to allow the theoretical rotation to occur on the mesial rest.

The assumption with this stress relief debate is that the forces of mastication generally torque the distal abutment toward the distal. Most RPD textbooks take this idea for granted and use it as the argument to create stress relief in the first place. However, there is evidence showing that masticatory forces actually tend to push the distal abutment tooth to the mesial.[9,10] This explains the inconclusive nature of clasp design comparisons and highlights the importance of evaluating the residual ridge anatomy. It is the ascending ramus and base contact with the retromolar pad in particular that creates the downward and therefore mesial direction of this force.

In either approach, the parallel guiding planes, contacted by the guide plates of the casting, restrict the path of insertion/removal to whatever angle of divergence was established in the mouth preparation phase of the treatment. The closer to 90-degree parallelism, the greater the frictional resistance to dislodgment of the denture with the potential for stress relief still viable. For the Class I partial denture, parallelism must be considered in another plane of space. In order for the partial denture to rotate freely around its fulcrum, the guiding planes must be parallel to each other from the occlusal view as they are in the sagittal (Fig 3-6). In other words, they must lie on the same plane across the arch so they can act in an identical fashion under occlusal load.

This need to consider the cross-arch parallelism invalidates unilateral diagrams for Class I design philosophies. For the other classes, the effect of the planes is enhanced by being in different planes as seen from the occlusal view. When the distal slopes of the two prime abutments cannot be made parallel through subtractive mouth preparation, usually when the canines are the prime abutments, the best option is to favor the weaker of the two. The other stronger abutment will be recontoured with additive mouth preparation to allow both sides to be parallel.

These design concepts work well with standard Class I situations. However, is stress relief still possible or advised when a modification space is present? This likely depends on tooth height, location of the modification space(s), and design of the framework. If rotation is still desired, guide plate contact will need to be limited or not present in tooth-bound modification spaces. If this modification space is for a lateral incisor and rotation is allowed, the tooth in this modification space will necessarily lift during function, creating food impaction and displacement issues. This is another argument for preferring fixed partial dentures (FPDs) for these spaces. This leaves the RPD to restore the posterior bilateral distal extensions in a fashion that allows freer rotation and limits food impaction issues to the major connector.

Connectors

As stated before, whenever possible, the maximum amount of soft tissue should remain uncovered by the RPD. This

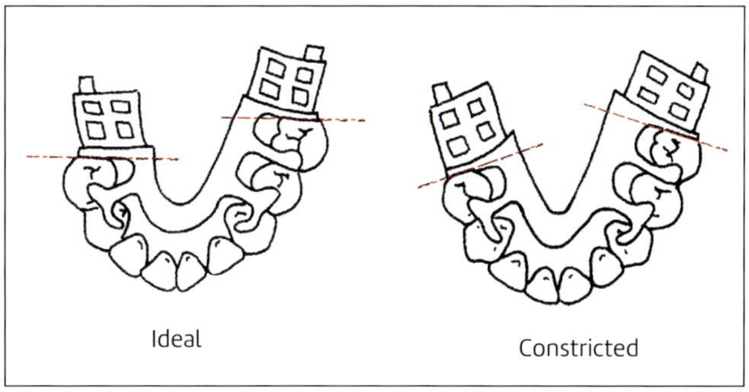

FIG 3-6 Ideal parallelism of guiding planes to allow unrestricted rotation.

would require, for example, the use of the lingual bar over the lingual plate. If, however, there is inadequate space or if there is the potential for loss of some remaining anterior teeth during the life of the partial denture, a lingual plate or a dental lingual bar will be the proper choice so that additions can be made easily. It may be possible to combine a lingual plate in the incisor area with a lingual bar distal to the canines instead of covering all the lingual surfaces. When space permits, this design is preferred because it offers the potential for lingual retentive clasping and no show of metal on the buccal surfaces of the abutments.

The maxillary Class I major connector varies in the placement of both the anterior and the posterior borders. As the number of teeth to be replaced with the partial denture increases, the natural inclination will be to increase the coverage of the major connector so that it approaches a complete denture outline. Because there can be no peripheral seal on the partial denture, there is little value in extending the posterior border to the vibrating line. The glandular portion of the posterior soft palate offers no real support to the partial denture and therefore should be left uncovered. The edentulous ridges, however, do support the partial denture and should always be covered to the pterygomaxillary (hamular) notch, either in resin or with metal.

Anterior coverage is dependent on the teeth remaining. If only six anterior teeth remain, going to full lingual coverage offers the option of easy addition of teeth should some be lost, and this option also provides the potential for additional stability on any guiding planes that can be established. Finding tooth structure on the lingual of maxillary anterior teeth that can be prepared to parallel guiding surfaces is, unfortunately, uncommon. When the remaining six anterior teeth are healthy and not mobile, it is certainly feasible to open the anterior area by projecting a cingulum rest onto a prepared acute cingulum rest from the distal of the canines. The anterior border must then blend into the anterior slope of the rugae area and end posterior to a major rugae. For

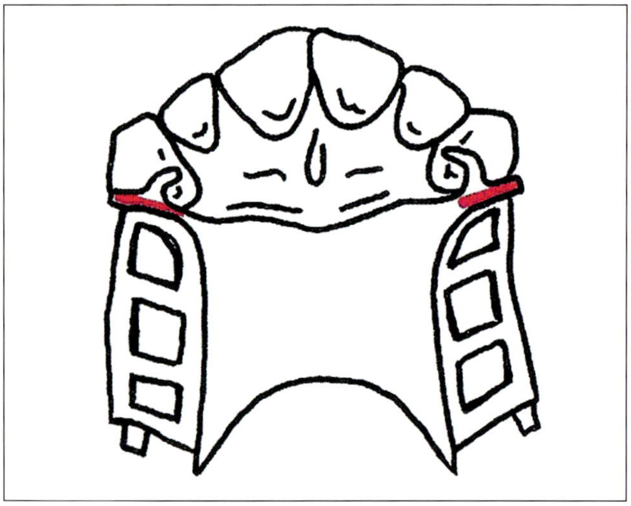

FIG 3-7 Minimal coverage of the anterior palate requires large guiding planes for positive results. Note also the cingulum rests extending off the distal minor connectors.

this approach to be dependably successful, the canines must have sufficient distal structure to allow for guiding planes of at least 3 mm (Fig 3-7). As previously noted, if covering the anterior and posterior palate can be avoided, the comfort of the RPD is much improved. Minor connectors will be of standard dimensions with care taken to see that at least 1.5 mm of metal thickness at the marginal ridge is available to support the rests and resist fracture.

Resin retention

Because the need for periodic reline of the distal extension base is expected, especially on the mandible, the resin retention of choice is a raised mesh with > 1 mm of space for resin below the mesh. In some maxillary situations, where there has been minimal resorption of the edentulous extension and therefore minimal room for the casting and the replacement denture teeth, a metal base with retentive beads as an integral part of the casting is the only viable option. Obviously, this base cannot be relined, but in the mature edentulous ridge, with the support of the palatal coverage, no reline may be needed during the life of the partial denture. The need to cover the maximum amount of available supporting tissue is more critical in Class I situations than in any other classification. The primary landmarks required on the definitive cast are the retromolar pads on the mandible and tuberosities on the maxilla.

Modification spaces are managed with metal bases and bead or post retention wherever possible. Only very recent extractions can be considered for mesh retention, but caution must be taken for a single-tooth replacement because the amount of mesh retention available for the single tooth is often inadequate. It is generally wiser to add a tooth to the existing partial denture temporarily or to construct an interim partial denture for the initial healing period. Once healed, the new RPD can be constructed with either a reinforced metal post or a veneered pontic form for the single tooth.

Clasping

The type of retentive clasp to be used is determined by two factors: *(1)* the availability of a retentive area on the tooth and *(2)* the clinician's preference. The options may be classified as follows:

- *Only a mesiobuccal retentive area:* Wire circumferential clasp to 0.015 inch.
- *Midfacial retentive area:* Cast or wrought I-bar to 0.01 inch (assuming appropriate gingival contour).
- *Only a distofacial retentive area:* Preferably wrought L-bar to 0.01 inch.
- *When no facial retentive areas are present or if esthetics is a real consideration:* Lingual wire circumferential clasps to 0.01 inch or recontour the abutment with subtractive or additive preparation.

In either arch, one retentive clasp per side will provide adequate retention if the support and stability are maximized through mouth preparation and careful fitting of the casting.

In choosing the retentive clasps for the mandibular Class I RPD, consideration must be given to establishing stress relief because the partial denture will always rotate in function. The maxillary RPD may show very little rotational movement due to the support of the hard palate and the generally superior ridge contour. The weaker the abutment teeth and the supporting ridge, the greater the rotational movement that must be allowed in the fit of the casting. This relief can be obtained in the blockout of the definitive cast or in the intraoral fitting of the frame, to be discussed later (see chapter 7).

Along with the fit of the frame, the flexibility of the retentive clasp arms selected plays an important role in stress relief so that a light wire retentive clasp in any of the appropriate clasp forms is indicated when the support is poor. This decision may sacrifice some retention and stability to relieve the abutment teeth from the full load of mastication.

In the Class I RPD, there is no need to consider the use of a so-called "bracing clasp" because the combination of rests, minor connectors, guiding plates, and opposing tooth contacts will provide any necessary reciprocation. Even if lingual circumferential clasping is chosen, it is not necessary to complicate the casting and show unsightly metal with a buccal reciprocal clasp arm (Fig 3-8).

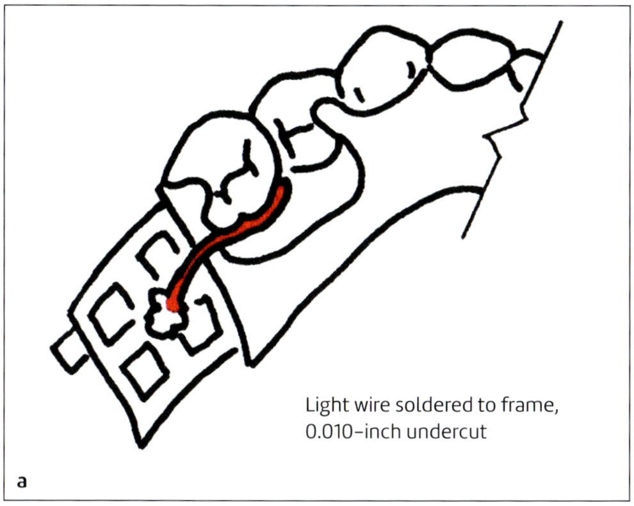

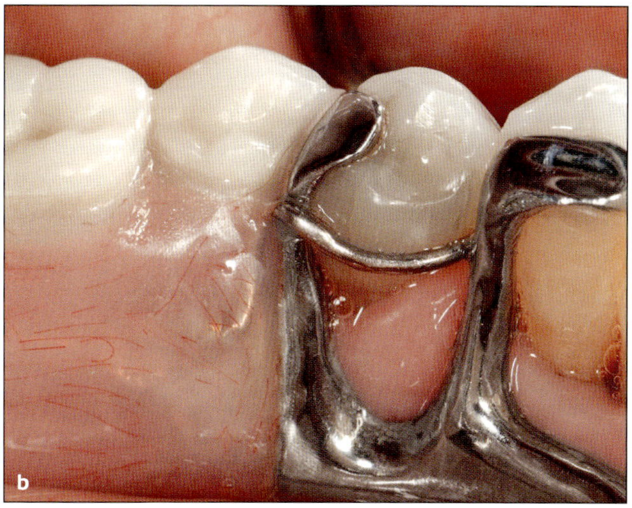

FIG 3-8 *(a and b)* Elimination of buccal reciprocal arm with lingual retentive wire.

Class II RPD

Abutment selection and rests

While the Class II partial denture design is often considered a mixture of the principles of Class I design and those of the Class III partial denture, special consideration must be given to the potential for rotation at the fulcrum line that will run from the distal-most rigid contacts of the partial denture with the abutment teeth on each side of the arch. One might imagine that rotation and the resulting stress relief will occur naturally without any effort. In truth, a decision as to the desirability of allowing motion around the fulcrum line must be made before mouth preparation begins. For the most part, there is no need to plan for stress relief for the Class II RPD because the remaining teeth will be able to support the teeth being replaced as a cantilever if the RPD properly contacts prepared surfaces—in particular guiding plane surfaces (Fig 3-9). This is certainly the case when a modification space is present on the dentate side. Mastication will most often occur on the dentate side due to increased efficiency in managing food particles, so the distal extension side will receive minor loading only.

Only when the abutments are weak and few in number must we consider functional relief of the casting and reducing the length of the guiding planes to allow limited rotation and partial loading of the edentulous ridge. When the casting has been relieved, the support of the edentulous area can be maximized through the altered cast impression. In the maxillary arch, additional support for the weakened teeth is obtained by covering a greater portion of the palate, and an altered cast impression is normally not needed. In practical terms, however, rotation can occur only if the casting does not contact the abutments, a situation clearly not desirable from the standpoint of support and stability.

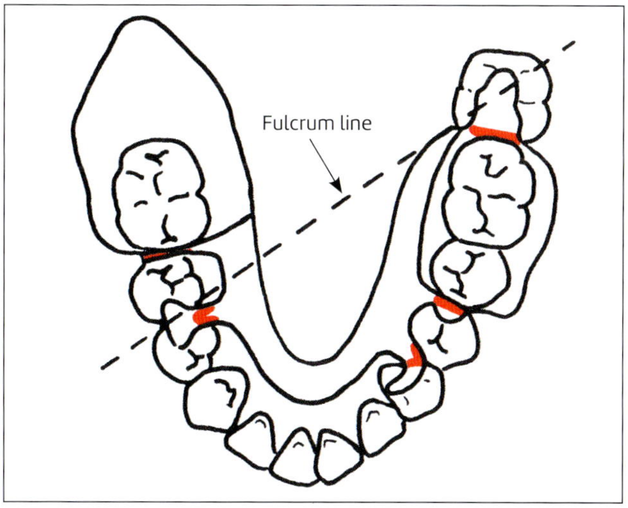

FIG 3-9 Guiding planes restricting rotation in the Class II partial denture. A traditional drawing of the fulcrum line using the mesial rest on tooth no. 29 as a rotation point. If the multiple (colored) guiding planes function as designed, the proposed rotation cannot occur.

For abutment selection, the distal extension side of the partial denture is treated exactly as in the Class I situation, with no exceptions. The management of the tooth-supported side offers a few options usually dependent on the number, strength, and position of the available

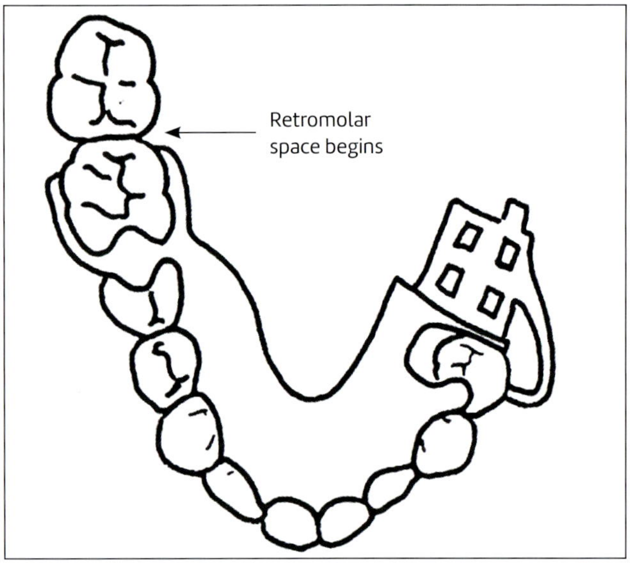

FIG 3-10 Stopping major connector short of the retromolar space.

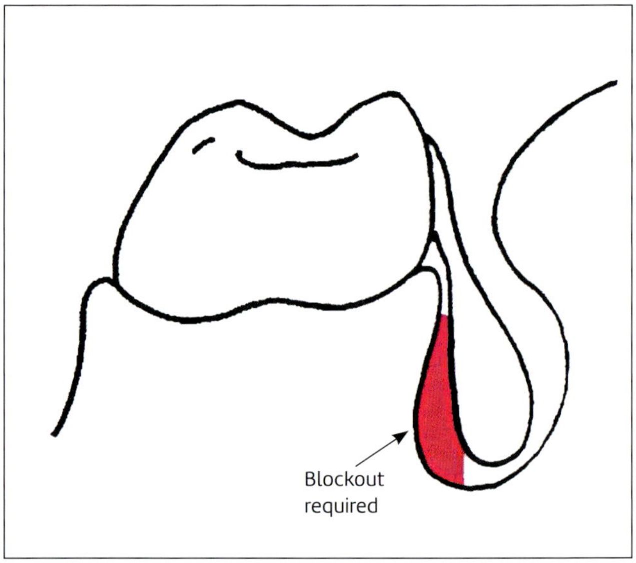

FIG 3-11 Major connector forced to stand away from the tissue in the retromolar space.

abutments. When the dentate side is complete (ie, no modification spaces), then an embrasure clasp on the first molar is the retention of choice. This clasp must be cast because the construction of an embrasure clasp made of wire is technically very difficult, and the long-term dependability of such a clasp is very much in question. The embrasure clasp is placed upon the first molar rather than the second molar because the mandible curves to the retromolar space starting at about the second molar (Fig 3-10). If a major connector extends back to a second molar, it tends to stand far away from the tissue, creating a food trap that patients do not appreciate (Fig 3-11). The first molar is more apt to allow the placement of the major connector in a comfortable position. Under no circumstances should a premolar be used in place of the molar because any clasp placed upon it will be shorter and more rigid and is often unesthetic as well.

The need for additional abutments on the tooth-borne side must be considered. At the very minimum, an additional minor connector and rest must be placed as far forward from the embrasure clasp as possible. This rest and connector combination has been called an *indirect retainer*, and it was assumed that it would counteract the upward rotation of the edentulous base. This antirotation device springs from dentistry's past, as far as partial denture design is concerned, when no mouth preparation for guiding planes was done. In the modern RPD, the guiding planes and the intimate contact with the casting through the guide plates prohibits rotation until the partial denture has moved beyond the contact of the guiding plane and the associated guide plate.[11] Only at that point could the denture rotate and the "indirect retainer" come into antirotational contact. Therefore, while true indirect retention is a thing of the past, the use of an additional rest/minor connector some distance from the embrasure clasp is essential to distribute support, provide a third point of reference for seating the framework during fitting of the frame, making the altered cast impression, and relating the framework again during future relines of the distal extension base. For these reasons, the term *auxiliary rest* should be used instead of the misleading *indirect retainer*.

The cingulum of the mandibular canine and the distal of the maxillary first premolar are often used for this third point of contact. Resting the canine makes sense from an abutment value standpoint as this tooth is typically superior in this regard. The mesial of the mandibular first premolar might be more ideal from a geometric standpoint, but unfortunately, the amount of tooth structure at the marginal ridge often does not allow the preparation of an ideal, acute occlusal rest. The mesial of the maxillary first premolar would also be ideal, but disclusion often occurs at the contact of the premolar and the canine, limiting the available space for minor connectors and rests.

When a modification space is present, the potential exists to develop additional frictional retention and reciprocation by maximizing the guiding plane surfaces adjacent to the edentulous space through either subtractive or additive tooth preparation. At the very minimum, a rest and guiding plane would be placed upon the isolated molar abutment and the tooth at the anterior extension of the edentulous space. Additional abutments would be added as required if the support from the two original abutments appeared

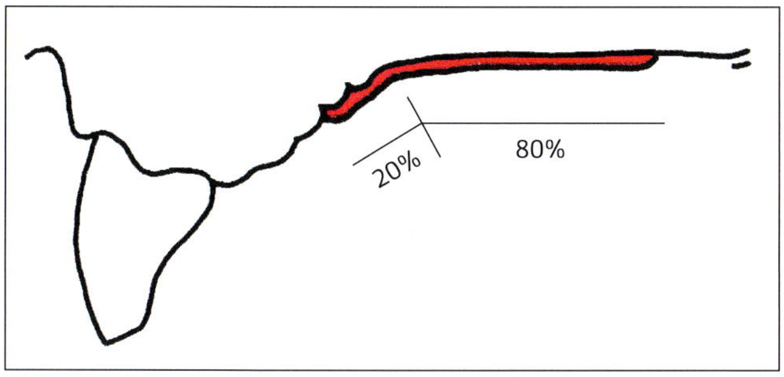

FIG 3-12 Configuration of broad palatal strap in cross section.

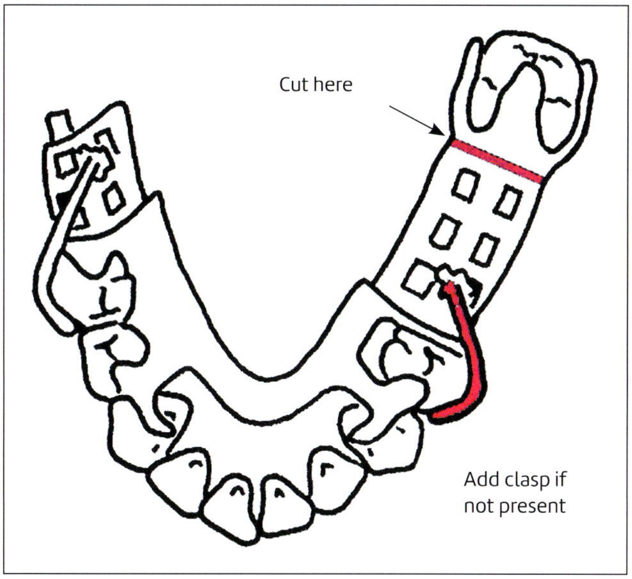

FIG 3-13 Conversion of Class II to Class I with loss of molar distal abutment.

to be inadequate. Guiding planes for the Class II partial denture should be as long as possible, provided that the casting is planned as a cantilever. If stress relief is indicated, the casting will be adjusted intraorally.

Connectors

Major and minor connector design on the dentate side of the partial denture will be that of the Class III RPD. Every attempt is made to cover as little gingival tissue as possible. The dimensions of the castings and their relation to the soft tissues are the same as for the Class I situation, while the third point of contact (auxiliary rest) may require it to be moved toward the anterior. In the maxilla, the minor connector to that rest must blend into the rugae area so that the speaking area is not compromised. Placing a small part (one-fifth) of the major connector onto the slope of the anterior palate and the remaining four-fifths on the more posterior horizontal palate will strengthen the casting as the corrugation allows for a thinner casting with the same rigidity (Fig 3-12).

Resin retention

The resin retention for the tooth-borne side of the Class II RPD favors the use of metal coverage of the ridge whenever possible according to requirements mentioned earlier. If only a single tooth is being replaced, special consideration must be given to metal retention because the space is often restricted. Usually some form of a retentive post is designed to fall within the denture tooth. When the desired tooth position is obvious, then the post can be randomly placed by the technician. When the tooth needs to be in some irregular position due to esthetic requirements or abnormal occlusal relations, then the denture tooth must be ground into place by the clinician, verified in the patient's mouth, and sent along with the definitive cast in some sort of matrix so that the technician knows exactly where the tooth must be placed.

A final consideration for the Class II mandibular RPD is the potential for conversion after additional tooth loss. The isolated posterior abutment on the tooth-borne side is often a weakened tooth, both restoratively and periodontally, and it may not last the life of the partial denture. In anticipation of the loss of this tooth, the partial denture should be designed as if it were a Class I RPD, ie, with raised retentive mesh and rests on the canine and premolar. This readies the premolar to become the prime abutment on that side of the arch with the potential for flexible clasping by adding a wire. In addition, the internal and external finishing lines must be positioned as if the posterior abutment did not exist, ie, at the distal and lingual of the premolar that will become the prime abutment. The retentive mesh, suitably reinforced, then runs distally to the isolated molar and its clasp assembly (Fig 3-13). When the molar is lost, the rest, clasp, and guide plate are cut off and the resin base extended to cover the total denture space during reline/rebase procedures.

Unfortunately, the maxillary arch cannot be treated in the same fashion for conversion because the major connector in the maxilla will not have a finish line assembly that can be converted to a Class I partial denture. Attempts to solder on finishing lines and associated meshwork are technically very complicated, and the cost seldom justifies the conversion.

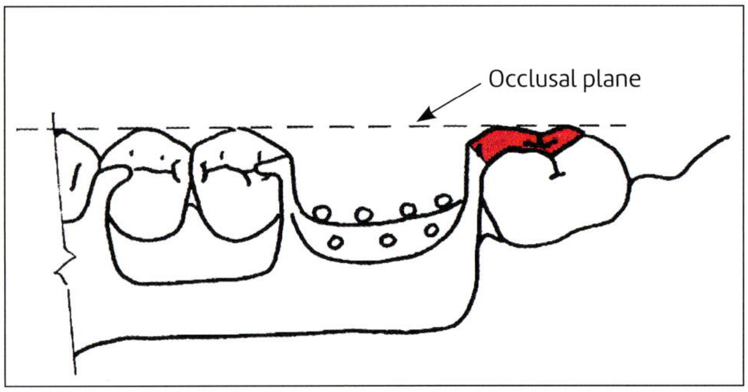

FIG 3-14 An overlay rest on a tipped molar restores the occlusal plane for an opposing complete denture.

Clasping

The clasp requirements for the distal extension side of the Class II are identical to those of the Class I. On the tooth-borne side, there is a major decision to be made. Because it is rare to find a mandibular situation where more than one clasp per side is needed for retention, the clinician should choose between clasping on the fulcrum line or anterior to it. In most cases, the posterior abutment on the tooth-borne side will be a molar because if it were a premolar, the case would be considered a Class I. The advantages are clearly on the side of clasping on the fulcrum line, ie, the molar on the tooth-borne side and the terminal abutment on the other side. Clasp selection for the molar is generally limited to a circumferential clasp, either cast or wire, with the lingual arm being retentive because the retentive area is most apt to be found on that side of the tooth due to its natural inclination in the arch. Because this clasp will be the terminal of the RPD, some reciprocation will be required to maintain the tooth in the arch and prevent it from moving away from the partial denture. This can be done in two ways: either with a conventional guide plate/rest and reciprocal arm combination or with the use of an extended guide plate (one that extends slightly from the mesial to the buccal and lingual surfaces) combined with an oversized occlusal rest that extends to the distal fossa. This long rest has the additional advantage of restoring a more ideal plane of occlusion if the distal abutment has indeed migrated mesially and lingually. This design is often described as an *overlay* and will be discussed further in chapter 12 (Fig 3-14).

Should the molar be so severely tilted that the retentive area is very deep and very near the occlusal surface, and minor orthodontics is not an option, consideration should be given to not clasping that tooth but retaining the guiding plane and the extended occlusal rest and moving the retentive clasp anterior to the fulcrum (to the premolar). The clasp choice in this situation can be either a circumferential clasp or an infrabulge clasp. The retentive arm will be anterior to the fulcrum, so a wire circumferential clasp arm is selected over a cast one because the potential for greater movement of the partial denture in function in that area dictates a more flexible clasp. As in other esthetic areas, a wire I-bar clasp, set to the distal, may be the best choice. Lingual retentive circumferential wire clasps offer the option of eliminating the visible clasp arm.

In the maxilla, a case can be made for the use of three retentive clasps because the force of gravity adds another dimension to the retentive requirement. Here, the molar clasp will most likely be a cast circumferential and the clasp on the distal extension side an I-bar, because this clasp is less likely to be visible when the patient smiles and speaks. The I-bar clasp has been presented as having to be placed midway on the tooth mesiodistally in order to function with minimum stress on the abutment. While this may be true on the mandible, there is not enough movement possible on a well-fitting maxillary casting to make any clinical difference. For this reason, the I-bar clasp can be set as far to the distal as possible as long as there is a mesial rest and a distal guide plate. If a wire I-bar is used, it is possible to place the clasp almost in contact with the buccal extension of the guide plate because this clasp is added to the framework after the frame has been finished and polished. A cast infrabulge clasp must be placed farther away from the guide plate so that space is available to finish and polish the clasp, making the clasp potentially more visible on the tooth. The third clasp, placed on the anterior abutment on the tooth-supported side, should also be a wire I-bar for the reasons given.

Class III RPD

This classification of partial denture could really be called a *removable fixed bridge*. In most situations, it uses the same abutments as would an FPD replacing the same missing teeth. The design options, at first glance, might appear to be endless but in truth can be reduced to only a few basic options as long as the clinician is willing to prepare the mouth ideally. The reasons for choosing the RPD in the Class III situation rather than an FPD can be reduced to

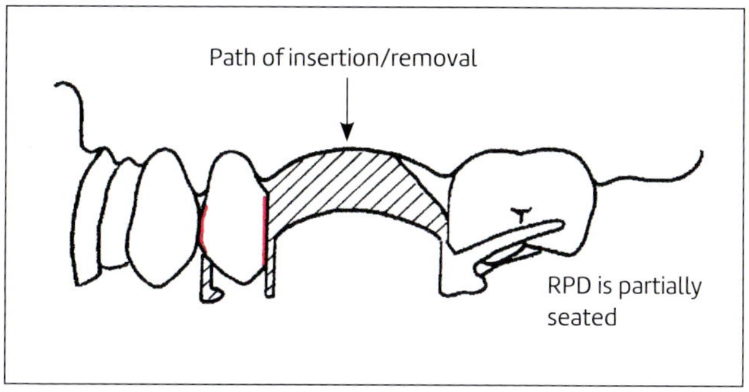

FIG 3-15 This partial denture cannot rotate out of the mouth but must travel down the guiding planes until the posterior retention is no longer effective.

four obvious treatment considerations. The first and most powerful reason is financial. The second relates to those situations where the length of span of the edentulous area and the periodontal support of the remaining possible abutment teeth combine to bring into question the long-term success of an FPD. The third reason to select the RPD over the FPD is strictly esthetic. The need to replace the interdental papillae in the anterior of the mouth may make an FPD a questionable solution. While it is true that ridge augmentation in any of its many forms can create an adequate gingival base, the restoration of the papillae is not always realistic in the hands of the average clinician. Finally, there will always be those situations where the loss of teeth was accompanied by traumatic loss of the alveolar process. In these cases, the need to replace missing soft tissue requires the use of a flange of such dimensions that the appliance be removable to allow the patient access for proper hygiene. The goal of RPD treatment for the Class III patient must be to make the appliance conform to the principles of FPDs as much as possible.

Abutment selection and rests

The choice of abutments is generally obvious: one abutment on each end of an edentulous area. This general statement is modified by adding abutments when the potential support of the teeth is in question. Whenever this question arises, it is better to add another abutment because additional frictional retention can be obtained. Unlike the case of the FPD in which splinted abutments bring potential problems of embrasure access and connector rigidity, double abutting in the RPD situation causes no particular problems. Remember, abutments must have positive rest preparations to maintain contact between the partial denture and the teeth over the life of the partial denture. These ideal rest shapes can usually be created with subtractive mouth preparation in the posterior of the mouth, but additive mouth preparation is often required for the anterior teeth.

As well as selecting the abutments and planning their rests, the potential for parallel guiding planes must be evaluated through careful consideration of the path of insertion/removal. The goal of the mouth preparation for the Class III case is to maximize the frictional retention of the guiding planes/guide plates to totally eliminate the need for any anterior clasping (Fig 3-15). Posterior clasping, one clasp on each side, is more than sufficient when the anterior portion of the partial is controlled by the guiding planes. For this reason, the guiding planes created on the abutment teeth must be as long as possible in the all tooth-borne case.

Connectors

Major connector design for the mandibular Class III RPD remains basically the same as for the other classes. Again, whenever possible in the mandible, the lingual bar is selected over the lingual plate to reduce the amount of soft tissue coverage. As in the Class II, consideration must be given to the conversion of the casting to a distal extension base when the choice of a posterior terminal abutment is questionable.

Selecting a design for the maxillary connector that will provide adequate strength and maximum comfort without bulk is more of a challenge. This is why the palatal strap design forms the basis of all maxillary major connectors. Modifications will depend on the number and position of the edentulous areas. Major connectors can be kept to a thickness of 0.5 mm if they are planned with the bend described previously (see Fig 3-12). This increased rigidity often allows a reduced length within the palate at the same time.

Modification spaces for missing anterior teeth present a special problem in that they complicate the design of the casting and often require that metal be placed in the speaking area of the anterior palate. When a lateral incisor is missing and must be replaced by the RPD, it may be possible to cantilever it off the rest and minor connector on the canine (see Fig 2-10). However, when a central and lateral incisor or two central incisors are missing, a full anterior casting will be required. A veneered incisor replacement can be made in a number of ways. A reinforced acrylic

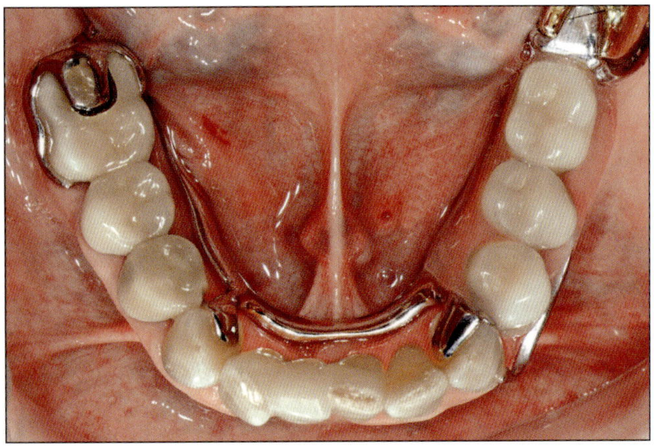

FIG 3-16 Tooth no. 25 is replaced with a lithium disilicate bonded pontic, leaving the RPD to replace teeth nos. 19 to 21. Note the minimal tissue coverage while still utilizing all molar and canine abutments. Short abutment teeth resulted in the need for an anterior clasp.

pontic (RAP) is a denture tooth with a custom post or backing and tends to be the most common. A laser-welded custom component is another option. A custom casting is made and veneered with composite or porcelain prior to being laser welded to the major connector. As noted previously, the better solution to the problem of an anterior modification space is to replace the tooth with a fixed or bonded partial denture and leave the RPD to replace only posterior teeth (Fig 3-16).

Resin retention

Because there is seldom any need to reline a Class III RPD, ideal resin retention will be metal ridge coverage with retentive beads, loops, or posts as well as the occasional metal pontic. These metal pontics can be veneered or, in the posterior region where they will not be visible, left in metal. The full metal pontic should not extend as far to the buccal as if it would if it were being veneered. By keeping the metal tooth lingual to the buccal line angle, its presence can be disguised.

Clasping

Clasping is limited to the posterior abutments of the Class III RPD whenever possible because the potential for parallel guiding planes adjacent to the edentulous spaces is great and will eliminate the need for anterior clasping in all but those situations where the clinical crowns are so short that no adequate guiding planes can be created. As the crowns get shorter, the need to have very parallel planes increases the challenge in subtractive mouth preparation. Guiding planes that are additive have the advantage of allowing machined milling to create "perfect" parallelism. The clasp of choice for the posterior area will be the cast circumferential placed into a 0.01-inch undercut for the terminal third of the active clasp arm. The need for anterior clasping can best be determined after the casting has been fitted. Should retention appear inadequate at that time, one or more distal wire I-bars can be added to the framework into a 0.01-inch undercut.

Class IV RPD

The Class IV partial denture patient classification represents a group of patients for whom the advent of osseointegrated implants has greatly reduced the reliance on the RPD. Many of these patients go through a stage of treatment where a cast partial denture may be employed even though the definitive prosthesis is supported and retained by implants. The cost of a casting is insignificant when compared with the possible problems of long-term resin-based provisional restorations. For these patients, as well as for those for whom no implant support or fixed prosthodontics is possible or affordable, the Class IV RPD represents a challenge both in design and construction. Some special types of partial dentures that are used almost exclusively in the maxillary Class IV, namely the rotational path of insertion partial denture, have great potential in this situation and will be addressed later (see chapter 12).

Abutment selection and rests

For the most part, the patient with an extensive anterior edentulous space will need the support of all the remaining teeth. Those with smaller edentulous areas will require at least the teeth adjacent to the edentulous area and the first molars. Again, the more teeth being replaced on the partial denture and the weaker the quality of the abutments, either periodontally or restoratively, the more teeth that must be involved as abutments. For the other classifications, the path of insertion/removal was planned to be in the long

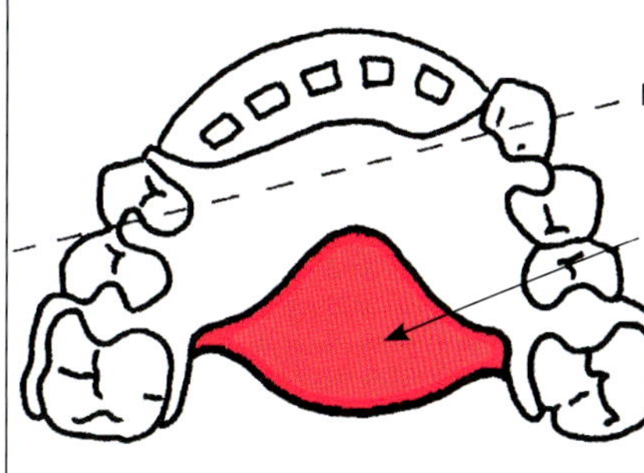

FIG 3-17 Extension in the palate *(red)* may rotate away from the tissue in function, creating discomfort and food impaction issues.

axis of the abutment teeth so as to load them vertically as much as possible and to reduce the amount of tooth structure lost to mouth preparation for guiding planes to the very minimum. For the Class IV situation, consideration must be given to the undercuts in the flange area because, if a full flange is desired, these soft tissue undercuts will have to draw with the posterior guiding planes. It is often impossible to make this alignment without crowning the abutment teeth. Another solution is to plan on a short flange only, one that extends just to the height of contour of the edentulous ridge when the path of insertion/removal favors the abutment teeth. Decisions on this dilemma are often based upon the need for a full flange to restore lip support. Clasping the posterior abutment on both sides with a conventional circumferential cast clasp that extends distally from a mesial rest is the norm.

A more dependable option is to utilize the distal surface of the most posterior teeth with a guiding plane that is parallel to the plane on the mesial of the most anterior remaining teeth. These parallel planes/plates effectively lock the remaining posterior teeth together and offer positive resistance to the tendency of the edentulous area to drop. This approach is indicated when the remaining posterior teeth are mobile. Stability can be increased if a continuous occlusal rest (strut rest) is used. This rest will run, usually through the central fossae, from the distal of the most posterior tooth to the mesial of the most anterior. A lingual or buccal circumferential cast clasp, approaching from the distal, is usually the only retention that is required due to the restriction of the path of removal generated by this system of connected guiding planes.

Connectors

Maxillary major connectors will often differ somewhat from those used for other classifications. Because the edentulous area is apt to be extensive, ie, greater than that which would normally be replaced with an FPD, rotational movements around an axis that will run between the most mesial rigid contact of the framework and the anterior abutment on each side can be expected. As rotation of the base toward the tissue takes place, any portion of the major connector that is posterior to this fulcrum will have a tendency to move away from the tissue (Fig 3-17). The further posterior the casting extends, the greater the potential for breaking contact with the soft tissue. The space that may be opened up here can act as a food trap during mastication. To reduce this rotational opening, the posterior extension of the major connector should be limited and should never extend beyond the posterior clasping.

While it may appear that the open oval or anteroposterior palatal strap configuration is appropriate for the Class IV situation, the palatal extension of the anterior segment can still interfere with speech unless it is carefully blended with the contour of the anterior rugae area. The special design options such as rotational path require additional decisions on major connector design (see chapter 12).

Mandibular major connectors for this classification offer the same options as the other mandibular designs. They are more apt to be full lingual plates because the necessary additional frictional retention can be obtained from the preparation of parallel guiding planes on the lingual surfaces of the remaining teeth. The continuous lingual plate facilitates the maximum contact with these surfaces.

When the remaining teeth are crowned, the lingual plate can lie on gingival rests milled into the lingual surfaces of the crowns. This brings the major connector entirely off of the gingival tissue, so it is now more properly called a *dental lingual bar* (see Fig 2-12). Clinically tall periodontally involved teeth are amendable to this design and may also benefit from the lack of tissue coverage. The transition from the bar to the edentulous area begins at the distal of

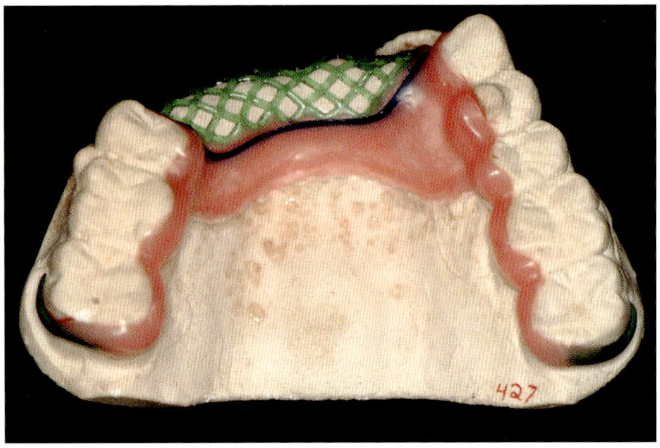

FIG 3-18 A refractory cast wax-up of a dental lingual bar. Properly designed crowns allow the bar to run along a lingual rest, further increasing support and stability. Note the thickness of the transition from the bar to the edentulous area.

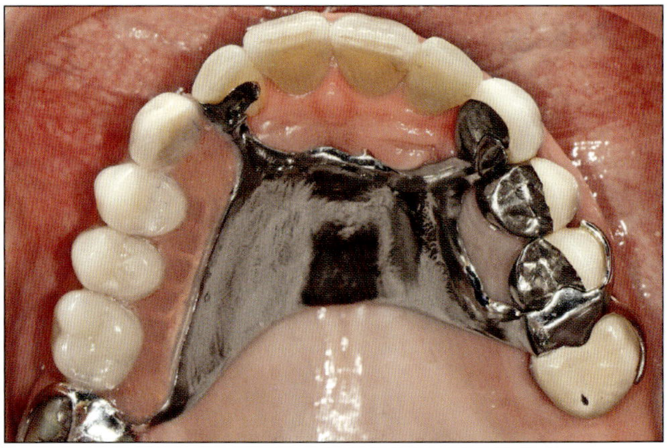

FIG 3-19 A Class V arch, according to the Applegate modification of the Kennedy classifications. Note the tooth-bound situation with maxillary lateral incisor abutment.

the tooth adjacent to the edentulous area to allow enough metal for a proper external finish line and to more precisely control the area of most flexural concern (Fig 3-18).

Resin retention

Most Class IV cases will require raised mesh retention because the edentulous spans are apt to be extensive and therefore may need future relines to keep the partial denture stable. Situations with limited interocclusal space or short flanges would of course be best suited with bead or post retention. The external finishing line of the maxillary partial denture will lie in the speaking area, so some consideration should be given to blending the junction of the metal and the resin in such a way as to eliminate a ridge in the area where speech is formed. This may require moving the finishing line posteriorly or bringing it almost to the denture teeth, depending on the palatal contour.

Clasping

A conventional Class IV partial denture will have its primary retention on the molar teeth (usually the first molars), one on each side. These clasps will often be cast circumferential, either coming from a modification space or as an embrasure clasp. In the maxillary arch, the anterior edentulous area often requires an additional clasp to offset the pull of gravity and sticky foods. When long parallel guiding planes are obtainable adjacent to the edentulous area, the casting may be retentive without the third clasp. The anterior clasp is likely to be visible and possibly unesthetic, so the casting should be evaluated without the anterior clasp. Should additional retention be required, the third clasp is added as a wire I-bar soldered to the casting or placed on a palatal surface as a circumferential wire.

The mandibular Class IV partial denture will not usually need a third clasp if guiding planes are well-planned and well-executed. If the guiding planes are inadequate, the same approach for the third clasp or the distal guiding plane options is indicated.

A final consideration for situations when the incisors are missing but the canines remain as an option for an FPD is to crown the canines and run a bar between them. The bar can be milled on its lingual surface to gain additional parallelism for the RPD. This design eliminates the need for anterior clasping and reduces the anterior cantilever on the canines while still splinting them together. The bar will facilitate maximum support and stability, which often eliminates the need to utilize a retentive clip on the bar. Lack of space in difficult Class II, division 2 malocclusions may preclude this option.

Class V RPD

Applegate suggested the Kennedy Class V is a Class III with a very weak anterior abutment tooth (Fig 3-19). A common example is a lateral incisor with small root form. The concept of a Class V RPD is not standardized within the profession. It is included here for consideration but more importantly to highlight the need for design modification with anatomically weak abutments. Therefore, while it was proposed specifically for tooth-borne situations, the modifications discussed in this section should be considered for distal extension cases as well.

Abutment selection and rests

The abutment and rest decisions are the key to the Class V situation. The fact that a critical abutment is too weak to withstand the forces the prosthesis will place on it cannot be ignored. Applegate's solution was to not rest or even contact the tooth in question. However, all benefits of Class III designs are lost when this is done. The clinician must remain committed to the rule of resting all teeth adjacent to edentulous spans.

The best way to manage the Class V dilemma is through treatment planning. Restoratively debilitated teeth with healthy root forms are frequently removed simply due to their inability to reliably retain a crown. Retaining the root as an overdenture abutment can effectively maintain the support that would otherwise be lost. Retaining these roots is often facilitated by a previous root canal treatment. The common scenario is a canine root maintained to help support the lateral incisor that is now the next abutment (see Fig 12-17a). If a root is not present or cannot be maintained, another option is the use of a strategic implant. If replacing a canine abutment would reclassify the arch to a Kennedy Class III arch, per Rule 9, it should be strongly considered. This is all the more logical as this is a strategic location for implant-retained tissue-supported overdentures, should disease claim the remaining natural teeth. More information regarding implant abutments is found in chapter 13.

If implants are out of the question and any potential overdenture roots have already been removed, then splinting the weak abutment to adjacent teeth is advised. If the teeth require full-coverage crowns for restorative reasons, this is a straightforward solution that also allows improved guiding planes and lingual clasping. In essence, we create multirooted abutments using splinted crowns. However, what if the natural teeth are unrestored? This is common in periodontal disease and tumor resection cases. Splinting these teeth can be accomplished conservatively with lingual bonded splints in either metal or pressed/milled ceramics (see Fig 4-20). The splint should also modify the lingual and proximal surfaces to allow ideal rest and guiding plane form. For maxillary situations, finding the interocclusal space to accomplish the splint can be a challenge.

If none of these options are readily available, then the splinting and/or sharing of support must be achieved through the use of multiple rest seats in the casting. In the lateral incisor situation mentioned, this would mean resting the lingual of the central incisor. The anatomical situation dictates whether one can rest both the lateral and central incisors with an extended rest arm coming from the minor connector on the distal of the lateral incisor.

Connectors

To allow resting of the additional abutments, lingual plating with a horseshoe major connector or the anterior equivalent of the strut rest, called a *Kennedy bar*, can be considered. The technical challenge of Kennedy bars is achieving an acceptable fit against multiple abutments. While laser welding can help accomplish this, one must be ready for the extra effort. Remember, the lingual plating or bar must be fit into positive rest forms rather than just being laid over unprepared teeth. The plate or bar itself does not transmit controlled force; it is the positive rest on the tooth that does. The dental lingual bar can be another viable option when the vertical space exists because it allows resting of the teeth while avoiding the periodontal consequences of tissue coverage.

Resin retention

In contrast to a Class III RPD, the risk of abutment loss in a Class V is implicitly high. Therefore, while resin retention would best be a metal base with beads, there is now an argument for mesh to facilitate a more effective reline. Should the weak abutment be lost, the reline is often needed for what is now becoming a lengthy edentulous span. If a root is being maintained, limited space and gingival health will supersede the future need for a reline, and metal base with bead retention is used.

Clasping

As with Class III situations, clasping should be limited to the posterior regions. However, this is more challenging in the Class V, as the edentulous span is often long. The longer the span, the greater the challenge to create parallel guiding planes and thus achieve the stability necessary to retain the prosthesis without an anterior clasp. Splinting the weak anterior abutment is an opportunity to maximize the guiding plane effect but also allows the lingual to be contoured for the addition of a short wire clasp. Clasping of incisors on the facial is rarely considered, as the additional stress on an unaided weak anterior abutment is best avoided. The various support alternatives of overdenture roots or strategic implants can also serve in a retentive capacity if space allows for attachments. When a single modification space exists, the edentulous span is long, and the weak anterior abutment is short or flared to the facial, it may be impossible to achieve adequate anterior retention. A lateral rotational path design can be very effective and esthetic in this situation.

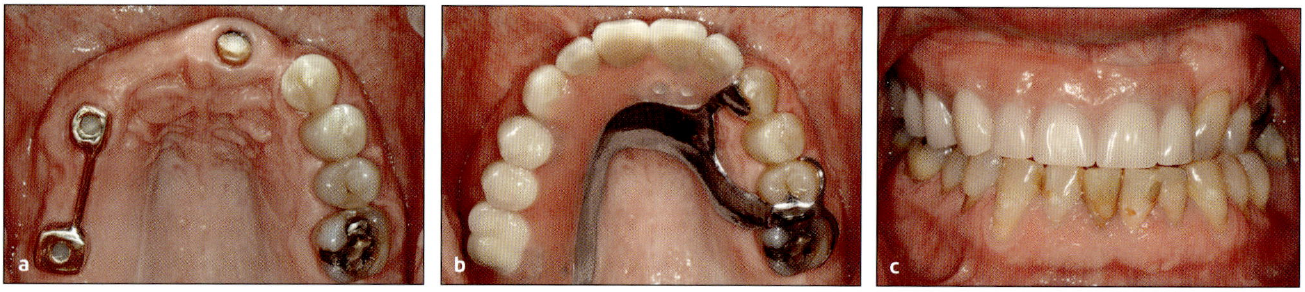

FIG 3-20 *(a to c)* An extreme Class II unilateral situation modified with the strategic use of implants. Six of the seven possible abutments were used. Not resting tooth no. 12 allowed the lingual of the tooth segment to remain unplated. The prognosis of the teeth was such that conversion to a complete denture is not expected in the future. A lateral rotational path retention method was utilized on the implant bar to maintain attachment-free retention of the prosthetic segment.

Unilateral and Limited Abutment Situations

There are several "extreme" examples of certain classifications that deserve special consideration. In many ways, these situations constitute their own classifications. While this may be true, from an educational and practical point of view, Kennedy's system remains the reference. These cases often begin to delve into the maxillofacial prosthetic realm, and indeed many of the techniques used with RPD/obturators are focused on managing the lack of support and stability inherent in these unfortunate situations.

Unilateral partial denture

The unilateral partial denture situation seldom occurs, and as a result, the dentist is usually at a loss as to the design and construction of the RPD. When teeth remain only on one side of the arch, the dentist is faced with unique and often insurmountable challenges. These situations, while technically either a Kennedy Class I or II, cannot be managed with those design principles alone. When a unilateral group of mainly posterior teeth remain with no other teeth left in the mouth, the dentist must strongly consider edentulation as a better long-term option. This is dependent upon all the disease, anatomical, and adaptability factors discussed in chapter 1. When a complete denture is strongly contraindicated or adamantly refused by the patient, the dentist may be obligated to proceed with an RPD.

ABUTMENT SELECTION

With so few abutments, the need to rest all remaining teeth is obvious. Next, the soft tissue support must be maximized. In this way, a unilateral arch is similar to a Class I with hard and soft tissue support requirements. The unfortunate asymmetry in support for the unilateral situation is impossible to control long-term without the use of strategic implants. While the use of strategic implants to modify the unilateral situation into a more manageable Class III or IV arch at first seems logical, it must not be undertaken lightly (Fig 3-20). Doing so is complicated and costly for the patient and dentist. The dentist must first consider what would happen to such a complex RPD if the few unilateral teeth that were maintained were lost to caries or fracture after a few years: Was the effort and expense of the implants worthwhile? How will the implant components be utilized now that the teeth are lost? Have you just gone from a unilateral tooth situation to a unilateral implant situation? If this scenario is anything near possible, the rehabilitation is probably best done with properly distributed implants after removal of the remaining natural teeth.

CONNECTORS AND RESIN RETENTION

Due to the need for maximum soft tissue coverage and the possibility of converting to a complete denture, full palate connectors are typically the first choice. Lingual plates for the mandibular arch are typically also necessary to maintain rigidity across a narrow arch or at the most anterior abutment. The lingual contour should be as symmetric as possible for comfort, which means lingual plating rather than open-spaced minor connectors. Because relines will be required to maintain adequate soft tissue support, the edentulous segment of the unilateral RPD should be mesh or lattice work raised 1 to 2 mm off of the tissue. As usual, when mesh is used, a 2- to 3-mm area of highly polished metal must exist at the gingival margin of the abutment teeth.

CLASPING AND RETENTION

As in obturator designs, the use of embrasure clasping on the dentate side with soft tissue undercuts on the edentulous side is the only conventional way to achieve retention.

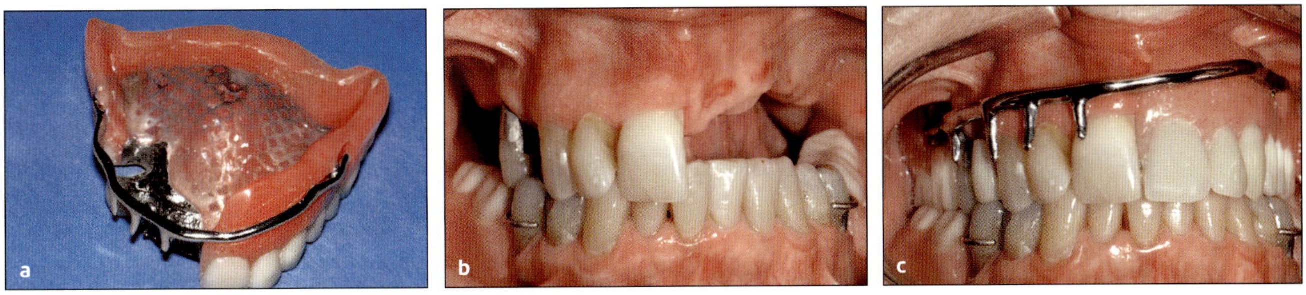

FIG 3-21 *(a)* Unilateral situations require full coverage of the available denture-bearing tissues to maximize support. Note the resin retention design. *(b)* A classic maxillary unilateral Class I situation that needs both support and retention on the edentulous side. *(c)* A swinglock framework will provide both support and retention.

Until the advent of the implant, the only more effective option for a stable and retentive restoration was to employ a swinglock partial denture (Fig 3-21). This hinged major connector design, discussed in chapter 12, is costly from a laboratory perspective yet has been somewhat successful in these situations.

While the swinglock partial denture is certainly effective in replacing teeth in the unilateral situation, the use of implant-supported bars that are milled on the lingual surface to be parallel with the lingual surfaces of any remaining teeth will allow a more conventional design that has limited major connector coverage. This concept will be demonstrated later in this text (see chapters 13 and 14).

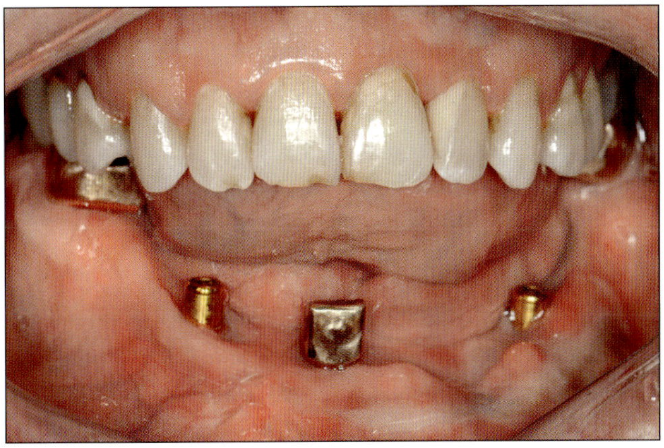

FIG 3-22 An extreme Class IV arch modified with three anterior implants. Support is now that of a Class III situation, and conversion to a hybrid or conventional implant overdenture is straightforward should the teeth be lost.

Limited abutment situations

Even beyond the extreme Class II situations are those with limited abutments. There really is no reasonable argument for maintaining an individual natural tooth in an otherwise edentulous arch. The results are typically uncontrolled resorption patterns that make the eventual complete denture less likely to be successful. Therefore, limited abutment situations, other than the unilateral situations just discussed, tend to be extreme Class IV cases. This could include retained mandibular third molars in an otherwise edentulous mandible. In general, this situation appears to be the reverse of a Class I arch with the resorption of the typically delicate anterior mandible and mentalis muscle contributing to the need for frequent relines. The persistent resorption and associated depression of the anterior segment of the prosthesis makes management of a reasonably stable occlusion nearly impossible. For this reason, it again is advised to either edentulate or consider implant modification. The implant modification here is safer in the long term because the implants would be positioned as if the prosthesis was to be a conventional tissue-supported implant-retained overdenture. Only now, the retained third molars create a Class III hard tissue support situation that tends to be very stable (Fig 3-22). These teeth are always rested, oftentimes with overlays to level the occlusal plane. The combination of contralateral mesial and lingual guiding planes can improve support but are very challenging to cast accurately due to the distance in arch length from one to the other. This type of RPD is nearly an implant-retained tissue-supported overdenture, and it often transitions into one over time. These design aspects are discussed in more detail in later chapters.

CASE STUDY:
Managing a unilateral limited abutment situation

When partial dentures are not managed well, it is common for the patient's condition to deteriorate. In this example, unmanaged residual ridge resorption, a poorly fitting partial denture, and a persistent malocclusion contributed to further tooth loss. The patient's previous provider recommended dental implants. However, two mandibular implants had previously failed, and the remaining anatomy was not amenable to adequate implant sizes or positions. The patient therefore sought an alternative. A hinged major connector was suggested after more focused attention to the aforementioned etiologic factors. Among the arguments for partial denture therapy was that the more aggressive dental implant therapy could be reserved as an option in the event the remaining abutment teeth were to fail. If implant therapy was attempted at this time and failed, there would be no reasonable alternative plan.

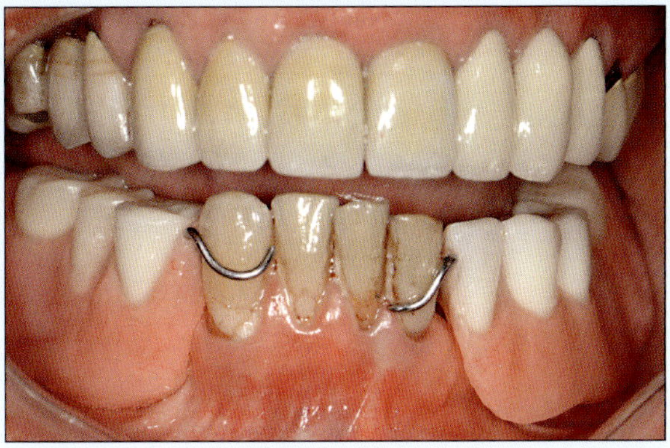

FIG 1 The step between the mandibular incisal edge and posterior occlusal plane indicated that continued residual ridge resorption allowed the base, and therefore teeth, to seat further apically. The lack of posterior support was detrimental to the patient's remaining anterior teeth. Her maxillary teeth had all been previously crowned. Fortunately, they were in a reasonable alignment and free from disease.

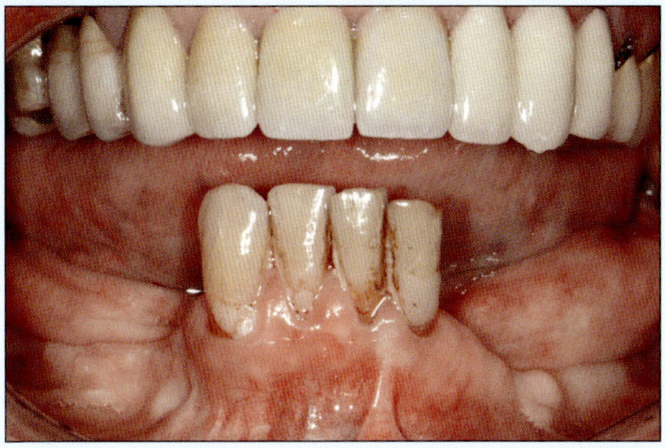

FIG 2 Severe residual ridge resorption is obvious on both edentulous segments. Note how the floor of the mouth now folds over what remains of the residual ridge. Migration of the remaining teeth and degenerative changes of the patient's temporomandibular joints have contributed to the mandible now being offset to the patient's left when in centric relation.

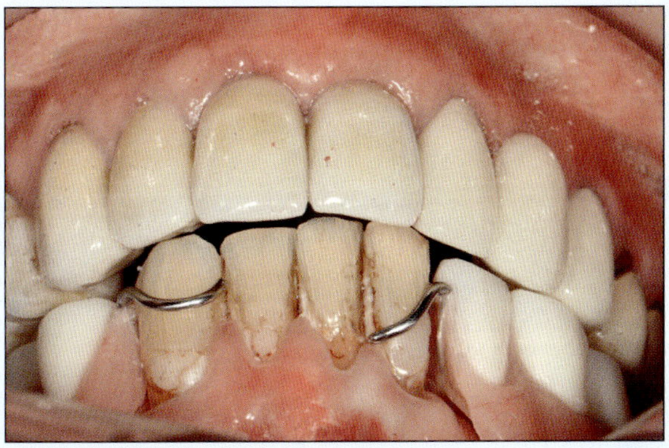

FIG 3 An inferior view of the patient in maximal intercuspal position confirms excessive contact on the mandibular left central incisor. This tooth was class 3 mobile, nonvital, and had an apical radiolucency. Mandibular central incisors are inadequate abutment teeth, especially when clasped as distal abutments.

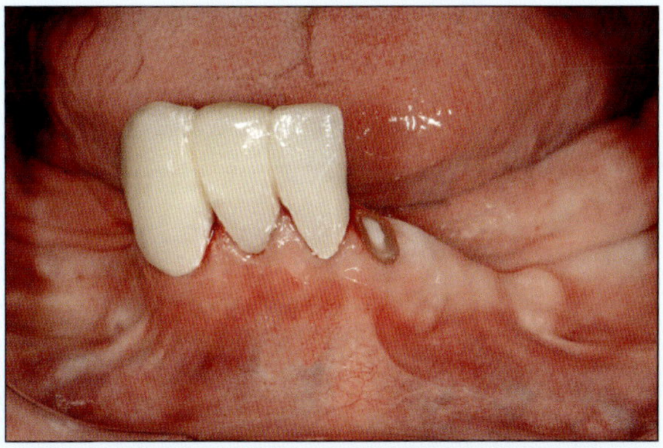

FIG 4 As with all uncontrolled debilitated situations, initial therapy included interim rehabilitation. After root canal therapy, the mandibular left central incisor was decoronated and maintained. This root will help maintain bone on the distal of the mandibular right central incisor and provide support as an overpartial abutment. Due to restorative concerns, the remaining teeth were then splinted with full-coverage provisional crowns.

FIG 5 The patient's existing partial denture was relined to restore both the tissue-base and tooth-frame relationships. Clasps were removed to test whether the improved support and stability would be adequate for patient comfort and function. Disease-control measures were also instituted at this time; note the mandibular gingival inflammation at the time of provisionalization.

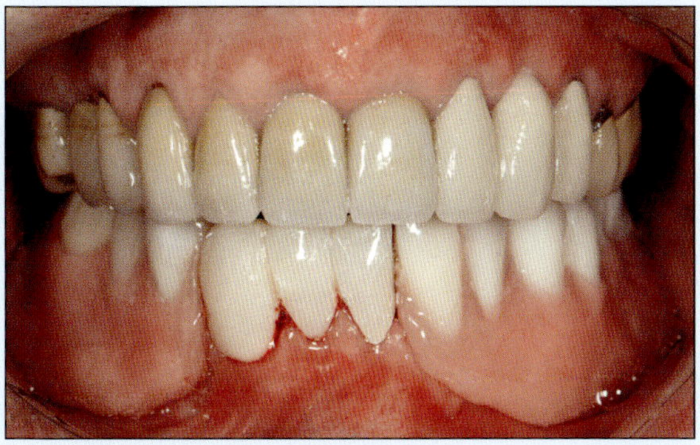

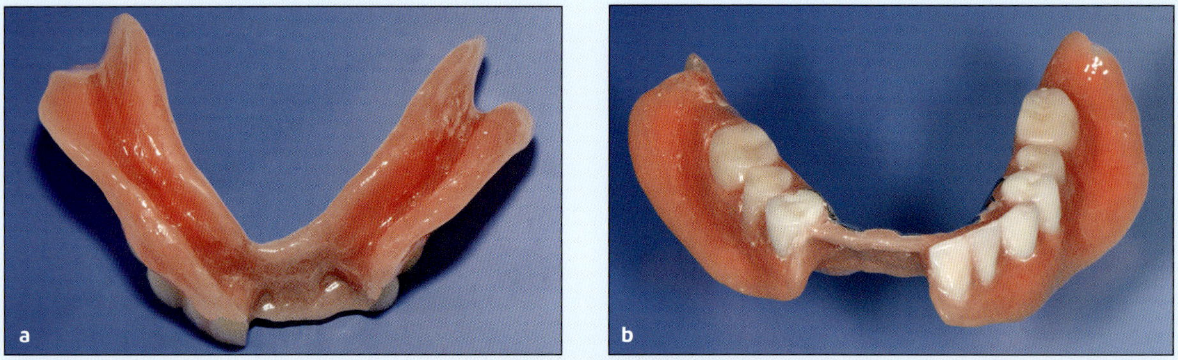

FIG 6 *(a and b)* An anatomically correct contour of the bases has been reestablished. The partial denture adapts to guiding planes that had been diagnostically waxed, replicated in a pull-down shell, and then created in direct temporary crowns. Note also the well-defined cingulum rests replicated in the relined partial denture. Major occlusal modifications and the addition of the mandibular left central incisor completed the rehabilitation. The result was even and simultaneous bilateral contact with limited anterior contact when this skeletal Class II patient was in centric occlusion. The interim rehabilitation allowed an assessment of the treatment plan and a more accurate prognosis. There was a demonstrated improvement in gingival health, in large part due to renewed daily hygiene effort. Functionally, she was able to eat most of her favorite foods, was comfortable, and was convinced that an RPD would meet her expectations. This allowed the treatment plan to proceed with confidence.

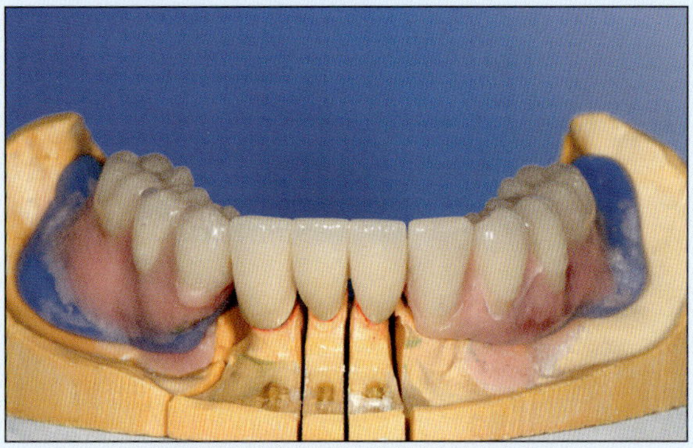

FIG 7 The final diagnostic tooth arrangement was confirmed intraorally and then used to facilitate creation of the definitive splinted porcelain-fused-to-metal crowns. Symmetry was recreated by designing four incisors and no canines. Note how the incisal and posterior occlusal planes are now level.

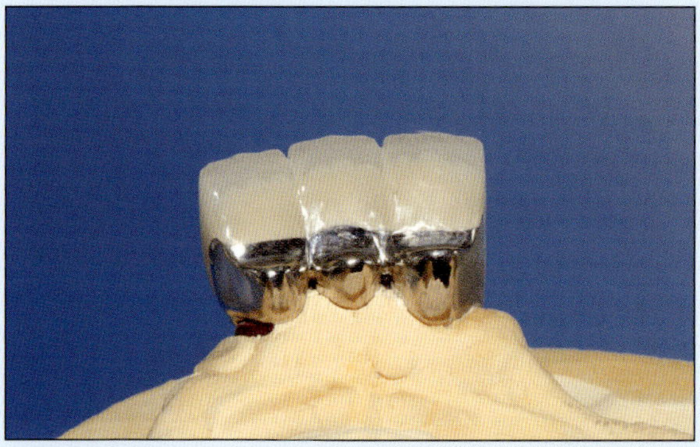

FIG 8 A pickup cast was created after the fit and appearance of the splinted crowns had been confirmed. The milled guiding plane surfaces and broad cingulum rest seats mimic the provisional. Metal was preferred in this situation due to the expected stresses on, and between, abutment teeth. It also allowed for more conservative metal collar margins to be used on the facial.

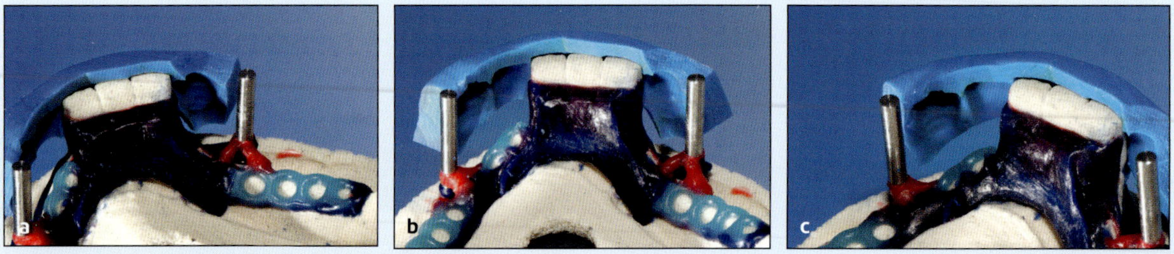

FIG 9 *(a to c)* The waxing of the hinged major connector must include evaluation of the space for both the hinge and the latch. These images demonstrate that both the hinge and the latch should be moved slightly to the mesial. This will place them within the interproximal space, leaving more room and resulting in a better contour of the acrylic around both. This matrix also confirmed that there is enough vertical distance for the components to function freely.

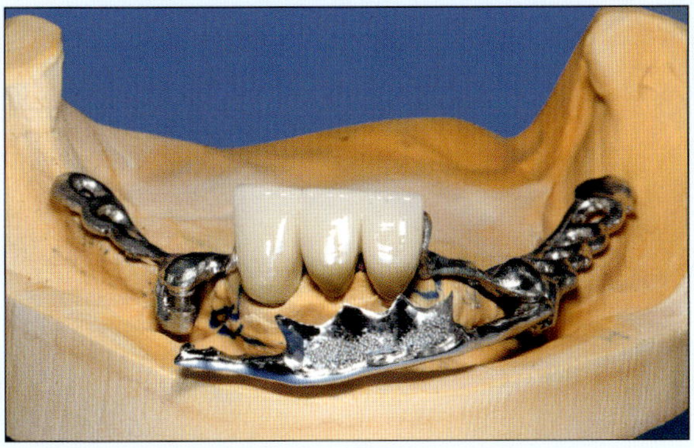

FIG 10 The hinged major connector at maximum opening. If the labial bar is opened any further, the components will bend or break. It is designed to open just enough to release and be removed.

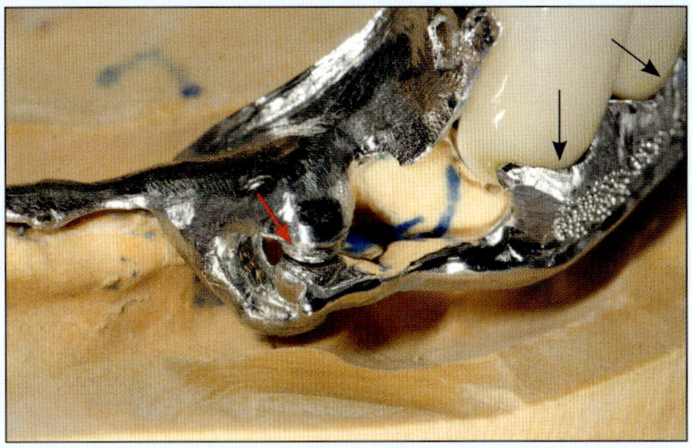

FIG 11 The hinge in closed position with the latch engaged *(red arrow)*. The *black arrows* indicate the labial plate in contact with the abutment teeth below the height of contour. This broad, solid contact will provide extensive support and stability, as it is opposed by the rests and guide plates.

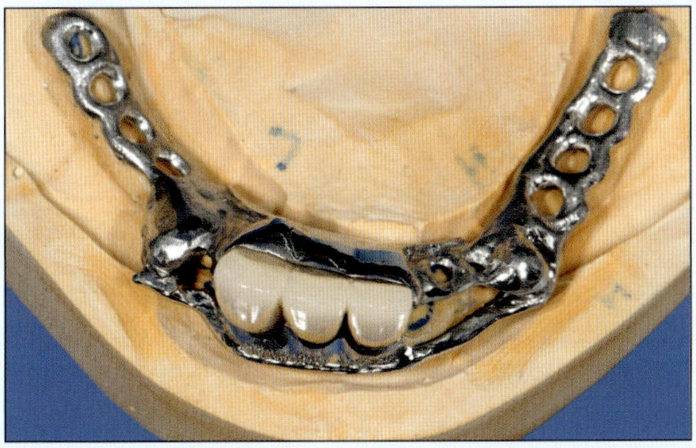

FIG 12 Note the size and position of the various components. The labial bar must swing open enough to disengage from the contact area farthest from the latch. If the latch or hinge is too far to the buccal, it will irritate the patient's lip and interfere with muscle function. The labial plate design also tends to create excess bulk facial to the abutment teeth.

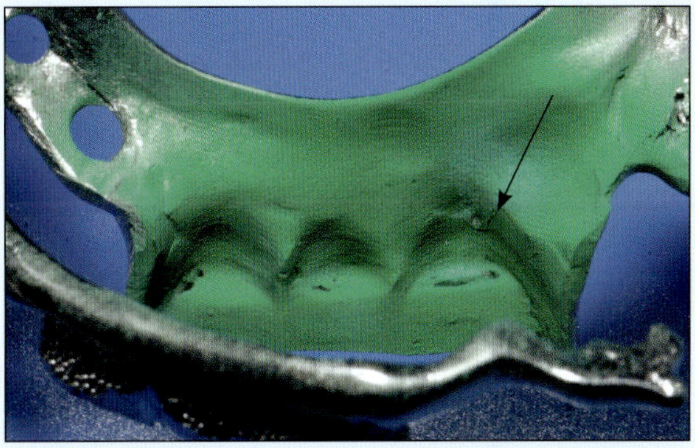

FIG 13 Final framework fitting was completed on a pickup cast. Marks confirm contact on the cingulum rest seats. The contact on the lingual of the mandibular right canine *(black arrow)* must be adjusted to ensure complete seating and a degree of stress relief. Some movement must be allowed when pressure is applied to the distal extensions in Class I situations.

FIG 14 A fluid wax altered cast impression was made. This was selected due to the challenging patient musculature. It is typically very difficult to record proper extensions when there has been significant residual ridge resorption. In addition, maximum support from the soft tissue is required in limited abutment situations.

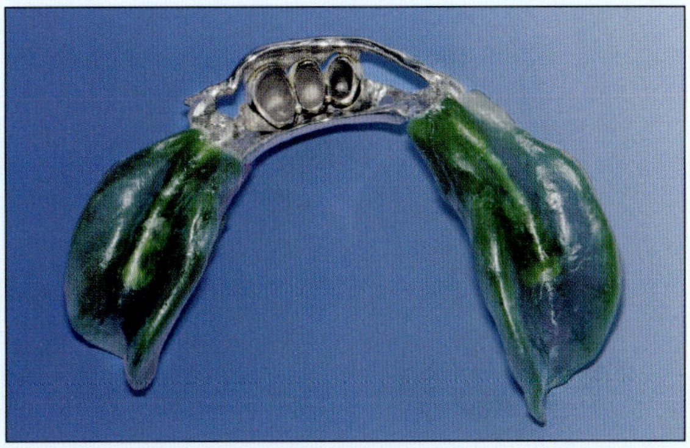

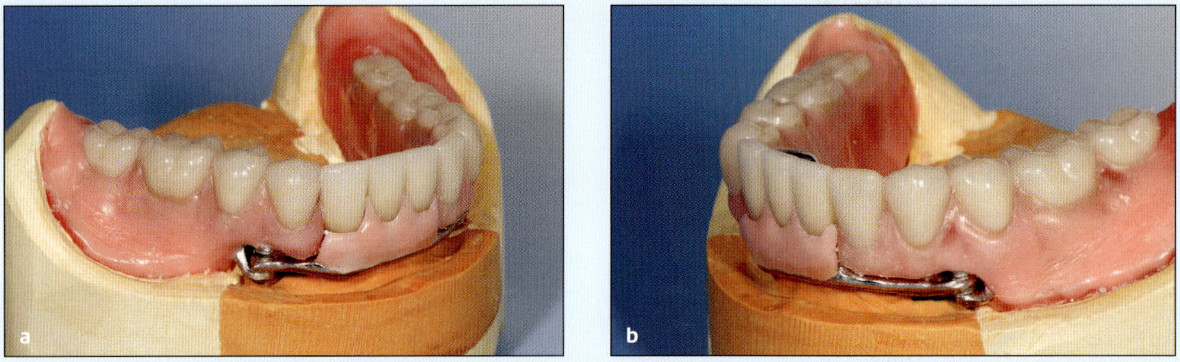

FIG 15 *(a and b)* After altered cast creation, a final arrangement with fully contoured waxing is completed. Note the coverage of the retromolar pad and contouring around the hinge and latch. Excess waxing of this area will tend to interfere with movement of the hinge or labial bar.

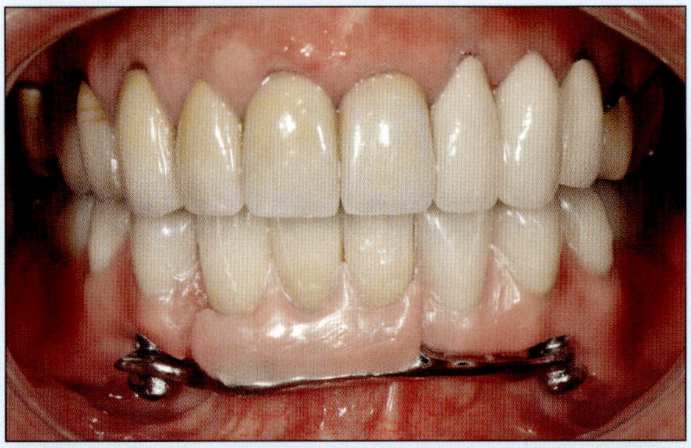

FIG 16 With such complicated contours, a final full-contour intraoral evaluation is critical. Note how the components are positioned as apical and lingual as the anatomy will allow. The goal is to have the hinge and latch hidden within the contour of the flange.

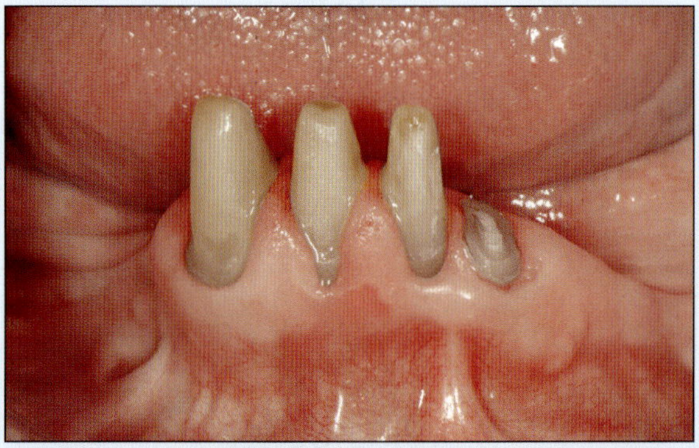

FIG 17 Gingival health has been restored. The effectiveness of the patient's daily plaque removal has been improved. In addition, the patient has had professional oral hygiene instruction and prophylaxis appointments every 3 months. This will continue after placement of the RPD.

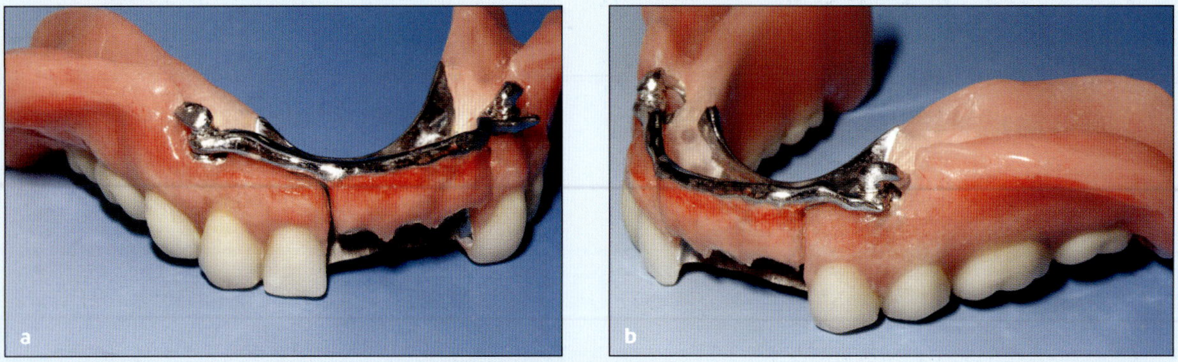

FIG 18 *(a and b)* After processing of the RPD, the labial plate was sandblasted, and pink opaquer was bonded to it to hide the metal color. A direct composite (Pala cre-active, Kulzer) was used to layer and color match the plate to the custom-stained denture base. After processing, the labial plate must be allowed to freely swing open and close. Any contact caused by excess acrylic or composite will interfere with the fit and is likely to fracture off.

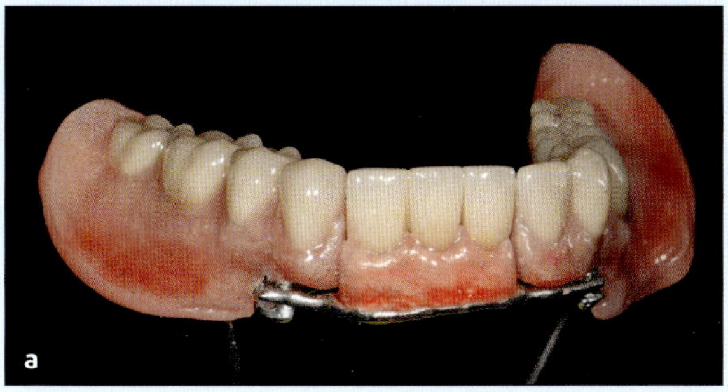
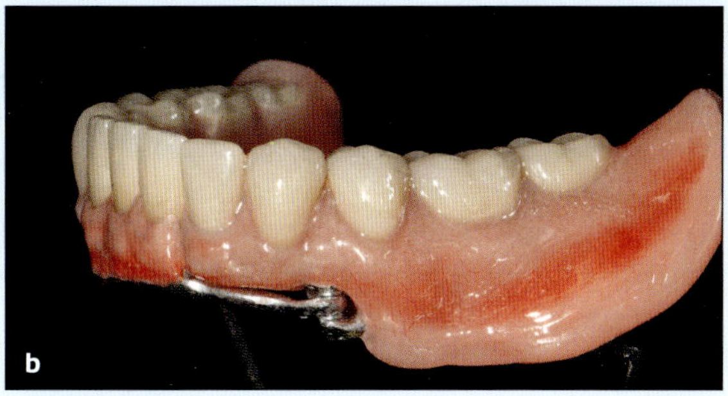

FIG 19 *(a and b)* The completed RPD and crowns ready for placement. Contact with the crowns occurs only on the metal portion of the plate. The composite extends slightly coronal to the metal margin of the plate in order to hide the metal and to create the appearance of papillae. If the composite is actively contacting the crowns, it is likely to chip off when the latch is closed or when the RPD is placed in function. The extent to which the composite can be contoured interproximally is further limited by the draw of the gate. This is because the movement away from the abutments occurs on a curve rather than directly toward the facial.

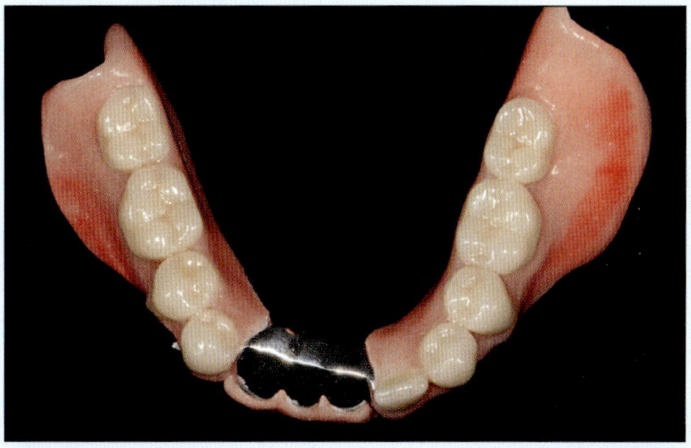

FIG 20 A symmetric contour along the labial surface is confirmed after completion of the RPD. The bulk of the labial plate was minimized.

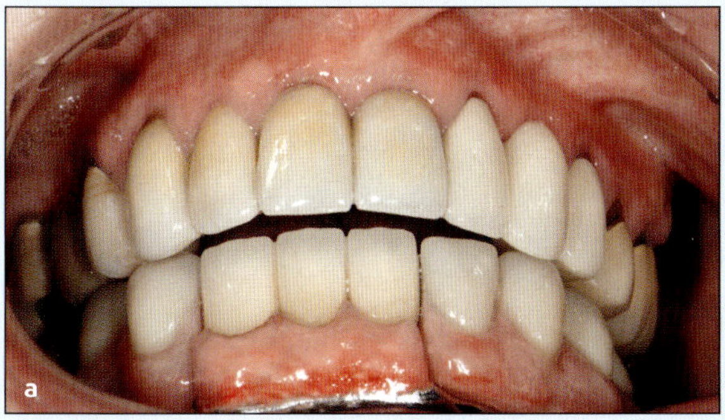
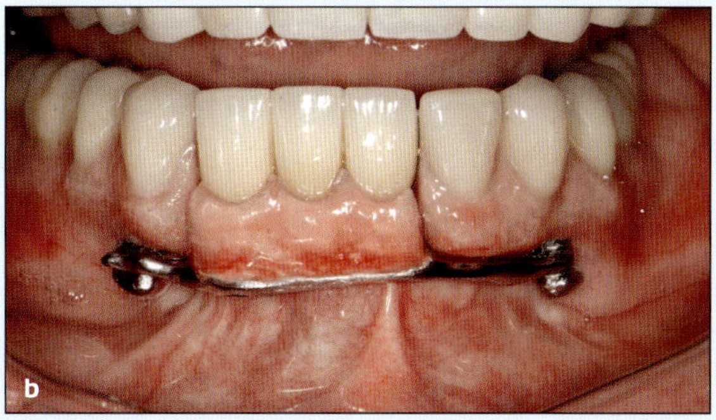

FIG 21 *(a and b)* A corrected occlusal scheme with level occlusal plane and anterior open bite. The case was designed in centric occlusion rather than the postural position that was resulting in excessive contact on the weak abutments. The open bite is due to the significant skeletal Class II relationship; anterior contact occurs in postural and functional positions. This scheme helps limit the force on the remaining natural teeth, assuming stress relief is built into the RPD.

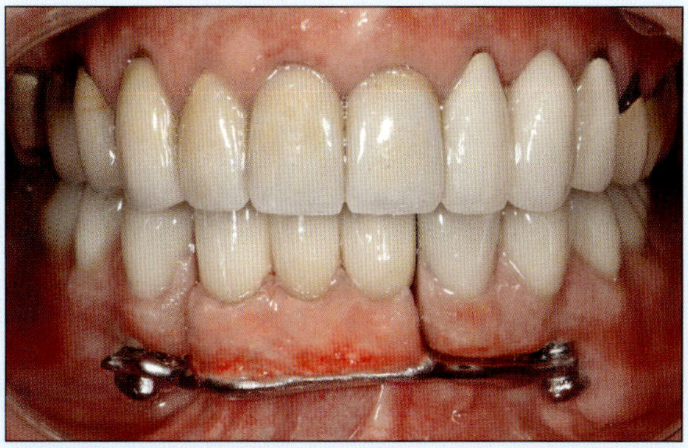

FIG 22 The completed RPD: functional, cosmetic, and comfortable. Note the "knob" on the end of the latch. This is the purchase point the patient uses to unlatch the RPD. This requires some degree of dexterity and strength. Time must be spent to train the patient to completely lock the latch upon insertion. If the latch is not completely closed, the knob will irritate the lip, and the plate will not be completely closed.

Conclusion

The basis of RPD design has been covered in this chapter. The keys to success are careful and exacting preparation of a healthy mouth and control of the tooth-frame relationship through attention to detail in the laboratory. The clinician who follows the principles established here will find design decisions reduced to a minimum. The anatomy of the mouth and the number and location of the missing teeth will greatly influence the decision, leaving personal preference as only a minor modifying factor. Prosthodontists do not, as a rule, wear RPDs and so have no feeling for the patient's response to the addition of so much material in the mouth. The clinician can, however, make a casting or two to fit their mouths and at least evaluate the placement and configuration of the major connector. Many of the ideas expressed here have come from just that experience.

References

1. Kennedy E. Partial Denture Construction. Brooklyn: Dental Items of Interest, 1928:3–8.
2. Applegate O. Essentials of Removable Partial Prosthesis, ed 1. Philadelphia: Saunders, 1954.
3. Curtis DA, Curtis TA, Wagnild GW, Finzen FC. Incidence of various classes of removable partial dentures. J Prosthet Dent 1992;67:664–667.
4. Pun D, Waliszewski M, Waliszewski K, Berzins D. Survey of partial removable dental prosthesis types in a distinct patient population. J Prosthet Dent 2011;106:48–56.
5. Applegate OC. The rationale of partial denture choice. J Prosthet Dent 1960;10:891–907.
6. Roach FE. Mouth survey and design of partial dentures. J Am Dent Assoc 1934;21:1166–1176.
7. Kratochvil FJ. Influence of occlusal rest position and clasp design on movement of abutment teeth. J Prosthet Dent 1963;13:114–124.
8. Krol AJ. RPI (rest, proximal plate, I-bar) clasp retainer and its modifications. Dent Clin North Am 1973;4:631–649.
9. Ceconni BT, Asgar K, Dootz E. The effect of partial denture clasp design on abutment tooth movement. J Prosthet Dent 1971;25:44–56.
10. Maxfield JB, Nicholls JI, Smith DE. The measurement of forces transmitted to abutment teeth of removable partial dentures. J Prosthet Dent 1979;41:134–142.
11. Frank RP, Nicholls, JI. An investigation of the effectiveness of indirect retainers. J Prosthet Dent 1977;38:494–506.

MOUTH PREPARATION 4

Failing to prepare is preparing to fail.

Mouth preparation, as described earlier, covers everything done to prepare the mouth for the actual construction of the RPD. Restorative procedures associated with the remaining teeth are a responsibility of the primary clinician, but most other areas of mouth preparation fall under the management of surgical, orthodontic, or endodontic specialists.

In most general practices, mouth preparation is looked upon as preparing a few rest seats, perhaps a surveyed crown or two, and then getting on with the final impression for the casting. This is woefully inadequate for the majority of partially edentulous patients. The disease experience of the average partial denture candidate not only leaves teeth in poor condition but also often in a poor location. Having reviewed disease control in chapter 1, this chapter assumes a healthy dental patient with reduced risk of disease recurrence. The clinician can therefore prepare to proceed with definitive partial denture therapy. Because mouth preparation is the foundation of all that the clinician plans to do later on, it is essential that a planning phase be developed. This planning phase will make final determinations regarding occlusal, structural, and periodontal factors (Figs 4-1a and 4-1b). All possible changes required to maintain the state of health achieved during initial therapy must be identified. In addition, the remaining dentition must be properly aligned and positioned so that ideal occlusal and esthetic results can be achieved. Mouth preparation for the state-of-the-art RPD therefore requires diagnostic procedures that include, but are not limited to, the following:

- Centric relation records and articulated diagnostic/opposing casts (where indicated).
- Impressions, records, and wax-up of opposing arch (if completely or partially edentulous).
- Survey of the diagnostic cast with selection of the path of insertion/removal.
- Orthodontic setup for teeth requiring minor tooth movement.
- Ridge mapping for gingival surgery and implants.
- Reshaping of stone abutment teeth to ideal contours for subtractive mouth preparation.
- Diagnostic waxing of any areas requiring additive mouth preparation.
- Diagnostic setup of teeth to be replaced by the partial denture.
- Creation of a preparation guide for guiding planes needing subtractive preparation.
- Creation of a matrix for additive composite modifications.
- Creation of a preparation guide (vacuum formed) for surveyed crowns.

As can be seen, this phase requires active involvement by the treating dentist. Despite the fact that these procedures are conducted on diagnostic casts, they are the basis of clinical treatment planning (Figs 4-1c and 4-1d). If delegated to a typical dental laboratory, it is unlikely that the decisions made

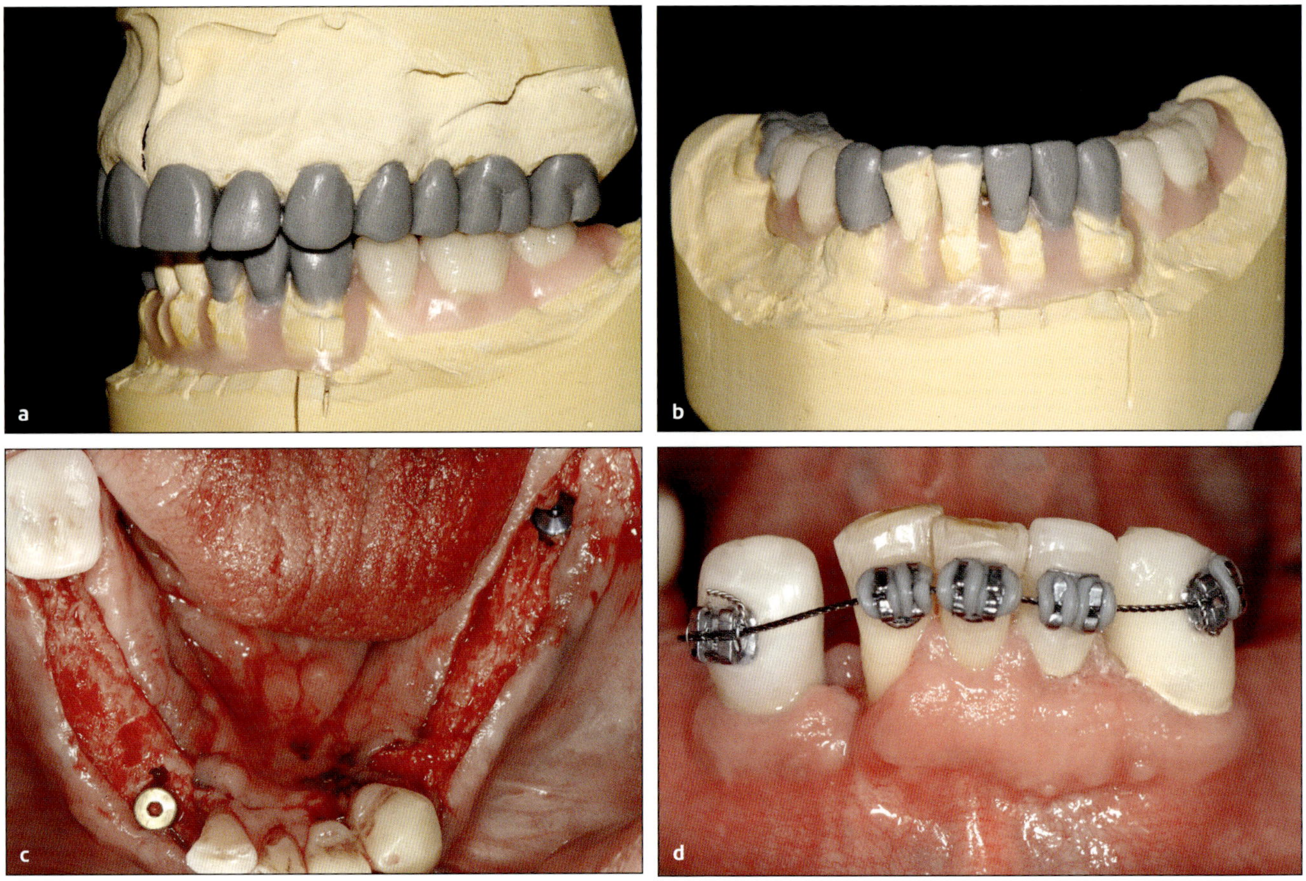

FIG 4-1 *(a and b)* Complete diagnostic mouth preparation is required for a definitive treatment plan. *(c and d)* The diagnostic mouth preparation leads to treatment planning decisions such as the implant placement, tori removal, and subsequent minor orthodontics shown here.

will be appropriate. When these extensive diagnostic procedures have been completed and all consultations finished, the definitive treatment plan can be finalized. A treatment plan letter for informed consent is then written and signed by the patient. Only once informed consent is obtained should the actual irreversible mouth preparation begin.

Surveying the Diagnostic Cast

Once the diagnostic cast has been mounted in the survey table, the easiest way to begin the survey process is to stand over the cast and, using the parallax of your eyes, attempt to look down the long axes of the abutment teeth. The prime abutment(s), should they exist (as in Class I and II situations), will determine the path of insertion/removal for the partial denture because the guiding plane established on the distal surface of the prime abutment will be the key to the remaining mouth preparation. This position is found by tilting the cast in the sagittal plane. Once the anteroposterior position has been determined, possible retentive areas can be equalized by tilting the cast in the frontal plane. Before tripoding the cast, all proximal surfaces that will have guiding planes and all potential retentive undercuts are verified using the analyzing rod in the surveyor. Minor adjustments to the tilt are then made and tripod marks placed on the cast. The tripod marks should be in such a position that they can all be seen at one time. Vertical markings on the sides of the land areas, while they do allow accurate repositioning, are much more difficult to use since they cannot all be seen at one glance. When the marks are widely spread out, one on the lingual of the anterior area and the other two on the lingual lateral surfaces of the retromolar pads or tuberosities, the cast can be easily repositioned by clinician and technician alike.

At this point, the lead is placed in the surveyor and the entire height of contour of all teeth that will possibly be contacted by the partial denture is marked. The height of contour of edentulous and soft tissue areas must also

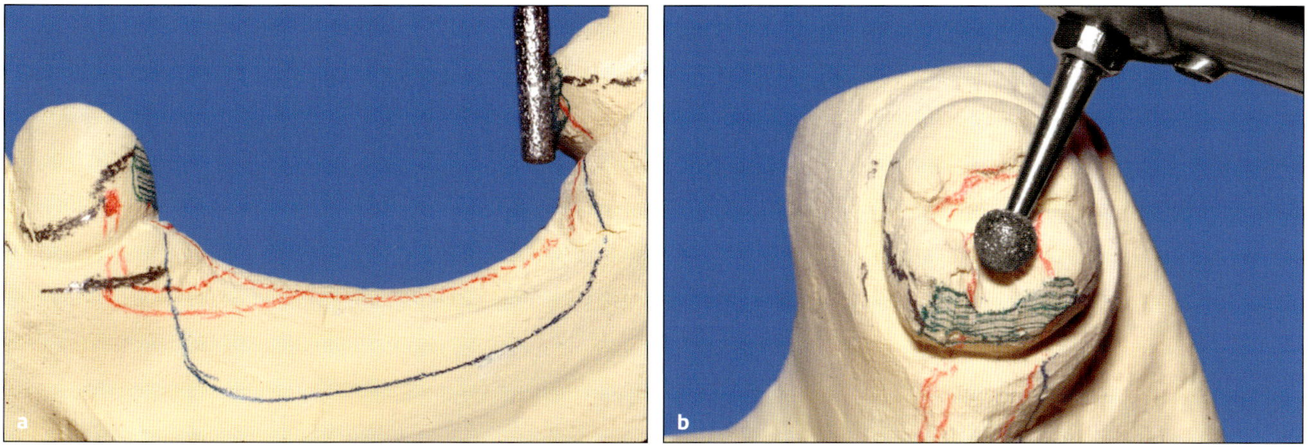

FIG 4-2 *(a and b)* A surveyed diagnostic cast with design drawing is modified with the same diamond burs that will be used clinically.

be surveyed. Without information on both hard and soft tissue undercuts, there is insufficient data on which to base the design and the mouth preparation that will be needed.

A reasoned design needs to be carefully drawn on the diagnostic cast before diagnostic mouth preparation can begin. It makes sense to use a color code that is familiar to your laboratory. Making a neat and precise drawing on a stone cast is not as easy as it would appear, and most diagnostic casts seen in the dental laboratory will have drawings that are childish at best. None of us has a natural talent for drawing in three planes: All our previous efforts in drawing have been done on the two dimensions of a piece of paper. In order to simulate the two-dimensional drawing with which we are familiar, the cast is braced against the clinician's stomach and rotated with one hand while the other hand draws. In this way, the pencil stays in the comfortable two-plane position while the third plane is managed via the rotation of the cast. Just a little practice will allow even the non-artist to make a credible drawing. There is an added value to having a neatly constructed design drawing—technicians are much more likely to give their best effort when the materials submitted to them are of the highest quality. The well-drawn design on the diagnostic cast reinforces the level of quality desired in the final prosthesis.

Diagnostic Mouth Preparation

Perhaps the most important yet forgotten step in the construction of an RPD is the preparation of the diagnostic cast. The process is broken down into *subtractive mouth preparation*, the reduction of existing tooth contours to some predetermined ideal state, and *additive mouth preparation*, the diagnostic waxing of contours that must be altered with restorations (either bridges, crowns, or bonded contours).

Subtractive mouth preparation is done first. This keeps reduction conservative and sets the path of insertion/removal for all additive restorations, which can more conservatively correct for tooth malalignment. The same instrumentation that will be used in the actual tooth recontouring should be used in the laboratory. The armamentarium will include the following:

- Preparation guides (reduction copings) to parallel guiding planes
- Tapered and nontapered diamonds of medium/fine grit for guiding plane preparation
- Round diamonds for occlusal rest preparation in either 8D, 10D, or 12D size
- Inverted cone for cingulum preparation in 37 or 39 size

Using the actual clinical diamonds on the stone teeth does not harm the diamonds and offers the opportunity to actually practice the preparations (Fig 4-2). The stone teeth are to be prepared to ideal contour even though it may not be possible to do so in the mouth. Once the practice subtractive mouth preparation is completed, a decision is made on a tooth-by-tooth basis on the clinical possibility of creating the same preparation on the natural tooth. Obviously, there will be many instances when compromises will have to be made between the ideal and the possible. For some of these situations, the actual design may be changed, orthodontic minor tooth movement required, or additive mouth preparation undertaken in order to achieve the ideal situation.

The sequence of subtractive mouth preparation must always be guiding planes first, other contour adjustments next, with rest seat preparation last. Once the stone teeth have been prepared, the design is redrawn to its original state. Dimensions and depths of rest seats should be ideal,

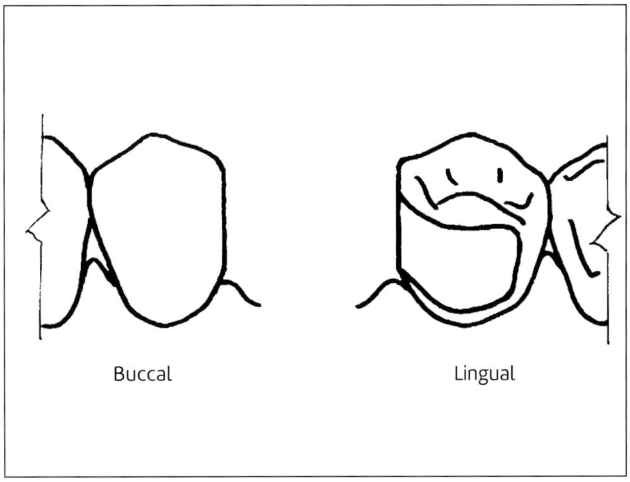

FIG 4-3 Guiding planes fully extended.

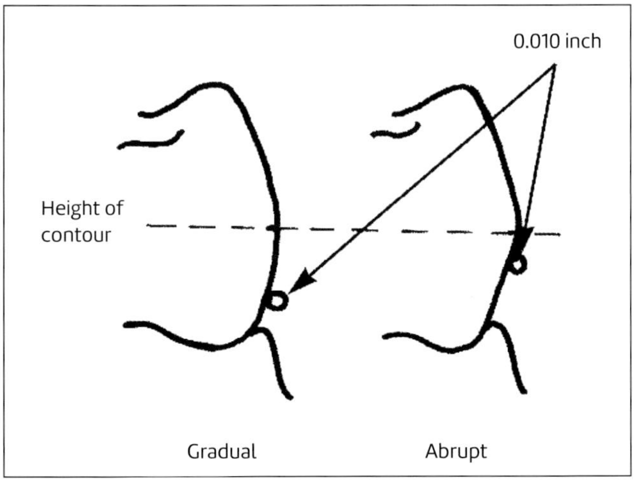

FIG 4-4 Quality and quantity of retention.

once again, with possible compromises or changes in design coming after intraoral reevaluation.

Additive preparation follows with the diagnostic waxing of crowns and bonded contours. The surveyor blade is used to create "milled" guiding plane surfaces on the wax-ups, again to ideal contours. When full crowns are desired for the abutment teeth in Class III and IV partial dentures, the proximal guiding planes will be extended as far as possible so that maximum frictional retention can be obtained (Fig 4-3). The contours of bonded restorations are waxed directly on the diagnostic cast. The design of the base of these units will be identical to those of the resin-bonded fixed partial denture (Maryland bridge or Rochette bridge). Retentive areas for clasps are to be brought as close as possible to the gingiva, leaving a minimum of 1 mm of space between the proposed clasp arm and the soft tissue, a task easily accomplished in the waxing of a crown but not always possible in natural tooth structure or bonded restoration. Because the crown gives us the potential for creating the ideal abutment contour, thought must be given to the timing of the undercut.

The relationship of the height of contour to the desired undercut depth determines the quality of retention that will occur when the retentive clasp dislodges from the tooth. If there is some distance (a gradual transition) between the height of contour and the desired undercut (0.01 inch to 0.015 inch), then the resulting retention will be weaker but last longer as the clasp moves toward the height of contour. If the undercut is steep (ie, with little distance between the 0.01-inch point and the height of contour), then the initial retention will be greater but not last as long (Fig 4-4). The gradual undercut is best suited for a distal extension situation (Class I) in the mandible. This will allow a certain amount of stress relief in the clasp-tooth relationship. The steeper undercut area is better for a tooth-borne situation in the maxilla where the patient will appreciate maximum retention against the force of gravity. These decisions on contour are made at this time so that a diagnostic record of the ideal contour of the abutment teeth will be available throughout the treatment phase and not have to be redesigned at each subsequent step in treatment.

The final step in the diagnostic preparation of the mouth is to position the replacement denture teeth (see Fig 4-1). Because the teeth have to be ordered from the manufacturer at some time during treatment, the earlier the better. The criteria for shade selection will be the same no matter when the selection is made. The mold can best be determined from an analysis of the diagnostic cast as soon as it is recovered. The definitive denture teeth can therefore be readily available to the clinician at the time of diagnostic mouth preparation. An alternative is to use teeth from a mold guide for diagnostic procedures and then use the actual denture teeth later on. However, as modifications are made, the continued recontouring of the mold guide teeth may be unacceptable.

A quick wax procedure for isolated missing teeth can be accomplished by selecting a tooth from the mold guide and impressing it in alginate. When the alginate is set, the denture tooth is removed and molten wax poured in the mold. The wax tooth is modified to fit the edentulous area on the cast and waxed to place.

With the denture teeth in position, the diagnostic procedure is complete, and the patient can be shown the recontoured cast as a means of describing the treatment plan. This is another reason to have a quality drawing and a clean and neat cast.

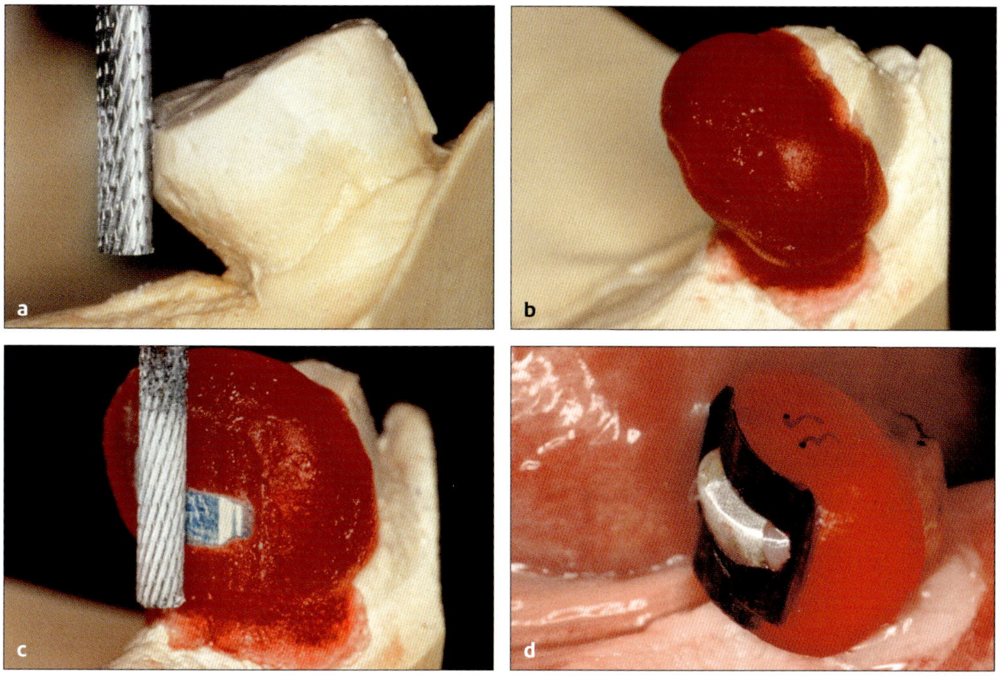

FIG 4-5 *(a to d)* Fabrication sequence for a guiding plane preparation guide.

Construction of Preparation Guides

With the patient now ready for abutment modification, the clinician must consider the challenge of how to transfer the diagnostic modifications to the actual clinical environment. Traditional dental education typically expects this be done freehand. While this can occasionally suffice in simple Class I situations, it is unrealistic to expect ideal results in most tooth-borne situations without some form of guide for accurate transfer. From the perspective of a busy clinician, preparation guides have great value in reduction of chairside appointment time. Compare a typical 5- or 10-minute guided modification time to the traditional process of freehand preparation, making a check cast, and repeating the modifications until they are found accurate. In this context, any time spent in the laboratory to create a guide is worthwhile.

The most challenging modifications to accurately complete are the guiding planes. Preparation guides, made in a similar fashion to crown and bridge reduction copings, are ideal in situations where the parallelism of the guiding planes is critical. This includes nearly all Class II and III situations and Class IV cases not using the rotational philosophy. The modified diagnostic cast, once determined feasible and ideal, may be duplicated for preservation purposes. Duplication is typically necessary anyway when multiple abutments will be indirect restorations in need of provisional crowns. Resin separator is applied to the stone cast on all primary abutments that will receive subtractive modification. In some instances, wax blockout is needed below significant heights of contour on the buccal and lingual to prevent the overlaying acrylic from engaging and breaking the stone tooth. The stability of the reduction guide must be maintained by maximum contact on the unmodified tooth surface. Indiscriminate blockout would be counterproductive and create an unstable and inaccurate guide. An autopolymerizing acrylic resin like GC Pattern Resin (GC America) or a composite material is placed over the lubricated stone tooth to create a pattern. Once the resin is set, the pattern is removed and rough periphery trimmed.

The cast is realigned on a surveyor along the diagnostically determined path of insertion. While still locked tightly on a surveyor table, the resin patterns are then placed back on the stone cast. A commercial dental milling unit, a drill press, or a device that clamps on to the vertical arm of a dental surveyor to hold a dental laboratory handpiece can all be used to cut through the resin pattern until the parallel guiding planes on the stone abutment teeth are met (Fig 4-5). The milling of the pattern is extended to the periphery of the resin. This creates a large, flat surface area that will guide placement of the bur during actual tooth reduction. Ideal parallelism of the surface is thereby transferred. The stone guiding plane surface can be colored (see Fig 4-5) prior to milling the preparation guide as an additional visual marker for when the bur begins to contact the stone surface. This would indicate that the reduction of the acrylic

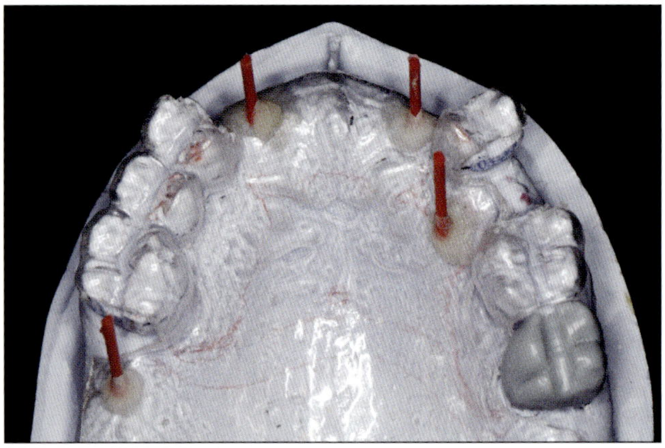

FIG 4-6 Paralleling reference markers on a pull-down matrix. The matrix is placed in the mouth, and the markers are used to orient the operator's bur as the guiding plane surfaces are modified.

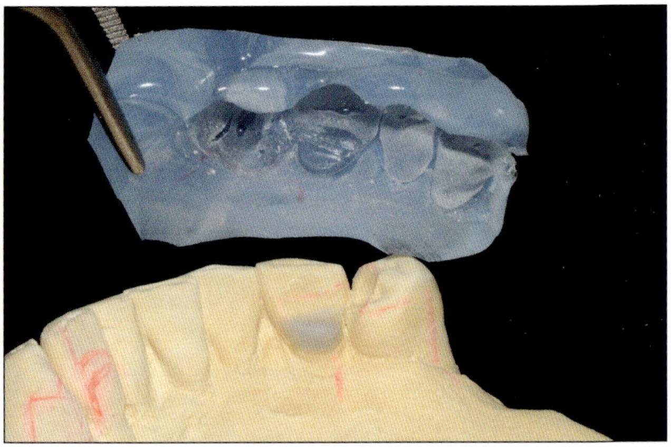

FIG 4-7 Diagnostic additive modifications like this cingulum rest can be easily transferred to the mouth using a transparent matrix. The composite is cured through this material once it is seated on the tooth.

guide is complete. If it is clear that the guiding plane modifications will be feasible and within the anatomical limits of the abutments, then the cutting of the preparation guide and the diagnostic guiding plane modification of the stone cast can be done simultaneously.

When these guides are placed on the natural tooth, the portion of the tooth to be removed in the creation of the guiding plane extends through the hole in the pattern. This makes it easy to remove the enamel parallel to the periphery of the pattern adjacent to the hole (see Fig 4-5), much like a traditional reduction coping. This periphery should be marked with a black felt-tip pen to identify bur cuts that are not parallel and to make the operator aware of when the reduction is nearing its planned end point. These preparation guides can be made digitally, although the overall efficiency when considering the necessary variety of diagnostic steps just discussed is limited.

While the reduction coping is the guide of choice for guiding plane modifications, additional types exist and are only limited by imagination. Most types include some sort of pull-down or jig that holds a paralleling reference marker, sometimes an old bur held by acrylic (Fig 4-6). These can be efficiently fabricated and will assist positioning of the handpiece. Unfortunately, they still require movement of the handpiece to and from the reference point, which is the source of different preparation angulations.

Additive modifications are also more accurate and efficient when they are completed with a preparation guide. Typically, in matrix form, these allow planned additive preparations to be transferred from the waxed additive modifications on the diagnostic cast. These are made in the same fashion as those for anterior composite veneers. In the case of an additive composite rest seat, this would mean a transparent silicone putty matrix (Memosil 2, Kulzer). The material is placed over the diagnostic wax-up of the rest (Fig 4-7). Once set, the putty is trimmed to allow it to be seated completely at the same time the rubber dam is in place. The bonding protocol for enamel is then followed, the light-cured composite material of choice is placed in the matrix, the matrix is seated on the tooth, and the composite is cured through the transparent matrix. This technique works just as well for bonded contours and dual-cured composites should they be preferred. In the case of a rest and guiding plane combination, as is typical with a mandibular canine, the reduction coping technique may still be preferred.

After final surgical and orthodontic modifications, the diagnostic mouth preparation steps are completed. Mouth preparation guides are readied as well. This sets the stage for the actual tooth modifications. There are three types, to be completed in the following order: subtractive, additive, and indirect. Regardless of the type, guiding planes are created first, followed by contour adjustments, and then lastly the rest seats.

Subtractive Mouth Preparation

The actual subtractive mouth preparation begins by using the diagnostic ideal mouth preparation from the cast as a template. The creation of parallel guiding planes without the use of custom preparation guides can only be accomplished with practice. Clinicians trained in the era of multiple pin ledge restorations will recall the paralleling devices that were attached to teeth not involved in the restoration so that the contra-angle handpiece could be kept in the same plane throughout the preparations. That type of device is not usable for the preparation of guiding planes because teeth on both sides of the arch are involved. The success and efficiency of the reduction coping method is such that we no longer need to discuss freehand guiding plane preparation. After all the guiding planes have been prepared, an alginate impression is made and poured in fast-set plaster to serve as a check cast. This cast, when recovered, is placed on the surveyor and the guiding planes are evaluated for parallelism. Any discrepancies are adjusted on the cast, and then the same correction is made in the mouth.

Guiding plane considerations

Remember, guiding planes for Classes II, III, and IV should be as long as possible vertically without compromising the enamel. In some situations, such as for elderly patients, the guiding planes can be taken into dentine. By preparing the teeth without anesthesia, the patient can indicate when the tooth becomes sensitive, and the extent of the guiding plane can be reevaluated. The buccolingual dimension of the guiding plane in these three classifications should extend just around the line angle in most cases. This slight extension, the turning of the "corner," will greatly enhance reciprocation and provide the bracing component formerly dependent on the bracing clasp arm that can now be eliminated (Fig 4-8). The only exception to the buccal extension of this plane would be on the mesial proximal surface of a tooth in the anterior portion of the mouth where the guide plate of the partial denture could be seen, most likely in a Class IV.

For the Class I RPD, the clinician will have to choose between the shorter guiding plane with the stress relief "built in" and the long guiding plane that will require functional adaptation of the guide plate on the casting for the same amount of stress relief. The Class IV situation has often been described as a "Class I in reverse," and if stress relief is indicated (when the remaining abutment teeth are less-than-ideal supports), the decision as to the prime guiding planes on the mesial of the most anterior teeth will have to be made on the same basis as for the Class I. However, when a rotational path RPD is planned, the proximal undercut must be maintained, thus eliminating the guiding plane adjacent to the edentulous area.

Contour adjustments

Once the guiding planes have been prepared, the final tooth contour adjustments are made. Additional reduction is often required on the buccal and lingual surfaces of posterior teeth to drop the height of contour closer to the gingiva, especially on lingually inclined mandibular posterior teeth. The approach arms of minor connectors will need a minor guiding plane gingival to the marginal ridge for additional frictional retention. When circumferential clasp arms are planned, the proximal two-thirds must lie at or slightly above the height of contour. Because the height of contour at the line angle of a tooth normally rises as it approaches the marginal ridge, reduction is required to bring the height of contour apical and thereby avoid a possible occlusal interference (Fig 4-9).

These contours are best reduced with a nontapered cylinder. As guiding planes enter the lingual embrasures on their way to the supplementary rests, it may be necessary to change to a finely tapered diamond cylinder just to get into the constricted space. The guiding planes can still be kept parallel to the proposed path of insertion by slightly tilting the handpiece so that the tapered bur cuts at 90 degrees and remains parallel to the other guiding planes. It is generally most efficient to verify the guiding plane and contour adjustments at the same time. Regardless, verification should be done prior to rest seat preparation in order to avoid a change in prepared rest seat form.

Preparing rest seats

Once verified, the occlusal rest seats are prepared. The tendency has always been to make the rest seats too small and to leave them with sharp angles or with undercuts to the path of insertion/removal. This is common with isolated mandibular molars, where the rest typically draws to the mesiolingual, but will not draw with the more vertical path of insertion of the overall casting. This difference means the rest will not seat due to an undercut at the buccal margin of a deep but narrow rest preparation. The rest seats are to be one-half to one-third the buccolingual dimension of the tooth. This same target dimension, one-half to one-third, is used for the mesiodistal rest seat length. Experience shows that if these reference lengths are met, it is much more likely that the reference width will be met as well. This is due to the desire to create a flared and rounded design. For this reason, the rest length is generally set with the first few bur strokes followed by refinement of the periphery. It is most efficient to select a round diamond that has the same diameter as the desired rest seat. The occlusal rest has historically been presented as needing to be spoon-shaped, meaning that the seat was deeper in the center of the tooth than it was at the marginal ridge. This, unfortunately, results in a marginal ridge without adequate space for metal. The resulting casting will be thin and may break at that point, leaving a difficult repair situation. The rest seat must be deep enough to allow for a minimum of 1.25 mm of metal at the narrowest portion of the rest. The rest seat on any isolated tooth, especially a single mandibular molar, should extend to at least the center of the

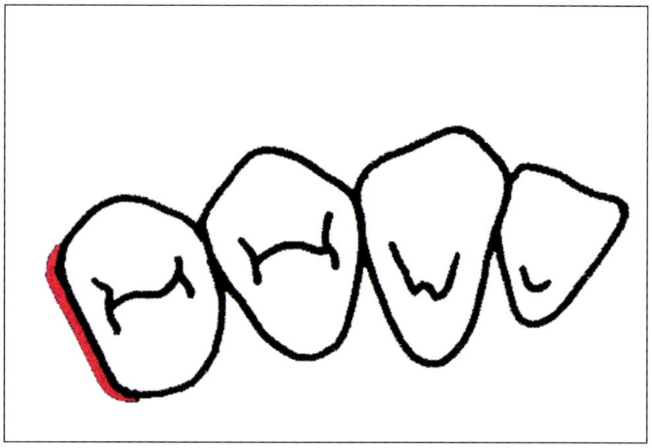

FIG 4-8 Buccal and lingual extensions of guiding plane.

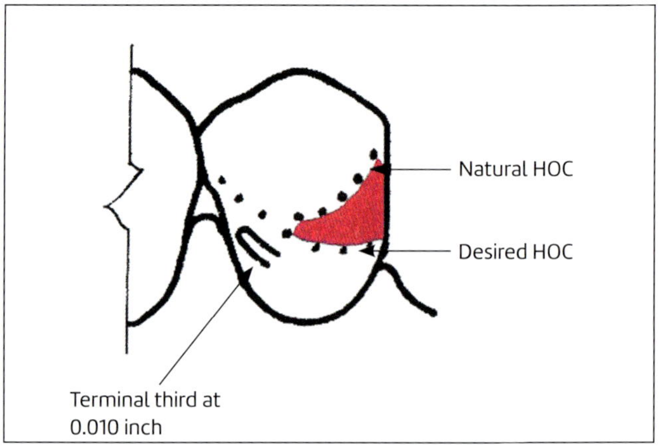

FIG 4-9 Required reduction for the proximal two-thirds of a retentive clasp arm. HOC, height of contour.

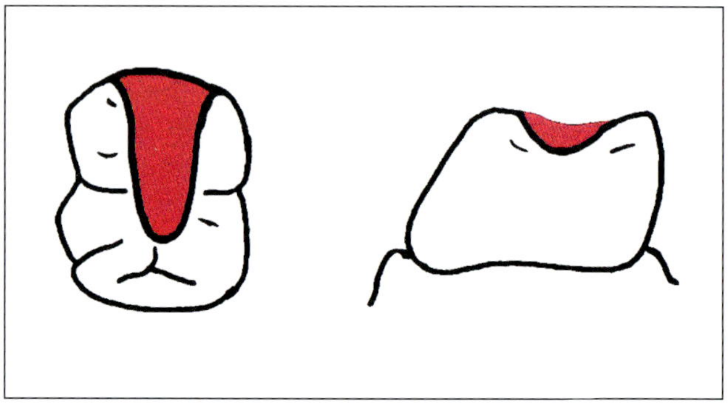

FIG 4-10 Ideal rest seat dimensions for the isolated mandibular molar.

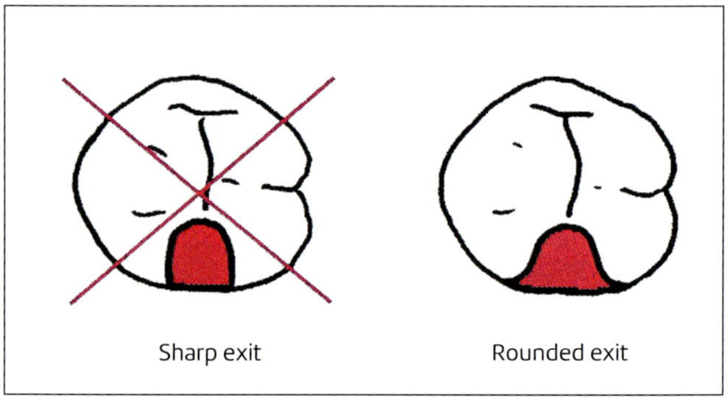

FIG 4-11 Proper rest seat contour at the marginal ridge.

occlusal surface, no matter the target dimensions, so that the rest can direct the occlusal forces down the long axis of the abutment (Fig 4-10).

The many minute clinical differences in tooth positions and relationships dictate variability in adherence to these references. However, failing to approach these dimensions in the name of conservative dentistry is almost always counterproductive. Undersized rest seats will be less likely to contact, less effective at distributing force, more difficult to fit, and more likely to break. Saving 0.5 mm of tooth structure in a cleansable occlusal area will not impact the biologic outcome. Likewise, the vast majority of RPD abutments will have previous restorations, and a rest modification often sacrifices nothing more than restorative material.

After the bulk of the occlusal rest seat has been prepared, attention must be paid to the junction of the guiding plane and the rest seat. The sharp line that results from the intersection of the two surface reductions must be rounded (Fig 4-11). To leave this sharp angle is to risk a casting that will not fully seat because the thin sharp edge is unlikely to stand up in the refractory or be milled precisely. If even a slight defect in this area is created during the formation of the refractory cast or in the waxing of the framework, a positive bleb will result. Clinical studies of the fit of partial denture castings indicate that the marginal ridge area is where the greatest amount of contact can be expected.[1]

When placing occlusal rest seats in amalgam restorations, there is always the possibility of weakening the alloy in the depth of the rest or along the vertical walls. If the amalgam appears to be compromised, it must be redone with greater extensions or composite. An alternative would be to consider a casting. If there is no opposing occlusal contact or if the contact is with a denture tooth, the rest preparation can be extended to go beyond the margins of the old alloy and the depth of the preparation reduced (Fig 4-12). The demands of the thickness of the rest remain, but this space can be developed at least in part at the expense of the opposing denture tooth.

Occlusal rest preparations in existing crowns are another area of concern because there is no way to evaluate the thickness of the occlusal metal or metal/porcelain. The patient must be informed that if a perforation occurs during mouth preparation, the crown must be remade. In rare instances, rest projections (see Fig 2-7) or overlays can eliminate the need to replace an existing crown. Often,

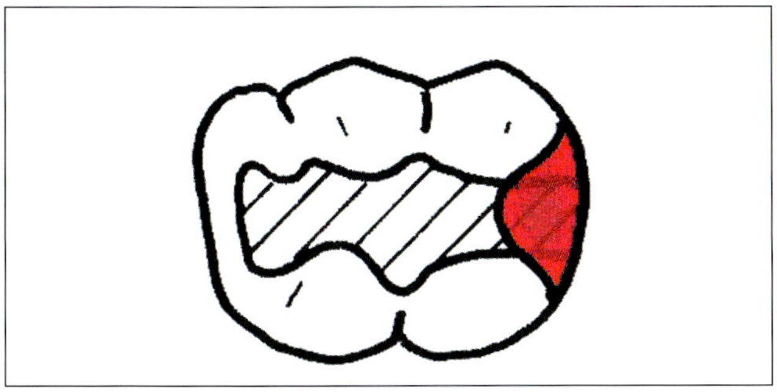

FIG 4-12 Rest preparation extended beyond alloy margin.

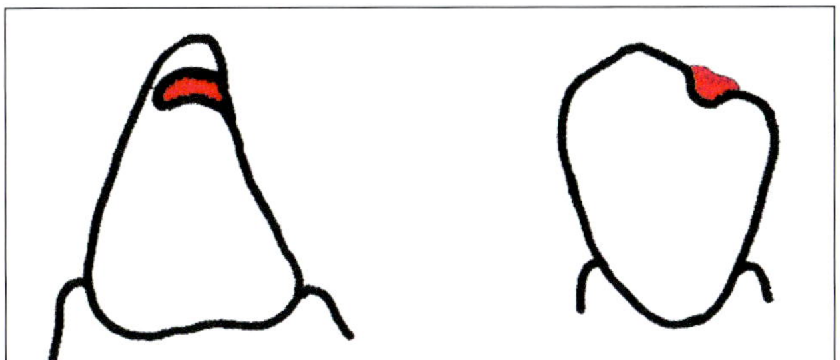

FIG 4-13 An incisal rest is used primarily on the distal aspect of mandibular canines.

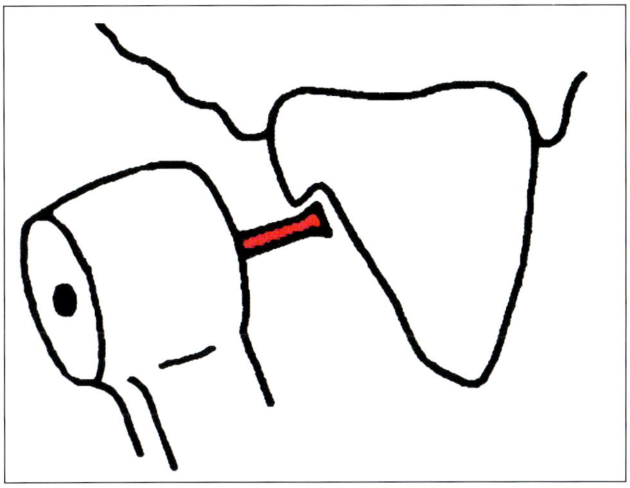

FIG 4-14 Proper angulation of an inverted cone diamond stone for a cingulum rest on a maxillary canine.

though, the treatment plan will have to include a new crown as a possibility.

Incisal rest seats are prepared in the same manner as for the occlusal rest, although they are now seldom used because of the public's increased concern about esthetics. The diamond of choice is the tapered cylinder rather than the round bur because the ideal incisal rest is one that is rounded both mesiodistally and buccolingually, without undercuts, to the path of insertion/removal. Here again, the junction of the seat with the guiding plane must be rounded (Fig 4-13). These rests are very effective and should be strongly considered when the anterior teeth do not show or if the patient is not overly concerned with a small show of metal.

Cingulum rests, mostly limited to maxillary canines, are prepared with a diamond inverted cone (Fig 4-14). The size of the cone is determined by the bulk of enamel in the cingulum. The greater the amount of enamel, the larger the rest seat can be. It is also possible to augment the rest seat with a bonded material to create a rest with a floor of 1.5 mm. The reason a diamond is chosen over a carbide inverted cone is that the diamond leaves a more rounded internal angle than does the carbide. The same problems can arise from having this sharp area as with the marginal ridge. The shape of the rest seat as seen from the lingual is one of an inverted "V" that follows the natural shape of the cingulum and requires the minimum reduction of tooth structure.

Cingulum rest seats on maxillary anterior teeth are often required, and if sufficient enamel exists below the contact of the mandibular incisors, they are prepared with the same inverted cone as the canine, the only difference being the shape of the rest. It is better for the rests to be straight or semilunar, as it follows the natural contour of the lingual gingival surface. These rests most often require augmentation.

Embrasure clasps and strut rests

Embrasure clasps require additional preparation beyond that of the rest seat. Depending on the contact area of the marginal ridges and the opposing occlusion, an access must be established for the clasp arm to both enter and exit the rest area. The exit to the buccal surface is usually the most critical. In either case, an absolute minimum of 1.5 mm of space, both vertically and horizontally, must

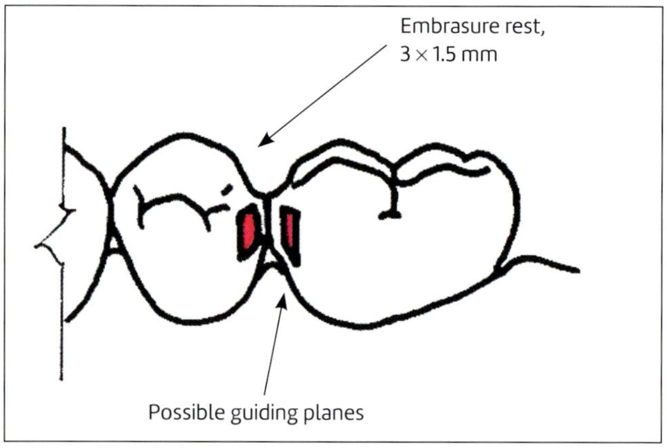

FIG 4-15 Lingual mouth preparation for embrasure clasps.

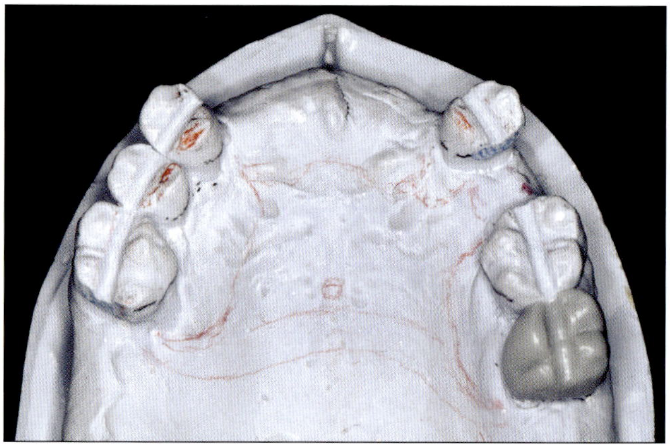

FIG 4-16 Diagnostic mouth preparation for strut rests. Note the continuous design.

be created. A tapered diamond cylinder is used to create the space, cutting at a dimension of 1.5 mm on the cylinder for automatic control of the dimension. With that as the minimum, remember that the maximum amount of space available should be utilized. This typically results in dimensions of 4 mm horizontally and 2 mm vertically. In situations with adequate interocclusal space, two adjacent occlusal rests can be created at the marginal ridges of the teeth through which the embrasure clasp is passing. This design serves to ensure adequate thickness and will help achieve positive contact with the abutments. The lingual approach to the marginal ridge offers the possibility of a minor guiding plane that should always be used, because the embrasure clasp assembly offers no other possibility of a guiding plane (Fig 4-15).

The rest seat area is to be shared between the two adjacent teeth to conserve tooth structure and still have adequate space for the rest. Under no circumstance should the contact actually be broken. If this occurs by mistake, a restoration will have to be placed on one of the teeth to restore contact. When a restricted space is left for the embrasure clasp, fracture of the retentive clasp arm can be expected. The dimensions of the plastic pattern used to wax the clasp have a cross-sectional measurement of approximately 1.5 mm. If any reduction is necessary on the occlusal portion of the clasp, an area of stress concentration will occur, and fracture can be expected after repeated flexure. Repair of a broken clasp arm in the embrasure area is difficult and will not be reliable.

A strut rest is a slot of metal running through a centrally prepared groove in a tooth. The strut typically comes off one guiding plane on the distal and connects to another on the mesial of a segment of teeth. It can also be on an individual lone-standing abutment. Strut rests can be very helpful when the need to splint mobile or periodontally involved teeth is a high priority (Fig 4-16). It is a very effective technique to achieve maximum support and positive rest contact because the strut runs from one side of the tooth to the other. This leaves no opportunity for the tooth or teeth with the strut to shift out of position. This type of rest will not rotate, meaning it should be avoided in Class I situations.

Preparing the strut is often made fairly straightforward due to the presence of restorations. Most commonly, the strut uses the buccolingual dimension of the existing restorations, leaving restorative material only below the strut rather than buccal or lingual to it. In this way, the restorations are left only in compression during function. This reduces the risk of restoration fracture beneath the strut. If a nonrestored tooth requires this design, a minimum recommended strut dimension would be 2 × 2 mm, with the occlusal portion of the preparation being wider than the apical portion. This taper, opposite to that of traditional amalgam preparation undercuts, is required to allow the strut to draw in and out with the path of insertion/removal. Rounding of all line angles is more critical than with other rest preparations in order to facilitate fabrication and fitting procedures. A more intricate and interwoven design created with the strut is difficult to accurately cast and adjust. Combine this with the fact that this design is often prescribed for mobile teeth that are a challenge to impress accurately, and achieving an ideal fit often requires alternative fabrication procedures like sectional construction.

The subtractive preparation of guiding planes on anterior teeth is not normally done because the reshaping of the proximal surfaces alters the shape of the tooth to the point where esthetics is compromised. Occasionally, a minor guiding plane can be created on lingual surfaces where gingival recession or crown lengthening leaves the full anatomical crown exposed.

When inadequate space is available for an anterior replacement, the adjacent teeth may be recontoured to equalize the pontic space with the adjacent teeth. When the space is so constricted that an esthetic result is not attainable, then orthodontics or a fixed partial denture replacement may be the only options.

At the completion of subtractive mouth preparation, the surfaces that have been recontoured must be finished and polished. Because these prepared surfaces should be the only areas where contact between the tooth and the frame takes place, there are significant advantages to having a surface that has been polished with either a fine diamond or fine white stone followed by rubber points and disks. The chances of alginate sticking and tearing are reduced. Because the refractory material for stellate alloys is large grained, the exact duplication of irregular surfaces is not possible. The smoother the surface to be duplicated, the easier it will be for the resultant casting to have an internal surface that is smooth and easier to fit.

Additive Mouth Preparation

Before any preparation is undertaken for additive contours, the subtractive component of the mouth preparation must be complete, including final polish. It should be obvious that it is much easier to create a crown casting that is in harmony with the contours already established on the teeth than to make the casting first and then try to create guiding planes on the teeth to match those on the casting.

Additive mouth preparation can be broken down into three different approaches to obtaining ideal contour: *(1)* indirect bonded contours, *(2)* direct composite bonded contours, and *(3)* more traditional surveyed crowns and pontics. The actual contours established using these modalities are the same; only the material or means of connecting them to the abutment teeth differ. Both indirect bonded contours and crowns require mouth preparation of enamel surfaces as a part of their construction. All bonded restorations require the presence of sound tooth structure, preferably enamel, to which to bond.

Bonded metal contours

Rest seat areas, guiding planes, and attachments all lend themselves to bonding to enamel. They offer a high level of predictability but are technique sensitive.[2,3] The more the attention to detail during the preparation of the enamel, the greater the long-term success.

The cingulum rest seat, to be placed on the lingual slope of a mandibular canine, is the most commonly used bonded contour. The mouth preparation for this restoration is limited to a horizontal notch cut in the enamel in the gingival third of the lingual slope.[4,5] This miniature cingulum rest serves as a vertical stop when seating the casting at cementation and as a positioning device to relate the restoration in its proper position. Because the enamel on the lingual of the mandibular canine is thin, this groove will not be more than 0.5 mm in depth to be certain to stay in enamel. Although not really necessary, one can reduce 0.2 mm of enamel overall and leave a finishing line so that the resultant casting, which will be approximately 0.4 mm, will have a smoother interface with the surrounding tooth structure.

When guiding planes are incorporated on the casting, microgroove preparations, as recommended by Marinello et al,[6] are placed in the enamel using the smallest-diameter slightly tapered carbide bur (Fig 4-17). These grooves offer lateral resistance to dislodgment and have been shown to greatly increase the successful bond between casting and tooth. Precision attachment castings will be discussed in chapter 11.

Final impressions for bonded castings are made in either silicone or polyether because they are poured in the refractory material that is compatible with the alloy to be used. These refractory materials do not, as a rule, set against alginate. The impression need not be full arch but must contain the other prepared abutments so that any guiding plane area on the casting can be made parallel with the existing guiding planes. If the base of the casting extends to the gingiva, a retraction cord should be placed to ensure accuracy in that area.

The borders of the casting are outlined, and a small piece of sheet wax, available from Kerr Dental at 0.5 mm thickness, is adapted to the outline and waxed to place by adding a small amount of very hot wax all around the border. The contours of the restoration are added to this wax base. For a cingulum rest, the base must have a width of 1.25 mm with a rounded internal angle. As usual, the rest must form an acute angle to the path of insertion/removal so that it will be positive. Decisions on the contour and extent of any guiding planes must be made relative to the classification of the edentulous situation and the established contours of the other abutment teeth. The wax-up receives a round wax sprue attached to the lingual surface of the cingulum. As a final addition for a metal rest, a plastic bristle from a toothbrush is attached near the incisal or occlusal margin to act as a holding device for the casting during finishing and cementation (Fig 4-18).

Because the pattern is waxed against a refractory cast, no attempt is made to remove the pattern. The refractory model is cut with a die saw so that only a minimum amount of stone is present. The sprue is attached to the base of a casting ring and the second stage of the investment poured. The material of choice for the bonded metal casting is some form of nickel-chrome alloy like Rexillium (Argen) to facilitate

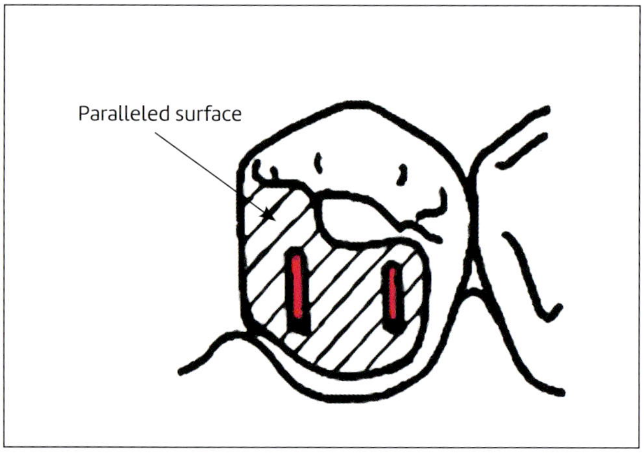

FIG 4-17 Microgroove preparation for bonded castings.

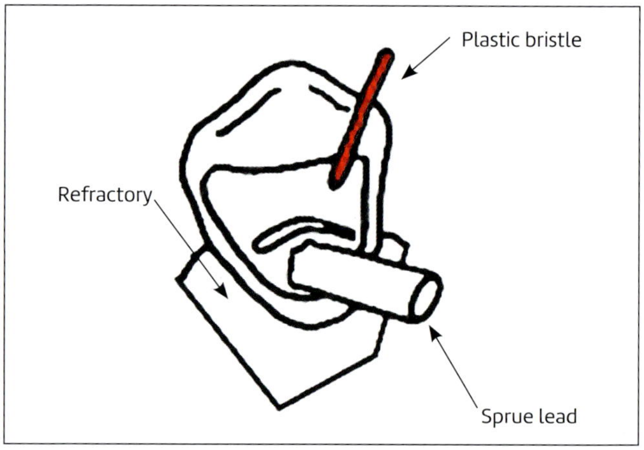

FIG 4-18 Wax pattern with sprue on sectioned refractory cast.

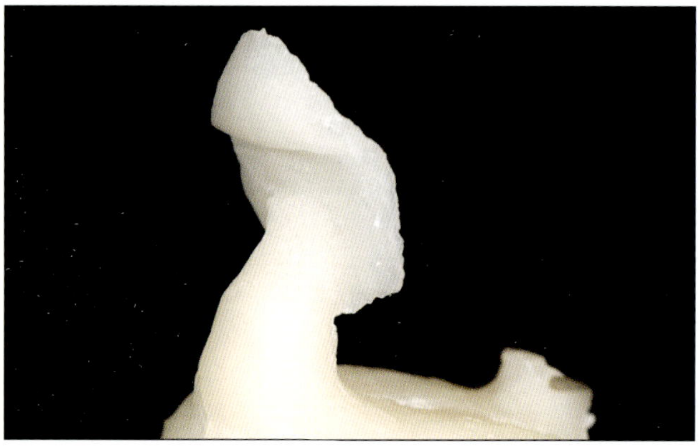

FIG 4-19 A pressed lithium disilicate cingulum rest that also modifies the distal guiding plane surface area. Note that the sprue remains on until bonded.

the etching process. The completed casting is finished and polished and, if it has a guiding plane, returned to a definitive cast for final milling using a milling machine. It is then prepared for either micro retention through an etching process (as for a Maryland bridge) or for macro retention using countersunk perforations (Rochette bridge). Electrochemical etching of the internal surface of metal is preferred. Care must be taken not to contaminate the etched surface once the etching is complete. The holding device, cast from the plastic bristle, is used to hold the casting during cementation with a chemically cured composite. Light-cured composites can be used with the perforated design. Once the resin is cured, under rubber dam, the holding device is cut from the casting and that area stoned and rubber wheeled to finish the restoration.

Bonded ceramic contours

Success with the pressed or milled ceramics for veneers and crowns has led us to consider using them for bonded contours to support the partial denture. The process of creating a pattern for a pressed ceramic contour is similar to that for a metal contour. Because of the extreme thinness desired in these units, it is difficult to control the wax pattern during shaping and investing if it is not supported. This requires either refractory cast investing or pattern resin cores to support the wax. Both of these techniques should include small sprues to handle the pattern after pressing. The sprue should be left in place during the finishing procedures and only be removed after the casting has been bonded. That area of the unit is then finished and polished (Fig 4-19).

One of the advantages with modern ceramics is the ability to create the pattern by milling. This is theoretically more efficient. Knowing that most ceramists will not be familiar with the specifications needed for RPD contours, communication with the computer designer will most likely be extensive. If the fabrication of these contours is not a regular event, it will be all the more difficult to train the technician to the point where you can confidently refer the fabrication process to them without intense detail. This means that those using digital impressions are likely better off designing the restorations themselves. Knowing the time spent is later recovered during the actual milling, this may still be a positive trade-off in terms of time.

All of these bonded options offer a relatively noninvasive approach to ideal mouth preparation with excellent reports

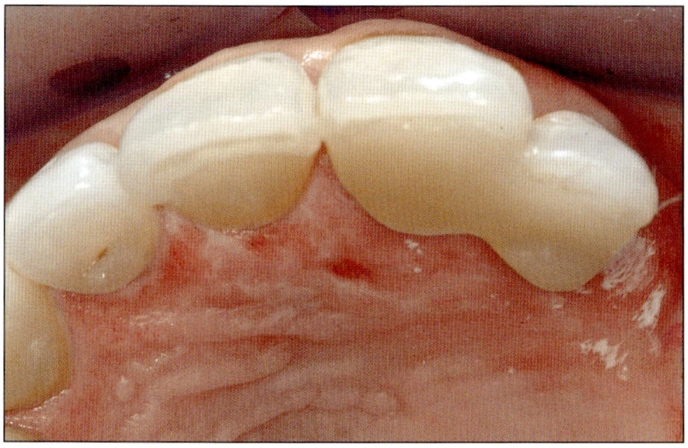

FIG 4-20 A lithium disilicate splint connecting weak incisors on the lingual. A positive cingulum rest and distal guiding plane were added to tooth no. 10.

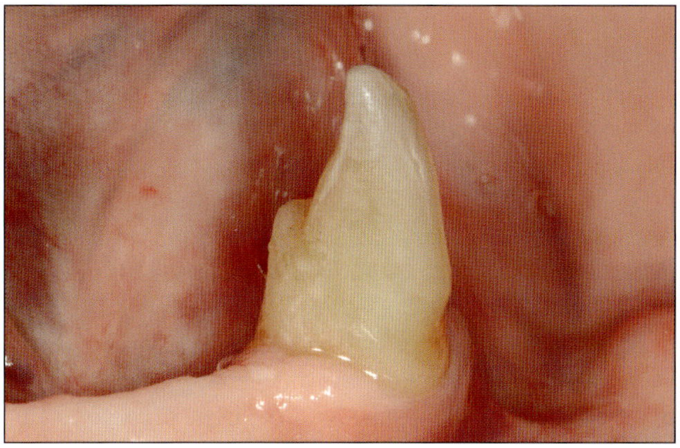

FIG 4-21 Directly placed and modified composite cingulum rest.

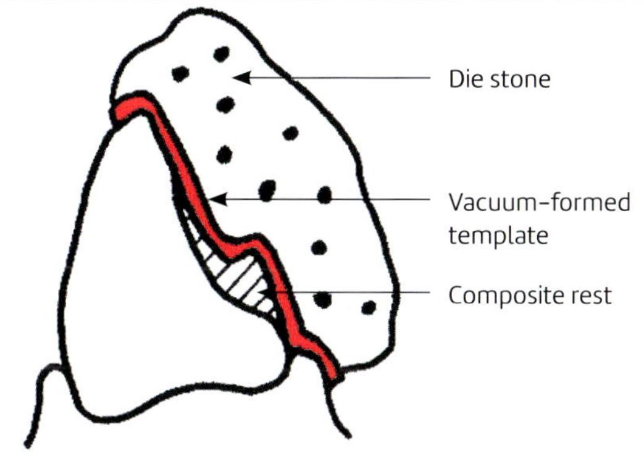

FIG 4-22 Traditional template method with stone positioner.

of longevity for low cost. As previously stated, they require ample enamel for quality bonding. However, the ceramic indirect bonded contours offer the additional benefits of maximized esthetics and reliable bonding protocols that fit into current everyday clinical practice (Fig 4-20). The ceramic, however, does not do well in tension and may fracture if used to splint mobile teeth. Likewise, it cannot be used like metal can for bonding on any sort of cantilevered extensions, such as an attachment.

Bonded composite resin contours

Rest seats and guiding plane contours can also be established in composite. While it may appear that a restoration formed in composite would be likely to fracture or debond when stressed repeatedly, several decades of clinical experience and laboratory research has shown this not to be the case.[7–9] The bond, in fact, is often the strongest element, as a rest may occasionally chip but not debond. Enamel bonding protocols must be followed exactly. When the abutment tooth has been properly etched, under rubber dam, and the composite placed according to the manufacturer's directions, this becomes a viable and less expensive alternative to the bonded metal or porcelain contours. For these reasons, the bonded composite cingulum rest seat has become the first choice for mandibular canines (Fig 4-21).

The rest and/or guiding plane can be created in a bulk of bonded composite, and then prepared as if it were enamel. For a single simple cingulum rest seat, shaping a bulk of previously bonded composite is the most practical way to create the desired form.

For more complicated additions, a precise design can be transferred from the diagnostic mouth preparation. As mentioned earlier, a template of the diagnostic wax-up can be used to mold the composite as it is being bonded to the tooth. Traditionally, a vacuum-formed clear plastic template was used (Fig 4-22). However, this requires a stone duplicate of the wax-up. With fairly rigid and transparent polyvinyl siloxane materials like Memosil 2 now available, a matrix can be made directly from the diagnostic mouth preparation or wax-up (see Fig 4-7). This eliminates the need for a duplicate cast and tends to be the most efficient.

After placement of the rubber dam, the tooth is etched and prepared according to the directions for the specific light-cured composite being used. The matrix is filled with composite to approximate the amount required to create the restoration. The matrix is forced to seat until contact with the unmodified surfaces of the teeth is achieved. This can be visualized through the transparent material prior to initiating the light-curing process. Large additions may require a vent in the direction of a noncritical area to allow excess material to flow out of the matrix. This excess is then trimmed away after curing. Small pieces of polytetrafluoroethylene tape can be used to prevent bonding to proximal surfaces of adjacent teeth while under the matrix.

After the composite is light cured, the matrix is simply peeled away. Additional curing time is recommended after the matrix is removed to be sure the light has reached all marginal areas and within the depth of the material. Only then is the excess composite removed and the borders finished and polished. Use of the matrix results in a superior finish since the bulk of the restoration will not need to be touched after curing.

The effectiveness of additive composite modifications has been such that it is used regularly for repairs and modifications to abutment teeth for existing RPDs. This includes replacement of fractured amalgam restorations and fractured cusps with undercuts. Complete reverse fabrication techniques, where the teeth are made to match a predesigned ideal framework by use of direct composite, is yet another application. These specific situations are discussed later in this text. They indicate the wide breadth of uses and benefits of composite.

Specific properties of the various composite types will have an effect on the wear and strength of the particular modification. Nanofilled, microfilled, and microhybrid all work well in specific situations with the details best reviewed in operative dentistry texts. When the composite modification is kept in compression and when there is little to no movement of the frame over the surface, the risks of material failure are very low. Unfortunately, all composites are somewhat brittle and do not hold up well with excessive abrasion or tension.

With that in mind, two primary contraindications are a mobile abutment tooth and an active clasp arm. When a tooth is mobile, a positively designed composite rest will tend to be held rigidly by the RPD while the tooth itself will pull away when in function. This puts the composite and bonding in tension, making it more likely to fail. If the mobility is controlled with strut rests or guiding planes, this may not be an issue, but a composite cingulum rest on a mobile maxillary canine in a Class III situation will often debond or fracture. This occurs as the frame remains rigid against all the other abutments while the canine is forced labially away from the frame–rest interface during function. In these situations, indirect metal or ceramic bonded restorations are more appropriate as the material is not as liable to fracture. Logically, components that move frequently over composite will tend to rapidly wear the relatively soft material. So, while composite used to create an undercut in a rigid Class III design holds up fairly well, the same composite undercut used in a Class I with appropriate stress relief will often wear away in a matter of months. This is due to the movement of the clasp arm as the distal extension bases rotate during function. In contrast, the wear from the retentive action of a clasp is limited to placement and removal in Class III RPDs.

Surveyed crowns

The third and final form of additive mouth preparation is with the surveyed crown. This descriptive term has long been applied to any crown or pontic specially contoured and placed in conjunction with and as an abutment for an RPD.[10] Unfortunately, the crown, as obtained from the dental laboratory, is very likely not to have the desired form, as far as the partial denture is concerned, even though it may be ideal as a single-tooth restoration. The technician(s) who construct the crown most likely will not have had partial denture experience and so will favor the contours of the natural crown. The modifications required by the ideal abutment may not be a part of that technician's training, and because the partial denture casting may well be constructed in a different laboratory, it will be the clinician's duty to control the contour of the crown. This typically requires review of the pattern or digital design so that it can be related to the path of insertion.

While listed here as an additive mouth preparation, a surveyed crown is decidedly subtractive as far as conserving natural tooth structure is concerned. The notion of crowning teeth for the sole purpose of achieving the desired contour should no longer exist. Teeth that are so far malpositioned as to require a crown for contour purposes should be managed with orthodontics or an alternative design. The additive and subtractive modifications just discussed are adequate in all instances where orthodontics is not required. This makes them the preferred method of contour modification when a crown is not indicated for restorative reasons.

The primary reason for the high frequency of surveyed crowns in practice is that most modern RPD patients come to us in a debilitated condition. A typical patient will have failing intracoronal and full-coverage dentistry. In this environment, new or replacement full-coverage restorations are typically indicated. Therefore, during the treatment planning phase, the clinician relies primarily on standard restorative decision-making algorithms such as whether marginal ridges remain and the size of intercuspal restorations. When a crown is indicated for structural reasons, the choice has been made. There are times when a crown may be indicated but not to such an extent that it is required. In these scenarios, the ability to create ideal contours or splint critical teeth together will often tip the balance toward the crown being the preferred treatment. While splinting can be accomplished with indirect bonded contours, it is more reliably accomplished with crowns. This is particularly true with mobile teeth.

Before beginning the mouth preparation phase of crown construction, the clinician must have gone through the diagnostic process of developing the ideal contour for the abutment tooth in question. The clinician must then prepare the tooth as if no crown were to be constructed; that is, to cut a guiding plane, prepare the rest seat, and make all other modifications of contour. Only then can the actual crown preparation begin. The initial subtractive mouth preparation will ensure that there has been adequate tooth reduction to allow the formation of the ideal contours in the final crown without compromising the restorative materials (Fig 4-23). If this additional preparation compromises the tooth, an error was made during the diagnostic mouth preparation phase.

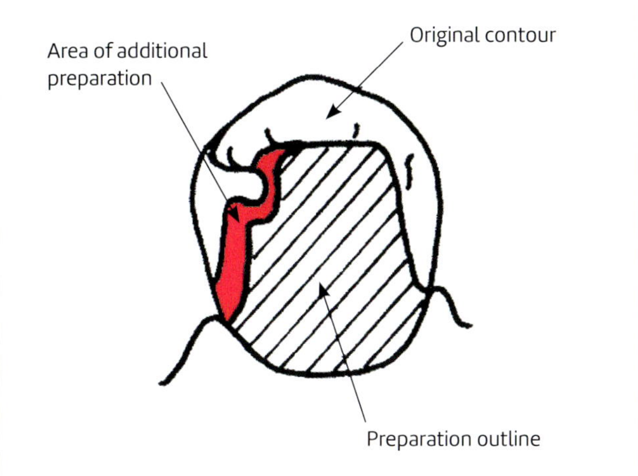

FIG 4-23 Subtractive mouth preparation before crown preparation.

As a general rule, for veneered crowns, a disappearing margin or a metal collar should be used rather than a porcelain butt-joint margin, since additional forces will be placed upon the crown by the partial denture. It is essential that all aspects of ideal soft tissue management be employed for the surveyed crown. Margin placement at or above the gingival margin, respect for the biologic width, and careful manipulation of the retraction cord must be a part of the treatment.

CROWN MATERIALS

Despite all-ceramic restorations, and in particular zirconia, becoming the crown material of choice in most general practices, the clinical survival of such materials when used for surveyed crowns has yet to be determined. Research on this issue is currently lacking, leaving only clinical experience to guide us.[11] The two primary driving forces for these all-ceramic materials are cost of fabrication and esthetics. When choosing materials for a posterior abutment, the esthetic argument is minimized. Remember that, in most designs, there will be metal occlusal rests, and elderly patients tend to not be overly concerned with dental appearance. Cost certainly is an issue, but what would the cost be to the clinician and patient if an all-ceramic molar abutment crown fractured 6 months after placement of a new RPD? These materials have not been tested or followed in the long term under RPD conditions. So, while the fracture rates appear to be very low, they are not zero. A full gold crown that costs an additional $100 or even $200 more measures as a valuable investment when compared with the cost of redoing an entire case.

Another factor to consider is that these all-ceramic crowns are typically created entirely digitally. Remember that crown and bridge technicians are notoriously uneducated with regard to RPDs. With that as a baseline expectation, imagine a young computer technician being asked to create a guiding plane surface parallel to the path of insertion. Not all software will make this clearly visible, even to the technicians who are aware of the specific goals. This forces the clinician to be hands-on if they wish to receive an appropriately contoured digitally fabricated all-ceramic crown. Metal lends itself to surveyor-based milling, so the clinician can easily take control of the final contouring. While zirconia can be handled similarly, it is not as user friendly to modify, and questions on crack propagation arise when extensive postprocessing adjustments are made. Time will tell if zirconia will replace metal-based surveyed crowns. For now, ceramics are not generally used for combined fixed-removable partial denture reconstructions.

FINAL IMPRESSION AND DEFINITIVE CAST REQUIREMENTS

The final impression for the crown will require more complete extensions than would the usual single-tooth impression. The entire denture-bearing surface area must be replicated on the definitive cast. This will ensure that the plane of occlusion can be established independent of the maxillary teeth in complete denture or RPD situations by using the junction of the middle and distal third of the retromolar pad as the posterior determinant of the plane of occlusion. The full cast will also allow the creation of a stable trial base for maxillomandibular relationship records, should that be required. Obviously, all the other abutment teeth must also be present on the definitive cast so that the additive mouth preparation can be in harmony with the previously completed subtractive preparation. The only restriction on the dimensions

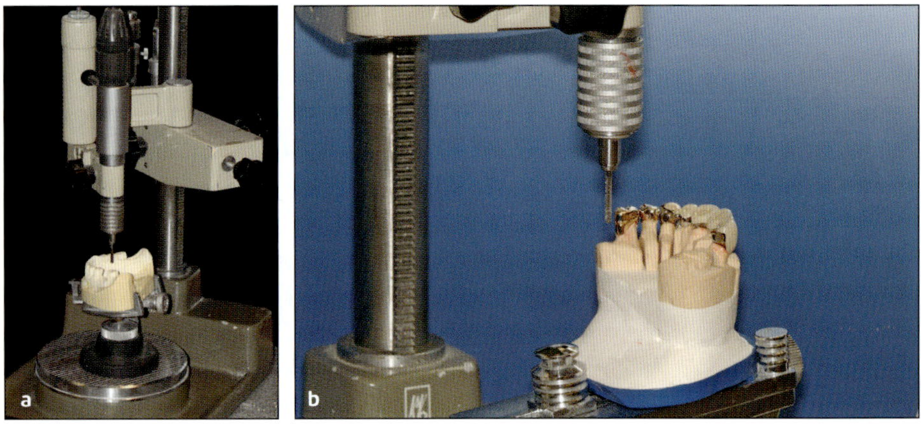

FIG 4-24 *(a)* A traditional milling machine has a movable arm that maintains the perpendicular position of a handpiece. *(b)* The milling machine acts as a functional surveyor. This image shows the machine completing the final contour of guiding planes on surveyed crowns prior to a pickup impression.

and contour of the definitive cast is that it must fit into the survey table. This demand often creates a problem when the distance of the base of the cast to the mounting ring is great. This makes the use of the dental surveyor and possibly the milling machine difficult if not impossible. Some modification of standard techniques is generally required, especially if the final impression is sent to the dental laboratory rather than being poured in the clinic.

There is a distinct advantage, however, to pouring the cast, trimming the die(s), and articulating this type of case in the dental office. It allows the repositioning of the definitive cast for final determination of the path of insertion/removal and the placing of the three tripod marks on the cast. To expect the dental laboratory to complete all these steps and not lose control of the case requires a high level of experience and excellent long-term communication between clinician and technician. Until such time that a specific dental technician has been suitably trained and has demonstrated compliance with the requirements of a specific clinician, the "surveyed" crown is to be waxed to full contour and returned to the clinician for the actual shaping of all areas of crown–partial denture contact. In this way, design of the critical tooth–frame interface remains under the control of the clinician.

Because the ideal contours of the surveyed crown have been established in the diagnostic waxing phase of treatment planning, it should be a simple matter to copy the contours. Due to the critical nature of the "surveyed" surfaces in the long-term success of the treatment, it is essential to review the modifications to the full contour wax-up usually required to create the ideal crown. The first step is to reposition the definitive cast in the dental surveyor and reestablish the tilt of the cast to the original path of insertion/removal. It is to this path that we must evaluate the contours of the crown as returned from the laboratory. Dusting the wax with zinc stearate or baby powder will allow the analyzing rod of the dental surveyor to create an easily seen height of contour.

Using the blade that is normally a part of the components available for the surveyor or a wax milling bur in a dental milling device (Fig 4-24), the wax guiding planes are established parallel to any previously prepared planes in the enamel of the noncrowned teeth. These milling burs come in various tapers and margin configurations (Fig 4-25). When in carbide form, they are available in both cutting and finishing forms. Guiding planes can be cut as flat planes with or without a gingival ledge. The advantage of using the lingual gingival ledge is that it functions as a rest and can eliminate the need for an occlusal rest preparation. This is of particular value when esthetic demands require full porcelain occlusals or when a deep vertical overlap of anterior teeth leaves limited interocclusal space. The guiding plane is not restricted to the proximal surface. In fact, the greater the extension of the guiding plane onto the lingual or buccal surface for reciprocation, the greater the frictional retention possibilities (Fig 4-26).

REST SEATS AND RELATIVE CONTOUR HEIGHT

Only after all guiding plane surfaces have been contoured can we proceed to the placement of rest seats and retentive contours. It is essential that the junction of the guiding plane and the rest be rounded and that sufficient wax has been removed to allow a minimum of 1.25 mm for any clasp/rest assembly. Rest preparations in crowns should be one-half the occlusal table, which will often make them larger than they would be if cut into enamel. The larger and smoother the rest preparation, the greater chance that the partial denture will be in solid contact with it. One of the problems we face with every crown that will have a conventional clasp arm or arms is the determination of just where the height of contour is to be located in the wax-up. It is most desirable that any circumferential clasp

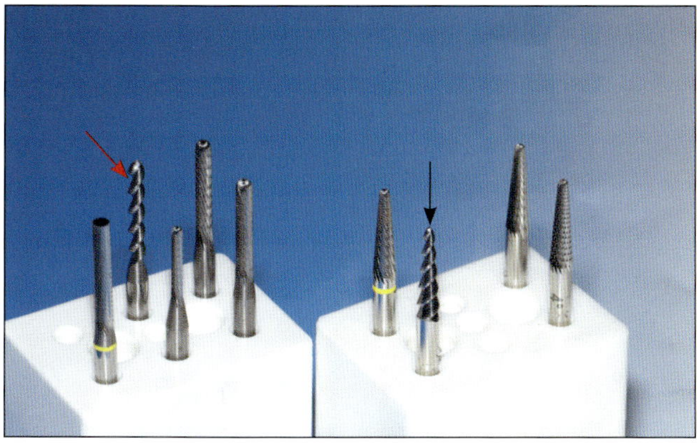

FIG 4-25 A selection of milling burs. The *red arrow* indicates a 0-degree wax miller, and the *black arrow* indicates a 4-degree wax miller.

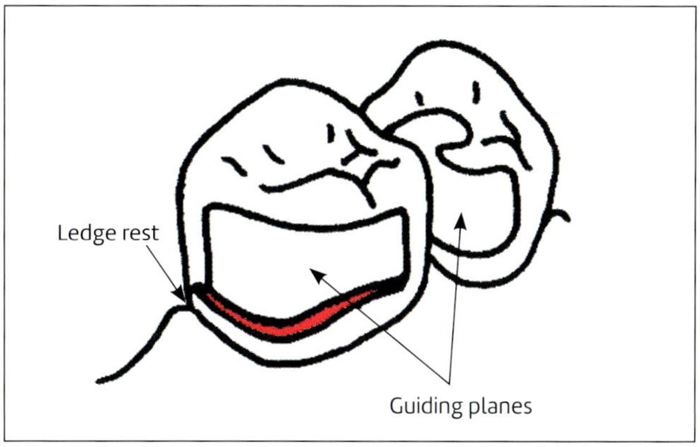

FIG 4-26 Guiding plane extensions.

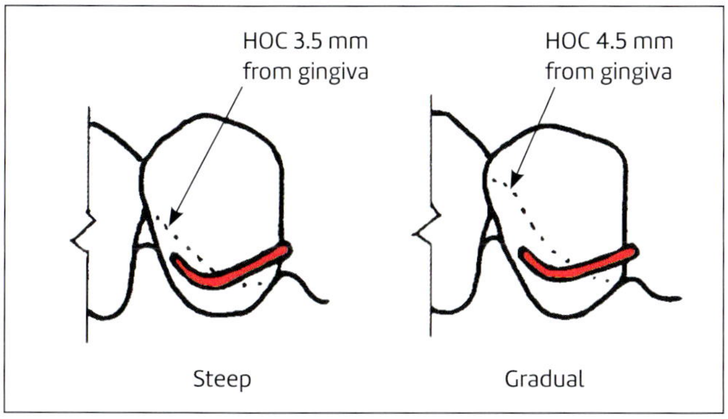

FIG 4-27 Options for retentive areas. HOC, height of contour.

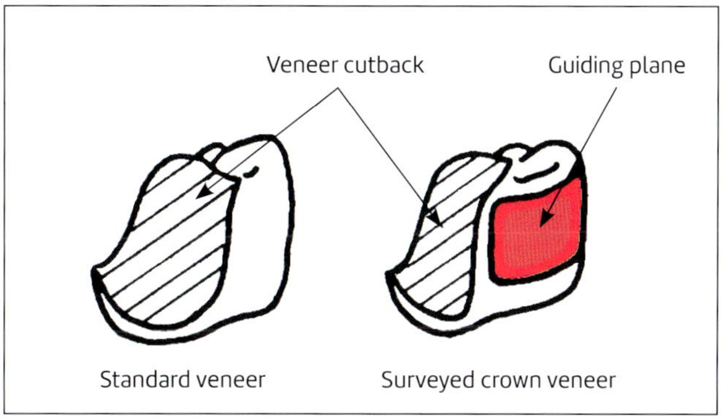

FIG 4-28 Options for cutback.

lie as low on the tooth as is possible, both for esthetics and to maximize the retentive nature of the clasp arm. Because the die stone that represents the gingival marginal tissues has been removed from the die, an untrimmed second pour of the definitive impression is needed so that either the clinician or the technician can know the relation of the margin of the crown to the gingiva. The inferior border of any circumferential clasp is placed a full millimeter above the marginal gingival tissue. The average cast clasp arm measures 1.5 mm occlusogingivally, so the height of contour must be at least 2.5 mm above the tissue.

Since we have the opportunity to make the crown contour truly ideal, a clinical—not laboratory—decision must be made as to the relation of the survey line to the final position of the clasp when the partial denture is fully seated. As mentioned earlier, the greater the distance of the height of contour from the final clasp position, the longer lasting the retentive effect of the clasp will be. The flexing of the clasp will be more gradual, both on insertion and removal, but the initial retention will be reduced. Therefore, for those situations where some level of stress relief is desired, the height of contour is raised to 4.0 to 4.5 mm from where the marginal tissue is known to be (Fig 4-27; see also Fig 4-4). In contrast, for all tooth-borne partial dentures, the height of contour should be close to the final position of the clasp, perhaps 3.0 to 3.5 mm from the marginal tissue, and therefore fairly abrupt. This position will give a retentive force that is shorter acting but of greater intensity.

In addition to the creation or verification of the height of contour, the clinician must also determine the margin of the cutback for porcelain application. It is essential that a margin of metal exist beyond any extension of the partial framework so that guide plates, rests, and minor connectors contact only the metal of the crown, not the porcelain. This margin need only be 0.5 mm. The resulting margin of the cutback will not be where it would be placed on a standard metal-ceramic restoration, so the technician needs to know exactly where to start the wax cutback. The clinician must outline the margin with an explorer so that there is no misunderstanding (Fig 4-28). Because the cutback will be a uniform reduction of the wax, allowing a uniform thickness of porcelain, it is essential that the wax crown has the exact contour desired in the final surveyed crown.

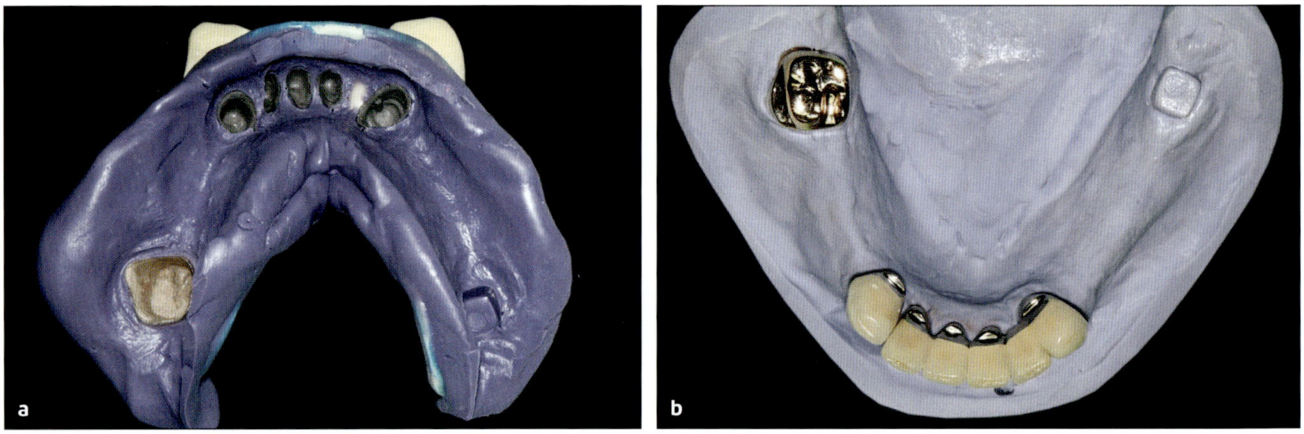

FIG 4-29 *(a)* A pickup impression prior to cast fabrication. A bridge for teeth nos. 22 to 26 and crowns for teeth nos. 27 and 31 are still within the polyether. *(b)* Resin dies support the crowns on a solid definitive cast. Final milling is now completed prior to partial fabrication.

Even if the original contour was ideal and the cutback properly done, the application of the porcelain veneering, which must be done to excess because of the shrinkage factor, offers another opportunity to alter the height of contour and potentially render the crown unusable. For that reason, it is advisable for the clinician to evaluate the crown after the porcelain is contoured at the bisque bake stage. Minor corrections of contour can easily be made by adding or subtracting additional porcelain before final stain and glaze. The porcelain must be very smooth from the height of contour down to the final position of the clasp. If it is not, a dark line often becomes visible as the porcelain wears the metal of the clasp through repeated insertions and removals. Obviously, once the clinician and technician really understand each other, the technician can simply create an exact copy of the diagnostic wax-up.

USING A PICKUP IMPRESSION

The clinician has two options relative to combining these crowns and the partial denture framework. The crowns can either be cemented permanently before the final impression for the framework, or they can be picked up in the final impression (Fig 4-29a). For the single surveyed crown, it is impractical to include the crown on the definitive cast, but for those situations where there are multiple surveyed crowns and bridges with precise milling of their guiding surfaces, it is essential that the crowns be present on the definitive cast (Fig 4-29b). The definitive impression in this situation will "pick up" the surveyed crowns or bridges.

For less obvious pickup situations, the clinician should consider the number and location of the crowns to be picked up as well as the Kennedy classification. In general, there is less indication to pick up in Class I situations, while the other classes are more likely to need it. Pickups are indicated in longer tooth-bound spans where guiding plane accuracy is more critical and more difficult to analyze in the mouth. Examples include bilateral mandibular second molar surveyed crowns on lone-standing abutments (Fig 4-30). Surveyed crowns not adjacent to edentulous spaces are generally safer bets to cement prior to final impressions because they tend to involve only auxiliary guiding plane surfaces.

Cases involving surveyed crowns typically have fairly complicated interim restorations. Cementing prior to final impression will therefore require sometimes complicated modification of the current interim partial denture. When a pickup impression is used, the surveyed crowns are cemented the same day the completed partial denture is placed (Fig 4-31). This eliminates the need for extraneous management of provisional restorations. From the standpoint of clinical efficiency, a pickup impression technique may actually save patient chair time.

When the pickup technique is chosen, the impression is made with a firm-setting elastomer like polyether (Impregum F, 3M). Resin dies must be constructed and are inserted into the crowns while they are still within the impression and before it is poured. The resin dies are thereby incorporated into the definitive cast. These dies are made by lubricating the inside of the crown, filling the

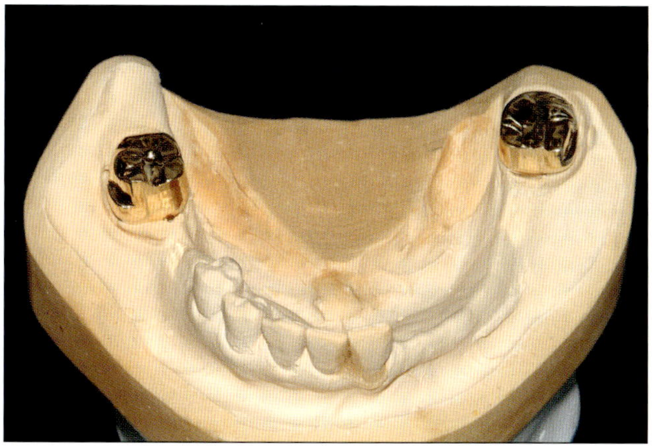

FIG 4-30 A pickup cast was made for this Class III Mod 1 situation because there were surveyed crowns on lone-standing second molars with a long edentulous span.

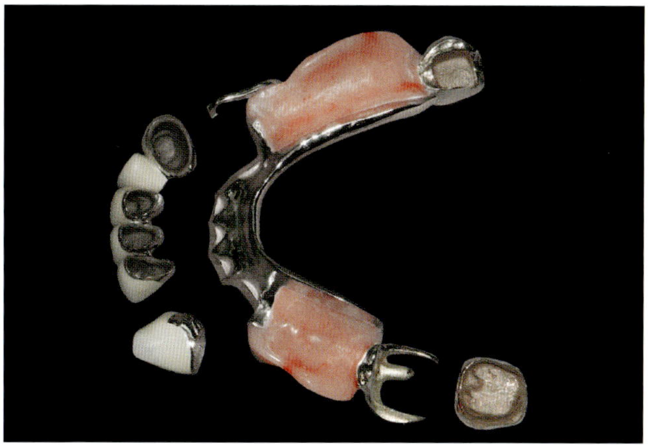

FIG 4-31 When the pickup method is used, the partial denture is completed and placed the same day that the surveyed units are cemented. Shown here is a completed combination case ready for placement.

crown with fast-setting resin, and adding a dowel pin prior to final set. Very retentive preparations may require confirmation of the ability to remove the die prior to pouring of the cast. Delicate margins should be protected by a thin layer of wax prior to pouring of the cast.

The resulting solid definitive cast will serve as the milling cast. This provides a stable and thereby accurate base on which the final milling of the guiding plane surfaces is completed. The accuracy of the refractory cast is increased because the actual crowns, not stone replicas, were available for duplication. The final fit of the partial framework to the milled surfaces should therefore be enhanced. In addition, having a stable, completed partial denture to orient the crowns during the cementation process facilitates a more ideal tooth–frame relationship. The cement thickness and physiologic tooth mobility of the crowned teeth therefore work as an advantage. These special impression procedures are essential to the use of fixed restorations with precision attachments and will be discussed further in chapter 11.

Mouth preparation, in the largest sense, when well-planned and well-executed, will simplify the actual construction of the advanced partial denture and ensure its long-term success. It is unfortunate that the great majority of RPDs are made with little or limited regard to this crucial component of care. Remember, it is essential to establish all aspects of the mouth preparation on the diagnostic cast before any attempt is made to go to the mouth.

References

1. Dunham D, Brudvik J, Morris J, Plummer K, Cameron S. A clinical investigation of the fit of removable partial dental clasp prosthesis clasp assemblies. J Prosthet Dent 2006;95:323–326.
2. Leupold RJ, Faraone KL. Etched castings as an adjunct to mouth preparation for removable partial dentures. J Prosthet Dent 1985;53:655–662.
3. Taylor TD, Gerrow JD, Brudvik JS. Resin-bonded components for maxillofacial prosthesis construction: A clinical trial. J Prosthet Dent 1988;59:334–339.
4. Seto BG, Caputo AA. Photoelastic analysis of stresses in resin-bonded cingulum rest seats. J Prosthet Dent 1986;56:460–465.
5. Seto BG, Caputo AA. Bond strength of etched-metal resin-bonded cingulum rest seats. J Prosthet Dent 1987;58:458–462.
6. Marinello CP, Scharer P, Meyenberg K. Resin-bonded etched castings with extracoronal attachments for removable partial dentures. J Prosthet Dent 1991;66:52–55.
7. Toth RW, Fiebiger GE, Mackert JR, Goldman BM. Shear strength of lingual rest seats prepared in bonded composite. J Prosthet Dent 1986;56:99–104.
8. Toth RW, Fiebiger GE, Mackert JR, King GE, Goldman BM. Load cycling of lingual rest seats prepared in bonded composite. J Prosthet Dent 1986;56:239–242.
9. Maeda Y, Kinoshita Y, Satho H, Yang TC. Influence of bonded composite resin cingulum rest seats on abutment tooth periodontal tissues: A longitudinal prospective study. Int J Prosthodont 2008;21:37–39.
10. Chandler HT, Brudvik JS, Fisher WT. Surveyed crowns. J Prosthet Dent 1973;30:775–780.
11. Manchester JA, Chung KH, Brudvik JS, Ramos V, Chen YW. Fracture resistance of cingulum rest seats in CAD-CAM tooth-colored crowns for removable partial denture abutments. J Prosthet Dent 2019;121:828–835.

5 RECORDING THE INTRAORAL CONDITION

No compromises.

With the preparation of the mouth completed, it is time to record the patient's intraoral condition so fabrication of the prosthesis can begin. It is at this point where minor errors in procedures will more quickly compound. Rudd and Rudd's list of 243 possible RPD fabrication errors begins on the definitive impression appointment, not because it is the first opportunity to make a mistake, but because this is when the chance and volume of possible errors increases significantly.[1]

Scanning and Digitization

There is little doubt that by the time the next edition of this book is completed, digital workflows for RPDs will be mainstream. Digital manufacturing of partial dentures has already been refined to the point of being used in commercial dental laboratories. Currently, the vast majority of RPD cases are still being made from a definitive cast that comes from an intraoral analog impression. The digitization of framework manufacturing still typically begins after scanning of a definitive cast rather than the mouth itself[2]; no change in chairside procedures is therefore required. Experienced clinicians, having controlled the case, know that it will be the technician spending time on fabrication after a definitive cast is created. This reduces the incentive for clinicians still using chairside analog methods to change. However, if the intraoral condition can be recorded digitally, the chairside procedures could potentially be more accurately controlled. In addition, patients with a severe gag reflex or limited opening may find the scanning process easier to handle.[3] Scanning is obviously the lead-in and final hurdle to a completely digital workflow. The latter half of this workflow, computer-aided manufacturing, is discussed in chapter 6.

Kattadiyil et al first reported the use of an intraoral scan instead of a final impression to fabricate an RPD framework.[4] Two significant hurdles for mainstream adoption of intraoral scanning for RPD cases are cost and accuracy. The financial investment required to change from analog to digital recordings remains significant. To begin at the entry level, a dentist will need a scanner (Fig 5-1a) and proper software to manage the digital data (Fig 5-1b). While the costs continue to drop, they can still approach $40,000. This does not include the monthly or yearly fees associated with some systems or the costs of building and maintaining the more complicated IT networks required. At this level of investment, the volume of cases treated will determine whether the expected efficiency benefits are worthwhile. Quality-over-volume practices may therefore not find adequate value for RPD-specific care.

Beyond the issue of cost, the accuracy of intraoral scanners is lacking when it comes to full-arch complex partially edentulous situations.[5] Several recent laboratory-based comparisons of a fully

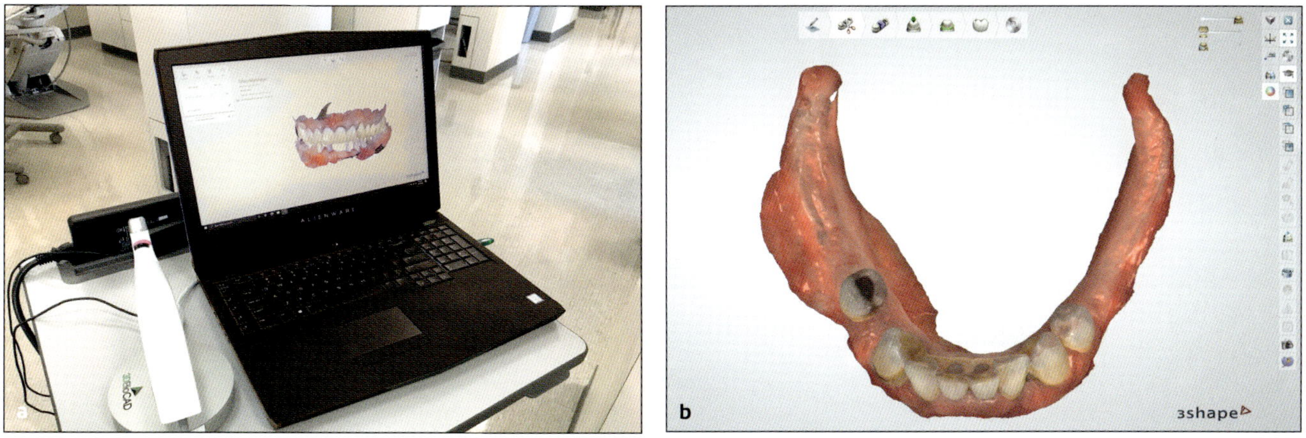

FIG 5-1 *(a)* A typical chairside scanner. *(b)* A digital impression eliminates the need for a physical cast.

digital approach found that conventional RPD framework fabrication was more accurate.[6,7] While there are reports in the literature that present a fully digital approach to RPD fabrication, this approach appears limited to simplistic and straightforward clinical scenarios. Even for straightforward frameworks, the inability of a scanner to accurately record a dynamic border, such as the lingual extension for a Class I situation, complicates a fully digital approach.[8] Clinicians using scanners, even for single crowns, typically have impression material available for those inevitable clinical scenarios that don't fall within the normal range. The technical details and clinical issues with this rapidly evolving area of dentistry are beyond the scope of this textbook. Considering the variability and complexity of the clinical challenges presented by advanced partial dentures, it is fair to say that an analog impression presents the most reliable method at this time.

Final Impressions

Final impressions for RPD frameworks are made with irreversible hydrocolloid in either modified stock trays or custom trays. Alginate, properly managed, is the impression material of choice for an RPD framework. It has the distinct advantage of tearing rather than distorting if it is forced to pull out of an undercut beyond its capacity.[9] In contrast, the silicone-type impression materials were designed for the impression of prepared teeth where minimal undercuts will be found. The RPD impression will often include unprepared teeth that may be severely tipped or rotated. These areas tend to have large undercuts that cause the stronger silicone or polyether material to pull away from the impression tray, creating a distorted area. Because the material does not appear outwardly damaged, the impression tends to be accepted until the casting does not fit the mouth. Because the contact surfaces between RPD and teeth are to be smooth, rounded, and well-polished, there is no need to reproduce minute detail with the fixed prosthodontic impression materials. When handled as described in chapter 1, an inaccurate alginate impression will be visible to the clinician, while with the other materials, it may not. A tear, rip, crease, or other form of visibly altered surface in the alginate signals a change in accuracy. In order to utilize this advantage, the clinician must carefully evaluate the final impression under good light. As discussed with preliminary impressions, the final impression should be relatively easy since the majority of potential problems were identified and managed during initial therapy.

Using the diagnostic cast, the adaptation of the stock tray can be evaluated. A minimum of 0.25 inch (6 mm) of clearance between the tray and teeth is mandatory (Fig 5-2a). In some instances, this 0.25 inch cannot be found with a stock tray. A custom tray is then made with adequate planned relief to ensure that the 0.25-inch space will exist (Fig 5-2b). Custom trays for alginate must have multiple retentive holes placed in them using a no. 8 or 10 round bur. These retentive holes combined with alginate adhesive will ensure retention of the impression material. Handling of the alginate is obviously more important when making the final impression than the preliminary. Proper measurements, mixing, placement, and control during setting were all highlighted in chapter 1. If the preliminary impression is taken seriously, however, there will be no difference in the techniques employed to obtain an accurate definitive cast.

A common source of frustration with RPD impressions can be the deep interproximal spacing seen with

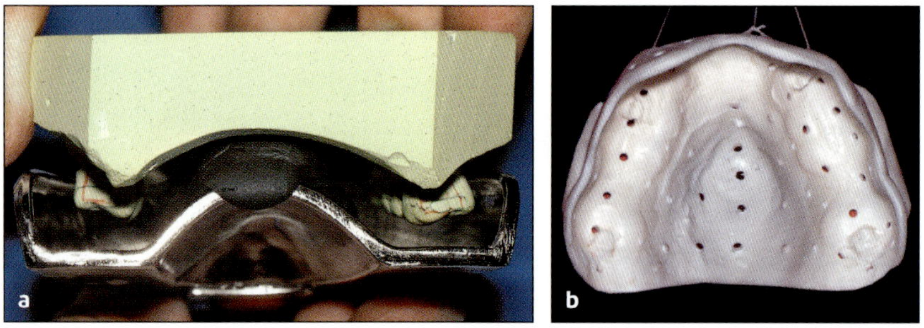

FIG 5-2 *(a)* Compound is used to modify the tray and guarantee a 0.25-inch space around teeth. *(b)* Custom tray with holes and 0.25 inch of wax relief.

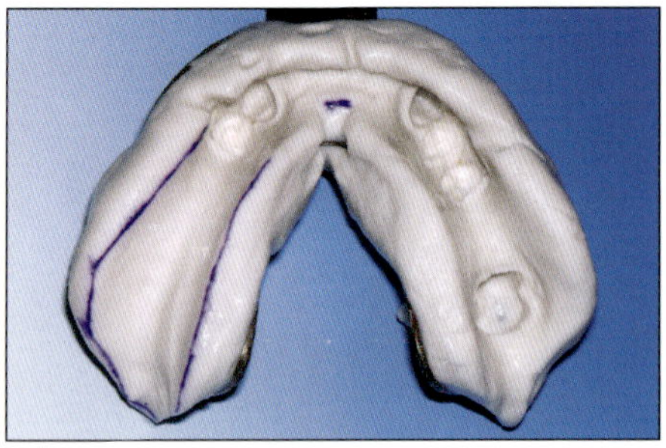

FIG 5-3 The extension of the critical border anatomy is marked.

periodontally involved teeth. Locking of impression material around these teeth will complicate removal of the impression. These areas are the most at risk of pulling and/or tearing. Because it is frequently impossible to remove these impressions without a tear, these areas must be blocked out. One way to accomplish this is to inject a small amount of alginate into the space with a syringe. After molding the injected area with a wet finger to ensure that it does not overextend onto any areas of tooth-frame contact, it is allowed to set. Because fresh alginate does not generally stick to set alginate, these areas are effectively blocked out. Dedicated blockout materials such as OraSeal putty (Ultradent) are generally avoided unless the undercut is far from any framework component because they may alter the set and texture of die stone.

Mobile teeth present a particularly challenging situation. Even with proper control of periodontal disease and occlusion, abutment teeth may remain mobile. It has been shown that these teeth displace as pressure from the impression material is inevitably applied.[10,11] This unseen displacement is a frustrating source of definitive cast inaccuracy. A two-stage impression is one option for this situation, but the seam between sections often proves an alternative source of error. Where possible, mobile teeth are best temporarily splinted with composite. The composite can usually be placed away from areas of framework contact, thus not interfering with the modified contours. This would be the facial surface, at the coronal half of anterior teeth. For posterior teeth, the temporary splint is placed high enough and far enough proximally to avoid any planned clasp or occlusal contact. If an I-bar is being used, there will certainly be adequate available surface to stabilize the abutment. To ensure effective stabilization of the tooth, spot-etching and bonding can be used. The temporary splinting is typically removed immediately following a successful final impression. In some situations, where it does not interfere significantly with hygiene or esthetics, it can be left in place until the framework fit is confirmed. This is one situation where a digital impression process may prove more accurate, as the tooth or teeth in question are in a static position during the recording.

Before pouring the final impression, an outline of the critical soft tissue contours is marked on the impression with an indelible pencil or color transfer applicator (Great Plains Dental Products) while the patient is still in the chair (Fig 5-3). The placement of this line forces the clinician to evaluate the accuracy of all extensions to be certain that all critical areas will be transferred to the definitive cast. Areas of possible overextension are measured in the mouth with a periodontal probe and transferred to the alginate. This is of particular importance for determining the extent of major connectors.

Definitive Casts

The final impression is poured using a double-pour technique. This approach offers the best chance of creating a definitive cast without distortion of the alginate. Because only a small amount of stone is added in the first pour, a minimum load is placed on the alginate as compared to boxing and pouring the entire cast at one time. The first pour must extend to cover the line placed on the alginate (Fig 5-4a). Once the stone has reached initial set, the addition of the base presents no opportunity for distortion (Fig 5-4b). The only potential problem arises when inadequate retentive blobs of stone are placed on the first pour (Fig 5-4c). Without this retention, there is a possibility that the definitive cast will separate in the flask during boil-out and flask opening. If a vacuum mixing device is available to the operatory, the clinician can pour the first pour right at the chair and thereby ensure that the impression has been correctly managed. The base can be added any time thereafter. A Type IV die stone is indicated for the definitive cast, not for any increase in accuracy but for greater resistance to abrasion.

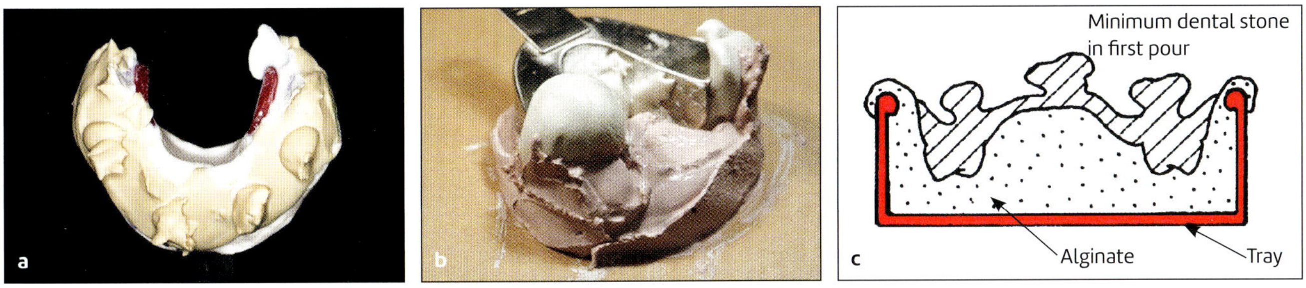

FIG 5-4 *(a)* The first pour is covering the line indicating critical border anatomy. *(b)* Addition of a base occurs after setting of the first pour. *(c)* Cross section of ideal alginate with a minimum of 0.25 inch of impression material. The first pour has retentive blobs.

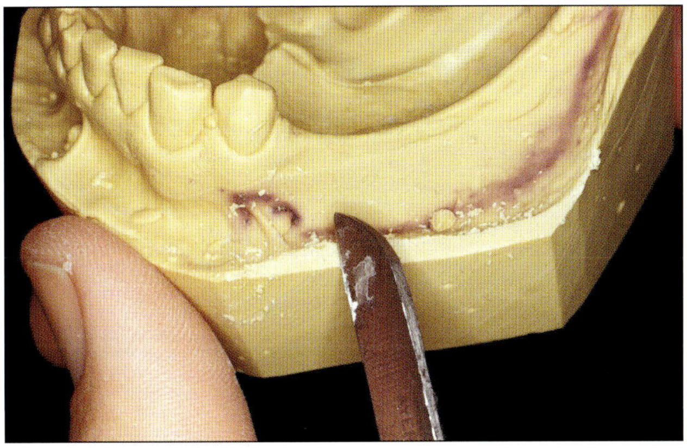

FIG 5-5 Land area being carved according to indicated border anatomy.

Separating the final impression from the now set stone cast can be a risky endeavor. Tall, thin teeth or those with significant undercuts may break. While these pieces can occasionally be super-glued back to place on diagnostic casts, any breakage in an area of tooth-frame contact eliminates any chance that a cast will have acceptable accuracy for framework fabrication. This highlights an additional benefit of using alginate. As long as alginate is not allowed to dry and harden, it generally retains enough flexibility to be safely removed. This is not the case for silicone or polyether materials. Even with the flexibility of alginate, very tall or flared teeth are easily broken off during removal of the tray. In these situations, it is best to cut and section the impression tray in order to separate and remove it from the underlying impression material. The unconstrained impression material can then be safely peeled away, thereby minimizing the risk of tooth breakage.

Once the cast is recovered, it should be trimmed as soon as possible so that any blebs can be removed easily. When the cast is shaped with the model trimmer, thin slurry inevitably covers the cast and, if it is not removed, will affect the accuracy of the cast. The slurry will adhere less if the cast is rinsed prior to trimming. Slurry that does stick can be removed with a soft brush and running water if done immediately. Dies or other critical areas can be protected from the slurry by covering them with a latex or silicone material before trimming the cast. The cast should be trimmed to the smallest possible dimension without compromising the critical anatomy as indicated by the marking (Fig 5-5). The smaller cast will allow a greater bulk of duplicating agar in the flask. Undercut areas, blebs, or other rough areas on the tongue side of the mandibular cast should be removed to reduce the possibility of tearing the agar. The distal extension edentulous areas that will require an altered cast tray were outlined as described so that the technician knows exactly where the borders of the tray will end.

A final task that is unique to the maxillary definitive cast is beading the outline of the major connector. To reduce the tendency for food to impact beneath the major connector, a

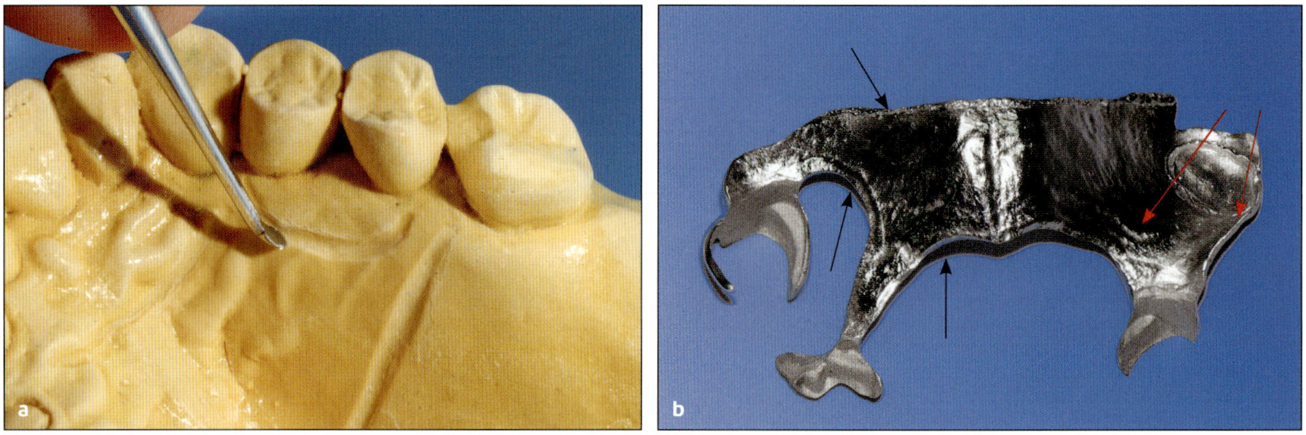

FIG 5-6 *(a)* Placement of a rounded 1-mm-deep bead according to connector design. *(b)* The positive bead line on the border of the major connector after casting. The *black arrows* indicate beading along the periphery. The *red arrows* indicate no beading.

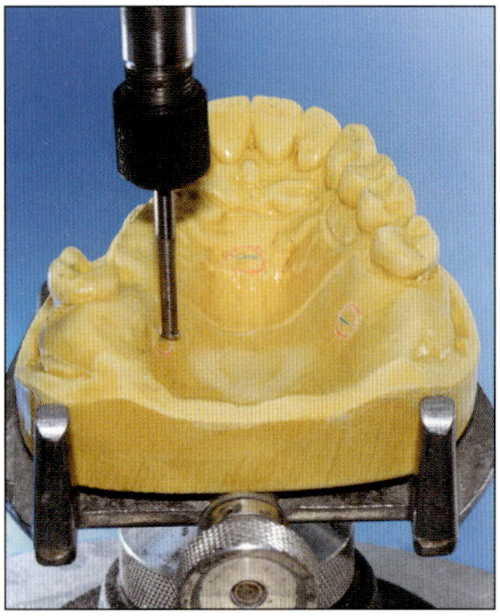

FIG 5-7 Definitive cast tripoded prior to final survey.

bead line is scraped into the cast following the outline (Fig 5-6a). In general, a width of 1.5 mm and a depth of 1 mm will suffice to ensure a positive contact with the underlying soft tissue (Fig 5-6b). The beading extends to within 4 to 6 mm of the marginal gingival tissues and phases out completely from there. The bead line is to be rounded rather than sharp and is usually created with a discoid carver or a rounded curette. The decision as to where to place the borders of the major connector should have been made during the diagnostic phase, and in the case of more complex reconstructions, it has already been tested with an interim restoration.

The definitive cast must be resurveyed and, depending on the arrangement with the laboratory, the design of the framework neatly drawn. If the clinician is unable to make a very precise drawing of the desired framework, then it is better to leave the definitive cast unmarked except for the tripod marks (Fig 5-7). The diagnostic cast is instead sent as the reference for the technician along with the work authorization form.

Maxillomandibular Relationship Records

For the most part, maxillomandibular relationship records are made on the framework after it has been fitted to the mouth. There will be occasions when the definitive cast must be articulated before construction of the framework can begin. These situations always involve occlusion, especially when the space available for denture teeth is limited or when components of the framework must be in contact with opposing teeth. When anterior teeth are being replaced with the partial denture and a steep vertical overlap exists without any significant horizontal component, articulated definitive casts are essential.

Whenever possible, the definitive cast should be related to the opposing cast by hand in maximal intercuspal position (MIP) without the imposition of any recording material. This of course assumes that any necessary occlusal equilibration has been completed. Any interocclusal recording medium would therefore only interfere with the accuracy of the cast relationship. The clinician is the ideal person to articulate the casts to ensure accuracy. If the definitive cast is sent to the laboratory without being articulated, then witness lines are placed between teeth of the definitive cast and the opposing cast while the casts are held in the desired occlusion. At least two marks per side are required to allow the technician to place the casts in the exact same position. As is standard, the casts must be rigidly stabilized during the process of articulation to prevent shifting or movement during the placement and setting of the mounting stone.[12] Any articulated cast must

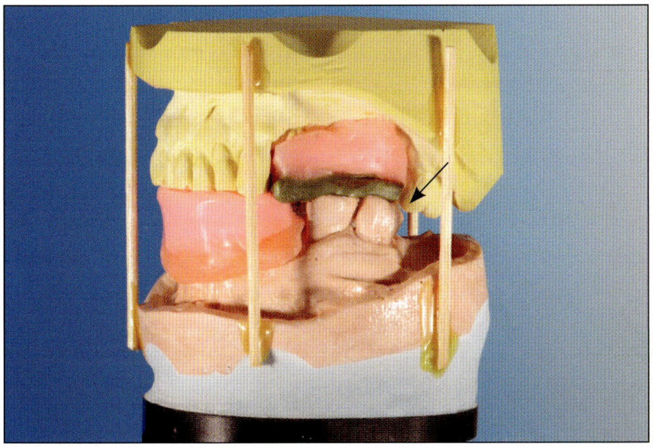

FIG 5-8 Casts with trial bases stabilized for articulation.[12] The *arrow* confirms that the record is made in centric relation, ie, prior to any tooth contact.

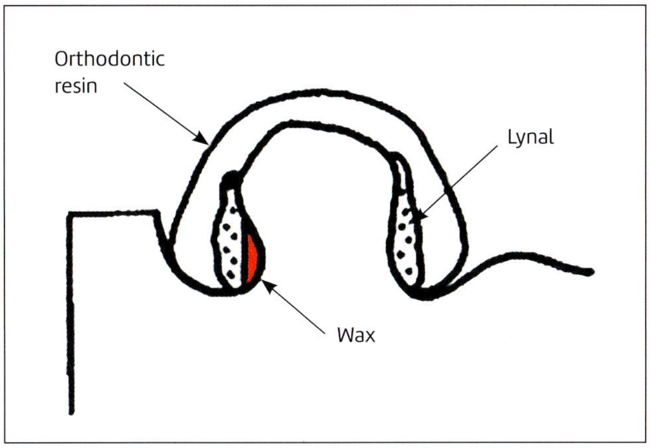

FIG 5-9 Blockout with wax and Lynal for sprinkle-on base (cross section).

have notches and separator placed on the base to allow it to be repositioned on the mounting, as it will have to be removed for blockout and duplication.

When insufficient teeth remain for positive positioning of the casts, a record base is constructed to support a record (Fig 5-8).[12] The construction of a record base for a partial denture definitive cast is not without some risk of damaging the stone abutment teeth. A combination of wax blockout, plasticized polyethyl methacrylate, and autopolymerizing resin, used with the following technique, will permit the construction of an accurately fitting base without injury to the definitive cast.

First, the definitive cast is surveyed, and soft tissue undercuts, if they exist, are identified and circled with a pencil line. The outline of the desired record base is also drawn. It is not essential that the base contact the remaining teeth, but some points of tooth contact are valuable: at least three, widely spread when possible. To reduce the risk of damaging a critical area, it is best to choose nonabutment teeth. A very small amount of baseplate wax is flowed into the gingival crevice of the teeth to be contacted. Any undercuts in the denture base area greater than 3 mm are partially blocked out with wax. The cast is then rehydrated by placing the base of the cast in water and allowing the moisture to penetrate the entire cast. The cast must not be submerged in water, as the accuracy of the tooth portions can be altered by dissolution of the stone. Once the cast is hydrated, tinfoil substitute, diluted two to one, is painted on the areas the trial base will cover. Lynal (Dentsply Sirona) or similar plasticized resin is added to any undercut areas and around the necks of the teeth that will be contacted by the record base. The Lynal is mixed thicker than is recommended by the manufacturer, to the consistency of peanut butter, so that it will stay where placed. Autopolymerizing acrylic resin is immediately added in a "sprinkle-on technique" to complete the record base (Fig 5-9). The autopolymerizing resin will bond to the Lynal, and the resulting record base will be retained by the plasticized resin, engaging the undercuts. There is no need to place the cast in the pressure pot for curing.

The base can be removed and trimmed as soon as the resin has hardened. A wax occlusal rim can be added with the intent of having a supporting table of wax 2 to 3 mm out of occlusion. The recording material is mixed and placed upon the table for the maxillomandibular relationship record. This record will provide accurate and stable support for those cases with limited opposing tooth contacts. For more complicated records involving bilateral distal extensions or edentulous opposing arches, see chapter 8. These records typically interface solidly enough that they can be reliably submitted to a trained and attentive laboratory for articulation. Once articulated, the laboratory technician can make an interocclusal record of the casts on the articulator to enable the cross mounting of the refractory cast to the opposing cast. This allows for the waxing of the occluding portions of the framework.

Altered Cast Impressions

Made only after the casting is finished, the altered cast impression has traditionally been presented as an attempt to combine the support of the abutment teeth with the support that can be obtained from the edentulous ridge. However, its true value exists in the fact that it is an effective means of recording anatomically accurate extensions and support after the difficult process of framework fitting has been achieved. If an altered cast impression is going to be made, the clinician need not be overly concerned with

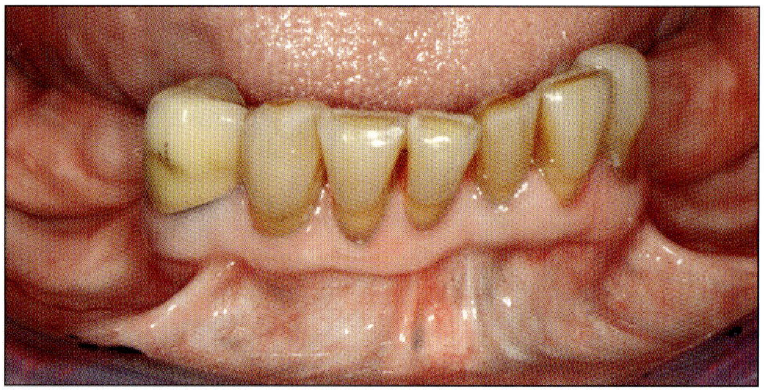

FIG 5-10 Note the excess lingual tissue below the tongue but above the severely resorbed residual ridges. Accurately impressing the teeth and tissue in a single impression is unlikely.

the accuracy of the edentulous areas and can concentrate instead on making the best possible final impression of the hard tissues. Originally, altered cast impressions were made on any edentulous area that had no posterior abutment, either maxillary or mandibular. Because the maxillary RPD is so well-supported by the easy-to-record and firm residual ridge and palate, little additional support is gained with an altered cast impression, especially if the final impression was made in a custom tray. In contrast, the difficulty of capturing the ideal denture space of the mandibular distal extension in the final impression has made the altered cast impression essential for many mandibular Class I and II situations (Fig 5-10).

The altered cast impression was proposed by a few prominent clinicians and is supported with several benchtop research studies.[13–16] While it is essential that the clinician master the technique of the altered cast, clinical studies have shown no difference in the health of the supporting tissues, hard or soft, after 1 year of use between an RPD with an altered cast and one made on the original one-piece definitive cast. Of course, the one-piece definitive casts in this study were all fully extended and had the ideal borders transferred by marking the impressions with an indelible marker.[17] There will be many clinical situations where this ideal final impression cannot be made. In these instances, it is essential that the impression of the abutments take priority over that of the edentulous ridges, which can be captured at a later date as described.

Tray construction

The altered cast tray is constructed on the definitive cast after the casting has been completed. The technician can return the framework with an altered cast tray in place, with its borders 2 to 3 mm short of the desired final extension of the denture base in the edentulous area. Guidance for the technician is required since they will be unaware whether the vestibule is overextended due to thick alginate or underextended due to a prominent and strong tongue. The desired altered cast tray must therefore be drawn as a part of the design. One thickness of baseplate wax, the same as for the relief for the retentive mesh, is adapted to the definitive cast to the outline of the desired altered cast tray extension (Fig 5-11a). The retentive mesh area is heated over a Bunsen burner and the framework seated onto the cast. The hot metal of the mesh must melt the relief wax and allow the casting to fully seat (Fig 5-11b). With the tip of a spatula, the wax that extruded up through some of the mesh holes is removed to allow the resin of the tray to lock onto the framework. The tray resin is mixed and a small amount removed from the mixing jar and immediately placed into the retentive holes that have been cleared of wax (Fig 5-11c). The fluidity of this resin would not allow it to be used as yet to form the tray, but it will flow into the retentive areas easily and provide the required retention. The remainder of the tray resin is added when it is no longer tacky and the tray is formed (Fig 5-11d).

The tray must be kept to the dimensions of the ideal denture base. In order to form the ideal denture border, the tray must be uniformly short and be slightly undercontoured to make space for the impression material to capture the border without becoming bulky. When the occlusal portion of the tray is kept thin, it will occasionally be possible to make the final maxillomandibular relationship record at the same appointment as the altered cast impression. If, at that time, the patient is unable to close into their previous unobstructed MIP because of the thickness of the tray or the general lack of interocclusal space, then the record must be made at a separate appointment.

The altered cast impression is made only after the framework has been fitted to the mouth and the full seating of the casting verified. (The actual fitting of the frame is discussed in chapter 7.) With the framework seated firmly on the abutment teeth, the extensions of the altered cast tray are evaluated. They are to be 2 to 3 mm short of the reflection of the border tissues. When the tray is properly extended, there is no need for border molding as a separate step. The wash impression will give ideal borders if the tray is in the proper position relative to the tissues.

Impression materials and taking the impression

The choice of impression material to be used for this impression does not appear to be critical. Early studies indicated that mouth-temperature wax impressions placed the denture base tissues in their most supportive state. This material is seldom used since it requires a good deal of experience to read the quality of the impression. Polyether impression materials offer the option of varying the

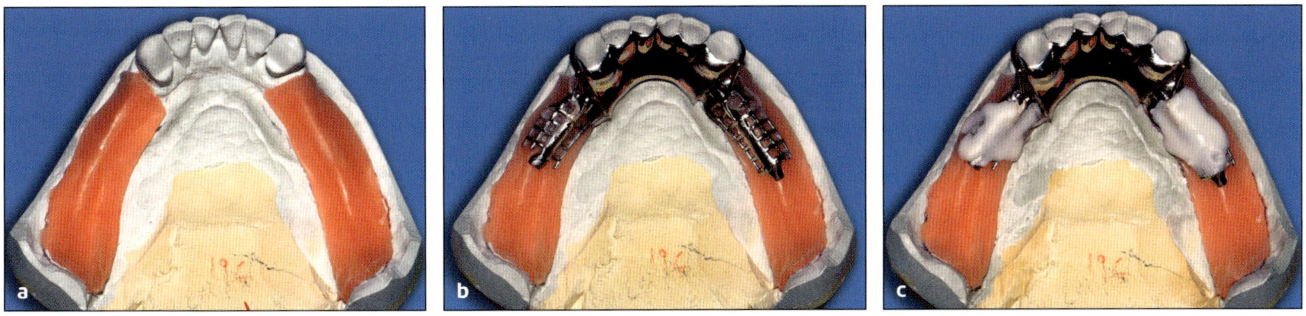

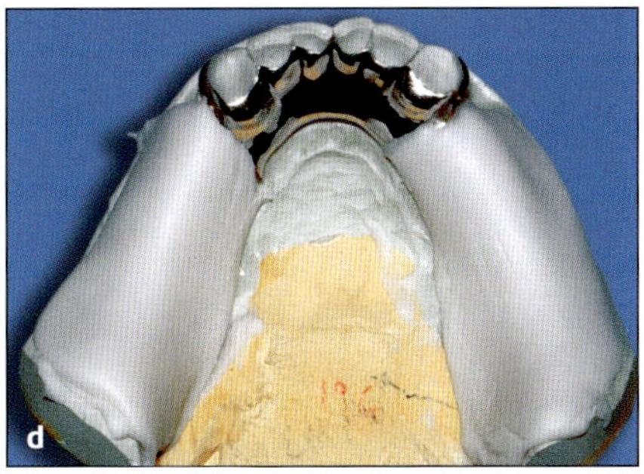

FIG 5-11 *(a)* One layer of baseplate wax is applied up to the anatomical markings. *(b)* The heated meshwork is seated completely; some wax is removed from the mesh. *(c)* Autopolymerizing resin is applied to partially engage the meshwork. *(d)* The set resin will be trimmed back to the anatomical markings.

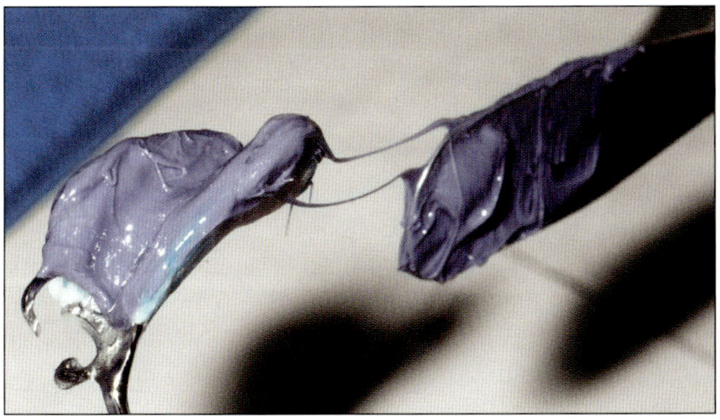

FIG 5-12 An altered cast tray loaded with fairly viscous polyether.

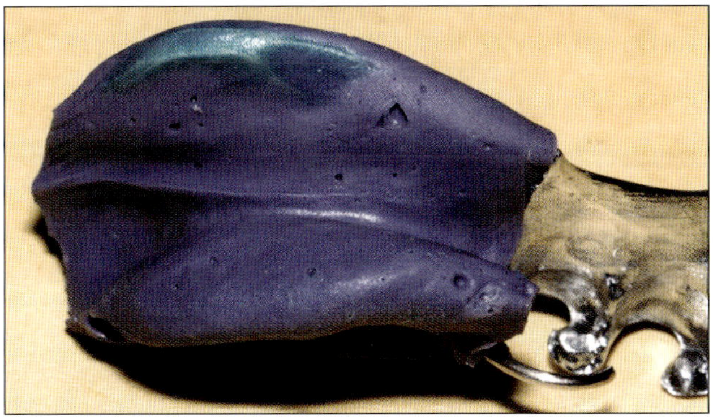

FIG 5-13 An altered cast impression.

viscosity by blending high- and low-viscosity material into one mix. The firmer the underlying tissue, the higher the percentage of high-viscosity impression material. When a good deal of unsupported or mobile soft tissue is found on the ridge crest, the mixture is altered to use a greater proportion of low-viscosity material. While a wash of all low-viscosity material will make an impression of this unsupported tissue with a minimum of pressure, it will tend to have poorly rounded borders since it is not thick enough to create the best border contours.

Excess saliva should be removed from the mouth, but there is no reason to have the mouth totally dry. The tray is loaded with just enough material to make up for the spacer plus an additional 20% to ensure full border contours (Fig 5-12). There must not be any excess material at the internal finishing line since it is likely to flow up into the guide plate area when the frame is seated. When placing the framework in the mouth, the clinician must make sure that the frame is fully seated and that no pressure is placed upon the tray itself. The fingers are placed upon three widely separated rests to maintain the frame in its optimum position while the borders are developed and the material sets.

When fully set, the impression is removed from the mouth and trimmed to remove any excess impression material (Fig 5-13). There will normally be a thin extension of the material into the retromylohyoid space on mandibular impressions and an extension of material onto the soft palate for the rare maxillary impression. Because it is almost impossible to fully border mold the retromylohyoid space on the altered cast tray, the determination of the extent of the resin border in this area is arbitrary. Remember that there is no need for full extension into the retromylohyoid spaces in the RPD as there would be for a complete denture. The retention of the partial denture is not dependent on this

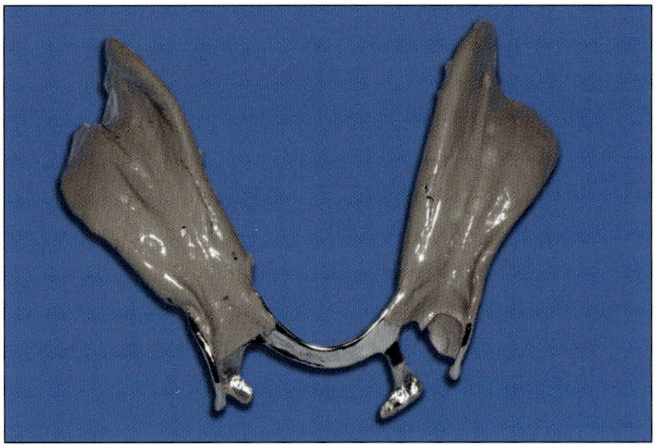

FIG 5-14 Impression material has flowed over the internal finishing line and must be removed with a sharp knife.

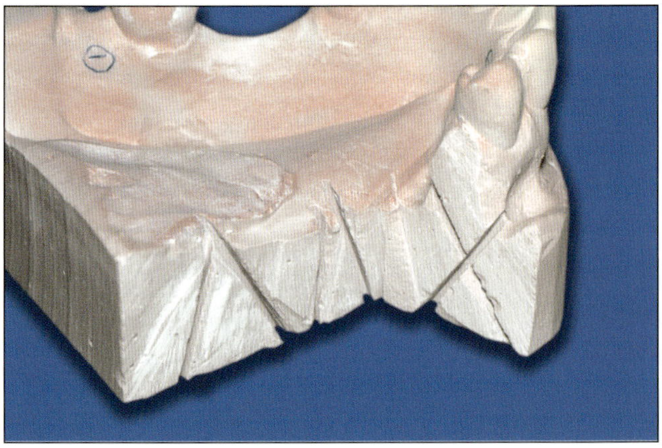

FIG 5-15 Previous distal extension is cut away, and retentive grooves are placed.

border. If a large undercut exists distal to the mylohyoid ridge, the denture base may be prohibited from entering the undercut, as it might in a complete denture, since the guiding planes determine the path of insertion. There is no reason for the lingual extension of the flange not to terminate at the soft tissue height of contour as determined by these guiding planes. The patient will be more comfortable with less resin in the mouth, and the support of the extension base will not be compromised since it is the ridge crest and the external oblique ridge that are the supporting structures for the distal extension.

Any borders of insufficient width can be recreated in wax if they are extended to the predetermined limits. Because this border width is arbitrary in the RPD, there is no need to confirm the width in the patient's mouth at this time. Should excess wax flow onto the internal surface of the impression when the borders are being created, the wax can easily be removed without damaging the accuracy of the impression.

Verification and pouring the cast impression

A final verification of the distal extension impression must be made after the base is trimmed and shaped. At this time, the clinician must be confident that the frame fully seats and that all impression material that has flowed onto the framework has been removed. Special consideration must be given to removing any material that extends beyond the internal finishing line (Fig 5-14). A very sharp blade should be used to trim the material in this area so that no pulling or tearing of the impression material occurs. At this point, a maxillomandibular relationship record can be made if required and if adequate space for the record exists.

Pouring the altered cast impression can be delegated to the technician, but the clinician must verify that the framework is fully seated on the definitive cast and that sticky wax has been added to hold cast and frame together during the boxing and pouring of the stone. This means that the original edentulous portion of the definitive cast must have been removed earlier and that adequate retention has been cut into the remainder of the definitive cast (Fig 5-15). Rather than go through an elaborate boxing process, the clinician may elect to pour the altered cast impression in two stages, much as was done for the definitive cast. The border roll of the altered cast impression must be preserved in the boxing and pouring of the impression. A line is drawn on the impression with an indelible marker just at the point where the border contour is complete. Boxing material is placed above and along this line to create a land area of 3 mm (Fig 5-16a). The impression is then filled with vacuum-mixed stone and retentive blobs placed (Fig 5-16b). The base can be added later after the initial set, without fear of disturbing the tooth-frame relation (Fig 5-16c). The altered cast impression is poured in standard buff stone rather than in die stone as was used for the original definitive cast. The softer Type III buff stone is far easier to remove from the processed denture base with the use of a walnut shell blaster and stone solvent.

When sufficient interocclusal space exists, it makes good sense to make the maxillomandibular relationship record before pouring the altered cast impression, thus saving the patient an additional visit. The recording material of choice is again one that is completely plastic to start and that sets hard quickly. The occluding surface of the tray is prepared by cutting a few crossing grooves in the resin or, when a great deal of space exists, adding a wax occlusion rim to reduce the space for the recording material. Since there will be natural teeth in contact in dentate cases, only a very small amount of recording material need be placed. Three well-defined and widely separated points of positive contact

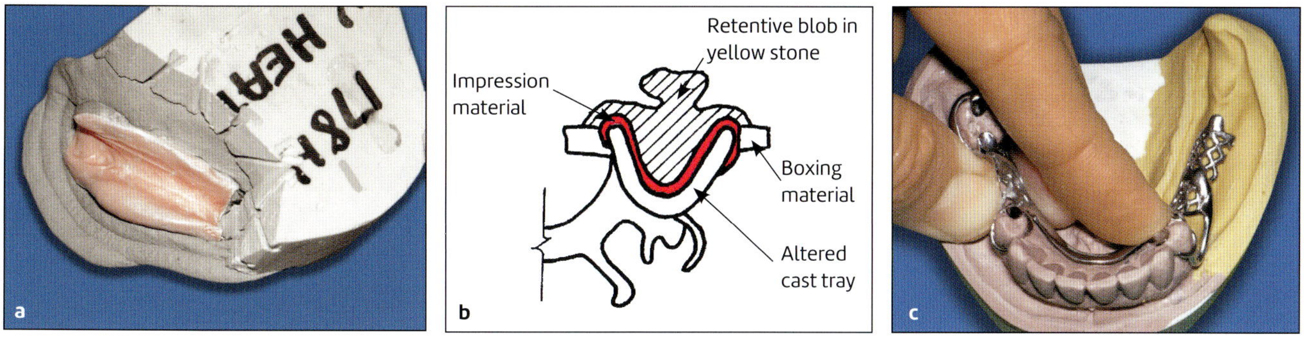

FIG 5-16 *(a)* The border roll of the altered cast impression is preserved. *(b)* Double pour for altered cast impression (base is added later). *(c)* Completed altered cast with framework fully seated.

will allow accurate articulation of the casts. Once the stone has set and the base has been trimmed, the cast with the framework and tray still in position is articulated against the opposing cast in the articulator. This is completed before the altered cast impression is ever separated from the cast. When the opposing arch is a complete denture, the maxillomandibular relationship records are made at a separate appointment because there are other procedures that must be completed as a part of this patient treatment.

No compromise in the quality of the final impression or that of the definitive cast can be allowed. The clinician must be prepared, and must prepare the patient, for the inevitable remakes that will occur. Once the patient understands that only perfection is acceptable at this critical stage, they will see that it is in their best interests to cooperate fully. Indeed, a repeated impression often demonstrates very clearly to a patient that the clinician is willing to uphold high standards even if it means more time and effort. In addition, the technician must feel comfortable telling the clinician that an apparent error has been identified on the definitive cast. Their advice must always be welcomed even if the natural reaction to a requested remake is one of some irritation. It is through this team approach that partial dentures of the highest quality are made on a routine basis.

References

1. Rudd RW, Rudd KD. A review of 243 errors possible during the fabrication of a removable partial denture: Part I. J Prosthet Dent 2001;86:251–261.
2. Williams RJ, Bibb R, Eggbeer D, Collis J. Use of CAD/CAM technology to fabricate a removable partial denture framework. J Prosthet Dent 2006;96:96–99.
3. Wu J, Li Y, Zhang Y. Use of intraoral scanning and 3-dimensional printing in the fabrication of a removable partial denture for a patient with limited mouth opening. J Am Dent Assoc 2017;148:338–341.
4. Kattadiyil MT, Mursic Z, AlRumaih H, Goodacre CJ. Intraoral scanning of hard and soft tissues for partial removable dental prosthesis fabrication. J Prosthet Dent 2014;112:444–448.
5. Chang TL, Orellana D, Beumer J III. Kratochvil's Fundamentals of Removable Partial Dentures. Chicago: Quintessence, 2019.
6. Soltanzadeh P, Suprono MS, Kattadiyil MT, Goodacre C, Gregorius W. An in vitro investigation of accuracy and fit of conventional and CAD/CAM removable partial denture frameworks. J Prosthodont 2019;28:547–555.
7. Chen H, Li H, Zhao Y, Zhang X, Wang Y, Lyu P. Adaptation of removable partial denture frameworks fabricated by selective laser melting. J Prosthet Dent 2019;122:316–324.
8. Wu J, Cheng Y, Gao B, Yu H. A novel digital altered cast impression technique for fabricating a removable partial denture with a distal extension. J Am Dent Assoc 2020;151:297–302.
9. Jasim FA, Brudvik JS, Nicholls JI. Impression distortion from abutment tooth inclination in removable partial dentures. J Prosthet Dent 1985;54:532–538.
10. Nishi Y, Hamano T, Kawahata N, Nagaoka E. Displacement of a mobile tooth during impression procedure: Effect of impression tray design. J Oral Rehabil 1998;25:553–559.
11. Nishi Y, Tsuru K, Kishita C, Hamano T, Kawahata N, Nagaoka E. Impression pressures against teeth in a partially edentulous model with a mobile tooth: Influence of impression tray design. J Oral Rehabil 2000;27:380–386.
12. Gunderson RB, Siegel SC. Cast articulation accuracy using rigid cast stabilization. J Prosthodont 2002;11:117–121.
13. Holmes JB. Influence of impression procedures and occlusal loading on partial denture movement. J Prosthet Dent 1965;15:474–483.
14. Leupold RJ. A comparative study of impression procedures for distal extension removable partial dentures. J Prosthet Dent 1966;16:708–720.
15. Leupold RJ, Flinton RJ, Pfeifer DL. Comparison of vertical movement occurring during loading of distal-extension removable partial denture bases made by three impression techniques. J Prosthet Dent 1992;68:290–293.
16. Maxfield JB, Nicholls JI, Smith DE. The measurement of forces transmitted to abutment teeth of removable partial dentures. J Prosthet Dent 1979;41:134–142.
17. Frank RP, Brudvik JS, Noonan, CJ. Clinical outcome of the altered cast impression procedure compared with use of a one-piece cast. J Prosthet Dent 2004;91:468–476.

6 LABORATORY CONSTRUCTION OF THE FRAMEWORK

The dentist must remain in control.

The laboratory phase of RPD construction is just as important as the clinical phase.[1] Because of the skill and expensive technology required to manufacture stellate alloy frameworks, the clinician is totally dependent on the dental technician for its construction. As a result of this situation, dental schools do not prepare their students to make frameworks. Unless the clinician has had previous laboratory experience, they will not understand the procedures necessary to create quality frameworks except in the most basic sense. Nonetheless, the clinician bears full responsibility for the quality of the prosthesis placed in the mouth and so must carefully interface with the laboratory to maintain this standard.

Laboratory Communication

While not as important as regular maintenance, much of the potential for RPD success rests with the quality of the laboratory phases of construction. Finding a state-of-the-art dental laboratory and building a working relationship with the technician has become a major logistical problem. As with dentistry in general, the dental laboratory industry continues to consolidate and become more corporate. Efficiency and profit often seem to supersede quality at larger factory-type laboratories. The smaller laboratory, which tends to facilitate more direct long-term interpersonal communication, is now a small and ever-shrinking minority of the laboratory industry. This trend is partly based on the belief that the efficiency and accuracy of digital fabrication will replace the need for hand-skill-based technicians. This transition is not likely to be easy. From the standpoint of the advanced partial denture, the more complex the RPD, the greater the need for technicians to be fully involved in the process. Besides the patient, it is the dentist who stands to lose the most from lack of adequate laboratory assistance. Without it, there is little hope of fabricating prostheses to the standards discussed in this textbook.

Finding, building, and fostering a cohesive clinical-laboratory team is the responsibility of the dentist. The clinician must work to keep their technicians current with what appears in the various prosthodontic journals and what is learned at conventions and study clubs. They should more regularly attend live continuing education events together. Not only will the information be received and therefore debated as a team, but it provides an opportunity to associate in a more relaxed nonclinical atmosphere. Almost without exception, the technicians are more than happy to reciprocate with what they learn from their journals and what comes to them from the dental industry. While it would be great if both sides of the "team" routinely read the same materials, it is not the current reality.

Clinicians have, unfortunately, often used the laboratory as a scapegoat for problems that arise during treatment. Problems in clinic–laboratory relations can most often be traced to a lack of communication and the unwillingness of the clinician to review the laboratory procedures at the appropriate stages in construction. For example, the clinician should always have the blocked-out definitive cast and the waxed-up refractory cast returned for evaluation before investing and casting the framework. This evaluation is well worth the delay, as there will always be cases where the clinician is unable to adequately describe what is desired in the final product. The interaction between the clinician and the technician is equally significant for the surveyed crowns discussed in chapter 4.

A dental laboratory cannot create a prosthesis for a patient without a specific work authorization coming directly from a licensed dentist. Likewise, the dental laboratory can only directly bill the dentist. Work authorizations vary depending on custom and jurisdiction but are typically approved by a state's dental examining board. From a medicolegal perspective, the dentist must therefore take any laboratory work authorization seriously. Studies and surveys continue to show that dentists spend little time and give little guidance when writing these authorizations.[2–4] Lack of clarity on what is expected will leave little recourse for the dentist if the laboratory produces inadequate work. It must be noted, in this era of delegation, that the work authorization also serves as a contract with the laboratory. In this way, if specific steps or procedures are not followed properly, the responsibility and therefore cost of remake will lie with the laboratory. On the other hand, the more thorough the design and instructions, the greater the likelihood that the technician will be encouraged to return a casting of the highest quality.

At a minimum, the work authorization for a typical RPD framework will need to include all design details, framework material to be used, specific handling instructions, time frame for completion of the requested step, as well as basic patient information (Fig 6-1). One benefit to a long-standing dentist–laboratory relationship is that the prescription may not need to include all minutia once specific procedures are established. With time, a quality laboratory partner will learn the specific handling details described in this textbook, leaving the dentist free to write a more concise authorization that focuses on the unique features and design of the individual case. A carbon copy of each work authorization must become part of the patient record. If the technical work produced by the laboratory does not comply or match that on the authorization, it is clear who is responsible. Past authorizations are also frequently referenced to confirm tooth molds, shade, and other information needed to make accurate repairs.

The communication of the specific design of the partial denture is facilitated by sending the diagnostically modified cast to the dental laboratory. This is an added value to the process described in chapter 4 (see Fig 4-2). If the clinical phases have proceeded according to plan, the definitive cast matches the diagnostically modified cast. The clear drawing and modifications will leave little doubt in a laboratory technician's mind as to the placement of the various components.

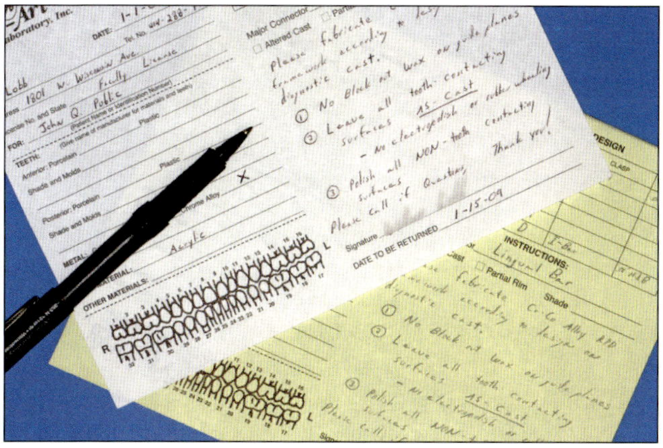

FIG 6-1 Laboratory prescription with carbon copy.

Analog Construction

The phases of RPD construction in the laboratory include the following (Fig 6-2):

1. Design transfer
2. Blockout
3. Duplication
4. Refractory cast
5. Waxing
6. Investing
7. Casting
8. Electropolishing
9. Metal finishing
10. Frame evaluation

The actual construction techniques and materials are usually proprietary, having been developed by the dental laboratory industry and the metal manufacturing companies. The alloys are generally chrome-based, although iron and titanium alloys have been proposed and are in use. Dentsply Sirona's Vitallium (65% Co, 30% Cr, 5% Mo) and Nobilium's Ticonium (72% Ni, 16% Cr, 5% Mo, 3% Mn, 3% Al, 1% Be) were for many years the most commonly used commercial alloys in North America. These two alloys use different investments and different duplicating agars but are otherwise quite similar in their construction techniques. They show similar results in materials testing as well. The composition and characteristics of various alloys

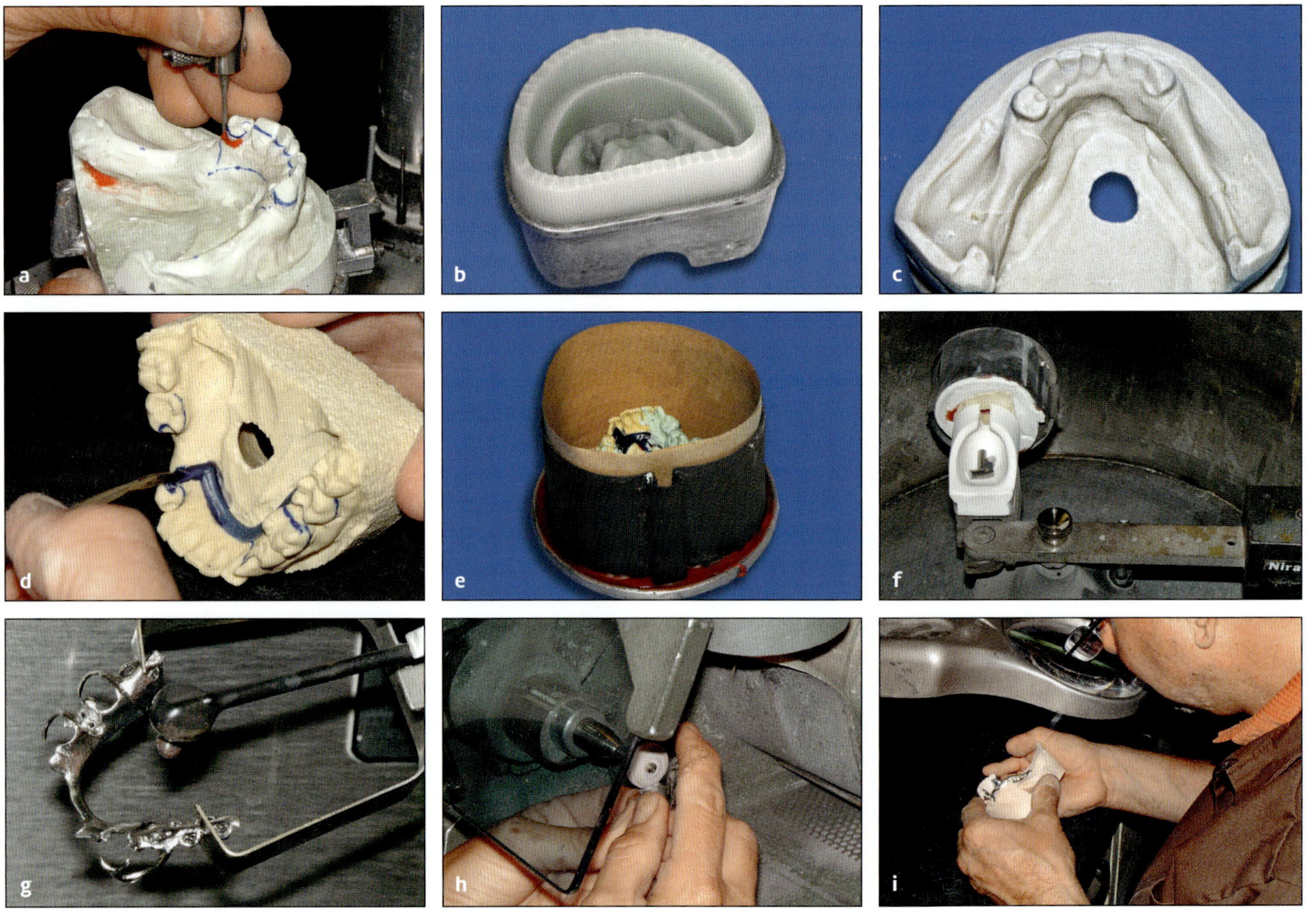

FIG 6-2 Phases of RPD construction in the laboratory. *(a)* Blockout according to path of insertion and design. *(b)* Duplication. *(c)* Refractory cast. *(d)* Waxing. *(e)* Investing. *(f)* Casting. *(g)* Electropolishing. *(h)* Metal finishing. *(i)* Technician evaluating framework.

are available in any text on dental materials and should be a part of the knowledge base of the clinician involved with prosthodontics at the advanced level. Advancing digital technology, to be discussed in this chapter, opens the door to alternative manufacturing techniques. Some of these techniques, such as selective laser melting (SLM), show great promise in both accuracy and material properties. Likewise, segmented construction and laser welding of components can also be expected to influence the construction methods for advanced RPD frameworks.

Construction in the laboratory begins with the transfer of the design from the diagnostic cast or the work authorization to the definitive cast. This completes the communication process between clinician and technician. Specialists who are comfortable with their ability to make a precise drawing on the definitive cast need to be sure that the color code they employ is known to the technician. By placing the design on the tripoded definitive cast, one area of potential error is eliminated. Special care must be taken in the outline of relief pads for retentive meshwork. The extent of the internal finishing line must be clearly marked 2 to 3 mm from the gingival marginal tissue to make clear that this area must be in metal rather than in resin (Fig 6-3). Heights of contour must be carefully marked with the surveyor lead on both hard and soft tissues so that no areas requiring blockout are missed.

Perhaps the most critical area of design transfer is the accurate drawing of retentive clasp arms. The terminal third of all circumferential cast clasps must be accurately placed at the desired undercut depth, almost always 0.01 inch (0.25 mm). Depending on the steepness of the undercut and the amount of mouth preparation, undercuts in the terminal third of the tooth surface may require blockout even though ideally the entire terminal third of the clasp should be contacting the tooth in the undercut area. A definitive cast must be rejected if the available undercuts are inadequate in depth or position on the tooth. Before deciding that the definitive cast will not be acceptable, the path of insertion/removal must be reviewed to ensure that the cast is, in fact, at the proper tilt on the surveyor.

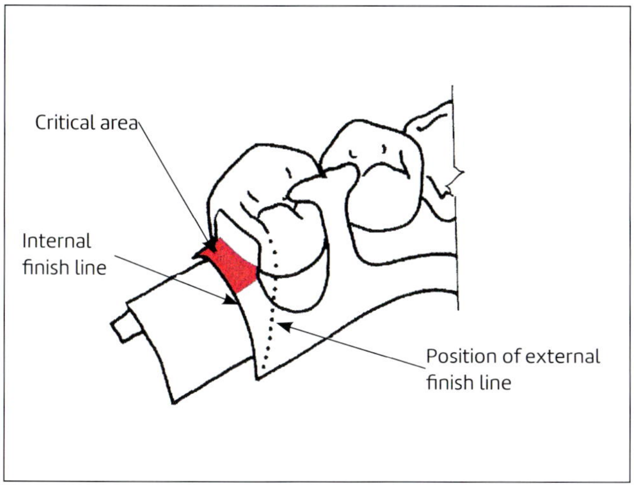

FIG 6-3 Placement of internal finish line.

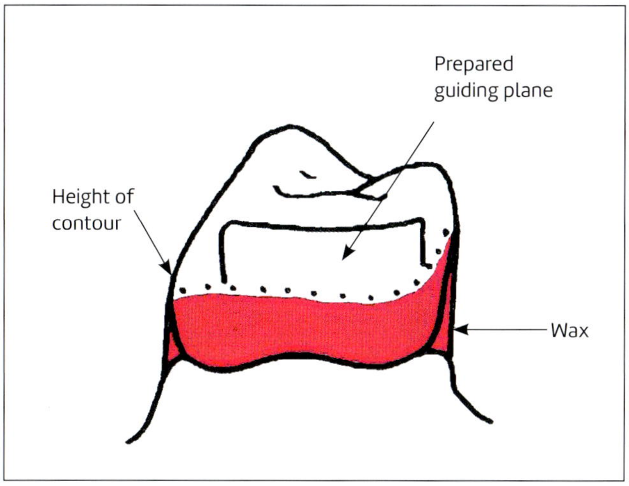

FIG 6-4 Relation of guiding plane and blockout wax.

Blockout and duplication

Depending on the proprietary techniques specific to the alloy being used for the framework, the designed definitive cast may be sprayed with a model gloss to seal the cast and preserve the drawn design. Obviously, care must be taken to not over spray since any accumulation of the protective coating would change the dimensions of the definitive cast and may result in an unusable casting. Most modern techniques have eliminated this process.

Blockout wax is then placed on the stone teeth to begin the blockout process. It is absolutely essential that no blockout wax be placed above the line indicating the height of contour on any areas where the casting is intended to touch the teeth (Fig 6-4). This includes, at a minimum, guiding planes, rest seats, and clasp arms. The reason for stressing this seemingly benign step is that the contours of the stone teeth will inevitably be changed by misplaced wax in areas where accuracy is essential to the final fit of the casting. The technician removes the excess blockout wax using a vertical blade in a surveying instrument, sometimes even one that is electrically heated to increase the likelihood of creating a smooth surface on the refractory cast. Wax placed above the height of contour in areas of tooth-frame contact must also be removed. In an attempt to do so, the technician will either *(1)* leave a small amount of wax, thereby making the definitive cast and resultant refractory slightly larger than it really is, or *(2)* in attempting to remove all the excess wax, scrape some of the stone and thereby make the definitive cast slightly smaller in that area. In either situation, the accuracy of the definitive cast has been compromised. It is far better to be very careful in the initial placement of the blockout wax and never have to deal with the problems that arise in its removal.

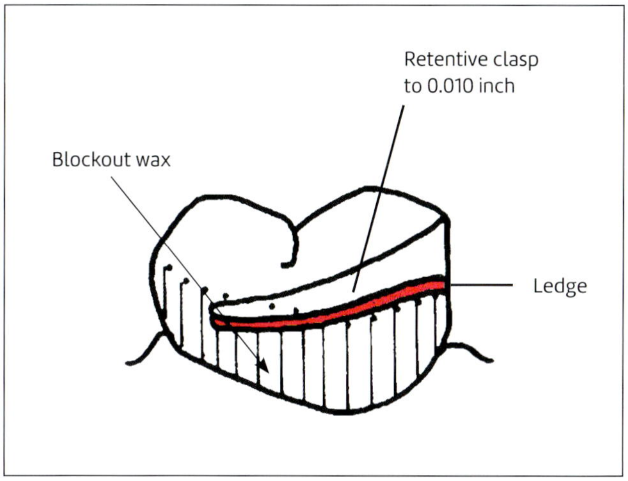

FIG 6-5 Blockout ledge for clasp placement.

Some laboratories use a technique where a ledge is created in the blockout wax at the inferior border of clasp arms. This ledge is duplicated in the refractory and serves as a shelf onto which the plastic clasp pattern is placed during the wax-up. It should be obvious that the ledge must be placed with careful regard for the underlying drawing of the clasp arm (Fig 6-5). Because the placement of the plastic clasp pattern to a precise position on the refractory cast is not an easy task, the ledge should be placed slightly (about 0.5 mm) below the line that represents the inferior border of the clasp. This will ensure that the clasp will reach the desired undercut position.

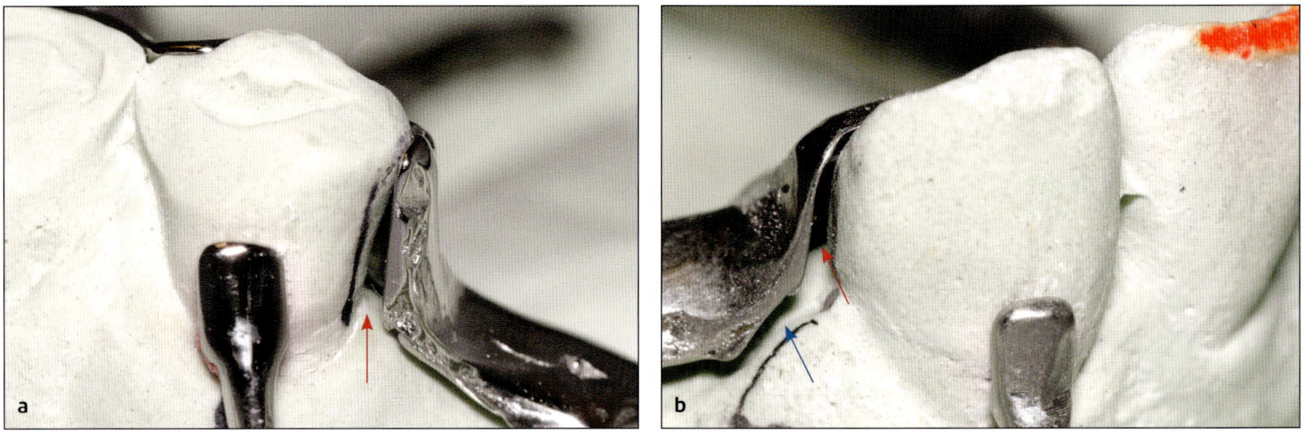

FIG 6-6 *(a)* Excess blockout wax results in a gap between the guide plate and the abutment tooth *(red arrow)*. This is often done intentionally to facilitate complete seating of the framework. *(b)* Excess blockout wax at guiding plane *(red arrow)* ran continuous with the relief pad *(blue arrow)*. The result is lack of guide plate contact and either acrylic over the gingival margin or space for plaque.

The blockout is generally done at 0 degrees, ie, parallel with the intended path of insertion/removal. It is possible to alter this angle by substituting a blade that has a 2- or 6-degree angle. This type of divergent blockout is used primarily for certain types of precision attachment situations. In using a blockout other than 0 degrees, frictional resistance to dislodgment is inevitably lost, forcing increased reliance on clasp or attachment retention. One must be wary of a laboratory that intentionally blocks out the guiding plane contact areas of teeth to facilitate uninterrupted seating of a framework (Fig 6-6). This is a common response by some laboratories to the majority of their dentist clients who simply want the frameworks to completely seat and who are not considering the fit of the framework as discussed in this book.

When the abutment teeth have been recontoured with the blockout wax to the extent prescribed, the relief pads are added to the definitive cast. A full thickness of baseplate wax (roughly 1 mm) is the minimum for the relief of the retentive mesh. Commercial laboratories often choose to use a thinner relief wax in the belief that by keeping the meshwork closer to the edentulous areas, there will be more room for the rapid placement of the denture teeth. While this is true, the thin relief leaves insufficient space for quality resin under the meshwork. If it is too thin, the acrylic resin will experience significantly more leakage and bacterial absorption. A thin relief pad also creates an internal finishing line that does not have adequate depth to retain the resin in the critical area next to the abutment tooth. The internal finish line is established by that portion of the relief pad that is adjacent to the abutment tooth. The pad in this area must be contoured to create an undercut wedge in the final casting in order to lock in the processed resin (Fig 6-7). The relief pad thickness also determines the amount of space that will be available for the impression material of the altered cast impression. Again, 1 mm is the minimum space for impression material. In addition, the recommended procedure for a reline of the distal extension base is to first remove a uniform amount of material to facilitate a good bond of the added resin to the old denture base. When less than 1 mm of resin exists under the meshwork, it will be exposed by the necessary grinding. The thickness of the relief wax pad must be prescribed by the clinician, not determined arbitrarily by the laboratory. This is especially true where overlay abutments and implants are involved (to be discussed in chapter 12). The relief pad must be sealed to the definitive cast so that it does not separate in the duplicating procedures to follow.

To complete the blockout procedures, wax or caulking materials are placed in all undercuts that are not part of the framework (Fig 6-8). Blockout of these nonessential areas is important, nonetheless, since the entire cast must be removed from the duplicating mold without tearing the agar. Any undercuts other than the 0.01 inch for the clasp retention have the potential to distort the agar. The fully blocked-out cast is placed in a saturated solution of dental stone to be hydrated before duplicating it in the refractory material.

The duplicating agar is commonly one that is provided by the manufacturer of the alloy system and is chosen for compatibility with the refractory material. For example, a phosphate-bound investment does not set against a water-based colloid, so a glycerin-based duplicating agar is used for the higher-heat alloys. The agar is usually kept

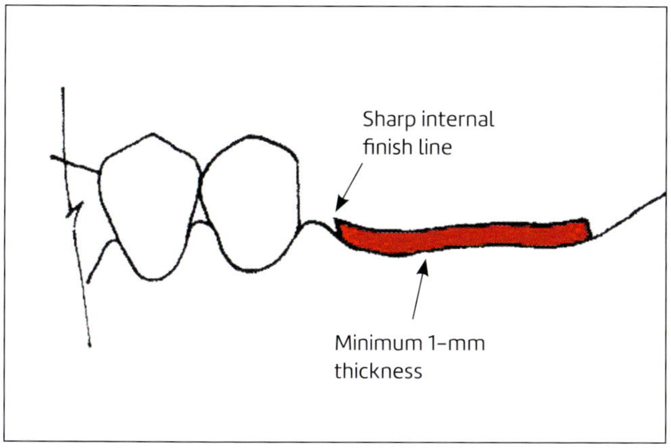

FIG 6-7 Proper location of wax relief pad to create a sharp internal finish line.

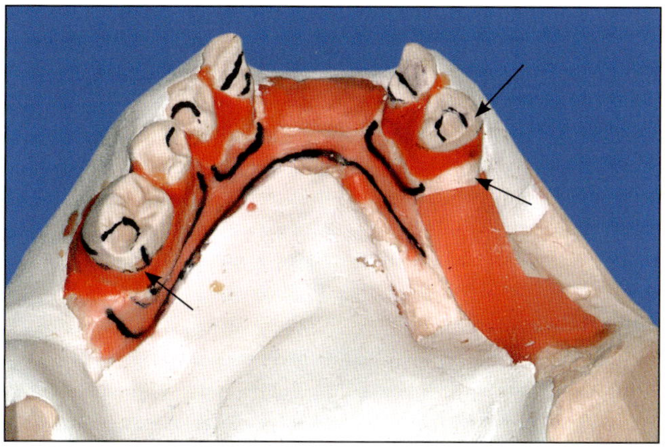

FIG 6-8 Completed blockout. *Arrows* indicate key unaltered tooth/tissue surfaces.

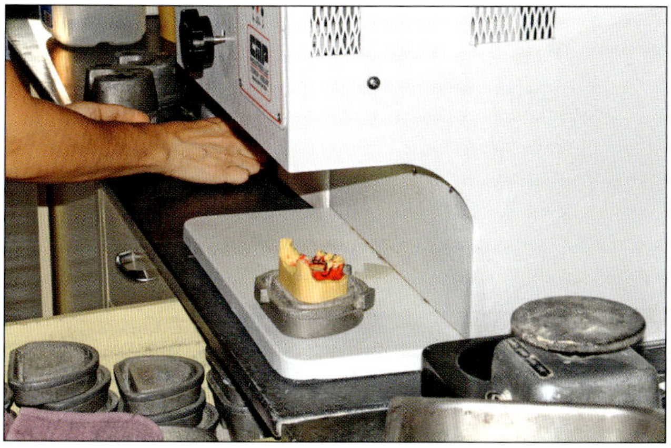

FIG 6-9 Duplicating machine with half of flask.

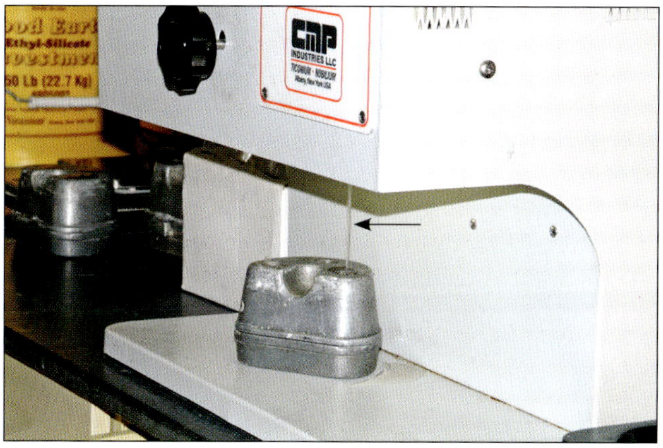

FIG 6-10 Fluid agar *(arrow)* being poured into metal flask.

in an electrically heated dispenser from which it is poured through a controlled valve into the duplicating flask at a prescribed temperature and to which it is returned after recovery from the set refractory at the end of the duplicating process (Fig 6-9). The duplicating material does have an expiration point based on the number of times it has been reheated. Clinicians need only assure themselves that the laboratory does indeed record the number of cycles and replaces the agar within the recommended time frame.

The flask used to contain the duplicating agar is designed with a metal base and a nonmetallic side ring that fits into a channel on the base. The blocked-out definitive cast is placed on the base and the hot (temperature depending on manufacturer) agar slowly poured into the flask up to the level of the top of the ring (Fig 6-10). The viscosity of warmed agar is very low, making it excellent for surface detail and accuracy reproduction (Fig 6-11). The entire flask is placed into a circulating cold-water bath where the metal of the base conducts the shrinkage of the cooling agar toward the base to result in an accurate mold. Once the agar is cooled

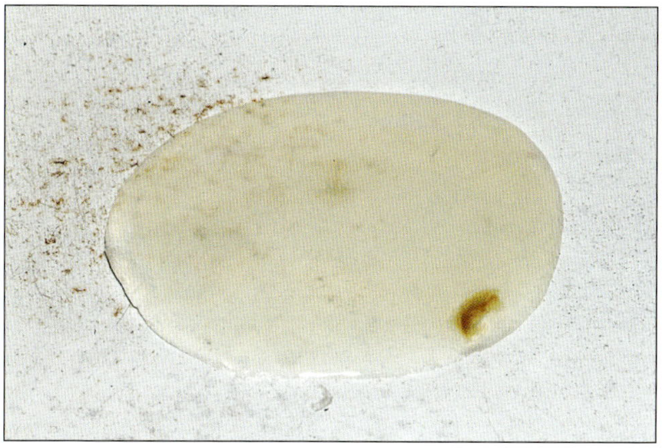

FIG 6-11 Agar is very fluid with a low viscosity.

to room temperature, the flask is removed from the bath. The definitive cast is carefully removed from the mold by placing a knife blade in the cast base at both sides and lifting the cast vertically out of the mold without stressing the agar. Having the sides of the base of the definitive cast trimmed

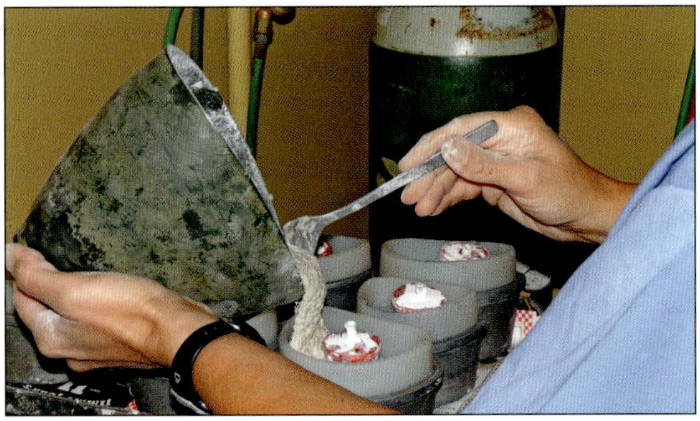

FIG 6-12 A vibrating table reduces air bubbles while the thick refractory is poured.

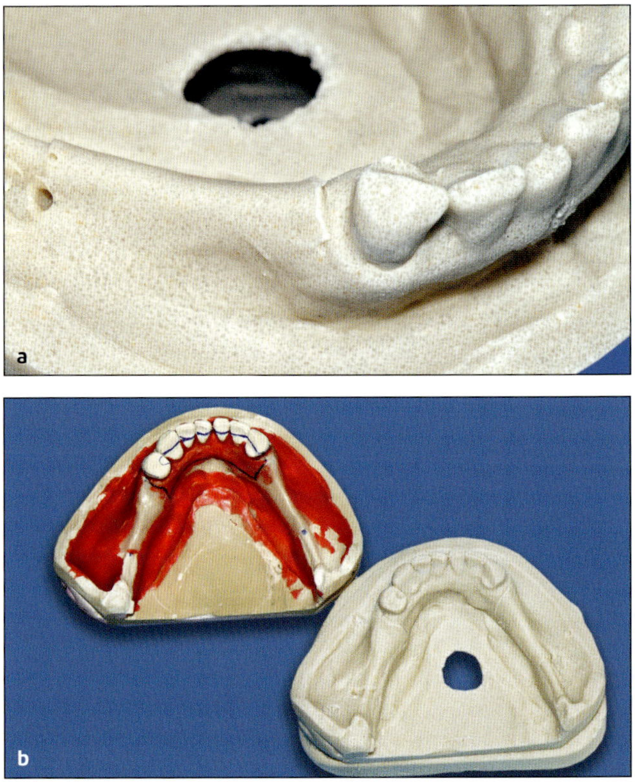

FIG 6-13 *(a)* Refractory cast with sprue former hole in base. Note the relief pad. *(b)* Blocked-out definitive cast next to its refractory cast.

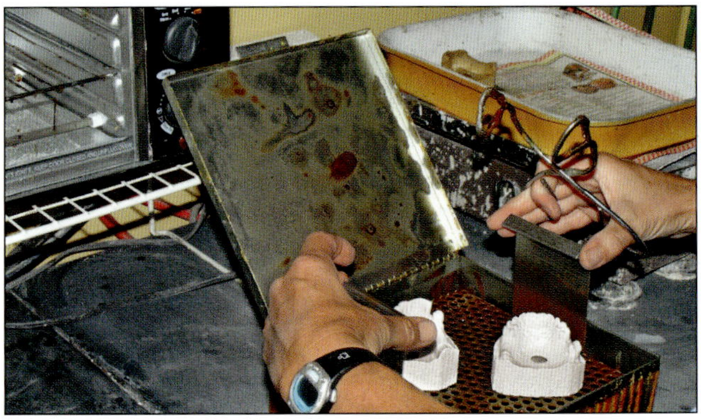

FIG 6-14 Dried refractory casts being placed into sealer bath.

to diverge slightly toward the base will make removal easier. More recently, silicone duplicating impression material has been advocated, and anecdotal reports indicate that a more routinely accurate tooth-frame relationship can be established with these materials. However, since they are not reusable, this potential accuracy comes with an additional cost.

The liquid-to-powder ratio for the refractory cast is critical for the accuracy of the casting. The density of the set refractory determines, to a great extent, the expansion of the investment mold.[5,6] It has been claimed that a change of as little as 1 mL of liquid in the liquid-to-powder ratio can affect the clinical fit of the framework. Research out of the University of Washington has shown that the addition of 1.4 mL of excess water to a 400-g mix will decrease the expansion of a phosphate-bonded investment cross-arch by an average of 50 μm. Because of the high casting temperatures of the stellate alloys, the thermal shrinkage with cooling is significant. Our ability to sufficiently expand the mold is limited. By decreasing the amount of liquid to powder, the expansion of the mold can be increased to offset the thermal shrinkage. Unfortunately, the thickening of the mix that results from the change in the ratio makes the mass too thick to pour into the agar mold without fear of trapping air. Even with exact measurements, extended vibrating times are used to release trapped air bubbles (Fig 6-12). The technician who uses the manufacturer's recommended ratio with exact measurements of both liquid and powder will generally produce a mold with adequate expansion. Beware the technician who is careless with the measurement of the liquid or perhaps overlooks water in the bottom of the mixing bowl. A mix that has too much liquid in the ratio results in a mold that cannot expand sufficiently to match the expected thermal shrinkage.

The porous and brittle nature of the large-particle refractory cast material is evident on close inspection (Fig 6-13a). If standard blockout procedures were followed, only the occlusal, tissue-contacting, and tooth-contacting surface detail will remain (Fig 6-13b). Most techniques for the casting of these RPD alloys call for the desiccation of the refractory cast in an oven to remove excess moisture, followed by dipping the cast in a bath of hot molten beeswax (Fig 6-14). This wax seals the porous refractory and makes it less susceptible to abrasion. It also eliminates the need to soak the refractory cast before adding the first layer of paint-on investment over the waxed framework. Commercial model spray can also be used for these purposes. For the spray, two light coats are required, with a 2- to 3-minute drying time between coats.

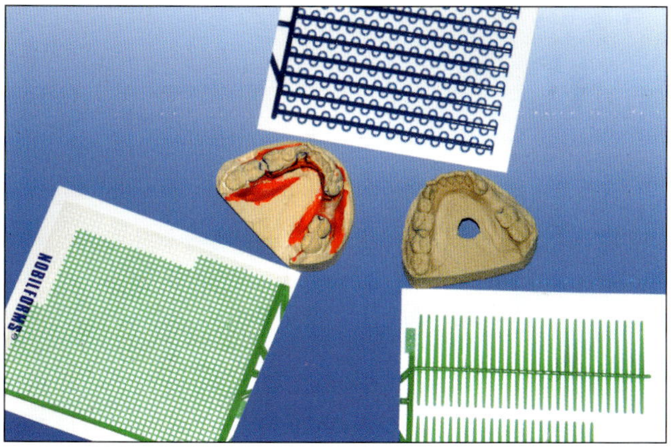

FIG 6-15 Several sheets of common wax patterns. The sealed refractory cast is on the *right*.

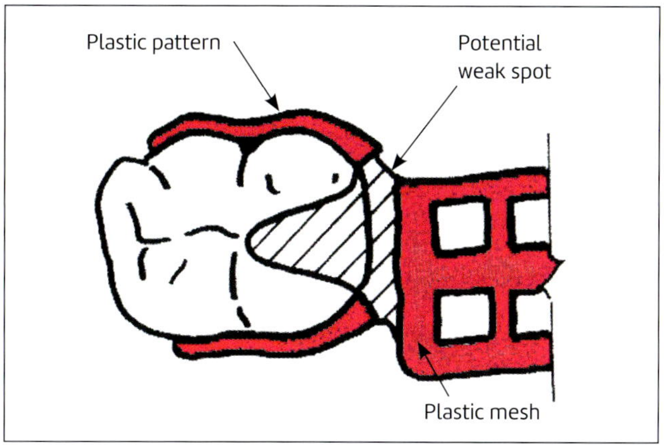

FIG 6-16 Junction of plastic pattern and hand-waxed minor connector.

Waxing

At this point, the design is again transferred from the definitive cast to the refractory cast to form the outline for the waxing of the framework. The clinician has every right to expect a casting that conforms to the design placed upon the definitive cast. Commercially available plastic patterns are used whenever possible to maintain standard dimensions for major connectors, clasps, and finishing lines (Fig 6-15). Rests are apt to be hand-waxed to blend in with the plastic patterns. The clinician needs to have seen the patterns and evaluated their shape and thickness to be able to truly prescribe the components of the framework. Because they have such a major effect on the performance of the cast clasp and come in such a variety of tapers and width/thickness ratios, clasp patterns must be selected with care.[7]

The plastic patterns are quite flexible and can easily be stretched when removing them from the cards on which they come or when adapting them to the refractory cast. They also have a memory, so they must be held in place with some sort of adhesive that is compatible with the entire process or with the addition of very small amounts of molten wax. A mixture of acetone and the plastic pattern material will create a tacky liquid that can be painted onto the refractory and to which the patterns will adhere. The tacky liquid should have only enough viscosity to glue the pattern in place. Excess material, painted on the cast, will change the dimensions of the resultant casting.

Once the tacky liquid has been applied, the patterns are cut to length and shape and adapted with either finger pressure or with a soft pencil eraser or a similar instrument. Sharp instruments may create cuts or grooves in the patterns that may influence the performance of the final casting. The sections of the plastic patterns will have to be joined with wax, trying to maintain the contours of the pattern. Because the resultant casting will not come out of the casting process as smooth and precise as a cast crown, the wax is always added in slight excess to allow for finishing and polishing of the surface. Where clasp arms join the minor connectors, care must be taken to ensure that there is a taper established that will not create a thin area in the active portion of the clasp or at the junction of the plastic pattern and the minor connector. This junction area will often be thinner than the pattern (Fig 6-16). This thin area, in between two thicker areas, can only act to concentrate stress, and a fractured clasp can be predicted in the future.

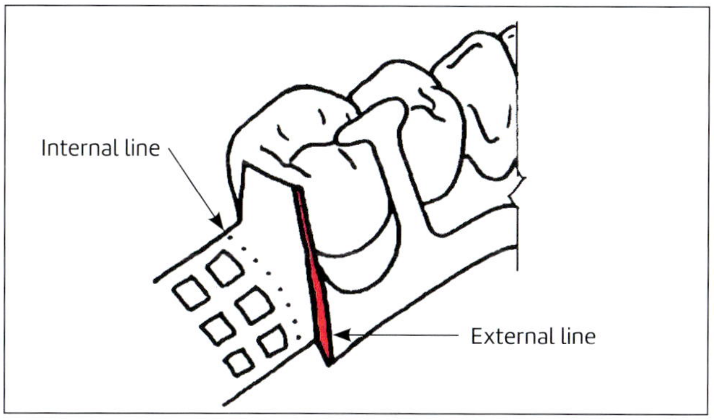

FIG 6-17 The location and extension of the external finish line.

Because the blockout/relief pad established the internal finish line, the technician need only worry about the accurate placement of the external finish line. This line, usually a portion of a plastic pattern, should extend to the occlusal portion of the line angle of the abutment (Fig 6-17). This position will permit a small amount of denture base resin between the denture tooth and the casting in the completed prosthesis.

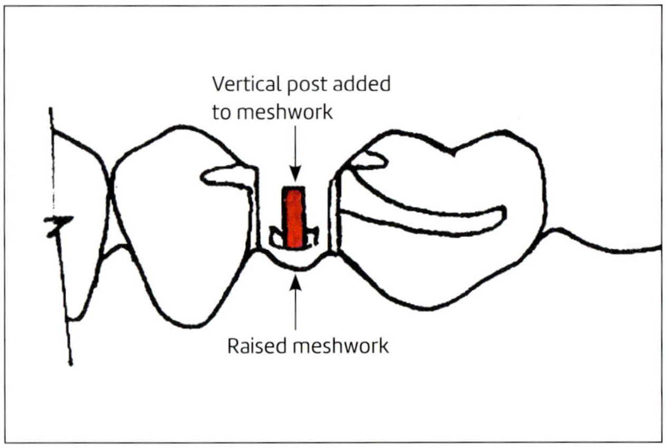

FIG 6-18 A vertical post is added to retain the denture tooth if mesh is inadequate.

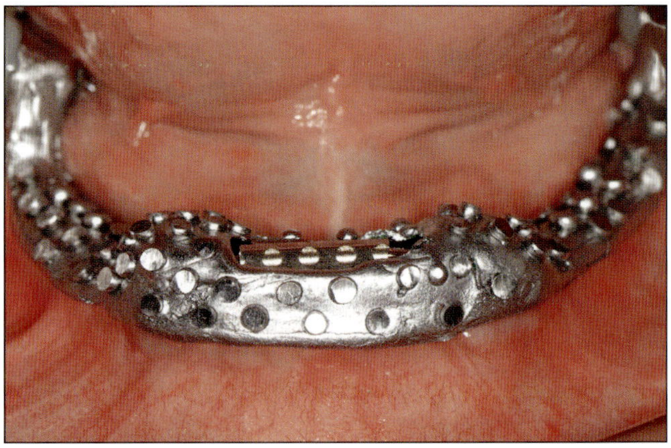

FIG 6-19 Half of the bead diameter is reduced, leaving only the retentive undercut.

The tips of cast clasp patterns should extend to just beyond the terminal extension of the transferred design to allow a small excess of metal for finishing, no more than 0.5 mm. To expedite waxing, there is a tendency for the laboratory to over-wax minor connectors and to plate technically challenging line angles. This additional tissue coverage and tooth-contacting surface area actually reduces the accuracy of the casting, makes fitting of the framework more time consuming, and has negative periodontal consequences. This is most commonly seen with cingulum rests that unnecessarily plate the lingual gingival margin of the canines.

Distal extension meshwork will require a tissue stop to be added at the end of the relief area of the refractory, either distal or mesial, depending on the situation. The stop should be roughly 3 × 3 mm and should be placed on the crest of the edentulous ridge or slightly buccal to it, wherever a relatively flat area can be found. The stop indicates a complete seating of the casting in that area for fitting and finishing. It should be removed as part of the altered cast procedure for those situations where this type of impression is required.

While a plastic pattern for the meshwork is adequate for the vast majority of situations, there are occasions when the resin retention should be created freehand in wax. Loops or strips of one-half round 8- or 10-gauge wax can be placed on the relief area of the refractory and waxed into the finish line area. This approach is most effective for maxillary tuberosity areas where space for resin is at a premium. The larger retentive areas of the hand-waxed resin retention may create a stronger link to the processed resin, although the shape of the commercial patterns appears to be adequate. However, the patterns do not provide adequate retention for resin in constricted spaces. In the very rare instance where mesh is required for a single tooth space, custom waxing is desirable, since the small lattice arrangement of the plastic patterns will not provide sufficient retention (Fig 6-18). These limited space situations are best managed with a metal base and bead retention, as previously noted, if the residual ridge is mature.

Bead retention, a term often used for metal coverage of the tissue with loops, beads, nail heads, or any solid retentive contours, is waxed by extending the major connector over the edentulous ridge with the addition of about 0.5-mm thickness of plastic pattern or wax and then adding an external finishing line in the same place as if retentive mesh had been used. The internal finishing line results from the butt joint formed from terminating the extension of the major connector buccal to the ridge crest and before any undercut is present. Bead retention can be formed from resin beads or by using round baking sprinkles. These beads should be separated by a distance of 2.5 times their diameter for the optimum resin retention. The beads are reduced to their circumference after casting using a cutoff disk (Fig 6-19). This leaves only the retentive undercut, saving some space for the placement of the denture teeth.

At this point, the refractory cast and the blocked-out definitive cast are to be returned to the clinician for review. It is essential that this review take place on every case until the technician truly understands the level of quality expected by the clinician. For complex cases and all precision attachment partial dentures, it must be standard practice. The technician sees that the clinician cares about quality and is knowledgeable about laboratory techniques. Misunderstandings that inevitably occur on design and construction are most often the fault of the clinician being unable to describe in words exactly what is required. It is only common sense that the wax-up should be reviewed

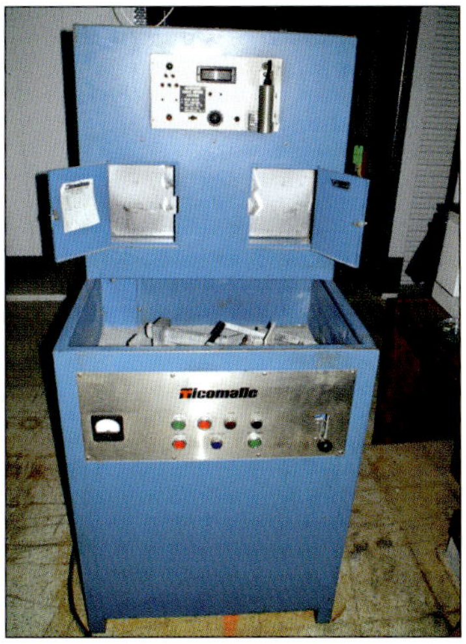

FIG 6-20 Ticomatic induction casting machine, circa 1990s.

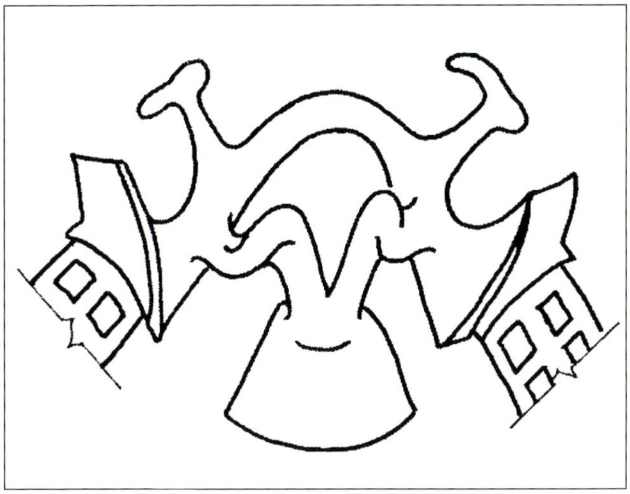

FIG 6-21 Helical sprue leads to reduce turbulence.

before the sprue is placed and the wax-up invested. Experience has shown that refinement will be needed to some aspect of the wax-up in around 25% of cases; this makes the inconvenience well worthwhile. In addition, if excessive blockout is found, it can be corrected and a new refractory made before a casting has been attempted. If all is well, the refractory is returned to the laboratory while the definitive cast is kept at the dental office. This will ensure that the definitive cast remains undamaged by fitting procedures.

Investing and casting

These steps in the laboratory construction of the RPD are industrial in nature and generally follow the proprietary instructions of the metal manufacturer. Induction casting machines are often part of the process (Fig 6-20).

These machines, when calibrated, improve standardization when compared with the art of torch-based casting. The clinician does not have a role to play here except to be aware of the process. This is especially true for sprue placement, since the variation in techniques is great, with every technician doing things just a little bit differently. As an example, the laboratory that has supported the University of Washington graduate program for over 30 years uses a helix in the sprue leads, usually two or three leads for a mandibular casting and four for a maxillary casting (Fig 6-21). The technicians feel that the helix does two things that dramatically affect the quality of the casting. First, the helix acts as a reservoir for the metal mass that reduces the potential for a suck back. Second, it slows the flow of the molten metal, however briefly, reducing the turbulence and thus reducing porosity. Sprue leads without the helix are sometimes used as an additional lead for complex casting configurations. These sprues are always slightly curved to slow the metal flow.

The clinician should always examine the resultant casting and any broken castings for evidence of porosity as a quality-control check on the laboratory. It is possible, but not practical, to make radiographs of a casting in order to visualize porosity. The persistence of casting shrinkage, and the clinical challenges that come with it, will be discussed in detail later (see pages 98–102 and chapter 7). While there is little, beyond showing interest, that the clinician can do about the casting of the partial denture framework, the treatment of the casting after it has been cast is a critical procedure that dramatically affects the ultimate success of the partial denture.

Metal finishing

Metal finishing is an all-encompassing term covering the steps from the actual casting of the partial denture framework to the fully finished and polished framework. It is an aspect of the process that historically has been left entirely to the discretion of the technician, with the clinician accepting the finished product without question. The most important phase of construction is in the finishing and fitting of the casting, and it is here where an accurate casting can easily be rendered unacceptable if the internal surfaces that contact the teeth are altered in any way. The standard means of finishing the casting, once the sprues have been removed with a cutoff disk, is to electropolish. This process will strip a small amount of metal from the entire surface of the casting electronically to improve the surface finish. Stripping or deplating occurs when a metal is placed in an acid bath attached to an electrode and a controlled amount of electrical current is passed through the metal via the electrodes and the bath. The framework is immersed in a temperature-controlled bath of electrolyte

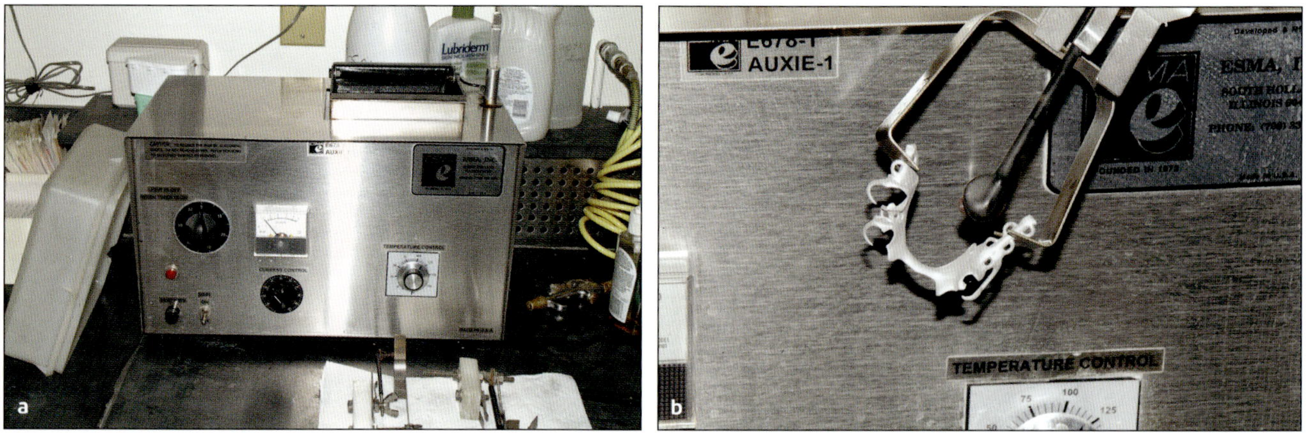

FIG 6-22 *(a)* Electropolishing unit. The bath is located on the upper right portion of the unit. *(b)* Casting attached to the anode with the cathode centered to the framework.

and serves as the anode. It is connected to the positive terminal of a DC power supply, and the negative terminal is attached to the cathode. A current passes from the anode, where metal on the surface is oxidized and dissolved in the electrolyte, to the cathode. A commercial unit with temperature, amperage, and time control is used (Fig 6-22a). A clamp is used to hold the framework on the electrode (Fig 6-22b). Obviously, all the ingredients of the system contribute to the rate of dissolution of the surface of the framework and so are susceptible to improper calibration or careless technicians. This system works in reverse as with a die-plating unit and is similar to the units used for micro-etching of bonded castings.

This process reduces the amount of fine finishing and polishing that will be required. Unfortunately, the removal of even this potentially very small amount of metal (40–50 μm at the very minimum) will reduce the frictional retention that could have been obtained with the parallel guiding planes established through mouth preparation[8] (Fig 6-23). The only way to control this electrochemical process is to not allow it to occur at all in areas that are critical to the tooth-frame relation. All tooth-contacting surfaces—guide plates, minor connectors, rests, and clasps—must be protected from the electrolytic polishing process by coating them with a high fusing wax or a substance like fingernail polish. This coating seals these surfaces from contact with the liquid acid bath. Once the contact surfaces have been protected, the frame can be safely placed in the bath and kept there until the normal dark color of the as-cast alloy is replaced by a clean and shiny surface. However, the areas protected from the electrochemical bath should appear in an as-cast condition with no surface polish (Fig 6-24).

The frame is now ready for preliminary finishing. Contrary to mainstream handling protocol, the clinician must insist that the contact surfaces are not touched in any way by the technician and that no fitting of the frame to the definitive cast takes place in the laboratory. This is best assured by having the clinician keep the definitive cast when returning the approved refractory. The technician is instructed to finish and polish all non-tooth-contacting surfaces of the framework in a standard fashion, leaving the fitting to the clinician. The reason for stressing this point is that in fitting the frame to the definitive cast, the technician will inevitably remove more metal from the contact surfaces than is required. This decreases the quality of the tooth-frame relationship. Once a casting has been placed on a cast, the cast surface will be abraded and no longer accurate. The subsequent fitting will therefore be done to a cast that does not represent the mouth.

If the casting is not fitted to the definitive cast in the laboratory, then this responsibility will rest with the clinician. The state-of-the-art casting will first be fitted to the teeth by the clinician, and only when an acceptable relationship has been obtained will the casting be placed on the definitive cast. Should the cast be scraped in the process, it will be of no significance since it will not affect the tooth-frame relationship. If it is not possible to fully seat the casting in the mouth, then the definitive cast must be remade since there is no way to accurately determine if the cause of the misfit is an inaccurate impression or a laboratory error.

After a level of trust has been gained between laboratory and clinician, it is possible to delegate some management of the tooth-frame interface to the technician. Specifically, the porous nature of refractory stone can result in small bubbles of metal cast into small stone voids. An experienced technician can, under microscope, remove these casting bubbles that would otherwise interfere with seating (Fig 6-25). Polishing of the clasp arms can also be allowed, with

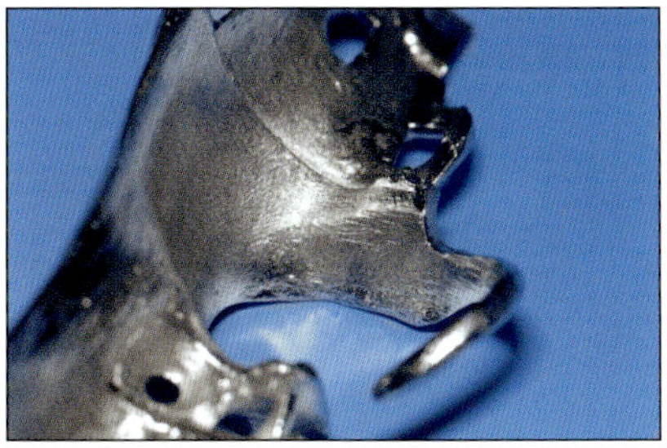

FIG 6-23 The guiding plane was left exposed in the electrochemical bath.

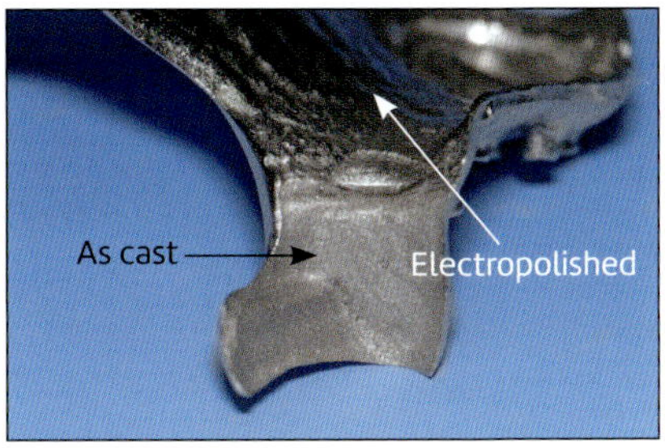

FIG 6-24 Tooth-contacting surfaces were protected from the electrochemical bath.

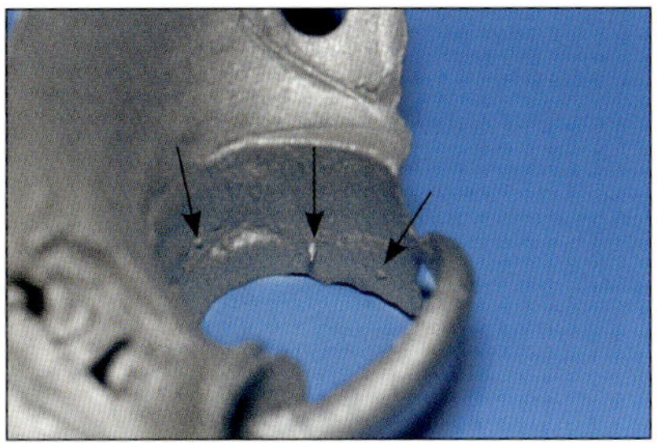

FIG 6-25 The *arrows* indicate casting blebs that an experienced technician can remove.

Table 6-1 Statistical average and range of metal loss under ideal conditions*

PROCEDURE	LOSS (mm)
Electropolishing	0.041
Stoning	0.024
Rubber/ polishing	0.062
Total	0.127
Range	0.413–0.425

*As found by Brudvik and Reimers.[8]

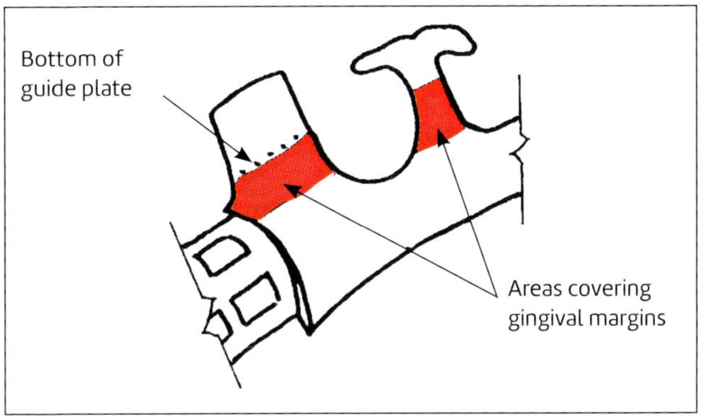

FIG 6-26 Internal view of casting indicating areas requiring high polish.

a minimum increase in flexibility to be expected.[9] If the blockout phase was handled accurately, there should not be need for adjustment to other inferences to the path of insertion. From there, the laboratory must be instructed to place the highest possible finish on the casting gingival to the contact area of the guide plate (Fig 6-26). This will require careful stoning and rubber wheeling so as not to abrade the contact areas. Statistically, it is this process of rubber wheel polishing that risks the greatest loss of metal (Table 6-1).[8] In a busy laboratory, using a high-speed lathe, this risk is greater still (Fig 6-27). This quality finish is required since plaque retention in this area has the greatest potential for tissue irritation. In fact, this is the only area of the partial denture for which there is a physiologic reason for polishing. All other surfaces could just as well be left in the as-cast state except that the technician, clinician, and patient expect the appliance to be highly polished as a customary finish for anything that goes into the mouth.

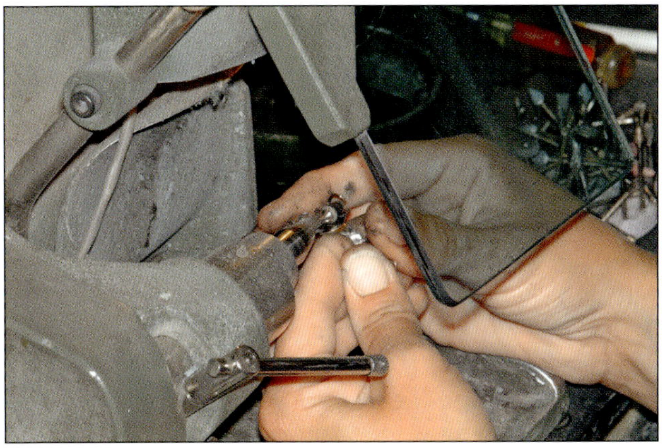

FIG 6-27 Due to the nature of RPD alloys, high-speed lathes are used for metal finishing.

The clinician has two options for seating the casting on the definitive cast when the framework requires the additional steps of adding wire clasps or altered cast trays. The casting can be returned to the clinician for the fitting of the frame and the fitted casting sent back to the laboratory on the definitive cast. Otherwise, the technician can be instructed to place the finished casting on a duplicate definitive cast while still at the laboratory, always at the expense of the stone teeth. The intraoral fitting of the framework can be done with the wires and the tray in place. However, it is generally easier to fit just the frame alone, as the wire clasps may interfere with the fit management process.

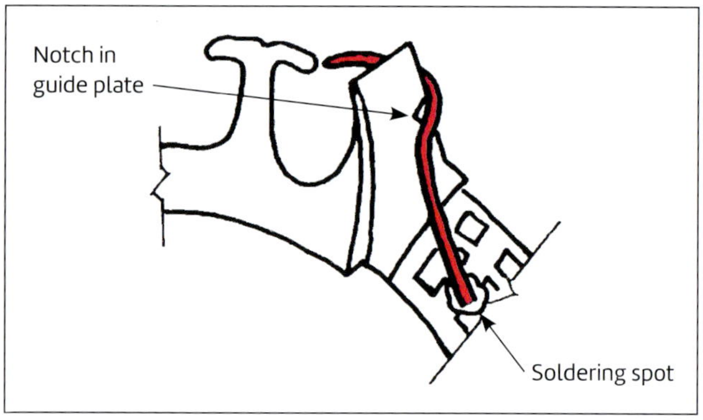

FIG 6-28 Position of the wire clasp on the framework.

While it is technically possible to cast to wires, this procedure is primarily used for gold base castings and wires with high gold content. When stellate alloys are used for the framework, the wire is best soldered to the finished framework some distance from the point of flexure. Casting a stellate alloy to a wire clasp or soldering the clasp directly to the minor connector will result in a more rigid and brittle clasp and increase the likelihood of subsequent clasp failure.[10]

Wires for retentive clasp arms are most often round in cross section.[11] It is possible, however, to use a half-round clasp wire. There is no clinical evidence that this form has any advantage over the simpler shape. In fact, the half-round wire is much more difficult to adapt to the tooth since any bend across the flat surface is a technical challenge. The desired position relative to the height of contour has been indicated on the definitive cast and marked with a single line. The technician should be able to contour the wire exactly to this line. For the wire I-bar, the clinician must indicate just how much of the foot of the clasp should contact the tooth. Usually a gentle bend 2 to 3 mm from the tip of the clasp will give sufficient linear contact to ensure a positive contact of clasp on tooth. The tips of either form of wire clasp should be rounded before they are soldered to the framework since access to the tip may be limited once the clasp is in place.

The wire clasp is adapted to the definitive cast with the framework in place. Occasionally, the guide plate is notched at the point where a circumferential clasp will exit the resin to position the clasp exactly as designed (Fig 6-28). The tang of the clasp is directed down the guide plate and onto the lingual surface of the casting. It will terminate in a positive contact area, either a retentive mesh square that has been filled in during the wax-up or to a retentive bead that has been flattened with a disk after casting. In either instance, the wire must make a positive contact with the casting for laser welding or brazing to be most effective. Laser welding, with minor power adjustments, will be effective regardless of the type of metal used for the wire or framework. The wire will also be physically retained by the resin, making debonding exceedingly rare. When using traditional resistance brazing, studies have shown that an 800 fine solder will produce the best joint with a nonprecious or a PGP (platinum, gold, and palladium) wire. Softer wires, such as those similar to the no longer available Jelenko Standard, are best soldered with a torch and 650 solder.

Sectional Construction

As will be further explained in chapter 15, frameworks were traditionally not cast in a single piece. Instead, in order to achieve acceptable passive fit, frameworks were made in pieces to be joined by some form of soldering. The one-piece casting technique, first proposed by Akers in 1925, was rapidly accepted primarily due to its economic benefits.[12] Unfortunately, one-piece castings are rarely able to achieve an ideal fit because of casting shrinkage. When the casting sprues are cut off, thermal-induced strains are released. Regardless of the management of the previous fabrication steps, a cast framework will always experience these distortions. The more complex the framework, the more likely casting shrinkage will have a significant effect. While this may not appreciably alter the functional fit of a Class I partial denture, a Class III partial denture casting with long edentulous spans, tall guiding planes, in a very wide arch, will almost certainly lack the ideal tooth-frame interface desired.

Sectional construction of RPD frameworks, more or less forgotten since the late 1930s, lived on only in the construction of precision attachment designs. These precision designs required very accurate interfaces, and in most situations, this meant that components were joined to the major connector using solder or acrylic resin. As technology has improved, the ability to economically and efficiently incorporate a sectional construction philosophy has returned. The major benefit of this concept is a

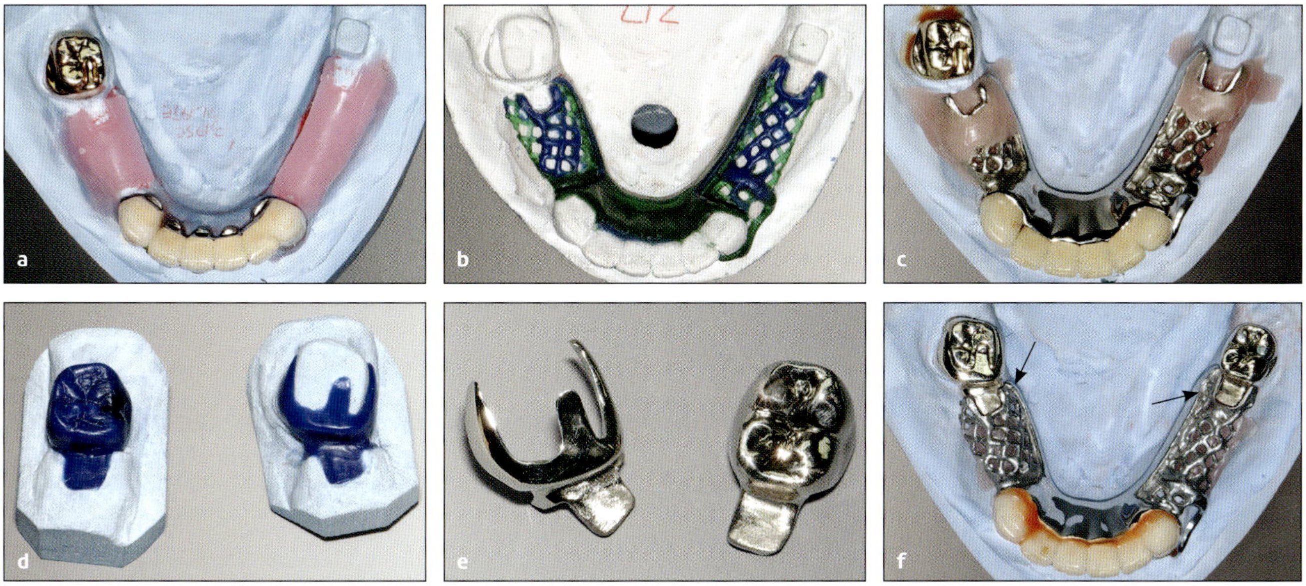

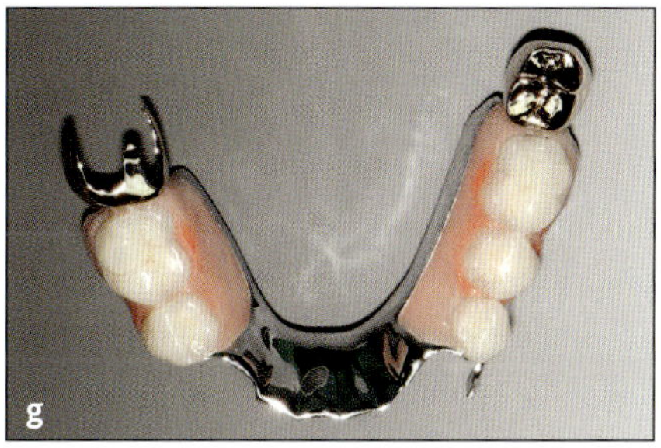

FIG 6-29 *(a)* Pickup cast ready for duplication. *(b)* Major connector portion of sectionally constructed mandibular Class III framework. *(c)* Anterior segment fit to anterior abutments and ready for posterior component fabrication. Note the recess created that allows beam access to the cameo and intaglio surface of the planned weld area. *(d)* Waxed distal components. *(e)* Cast distal components. *(f)* Distal components fit and ready for laser welding. The *arrows* highlight the intimacy of the joint seam. Pickup/weld will occur on the cast. *(g)* After welding, the partial denture is completed as normal.

more ideal tooth-frame interface and therefore a partial denture that functions as it was designed. Bert Cecconi described the return of the sectional construction philosophy when he wrote about the component partial.[13] He defined a *component partial* as an RPD whose framework is designed and constructed in separate parts. After fitting to the definitive cast, the components are joined during processing to become a single functioning unit. This technique originally used high-impact pourable acrylic resin. Now, however, component partials tend to be joined with laser welding (Fig 6-29).

While it is possible to section and solder a framework using resistance brazing, it is a challenging and technically sensitive procedure.[14] With the development of neodymium-doped yttrium-aluminum-garnet (Nd:YAG) and carbon dioxide lasers, this technology has taken the place of soldering and brazing in almost all applications. The accuracy and strength of this procedure has proven to be excellent.[15,16] The commercial laboratory that has supported the University of Washington Graduate Prosthodontics Program (Edgewood Dental Lab, Mukilteo, WA) used an Alpha ALC30 dental laser (Alpha Laser) beginning in 1998 (Fig 6-30). Back in 2005, using this laser to join the parts, the laboratory was averaging 8 to 10 component partials per month. Confidence with this technology has grown with time.

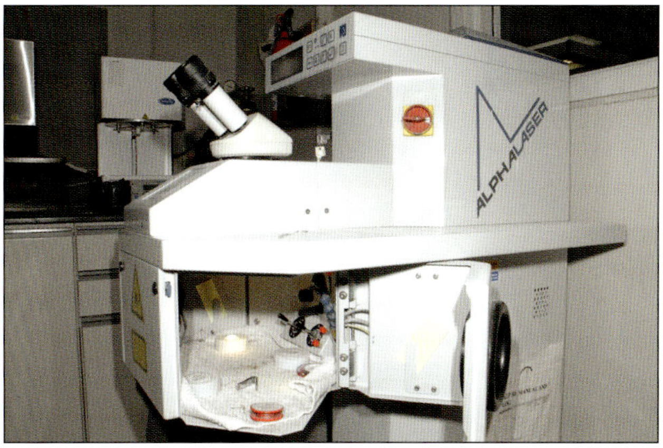

FIG 6-30 An Alpha Laser at a dental laboratory, circa 2008.

Research conducted at the University of Washington has shown that the influence of casting shrinkage and other aspects of the lost-wax technique can be resolved with

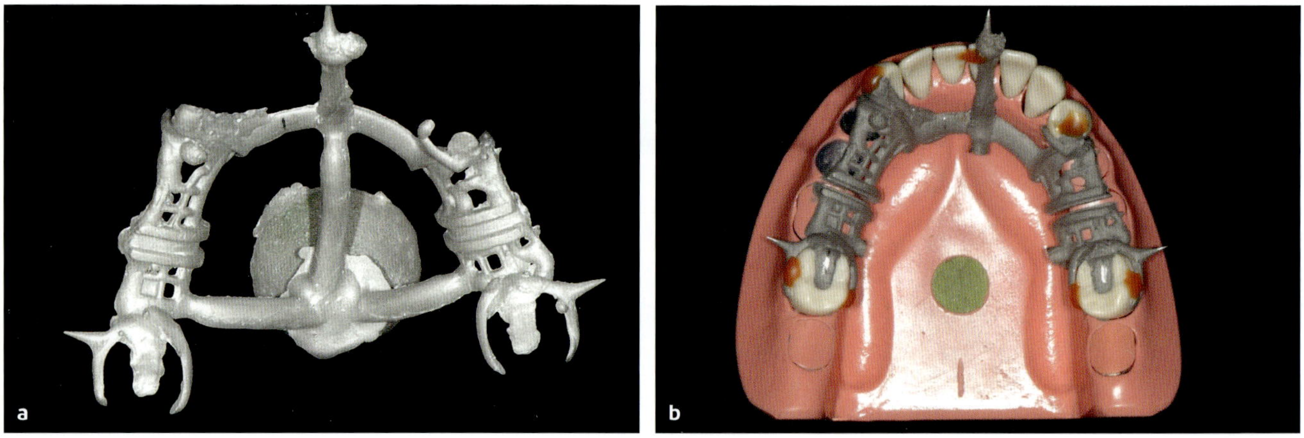

FIG 6-31 *(a)* Research casting with measuring points. After measurement, the sprue is cut off and the measurements are repeated. *(b)* Fit of casting measured again after sectioning and then again after the components are laser welded together. A secondary casting was used to minimize any gap at the weld.

sectional construction and laser welding[17] (Fig 6-31). The improved accuracy of fit demonstrated by this research, and two decades of regular clinical use, has proven that a higher level of tooth-frame interface accuracy can be efficiently achieved. Sectional construction using laser welding has become the preferred method of fabrication for any framework of significant complexity. These situations include, but are not limited to, precision attachments, custom housings, copings, overlays, Class IIs, Class IIIs, and Class Vs. Several clinical scenarios have been published and can be reviewed in detail.[18–20]

Access to laser welding has reached the point where benchtop units, meant for use within a dental office, are available at a reasonable cost. Despite this, it is still most common to delegate this step to the laboratory. The Alpha ALC30 laser uses the following manufacturer settings:

- *Volts:* 273 VDc
- *Pulse:* 3.0 Hz
- *Width of weld:* 0.8 mm, followed by 1.5 mm to smooth the joint

These settings are routinely used for the welding of cobalt-based alloys. Each manufacturer will have different recommended settings for different alloys. Standard laser welding procedure includes tack welding in four or more widely spaced locations. These tacks maintain the relationship of the components while the technician then returns to one end of the joint for the continuous weld of the seam. As the laser hits and melts the metal, the beam loses energy. This results in a triangular or wedge-shaped weld zone, with the wider part of the weld at the surface and the narrower portion at the interior. The deeper or taller the joint, the less effectively melted, and therefore weaker, the internal region of the joint will be.

The energy settings of the machine can modify the total width and depth of the weld, but the wedge shape will remain. This is managed in three primary ways. First, each laser weld beam or shot is overlapped with the one before it. By overlapping the wedge-shaped "effective zone," more of the internal surface area is welded. When there is no overlapping, the space between the welds at the narrower portion of the wedges remains unaffected and not welded. Second, the joints are best fabricated in close proximity. If there is a large gap between the two pieces, only the outer surface of the beam will touch and melt metal. This results in a weld with minimal surface area. In very large gaps, where the beam cannot affect metal on both sides at the same time, use of a filler material is required to bridge the gap. This filler material is weaker than the parent metals that preferably make up the weld. If a frame is made in a single piece and then sectioned, the gap between components tends to be fairly wide. This sometimes requires a secondary casting to bridge the gap and create an intimate fit between cast parts before welding. This additional step is typically avoided by creating one casting and then the other. The second casting can be made to fit intimately into a recess in the first casting (Fig 6-32). The close contact of the parts with this method facilitates a strong laser weld without the use of filler material.

The third technique to maximize weld effectiveness is to design the joint area in such a way that it can be welded from both sides. The laser beam should have access to the seam from both the cameo and intaglio surfaces (Fig 6-33). This doubles the surface area and depth of the weld, thereby increasing its strength. When mesh is the acrylic retention of choice, achieving access for the beam is an easy task. The joint or seam is best positioned away from abutment teeth, where minor connectors may interfere with direct access for the laser beam. For frame designs with metal on the

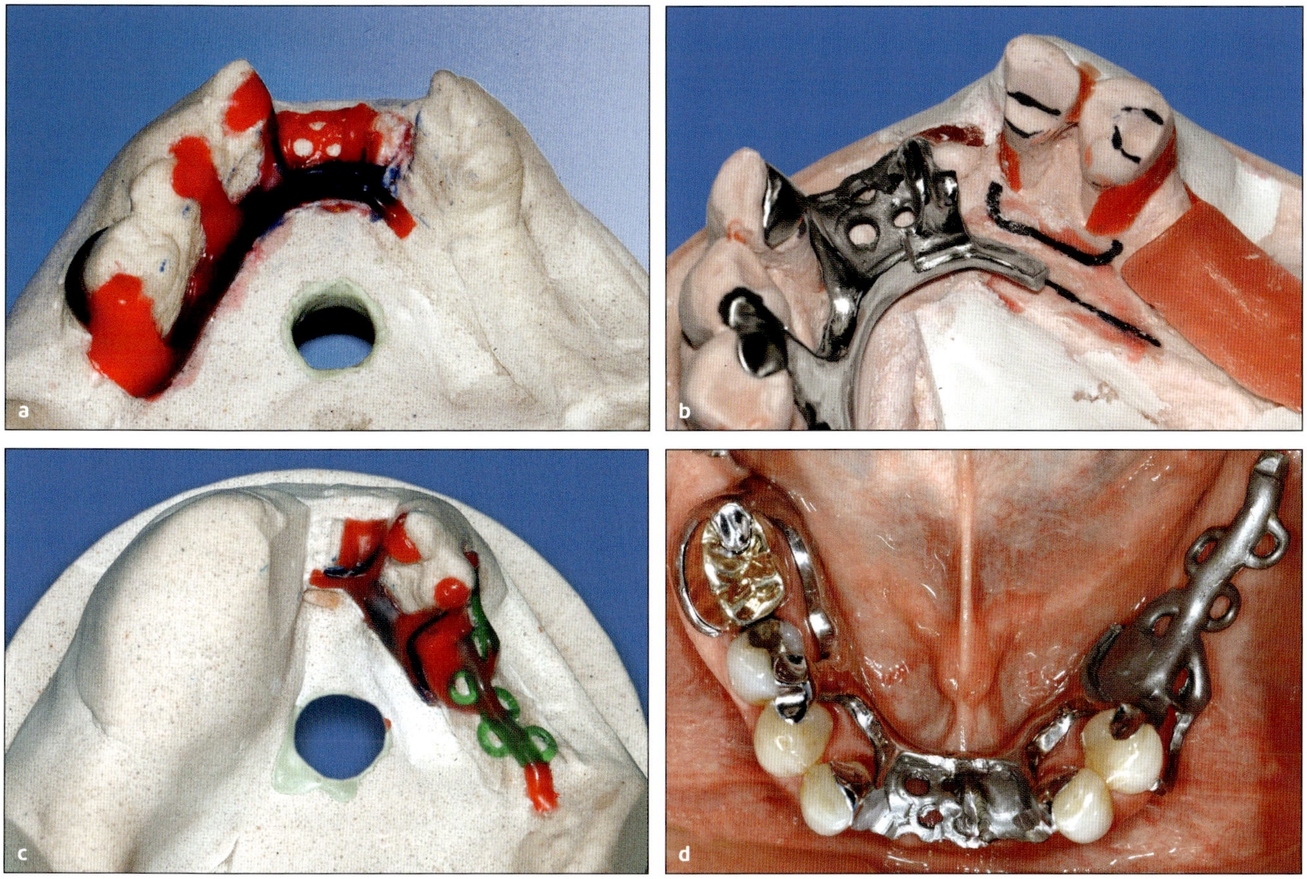

FIG 6-32 *(a)* First half of framework designed with multiangled interface for a strong weld. *(b)* First half cast, fit, and on cast. Note the lingual bar interface for the planned weld. *(c)* Refractory cast of first half, with second half of frame waxed. *(d)* Completed framework at clinical try-in appointment.

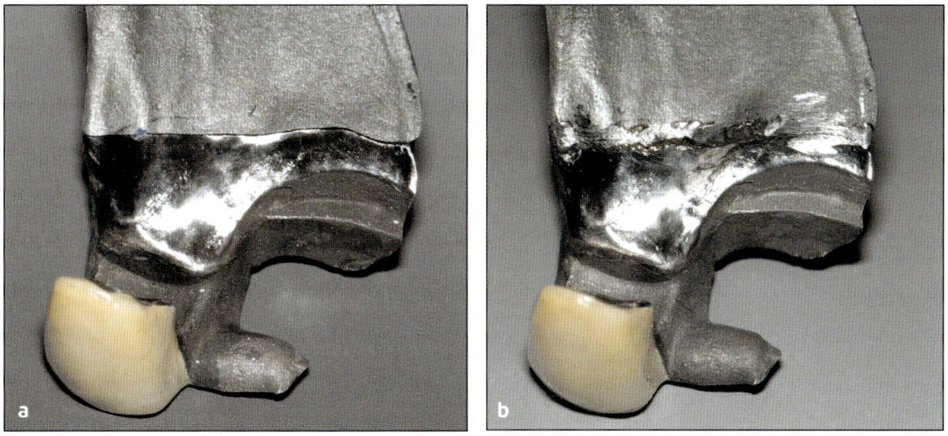

FIG 6-33 *(a)* Internal seam between as-cast palatal strap and polished custom overlay, prior to laser welding. *(b)* Same seam after laser welding. The component was also welded from the external surface.

tissue, some degree of accurate tissue contact may be lost. However, this is generally minimal and not detrimental in what is typically a tooth-bound situation (Fig 6-34).

There is a question for the clinician as to when and how to relate the components during sectional construction. Cecconi advocated for and reported excellent results when joining the components on the definitive cast.[13] This prevents the need for additional chair time, and if the cast is trusted, has the potential to eliminate the need for a framework try-in appointment. If a pickup impression has been created, discussed in detail in chapter 11, the components are best connected in the laboratory (see Figs 6-29f and

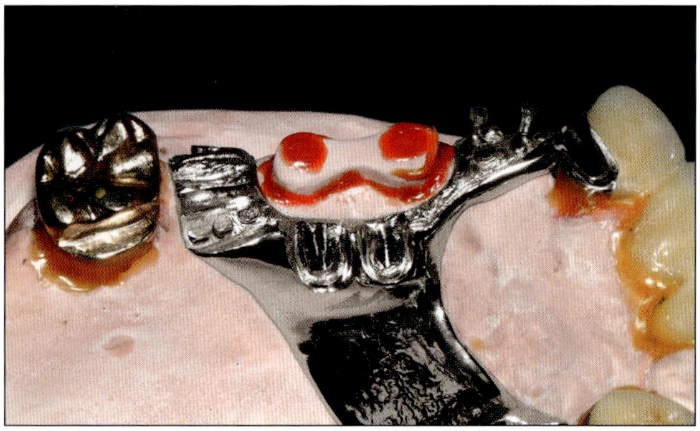

FIG 6-34 Component partial fit to pickup cast. Note the design of recesses for secondary components: a clasp assembly for tooth no. 2 and a housing over the implant bar.

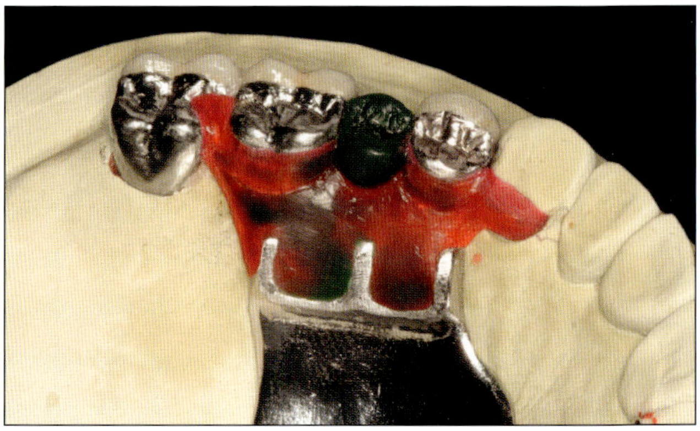

FIG 6-35 A custom overlay/rest assembly made from acrylic resin and wax. The pattern is removable and will be cast.[20]

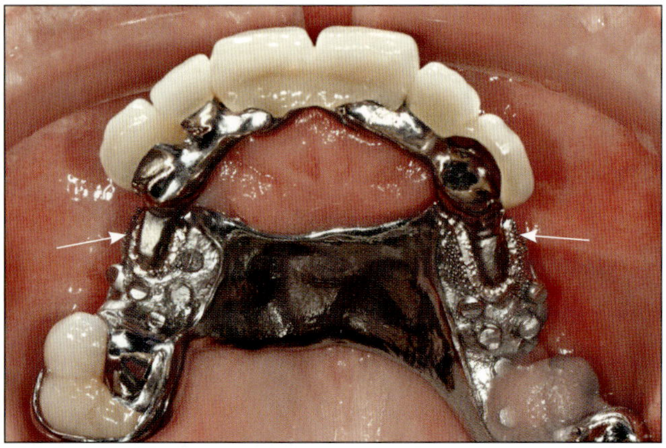

FIG 6-36 Due to mobile central incisors, the anterior components were picked up clinically. Once laser welded, the frame is tried in. Note that a locator housing at site no. 3 is picked up as well.

6-34). The accuracy of these casts, and the ability to relate the components directly to the abutment crowns on the pickup cast, facilitate an ideal fit of the component framework (Fig 6-35).[20] When the accuracy of the definitive cast can be questioned, as with mobile abutment teeth that tend to be displaced during the impression, relating the components clinically is the better choice. This is done by first fitting each individual piece. Once fit, the components are joined with an acrylic resin such as GC Pattern Resin. After setting, the joined parts can be removed and supported by a rigid index.[17] After removing the pickup acrylic, the parts are welded. A final try-in of the now one-piece framework will confirm the result. Due to the additional time and effort involved, clinical pickup of the components is generally reserved for situations where creating an accurate definitive cast is difficult to accomplish (Fig 6-36). This tends to include periodontally involved, mobile, malpositioned, or exceptionally tall abutments. If this is the case, it is more likely that a clinical pickup technique would save time and achieve a better result. This is why the clinician must make the decision on where to relate the components.

Once the framework is in one piece, with a confirmed fit, it is handled the same as a typical partial denture framework. Sectional construction, combined with the other fit management techniques described in this textbook, provides the ability to control all critical sources of misfit. Where it was once an unreasonable hardship, technologic advances have made it an efficient and everyday procedure in most laboratories. It therefore becomes one of the final pieces to the overall puzzle for the ideal functional results achieved with the advanced RPD.

Digitally Based Construction

The significant volume of critical and intricate steps for analog framework construction exists regardless of whether a one-piece or sectional technique is used. It is exciting to see that digital manufacturing has the potential to be more accurate than the one-piece casting technique and more efficient than sectional construction. Digital processes can be incorporated at several points in the provision of care (Table 6-2).

Due to the theoretical advantages, the ultimate goal is a fully digital workflow. Elimination of analog casts and casting shrinkage would result in significant chair time savings for the clinician. As noted in chapter 5, however, the digital scanning process has yet to match the accuracy, efficiency, and reliability of the conventional analog technique, at least for complex partially edentulous situations. This leaves the current discussion to begin at the point of having an analog definitive cast.

A laboratory benchtop scanner is used to digitize the analog definitive cast (Fig 6-37a). These units tend to be more accurate than intraoral scanners, in part because there is better access to all surfaces and contours. Once digitized, the data are managed

Table 6-2 Overview of analog and digital workflows for RPD fabrication

WORKFLOW	INTRAORAL RECORDING	FRAMEWORK DESIGN	PATTERN FABRICATION	FRAMEWORK FABRICATION
Traditional	Impression	Analog	Waxing	Lost wax
Semidigital 1	Impression	Digital	Printed/milled	Lost wax
Semidigital 2	Intraoral scan	Digital	Printed/milled	Lost wax
Fully digital	Intraoral scan	Digital	None	Printed/milled

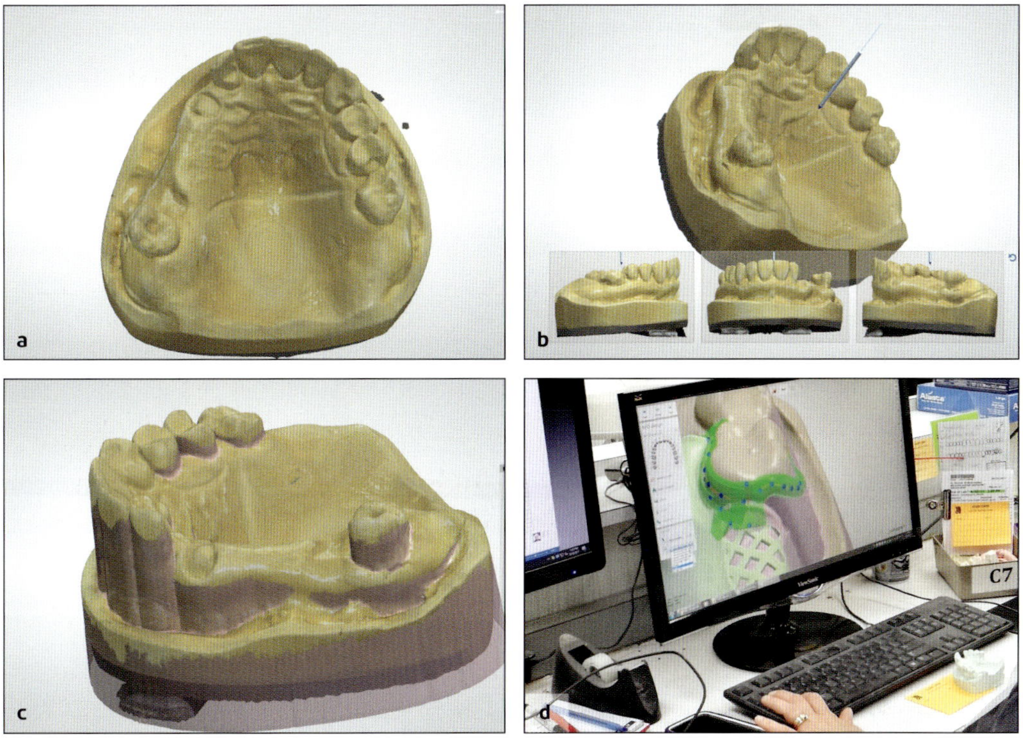

FIG 6-37 *(a)* Screenshot of a digitized cast. *(b)* Finding the path of insertion. *(c)* Digital blockout. *(d)* Design software on screen.

with some form of computer-aided design (CAD) software. It is here, within the software, where the same steps conducted during the analog process must occur on the digital cast (Fig 6-37b). This means, of course, that all undesired undercuts are blocked out just as previously described (Fig 6-37c). The RPD design can then be transferred from the analog cast to the 3D virtual cast on the technician's screen (Fig 6-37d).

It is a challenge for those experienced with analog fabrication to interpret changes and designs in digital format. Part of this is due to the limited ability of a 2D screen to demonstrate 3D form. Something as basic as determining and maintaining the path of insertion or heights of contour is a complicated formula for the design software to reliably execute. It is assumed, by both technicians and clinicians, that the precision of the digital representation on the screen is the same as that on the cast or in the mouth. Unfortunately, this is not necessarily the case. Just as water-powder ratios of stone must be constantly calibrated, so too must the data transfer process and data management software. As with any new technique, this creates frustration for those incorporating this technology without full and attentive technical support. Larger dental laboratories with extensive resources are more likely to have this support. Whether high-volume laboratories are able to maintain the highest standards necessary for the advanced RPD can be questioned.

After CAD is complete, a virtual framework exists within the design software (Fig 6-38). At this point, there are two basic ways to proceed. Either a pattern of the framework or the framework itself can be manufactured. With a semidigital workflow, a resin pattern of the framework (Fig 6-39) is printed by a stereolithographic printer. This pattern is then sprued, invested, and cast using the traditional lost-wax technique. When compared with traditional techniques, this process does not seem to incorporate dramatic benefits. It leaves casting shrinkage unresolved and may simply be trading issues with the blockout and waxing process for problems with resin pattern accuracy.

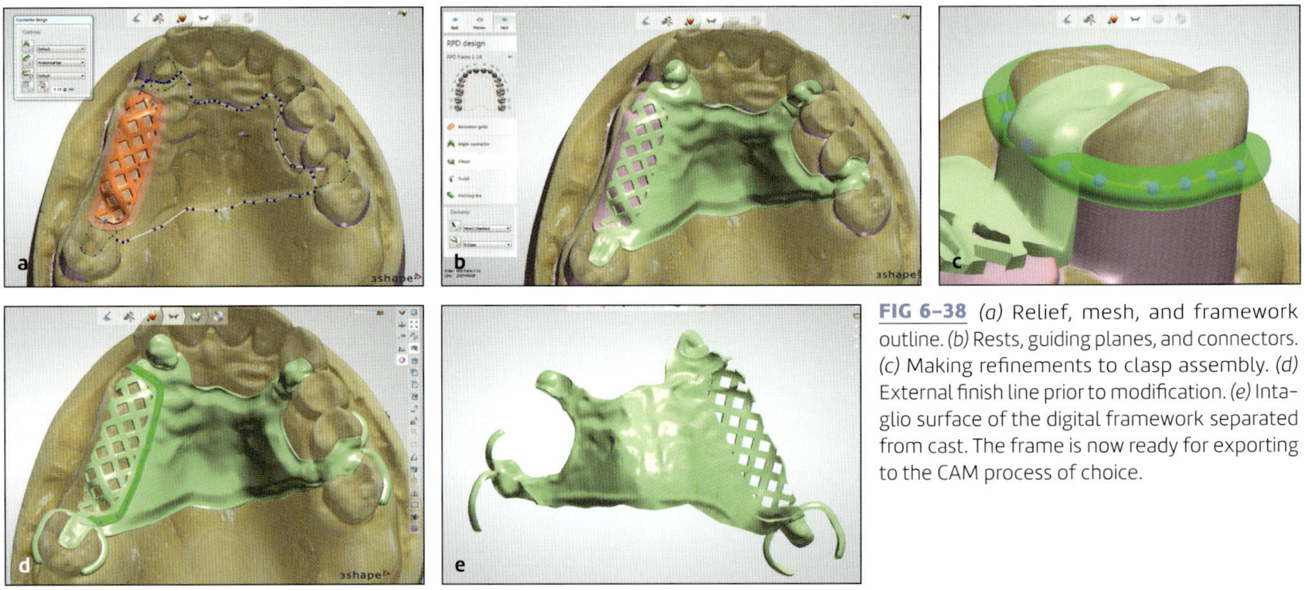

FIG 6-38 *(a)* Relief, mesh, and framework outline. *(b)* Rests, guiding planes, and connectors. *(c)* Making refinements to clasp assembly. *(d)* External finish line prior to modification. *(e)* Intaglio surface of the digital framework separated from cast. The frame is now ready for exporting to the CAM process of choice.

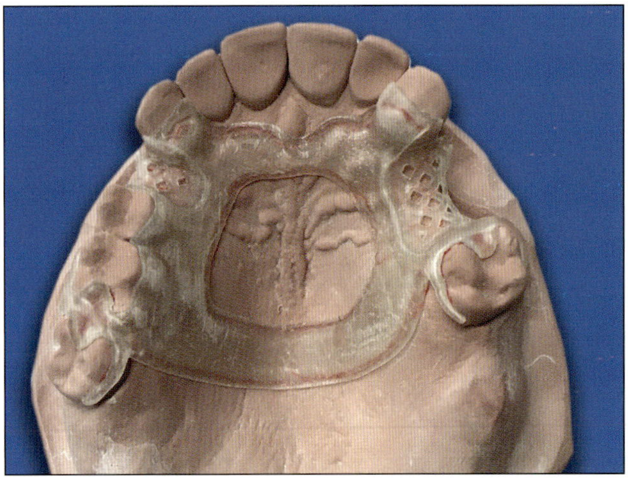

FIG 6-39 Printed resin framework pattern.

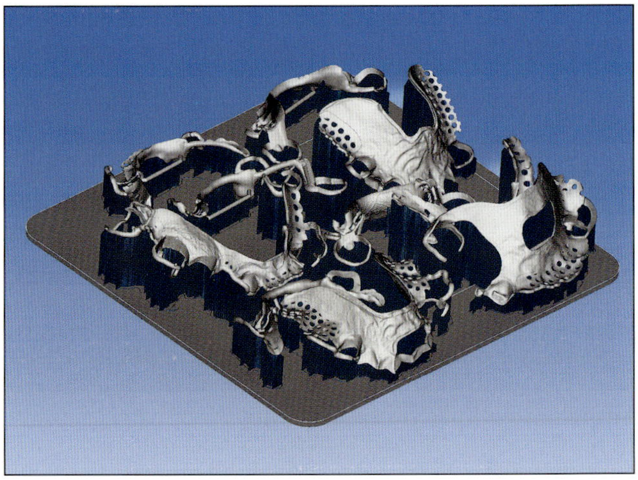

FIG 6-40 Multiple digital frameworks nested and ready for printing.

Instead of managing the inherent accuracy challenges of lost wax, computer-assisted manufacturing (CAM) processes, such as milling and laser sintering, could potentially create frameworks with fewer flaws, comparable accuracy, and greater efficiency (Fig 6-40). Fewer flaws can be expected since the frameworks come from either a manufactured block of material or powder that is melted with a laser. Milling, in particular, reduces the incorporation of voids when compared to the more random casting technique. Likewise, if the material is not cast, the problem of casting shrinkage will be eliminated. From a manufacturing standpoint, these methods could be more efficient since, once designed and programmed, machines are doing the actual fabrication (Fig 6-41). While milling has been applied with great success to crown and bridge dentistry, the size and intricacy of RPD frameworks is currently difficult to accurately mill and results in excessive material waste. Selective laser melting (3D printing), on the other hand, is being used successfully in practice for metal RPD framework manufacturing. This process appears to result in excellent mechanical properties such as improved fatigue resistance when compared with casting.[21] However, there are significant challenges with accuracy of fit and manufacturing imperfections.[22–24]

The preferred process for selective laser melting (SLM) is described well in a pilot clinical trial from McGill University in Montreal.[25] Definitive casts were scanned and the frameworks were designed digitally using the currently

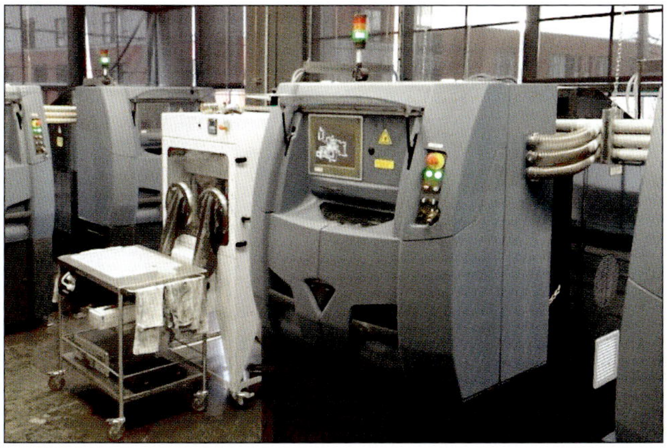

FIG 6-41 SLM printers.

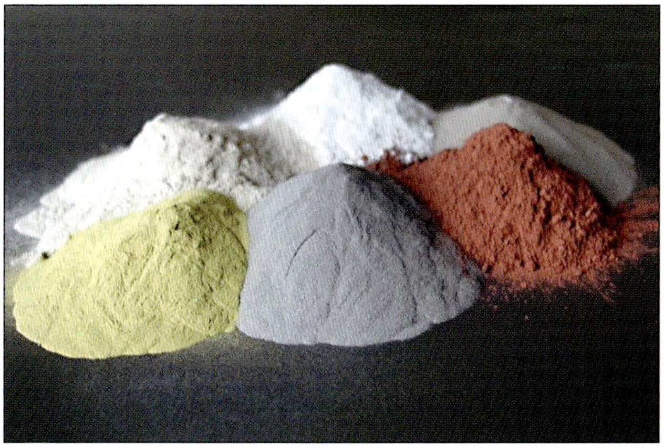

FIG 6-42 Alloy powders for SLM printing.

popular 3Shape CAD Points software, which has been further improved since this article was published. The STL (standard tessellation language) digital data were sent to a rapid prototyping machine where an SLM technique used cobalt-chromium alloy powder to create the framework (Fig 6-42). In a demonstration of how rapidly this technology evolves, the design software and prototyping machine used in this study have both been replaced by newer versions. While the results of this pilot study indicated that patients preferred laser-sintered framework partial dentures, the comparison appears to be moot. Only 12 partial dentures were followed up at a total of 4 weeks for each fabrication method, and most of the partial dentures were Kennedy Class I or II. More importantly from the standpoint of this book is the fact that these partial dentures do not appear to have been subjected to the dedicated detail and analysis of fit deemed so critical to a long-term functional result. As more is published on these developing technologies, it is hoped that the comparisons will be made with the proven principles of this book in mind rather than comparing a technology in the context of the everyday partial denture as it currently exists. In other words, a long-term randomized controlled trial to compare the outcomes of digitally fabricated RPDs with those of traditionally fabricated analog RPDs will be irrelevant unless standards of design and fit are stringently followed. This is because it wouldn't matter how a partial denture was made if it doesn't fit as described in this book. This is part of what makes these research projects so challenging.

While the current state of efficiency, cost, and accuracy are such that analog construction remains more common, it is obvious that the use of digital manufacturing will continue to rapidly increase. Regardless of this fact, the basic sequence, principles, and desired results highlighted in this book are not expected to appreciably change with a digital workflow. There will be little evidence-based guidance for clinicians until the fit of frameworks is compared and evaluated in the mouth, something that—truth be told—has rarely occurred even for conventional methods. Therefore, as clinicians or their technicians incorporate these technologic advancements, they must remain cognizant of whether digital recording, designing, or manufacturing will actually result in a better or less costly (but equally high-quality) prosthesis for the patient.

Nonmetal Definitive RPD Frameworks

As CAM processes have become more common, it has increased the ability to utilize newer materials. The lost-wax technique, by its very nature, is not compatible with materials that cannot be conventionally cast. Milling and laser printing both allow a greater variety of materials to be manufactured. In particular, nonmetal definitive framework alternatives are available with these methods. An alternative material could prove beneficial to better manage the challenging fabrication techniques, color, allergic potential, and, to a certain extent, weight of metal frameworks.

The majority of these newer materials lack the rigidity necessary for adequate cross-arch stability. These materials, namely polyamide and improved polymethyl methacrylate, are discussed in detail in chapter 10. However, high-strength polymers have been developed for RPD frameworks. These aim for an ideal combination of esthetics and mechanical properties. Many of these have been used in the medical field for some time, but with the mainstream use of CAM, have now been introduced to prosthetic dentistry.[26]

The polymer currently showing the most promise is polyaryletherketone (PAEK). These polymers are semicrystalline thermoplastics that typically have high temperature stability and mechanical strength. Within dentistry, polyetheretherketone

(PEEK) is the best known of these polymers. It was originally introduced for engineering purposes in the early 1980s and is currently used extensively in the aerospace, automotive, and chemical process industries. PEEK is also considered an advanced biomaterial and is used as part of medical implants for neurosurgical and orthopedic applications. In dentistry, PEEK has been used for dental implant components and as superstructures for prosthodontic appliances.[27,28] Modified PEEK is being used for RPD frameworks, buts it lacks any significant scientific comparisons.[29] Due to the reduced expense of the material, manufacturing waste from milling is less of a concern. The milling process appears to result in PEEK frameworks that fit more accurately than if made in cast metal or by an indirect technique.[22,30] A major limitation, however, is that these frameworks do not handle like metal and are difficult to precisely adjust. The material tends to melt and peel when adjusted rather than being simply cut away. This complicates the chairside fitting that is critical to achieve an ideal clinical fit, especially in Class III situations. PEEK also lacks the ability to be repaired or corrected. This means that if a fracture or poor clinical fit is found at trial evaluation, the framework creation process and recording of the intraoral condition will need to be repeated. Whether the benefits of this material will outweigh these negatives remains to be seen.

The advancements in manufacturing processes and materials make this an exciting time for RPDs. Regardless of these changes, the sequence, principles, and results highlighted in this book are not expected to appreciably change. This means the job, and its goals, will remain the same, while the process through which it is realized will gradually transition into a digital format. Once this does come to pass, it is hoped that the software and CAD programs incorporate the more sophisticated details and goals highlighted here rather than the limited poor-quality RPD philosophy that is pervasive in general practice. Herein lies the major concern and reason for slow adoption by advanced RPD practitioners. These clinicians know that the usual advanced RPD does not fit well within the "box" of current fully digital dentistry.

References

1. Rudd RW, Rudd KD. A review of 243 errors possible during the fabrication of a removable partial denture: Part II. J Prosthet Dent 2001;86:262–276.
2. Schwarz W, Barsby M. Design of partial dentures in dental practice. J Dent 1978;6:166–170.
3. Taylor TD, Matthews AC, Aquilino SA, Logan NS. Prosthodontic survey. Part I: Removable prosthodontic laboratory survey. J Prosthet Dent 1984;52:598–601.
4. Hardy F, Stuart LM. A critique of materials submitted by dentists to dental laboratories for the fabrication of removable partial dentures. Quintessence Dent Technol 1983;7:93–95.
5. Dootz ER, Craig RG, Peyton FA. Influence of investment and duplicating procedure on the accuracy of partial denture castings. J Prosthet Dent 1965;15:679–690.
6. Rantanen T, Eerikainen E. Accuracy of the palatal plate of removable partial dentures, and influence of laboratory handling of the investment on the accuracy. Dent Mater 1986;2:28–31.
7. Morris HF, Asgar K, Brudvik JS, Winkler S, Roberts EP. Stress-relaxation testing. Part IV: Clasp pattern dimensions and their influence on clasp behavior. J Prosthet Dent 1983;50:319–226.
8. Brudvik JS, Reimers D. The tooth-removable partial denture interface. J Prosthet Dent 1992;68:924–927.
9. Morris HF, Brudvik JS. Influence of polishing on cast clasp properties. J Prosthet Dent 1986;55:75–77.
10. Brudvik JS, Wormley JH. Construction techniques for wrought-wire retentive clasp arms as related to clasp flexibility. J Prosthet Dent 1973;30:769–774.
11. Brudvik JS, Morris HF. Stress-relaxation testing. Part III: Influence of wire alloys, gauges, and lengths on clasp behavior. J Prosthet Dent 1981;46:374–79.
12. Akers PE. A new and simplified method of partial denture prosthesis. J Am Dent Assoc 1925;12:711–717.
13. Cecconi BT, Campagni WV, Cecconi ML. The component partial: A new RPD construction system. Calif Dent Assoc J 1997;25:371–376.
14. Brudvik JS, Nicholls JI. Soldering of removable partial dentures. J Prosthet Dent 1983;49:762–765.
15. NaBadalung DP, Nicholls JI. Laser welding of a cobalt-chromium removable partial denture alloy. J Prosthet Dent 1998;79:285–290.
16. Bertrand C, Le Petticorps Y, Albingre L, Dupuis V. The laser welding technique applied to the nonprecious dental alloys procedure and results. Br Dent J 2001;190:255–257.
17. Brudvik JS, Lee S, Croshaw SN, Reimers DL. Laser welding of removable partial denture frameworks. Int J Prosthodont 2008;21:285–291.
18. Goto Y, Brudvik JS. Custom precision attachment housings for removable partial dentures. J Prosthet Dent 2002;88:100–102.
19. Ma PS, Brudvik JS. Managing the maxillary partially edentulous patient with extensive anterior tooth loss and advanced periodontal disease using a removable partial denture: A clinical report. J Prosthet Dent 2008;100:259–263.
20. Domagala D, Waliszewski MP. A maxillary laser-welded component removable partial denture—A clinical report. J Prosthet Dent 2009;101:1–6.
21. Alageel O, Abdallah MN, Alsheghri A, Song J, Caron E, Tamimi F. Removable partial denture alloys processed by laser-sintering technique. J Biomed Mater Res B Appl Biomater 2018;106:1174–1185.
22. Arnold C, Hey J, Schweyen R, Setz JM. Accuracy of CAD-CAM-fabricated removable partial dentures. J Prosthet Dent 2018;119:586–592.
23. Soltanzadeh P, Suprono MS, Kattadiyil MT, et. al. An in vitro investigation of accuracy and fit of conventional and CAD/CAM removable partial denture frameworks. J Prosthodont 2019;28:547–555.
24. Chen H, Li H, Zhao Y, et. al. Adaptation of removable partial denture frameworks fabricated by selective laser melting. J Prosthet Dent 2019;122:316–324.
25. Almufleh B, Emami E, Alageel O, et al. Patient satisfaction with laser-sintered removable partial dentures: A crossover pilot clinical trial. J Prosthet Dent 2018;119:560–567.
26. Campbell SD, Cooper L, Craddock H, et. al. Removable partial dentures: The clinical need for innovation. J Prosthet Dent 2017;118:273–280.
27. Bathala L, Majeti V, Rachuri N, Singh N, Gedela S. The role of polyether ether ketone (PEEK) in dentistry—A review. J Med Life 2019;12:5–9.
28. Najeeb S, Zafar MS, Khurshid Z, Siddiqui F. Applications of polyetheretherketone (PEEK) in oral implantology and prosthodontics. J Prosthodont Res 2016;60:12–19.
29. Zoidis P, Papathanasiou I, Polyzois G. The use of a modified poly-ether-ether-ketone (PEEK) as an alternative framework material for removable dental prostheses. A clinical report. J Prosthodont 2016;25:580–584.
30. Negm EE, Aboutaleb FA, Alam-Eldein AM. Virtual evaluation of the accuracy of fit and trueness in maxillary poly(etheretherketone) removable partial denture frameworks fabricated by direct and indirect CAD/CAM techniques. J Prosthodont 2019;28:804–810.

ESTABLISHING THE TOOTH-FRAME RELATIONSHIP

7

The fit is the thing.

Just as Dr Carl Boucher's quote highlights the impression tray as "the thing" in edentulous treatment, so too should the fit be "the thing" in RPD treatment. The accuracy of the tooth-frame interface will determine whether the partial denture will function according to its design. A well-designed partial denture that does not fit will fail to control forces. Therefore, it is here, during the process of fitting the framework, that the technical skill of the dentist will impact the clinical outcome of the RPD. Because the laboratory technician has not touched the tooth-contact areas of the framework during the recovery and finishing of the framework, the responsibility for fitting the frame devolves entirely to the clinician. While this may be interpreted by some as unnecessary and time-consuming, we see no other way to obtain the highest quality fit of the casting and to retain the frictional fit of the guide plates on the prepared guiding planes. This procedure is more or less the same regardless of how the framework was manufactured.

Removal of Casting Bubbles

There are three distinct phases of the fitting procedure. The first step is to examine the casting under magnification and to carefully remove all the blebs on the tooth-contacting surfaces (see Fig 6-25), primarily the guide plates.[1] These bubbles and blebs are a consequence of the porous surface and grain size of the refractory stone to which the alloy must be cast. Because stellate alloys are so much harder than gold alloys, adjustments are not easily or quickly accomplished. Special burs are available for these alloys. Several bur manufacturers make specific carbide cutters for nonprecious metals to be used in a straight handpiece and intended to run at 10,000–15,000 rpm. These burs come in a variety of sizes and in both regular and fine cut. There are also fully sintered diamond stones that are intended for use with chrome alloys. Both of these options will tend to cut smoother, last longer, and cut with less heat than standard burs and stones. The goal at this point is to remove the positive imperfections without changing the contact surface of the guide plate. Once the blebs have been removed, the contact surfaces are sandblasted to leave a uniform matte surface; this will make the identification of premature contacts easier. As noted in chapter 6, a skilled and trusted laboratory technician who is taught the need to maintain the surfaces in an as-cast condition can complete this step.

Static Fit

The second step is to obtain a static fit in the mouth where the framework fully and accurately seats on the prepared teeth. Using magnifying loops and a sharp explorer, this fit is verified first visually

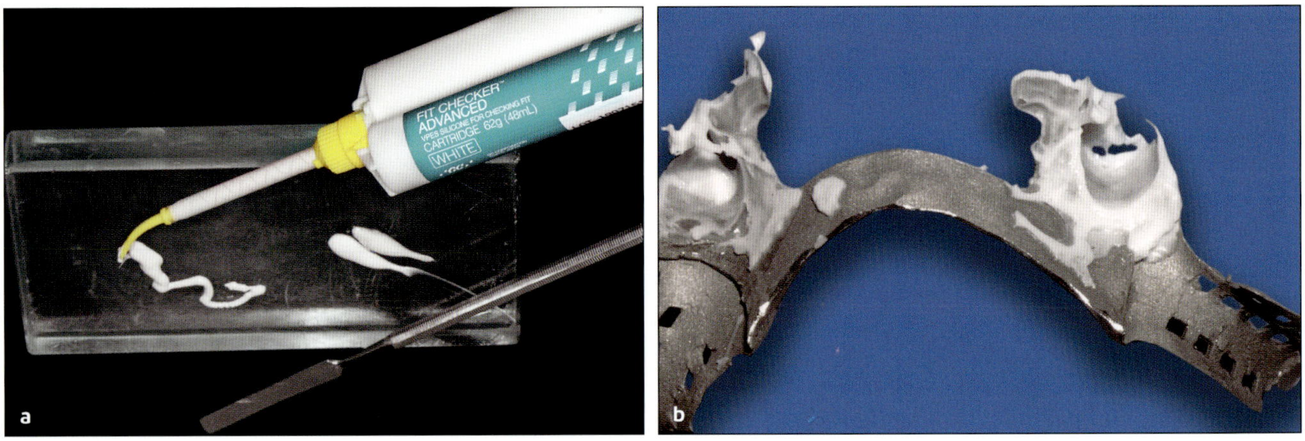

FIG 7-1 *(a)* Fit Checker hand-mixed silicone paste. *(b)* Checking the static fit with silicone.

and eventually with the aid of various marking mediums. The static fitting process should begin with an attempt to seat the framework without any marking medium. The initial focus is on the feel of the framework as it goes to place. With experience, the clinician will gain a sense of if and where the frame is binding. Class III frameworks made according the principles in this text will have a very specific path of insertion. It is common, even for an experienced clinician, to take several moments finding this exact path. Once it is found, it is also common that the frame will glide along this path until a point just short of complete seating. At this point, no further pressure should be applied and the frame should instead be removed so the marking process can begin.

Materials

Historically, disclosing waxes or a mixture of gold rouge in chloroform were used to identify premature contact areas. Both have been discontinued; the waxes because they were a mess to apply and to clean up and the chloroform-rouge mixture because of the concerns related to the volatility of the chemical and its toxic nature. Two convenient substitutes have been found in low-viscosity fast-setting silicone pastes like Fit Checker (GC America) and paint-on or spray-on aerosol marking powders like Occlude (Pascal International). Fit Checker is a quick-setting silicone, intended for evaluating the fit of crowns, that works equally well for frameworks (Fig 7-1a). It identifies contact points in a static fit only, since it sets chemically (Fig 7-1b). Spray-on powders, also used for evaluating the internal fit of crowns, can be applied in very thin layers and into the various tight corners and angles found within the internal portions of frameworks. Because the spray adheres to the metal surface, it tends to be easier to handle than the silicone materials, which may peel away from the frame as it is removed for evaluation. The spray-on powders work best in a moisture-controlled environment, as excessive amounts of saliva can distort the appearance. Another handling downside of the powders is that, with repeated applications, their thickness can increase to the point of altering the complete seating of the frame. If repeated checks are necessary, the excess must be removed prior to application of a new coat. This is easily accomplished with a steamer or in an ultrasonic bath.

A marking material that is cleaner, and in many instances more accurate, is articulating paper or tape such as Accu-Film II (Parkell). This product is a 21-μm-thick double-sided flexible plastic articulating tape. The thin, flexible material fits and adapts itself between the frame and the teeth as the frame is seated. A thin coating of petroleum jelly (eg, Vaseline, Unilever) applied to the tape facilitates marking of polished or wet surfaces. The material is also quite moisture resistant, making it a better choice than a spray-on powder when moisture control is not feasible. The different colors on each side of the tape improve identification of binding areas, as dye will be deposited on both the tooth and the point(s) of premature contact with the framework.

Having felt the proper path of insertion and initial binding point (Fig 7-2a), small pieces of the tape are placed between the framework and the abutments (Fig 7-2b). The frame is then seated with bilateral finger pressure along the path of insertion until the point of solid binding is felt (Fig 7-2c). It is best to use separate pieces of tape for separate abutment segments. The framework is then removed and the markings evaluated (Figs 7-2d and 7-2e). The tape will provide *positive markings*, meaning there will be color

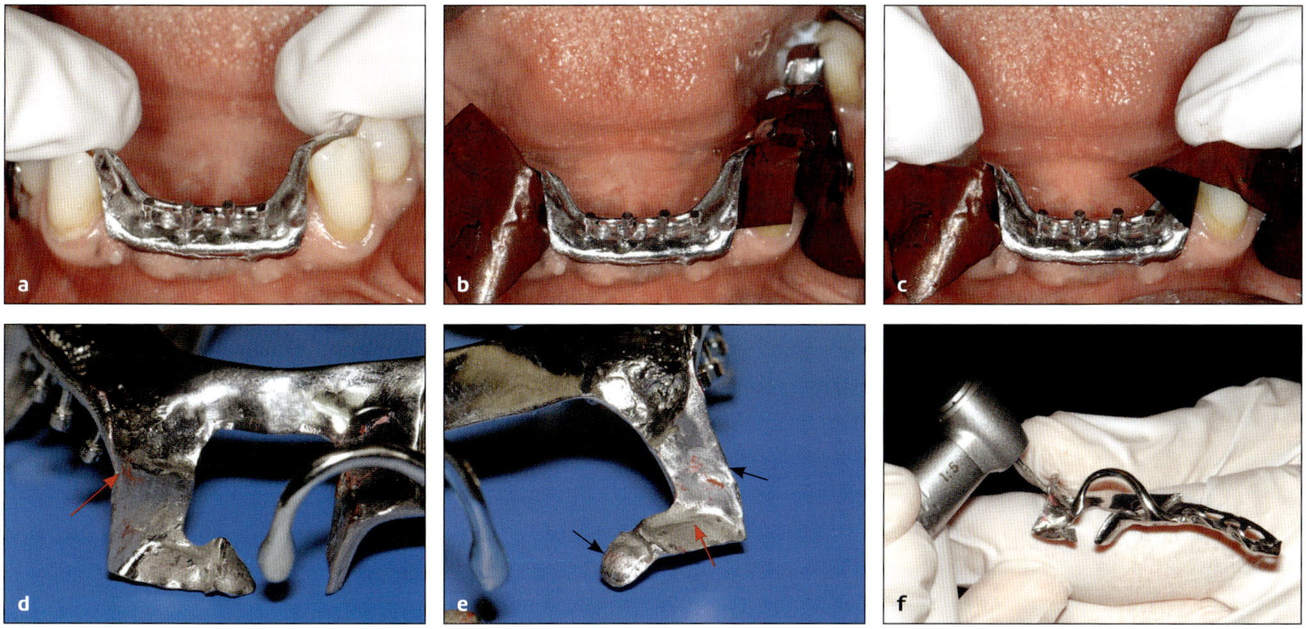

FIG 7-2 *(a)* Initial test seating of a framework stopping short of complete seating. *(b)* Articulating tape is placed between the tooth-contacting surfaces. *(c)* Slight finger pressure to feel and mark the premature binding areas. *(d)* Contact area limiting seating is highlighted by the *arrow*. The red marking further coronal on the guide plate will be maintained. *(e) Black arrows* indicate positive contacts in proper locations. The *red arrow* shows the rest area lacking positive contact. *(f)* Adjustment to area highlighted by the *red arrow* in part *d*.

present in the areas that are contacting. The silicone pastes and powder sprays will provide *negative markings*, meaning the areas that are rubbed away to show framework are the areas that are contacting.

Making adjustments

The marked areas of binding are now compared with the clinician's feeling of where the frame is being held up. The most likely match between these two factors is the point at which the clinician should first adjust (Fig 7-2f). Adjustments are generally made chairside with a high-speed handpiece and diamond burs. Finishing diamonds, despite their tendency to quickly lose grit, will not leave as rough a metal surface as more abrasive options. It is not advisable to adjust every area that marks, as a single point of binding can cause the frame to be displaced and therefore contact in other areas. If the point of initial binding is identified, and only that point is adjusted, unnecessary adjustment of these false positive markings can be avoided.

For the casting that is difficult to seat, it is good to remember those areas most apt to be in hypercontact. Studies have shown that the area most likely to have contact is the marginal ridge area where the transition from the guide plate to the rest occurs.[2,3] If the tooth preparation has left a sharp line angle here, the chances are excellent that the cause of the casting not seating can be traced to this area. Articulating tape tends to mark this area of interference more reliably than the other methods. It is also possible that there are still some minor blebs at this critical junction that were not identified in the first step. Another common area of binding is the initial one-third of circumferential cast clasps as they pass over the line angle height of contour.

As the marking and adjusting process proceeds, one must keep in mind the key areas of desired contact. These include the depth of all rest seats, the length of the guide plates, and the retentive tips of clasp arms. It is very rare that adjustment to the depth of a rest seat would be required. If significant adjustment is needed, this is a signal that there was a bubble in the rest seat or some error in one or more of the preceding steps. Adjustments to the guide plate surface are somewhat more common due to the precise path of insertion. Knowing this, they must be done conservatively to be sure that no overadjustment and subsequent loss of stability occurs.

Obviously, it is the frame that is adjusted, not the tooth. The process is continued until a satisfactory fit is obtained or it is determined that the framework will have to be remade. The ideal end point goals include contact at the depth of each rest seat, frictional contact along a maximum amount of the guide plate surface, and clasp arms that contact the abutment teeth as planned (Fig 7-3). It is

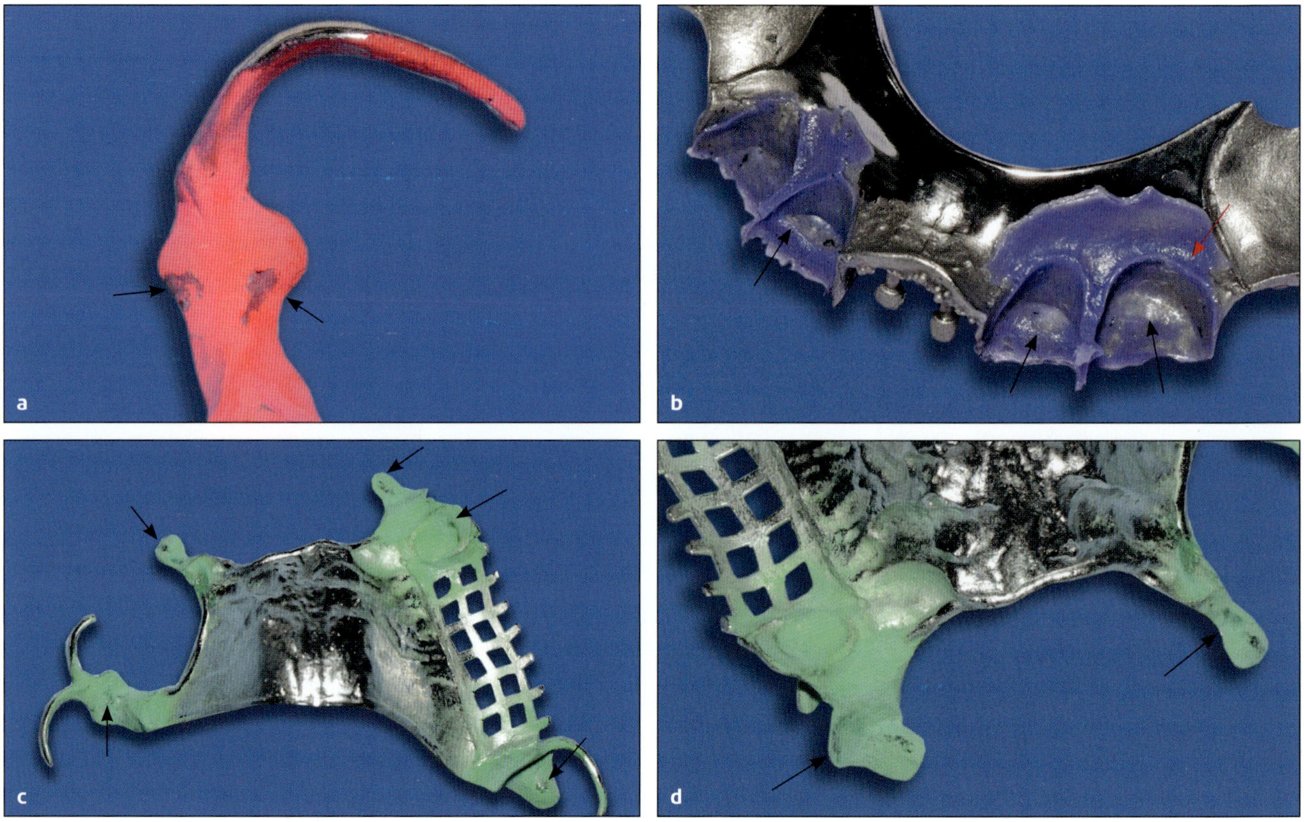

FIG 7-3 *(a)* The *arrows* highlight spray-on powder negative markings that confirm rest seat contact. *(b)* The *black arrows* indicate negative markings in low-viscosity polyether that confirm rest seat contact. The *red arrow* shows one area requiring functional evaluation. *(c)* The *arrows* confirm contact points on all support areas, including overlay of root no. 6. *(d)* The *arrows* confirm contact along guide plate surfaces for the same case as in part c.

important to note that these are the areas of the most solid and clear contact markings. Other areas of the framework, such as line angles and minor connector elements, may mark to varying degrees. As long as these areas do not interfere with accurate seating of the critical components, they need not be relieved, as this would increase space for plaque accumulation. Once the tooth-frame interface is confirmed, the cameo surface is considered in detail. A complete seating should result in a near inlay-fit with the periphery of the rest seat areas and along the margins of any plated surfaces. On occasion, slight adjustment of rest seat contact is required to allow the framework to seat further and thereby close any open margin areas.

With the framework now completely seated, it is brought into occlusal harmony with the opposing teeth. The clinician must evaluate the natural tooth contacts without the partial denture framework in the mouth and ensure that its presence has not altered this relationship. Because the occlusal and incisal rests are routinely overcontoured in the wax-up, it is to be expected that the cast metal may well interfere with complete closure to maximal intercuspal position. The clinician should first evaluate the thickness of the offending rest by measuring the thickness of the metal, both at the center of the rest and at the marginal ridge area. The rest should never be reduced beyond 1.2 mm for fear of subsequent fracture, which can occur months or years later. When this dimension is reached, further adjustment must be done on the opposing tooth. Obviously, careful mouth preparation will reduce the need for these adjustments.

The goals here are the same as with any occlusal equilibration. Articulating paper is used to locate where the contact point exists while 10-mm shim stock is used to feel if the contact is present. Once completed, the natural tooth contact points must hold the shim stock with the same intensity and in the same locations with the framework in as well as out of the mouth. Because the occlusal surface of the rest will have to be rubber wheeled and polished after adjustment, the metal should be sandblasted on those surfaces to make the identification of the dye marks from the articulating paper easier to spot. It is not easy to return the laboratory finish to the casting with standard chairside finishing stones and rubber points. The hardness of the metal requires that a high-speed dental lathe be used to quickly restore the metal to its original luster. The repolishing of these occluding surfaces is a laboratory function and should be completed before the positioning of the denture teeth begins.

Once a satisfactory static fit is obtained, the fitting of the frame is complete for all but Class I partial dentures. The combination of parallel or "milled" guiding planes, accurate final impression, and attention to detail in the laboratory should create a casting that can be fully seated without eliminating the frictional resistance to removal of the framework. Even the finest framework can be severely compromised by careless fitting. The clinician must get in the habit of treating the partial denture framework with the same care as would be given to a crown margin.

Functional Fit

Whether any further adjustment is conducted is based on the desire to allow movement of the framework while in function. For the bilateral free-end situation, functional relief is required if the clinician wants the supporting areas of the edentulous ridges to bear some of the load of mastication.[4–6] Remember, if no functional stress relief is created in the casting, either through the short guiding plane concept or the use of tapered blockout, the casting must be relieved to allow some rotational movement around the distal-most points of contact (see Fig 7-3b).

How much stress relief is desirable? There is no clear scientific answer to this question. It may be best to tailor the amount of movement to the displacement of the areas of major support for the denture bases. When the ridge tissue is firm and healthy, little relief is needed to protect the abutment teeth from luxation. However, when the supporting tissues are weaker, the amount of possible base movement in function is increased and the amount of stress relief should be increased to match. As a general rule, if 2 mm of rotational movement is possible at the distal extension of the retentive mesh without binding on the abutment teeth, stress relief will have been established. The longer the edentulous span or the fewer the number of remaining natural teeth, the greater the amount of stress relief that must be created in the casting.

In order to rotate the framework, the tissue stop must be removed from the distal extension of the meshwork. If it is not removed, it will quite possibly dig into the soft tissue beneath it and restrict rotational movement. Again, AccuFilm is cut and placed in the framework in the area of the guide plate(s). The frame is seated and rotated by placing a vertical load on the distal-most part of the meshwork or the altered cast tray (if one is attached at this point). The dye transfers to both the frame and tooth to identify the areas of heavy contact with rotation. These areas can be differentiated from the areas of static contact by repeating the transfer process with the reverse side of the AccuFilm and by not applying the rotational force. The color contrasting marks are thereby easily visualized. The framework is adjusted with the same instrumentation as used previously, always with care not to remove any more metal than is absolutely necessary, until the desired movement is obtained. The marking and adjustments are repeated by rocking the frame around the fulcrum until the desired amount of binding free rotation is allowed. This adjustment typically must sacrifice guiding plane contact, certainly in the apical half of the guide plate, to allow rotation. Any component anterior to the distal-most point of contact is also a potential interference to rotation. This makes single-tooth posterior modification spaces very difficult to manage since, at the very least, the functional relief at the mesial of the modification space will leave significant space for plaque accumulation. Anterior modification spaces are typically easier to adjust because they lift more vertically as the posterior area is depressed.

Framework Misfit

What do you do if the framework does not completely seat on the abutment teeth? In some instances, it may be possible to retrofit the casting to the abutment tooth by bonding on resin to contact the frame. The most obvious example of retrofitting is when the casting fits everywhere except for one or two rests that fail to contact their rest seats. When these rest seats are in enamel, it is both convenient and acceptable to etch, bond, and place the composite resin within the rest seat. Prior to curing, the framework is seated onto the uncured composite with the other accurately fitting areas controlling the relationship. In most instances, sufficient light can be transferred to the composite by varying the angle of the light source to achieve a stable mass of resin. Excess material that may have extruded over the casting is eliminated and the framework removed. Additional light curing is done before any finishing procedures are undertaken. The quality of fit of the new rest seat will be perfect since the seat was made to fit the existing casting.

Other areas of the framework are not as easy to retrofit, but guiding planes can be brought into contact with the guide plate using this process. Research has shown a dramatic increase in frictional retention with these retrofitted contacts.[7] This concept, discussed in more detail in chapter 9, can be used as an intentional fabrication process to achieve an ideal fit. These composite retrofits have stood up remarkably well over an 8- to 10-year period.

Inevitably, the clinician must face the problem of a casting that cannot be brought into an acceptable fit in the mouth. Often it will not be possible to determine the likely cause of the poor fit. The fit of the frame on the definitive cast will often show that the laboratory phase of construction has produced a frame that fits the cast in an acceptable manner. If this is true, one can only conclude that the error was not made in the laboratory. The clinician must then review the procedures for making the final impression. The inaccurate definitive cast can most often be traced to patient movement during the setting of the alginate gel or the separation of the alginate from the tray during removal of the impression. If one assumes that the alginate was prepackaged and mixed for the recommended length of time and that a careful double-pour technique was used to create the definitive cast, there really is no other place to look.

When a framework cannot be fitted to an acceptable level in the mouth, there are only two options open to the clinician. The first is to start over with a new definitive cast. It does not make sense to remake a framework without a new definitive cast since it is impossible to identify for certain the cause of the misfit. The second is to treat the RPD framework as one would a fixed partial denture framework. This is done by sectioning the offending area of misfit from the frame and attempting to fit the individual segments.[8,9] If you are lucky—and some luck is generally required—then the segments can be individually fitted to the abutments. They are then related in the mouth using some type of quick-setting and accurate pattern resin. Due to the geometry of more complicated frameworks, careful reinforcement of this type of pickup is often required. Some type of soldering cast is poured against the segments, and once set, the components can be laser welded. The newly reunited casting is then returned to verify the clinical fitting procedures before continuing on. This process is described in further detail in chapter 9.

Before proceeding in this manner, the clinician must weigh the cost versus benefit. For some castings, it is more efficient and cost effective to simply remake the frame rather than spend the extensive time and effort to try to save one that is significantly misfit. However, this clinically based sectional fitting procedure may indeed be worth the effort when dealing with mobile abutment teeth or a particularly complex casting. The principles discussed for sectional construction in chapter 6 highlight the possibilities with this procedure.

The RPD framework is not an easy casting to make with precision. The geometry of the frame and the variations that can occur just from differences in expansion based on placement in the casting ring make the framework far more complex than a crown. As has been noted, the accuracy of computer-assisted manufacturing (CAM) techniques is challenged by the framework complexity as well. One could well expect to find 1 out of 8 or 10 castings unacceptable if the standards of acceptance are high. Reviews of typical laboratory accuracy found extensive technical errors.[10,11] It only makes sense to reward the excellent technician if you are fortunate enough to find one. At the very least, the technician should be made to feel an essential part of the team and praised when things go well. Sending a photograph of a special completed case is an excellent way of keeping laboratory interest high and reminding the technician of the high standards that the clinician requires. Technicians involved with continuing education within the dental laboratory profession should be offered access to clinical photographs of the cases to which they have contributed.

The additional time and effort required to establish the ideal tooth-frame relationship must be added to the total cost of creating the very finest partial dentures. Without this level of attention to the final fit, the goals of esthetic tooth replacement without visible anterior clasping and the substitution of frictional retention for clasp retention cannot be achieved on a routine basis. As the partial denture becomes more sophisticated with the addition of precision attachments and implants, the ability to control the interface becomes even more essential to creating partial dentures of the highest quality.

This is not to say that these partial dentures need be extremely expensive. While very complicated situations involving special designs and dental implants will be costly for all involved, an experienced operator following the design parameters and clinical efficiencies outlined in this book will find that the clinical chair time is not significantly greater than industry standards. In fact, the philosophies outlined here are often more efficient. This is because the design philosophy outlined is one of simplicity. Which components are more time consuming to create and fit in the mouth—rests and guide plates, or clasps? Clearly, the more clasps on a case, the greater the challenge to the fit (Fig 7-4). Put another way, if the number of clasps is reduced, as outlined in this book, then the fabrication and fitting procedures will be less time consuming. An excellent example of this is the recommendation to not have wire clasps added to the framework until after the frame has been fit to the mouth. A frame with only rests, guide plates, and minor connectors will be very efficient to fit. It must not be forgotten that a simplified design with a reduced number of components will also result in a significant reduction in plaque accumulation.[12]

Why all of this attention to the fit? The vast clinical experience of the many authors cited throughout this book agrees that well-fitting partial dentures have the best chance of long-term success. The scientific evidence, as far as it exists in RPDs, supports this clinical experience and the philosophy of this textbook. Of the benchtop studies that have focused on the fit of an RPD, adjustments to and

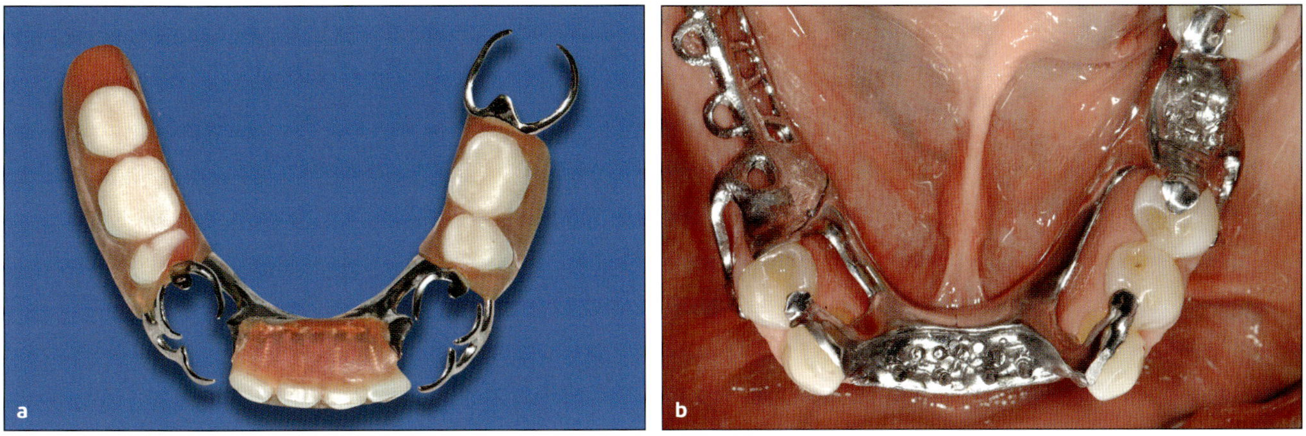

FIG 7-4 *(a)* This excessive amount of clasping complicates fabrication and fitting. *(b)* Limited clasping and strategic contact simplify fabrication and fitting.

accurate fitting of the partial denture reduces abutment tooth movement and directs forces apically and mesially.[13,14] Clinical studies have shown that one of the few mechanical factors for RPDs that have a direct statistical as well as a clinical effect on long-term tissue health is the requirement for a quality tooth-frame relationship.[15] This seems logical, as the support and stability goals highlighted in chapter 2 require accurate contact of the components for the expected benefits to be realized. Take for example the clinical reality that many rest seats do not actually contact.[2,3] This leaves other components, such as clasp arms, to bear the role of support.[16] The result is inclined plan contact, unplanned flexing of clasp arms, and unwanted torquing of the abutment teeth. This poor clinical fit explains the relatively high incidence of clasp arm breakage, mobile teeth, and marginal soft tissue inflammation seen with RPDs that do not fit well.[17] This chapter therefore highlights one of the main differentiating philosophies between the advanced and the everyday RPD. The standard RPD philosophies taught in most dental student–focused textbooks fail to describe the critical importance of framework fit. They tend to instead spend an extensive amount of time dealing with philosophical debate about designs and clasps that will lead to success. Whatever your preferred design philosophy, it is meaningless if the partial denture does not actually interact with the teeth the way that it was planned on paper. What the more clinically focused philosophy of this book is saying is that the accurate fit of the partial denture is more important than the design that has been chosen.

References

1. Brudvik JS, Reimers D. The tooth-removable partial denture interface. J Prosthet Dent 1992;68:924–927.
2. Stern MA, Brudvik JS, Frank RP. Clinical evaluation of removable partial denture rest seat adaptation. J Prosthet Dent 1985;53:658–662.
3. Dunham D, Brudvik JS, Morris WJ, Plummer KD, Cameron SM. A clinical investigation of the fit of removable partial dental prosthesis clasp assemblies. J Prosthet Dent 2006;95:323–326.
4. Hindels GW. Stress analysis in distal extension partial dentures. J Prosthet Dent 1957;7:197–205.
5. Kratochvil FJ. Influence of occlusal rest position and clasp design on movement of abutment teeth. J Prosthet Dent 1963;13:114–124.
6. Kratochvil FJ, Caputo AA. Photoelastic analysis of pressure on teeth and bone supporting removable partial dentures. J Prosthet Dent 1974;32:52–61.
7. NaBadalung DP, Nicholls JI, Brudvik JS. Frictional resistance of removable partial dentures with retrofitted resin composite guide planes. Int J Prosthodont 1997;10:116–122.
8. Ma PS, Brudvik JS. Managing the maxillary partially edentulous patient with extensive anterior tooth loss and advanced periodontal disease using a removable partial denture: A clinical report. J Prosthet Dent 2008;100:259–263.
9. Brudvik JS, Lee S, Croshaw SN, Reimers DL. Laser welding of removable partial denture frameworks. Int J Prosthodont 2008;21:285–291.
10. Firtell DN, Muncheryan AM, Green AJ. Laboratory accuracy in casting removable partial denture frameworks. J Prosthet Dent 1985;54:856–861.
11. Fenlon MR, Juszczyk AS, Hughes RJ, Walter JD, Sherriff M. Accuracy of fit of cobalt-chromium removable partial denture frameworks on master casts. Eur J Prosthodont Restor Dent 1993;1:127–130.
12. Brill N, Tryde G, Stoltze K, El Ghamrawy EA. Ecologic changes in the oral cavity caused by removable partial dentures. J Prosthet Dent 1977;38:138–148.
13. Thompson WD, Kratochvil FJ, Caputo AA. Evaluation of photoelastic stress patterns produced by various designs of bilateral distal-extension removable partial dentures. J Prosthet Dent 1977;38:261–273.
14. Eick JD, Browning JD, Stewart CD, McGarrah HE. Abutment tooth movement related to fit of a removable partial denture. J Prosthet Dent 1987;57:66–72.
15. Frank RP, Brudvik JS, Leroux B, Milgrom P, Hawkins N. Relationship between the standards of removable partial denture construction, clinical acceptability, and patient satisfaction. J Prosthet Dent 2000;83:521–527.
16. Keltjens HM, Mulder J, Kayser AF, Creugers NH. Fit of direct retainers in removable partial dentures after 8 years in use. J Oral Rehabil 1997;24:138–142.
17. Mojon P, Rentsch A, Budtz-Jorgensen E. Relationship between prosthodontic status, caries, and periodontal disease in a geriatric population. Int J Prosthodont 1995;8:564–571.

8 COMPLETION OF THE PARTIAL DENTURE

Accurate construction results in efficient placement.

Once the framework has been properly fit and found to be acceptable, the remaining steps in the construction of the advanced RPD are not all that different from the standard RPD. Certainly, attention to detail in the coloring of the denture base and perfecting the occlusal result merits our attention. The placement of the RPD should go smoothly if the level of quality has been maintained throughout the process. Because it is clearly in the maintenance of the partial denture where the long-term success of the treatment will be determined, educating and reinforcing this to the patient is among the most valuable uses of time and effort.

Maxillomandibular Relationship Records

Maxillomandibular relationship records are normally made only after the framework has been fit to the mouth and brought into the desired occlusal relationship with the opposing arch. Remember, if the definitive cast can be related to the opposing cast in maximal intercuspal position (MIP), simply hand articulating the casts in this position will prove the most accurate. Only when this stable relationship is not obtainable should an actual record be made. The best recordings are made in a material that is truly plastic for the recording and then rapidly and rigidly sets. Registration with zinc oxide eugenol (ZnOe), which has these properties, was traditionally the most reliable choice. However, modern polyvinyl siloxane (PVS) materials provide an alternative with equivalent accuracy and improved handling properties. Any material requires a base of hard wax, trimmed to be 2 to 3 mm out of occlusion, as a platform for the actual recording. Various versions of PVS allow the clinician to choose a setting time. Once set, these materials can be trimmed with a sharp knife or carbide bur so that only the tips of the opposing cusps are visible (Fig 8-1). This trimming is critical, since the opposing cast is typically not as accurate as the anatomy recorded by the PVS material. By reducing the record to only the cusp tips, the tiny grooves, embrasure spaces, bubbles, and indentations that interfere with an ideal interfacing of the record and cast are eliminated. Likewise, the record is more easily verified when using this technique. The hard wax base should not contact the soft tissue in a Class III situation. Only distal extension areas will require some support from the soft tissue.

Because ZnOe and most PVS pastes are truly flowable for a short time after mixing, the record could theoretically be made without any posterior support. Practically speaking, however, some (but not complete) support from distal extensions is advised. This can be made by placing an island of autopolymerizing resin under the place where the tissue stop is (or was) located. After the cast has been coated with a separating agent, the resin is added to provide surface contact about the area of a single molar with care taken to not engage any undercuts (Fig 8-2). This will reestablish the tissue

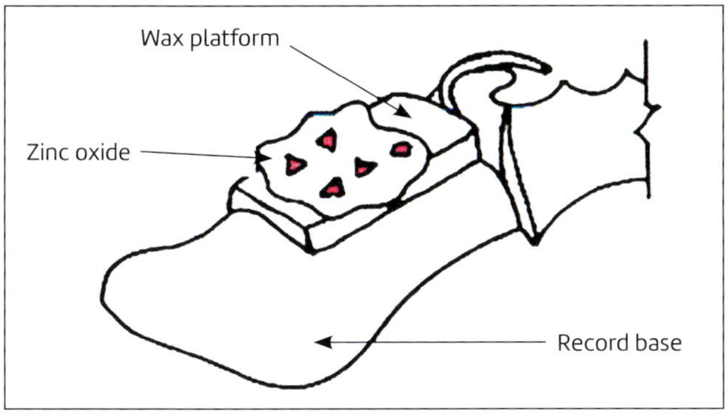

FIG 8-1 Recording material supported by wax rim with only cusp tip indentations.

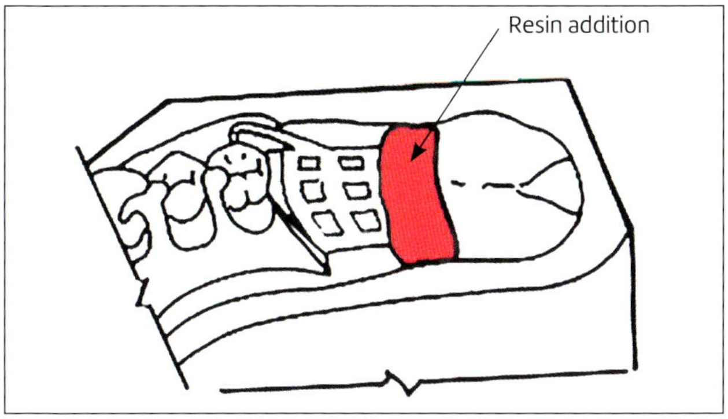

FIG 8-2 Autopolymerizing resin support for record is added to posterior meshwork.

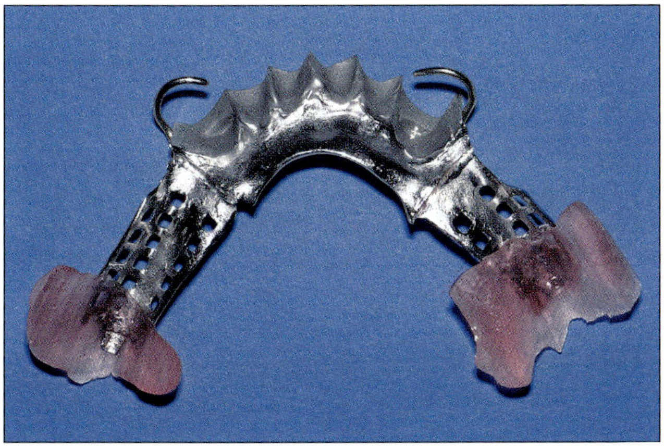

FIG 8-3 Resin supports for distal extension.

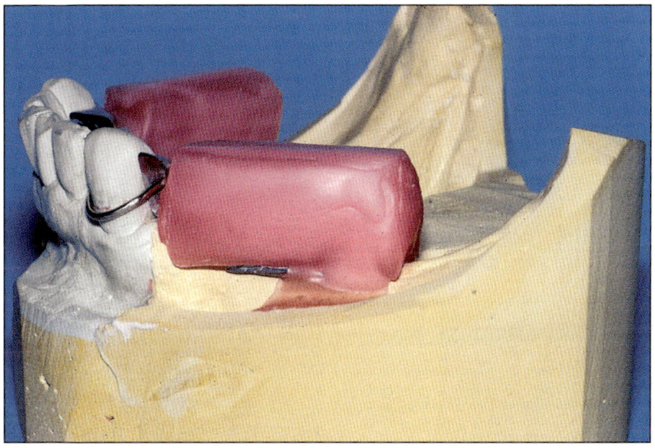

FIG 8-4 Wax rims improve the accuracy of the record by reducing its thickness.

support of the distal extension framework as well as serve as a base for the strip of hard wax that supports the recording material (Fig 8-3). The hard wax rim will reduce the vertical distance between the framework and the opposing arch; this greatly improves the accuracy of the record by reducing its thickness (Fig 8-4). In addition, flowable materials tend to slump away from contact if the distance is too great. When bead retention is present, a base is not required and the record rim or material can be directly applied to the frame (Fig 8-5).

There is little evidence to support the making of a facebow record for the RPD case with natural teeth in the opposing arch. Only when the opposing arch is a complete reconstruction could an argument be made for the use of a facebow or other more accurate spatial relationship record. The great majority of RPDs sent to a commercial laboratory for tooth arrangement and processing will use a nonadjustable articulator. The need for protrusive records to set condylar inclination is also of little use since the articulator is typically not adjustable. Keep in mind that, as discussed in chapter 1, any significant malocclusion has been previously addressed. The result at this point should be that the occlusion is stable, even, and nondestructive. The occlusal goals of most definitive partial dentures are therefore to integrate with this nonpathologic occlusion rather than to alter it in any significant way.

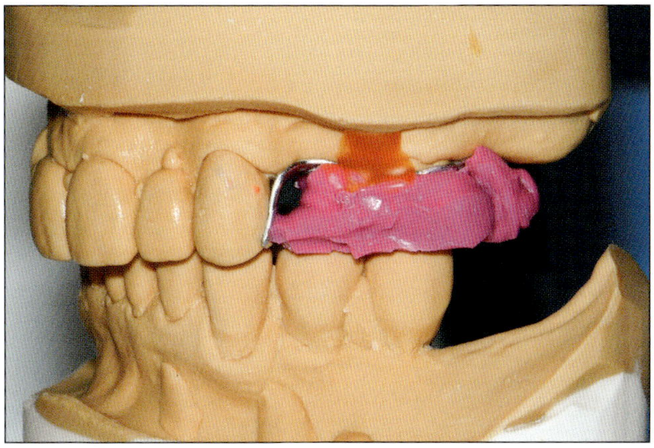

FIG 8-5 A PVS record supported by the metal base in a Class II situation.

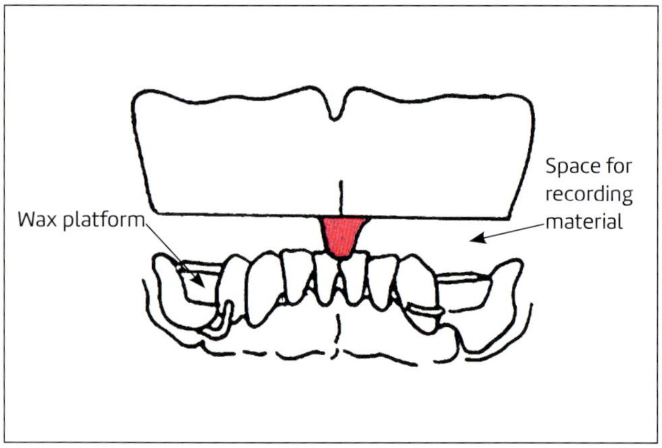

FIG 8-6 Use of a cone of wax or compound to establish the OVD.

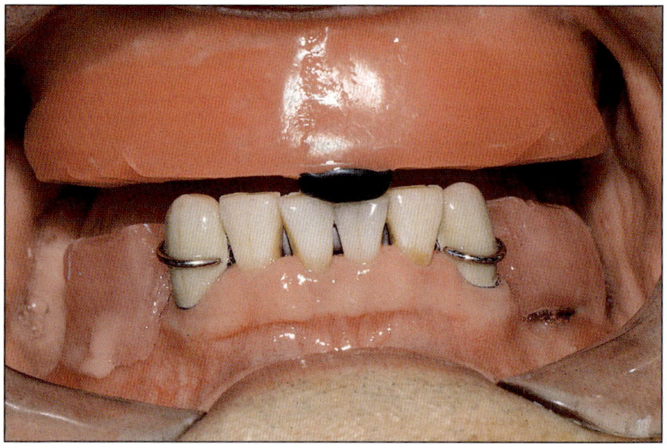

FIG 8-7 Cone method with compound.

There are times when more complicated maxillomandibular relationship records are required. For example, when a partial denture is being made at the same time as a new opposing complete denture (CD), the final occlusion has yet to be created. Maxillomandibular relationship records for these cases require more involvement. These records are most often made as part of a separate appointment where anterior teeth will be positioned as well as the basic records taken. When an altered cast impression is involved, that impression must be made before the maxillomandibular relationship record. On occasion, a suitable record can be made in conjunction with the altered cast impression as described earlier.

The relationship to be captured for the CD/RPD situation is centric relation (CR) rather than the MIP of other partial denture situations. Either a processed CD base for the opposing arch or one made with a combination of plasticized resin (Lynal, Dentsply Sirona, or similar material) and fast-setting orthodontic resin needs to be available for the CR record. The record must capture CR at an occlusal vertical dimension (OVD) that allows the establishment of an esthetically pleasing face height, adequate speaking space, and some interocclusal space at rest, the same as is required for CDs.

The first step in the records sequence is to establish the OVD. A quick and dependable method for finding and capturing the distance from the maxillary to the mandibular arches begins by establishing a length of maxillary wax rim that will extend just short of the length of the relaxed upper lip. The patient is instructed to close to first contact, and the face height is evaluated. The patient must appear obviously overclosed at this time. This does not in any way simulate the vertical position of the anterior teeth as tooth placement is independent of the maxillomandibular relationship record. A cone of wax or compound is added to the wax rim at the midline of the maxilla. This cone is directed to contact the incisal edge of one of the mandibular anterior teeth, usually a central incisor (Fig 8-6). When no natural anterior teeth are present in the mandible, a denture tooth (incisor) is arbitrarily placed onto the resin retention in the central incisor area. The cone is long enough to ensure that the OVD is exceeded at initial contact. The cone is warmed in a water bath so that once brought to the mouth, the patient can easily close through it. It is best to practice mandibular positioning with the patient prior to making the actual record. This practice helps ensure reliable positioning. The patient is instructed to close, in CR, into the cone until the clinician tells the patient to stop. This should occur when the face looks neither overopened nor overclosed. The clinician then evaluates the esthetic face height and repeats the procedure as necessary. The cone is allowed to harden to preserve the tentative vertical dimension record. After the cone has hardened so that it will not distort, it is run under cold water to confirm that it is set. Any excess material can now be trimmed away so that only the incisal edge indentation of the opposing tooth remains in the record.

The contact of the cone and the incisor tooth will normally be visible to the clinician so that the speaking space can be evaluated (Fig 8-7). The amount of space seen when sibilant sounds are spoken will usually give an indication that the necessary "speaking space" has been created. Unfortunately, speech is not a good measure until all the teeth are present in the dentures of both arches and the patient has had time to adapt to the new contours. The clinician can, however, easily evaluate the physiologic rest position by looking at the relationship of the tip of the cone and the opposing tooth, even if the lips have to be slightly parted by hand to gain a line of sight. This check must be done out of the dental chair with the patient standing in a

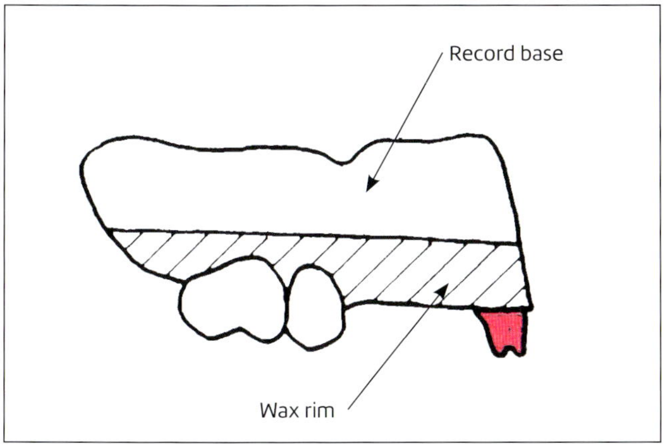

FIG 8-8 Lateral view of maxillary record base with cone and posterior denture teeth.

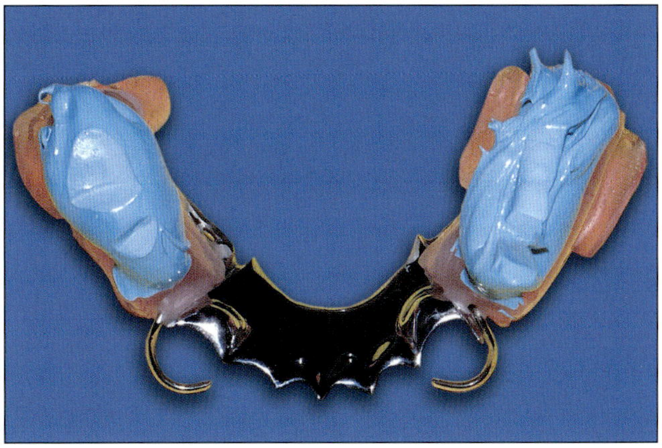

FIG 8-9 Record made opposing simple grooves. Note the limited interdigitation.

relaxed but vertical position since the head position in the modern dental chair will distort the vertical dimension of rest. One could expect to see anywhere from 1.5 to 6 or 7 mm of space at rest, with the Class III patient having the least and the Class II the most. Finding the ideal vertical dimension of rest requires the balancing of these different factors. Since it is quite clear that there is no exact OVD, the clinician need only find an esthetic and comfortable dimension and then verify that position later with the trial tooth arrangement.

As it contacts the mandibular incisor, the cone will also serve as a visual indicator of CR for the actual recording. To make the record as positive and as foolproof as possible for others to articulate, a molar denture tooth can be placed on each side of the maxillary rim in the area of the first and second molar (Fig 8-8). The cusps of these denture teeth will imprint the recording material with a minimum of pressure and leave precise indentations so that, with the cone as the third point of reference, a positive record can be easily verified visually, both in the mouth and when articulating the definitive casts. Instead of using a new denture tooth for this purpose, unused teeth, always available in the office, can be cut in half horizontally so that no interference will occur when placing the occlusal portion onto the maxillary rim. This method is always superior to cutting grooves in the rim and expecting the recording material to flow up into the grooves (Fig 8-9).

Tooth Arrangement and Final Waxing

The occlusion desired for RPD situations where the opposing arch contains natural teeth, restored in any manner, is one of contact in MIP only. Occlusal contact in eccentric positions should not occur on the denture teeth, if at all possible. When denture teeth must be involved in disclusion, as when a canine is replaced, some form of metal or porcelain coverage on the denture tooth must be considered to prevent the rapid wear that can be expected with resin against porcelain, natural teeth, or other restorative materials.

For those situations in which the opposing dentition is a CD, the partial denture occlusion should be similar to that of standard CDs: some form of working and nonworking contacts over a range of 1.0 to 1.5 mm from the centric position. Protrusive contacts are often not possible to obtain without drastically altering the vertical and horizontal overlaps of the anterior teeth, which will most likely be unacceptable esthetically.

Before placing the first denture teeth onto the partial denture framework, consideration must be given to the contour of the resin flange. Since severe resorption of the residual ridge is unlikely to occur immediately adjacent to an abutment tooth, the first denture tooth will be much more likely to appear natural if it is butted to the ridge and the flange begun in the interproximal area between the first and second tooth (Fig 8-10). A denture tooth with anatomically correct height must be used to allow a natural transition between the abutment tooth and the denture tooth. Often, this requires a tooth with a well-formed and well-colored root surface. Should the abutment tooth be clasped with a visible circumferential clasp, the denture tooth will have to be carefully contoured to create space for the clasp to exit without causing an esthetically unacceptable display of pink base material. If too much of the denture tooth will be removed, the resulting unnatural denture base can be removed with a cavity preparation and a microfilled composite placed. Done after processing and finishing the partial denture, this will simulate a proximal restoration (Fig 8-11).

In the CD/RPD situation, it is not always possible to position denture teeth as they would be in an ideal CD/

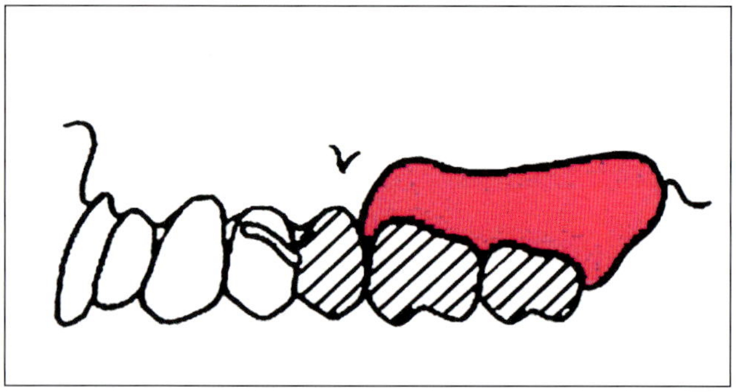

FIG 8-10 The denture flange begins distal to the most anterior tooth.

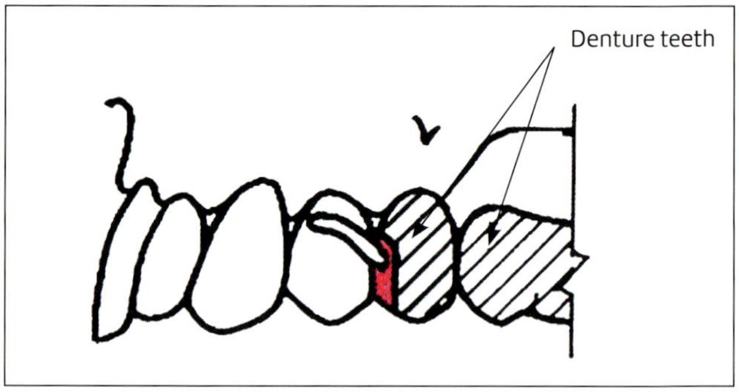

FIG 8-11 Use of composite restoration to disguise clasp exit.

CD situation. The position of the remaining natural teeth will often require the use of diastemas or crowding of the prosthetic teeth to properly interdigitate with the opposing CD. These mesiodistal spacing issues can also be expected to occur when the partial denture is opposed by natural teeth, with or without a partial denture. If possible, the guiding plane should stop just shy of the buccal line angle of the abutment tooth. The prosthetic tooth can then be adjusted to allow a slight overlap of the buccal surface with the metal of the guiding plane. This will maintain the mesiodistal dimension of the prosthetic tooth and help to hide any metal display. This adjustment of the guiding plane is normally only done toward the anterior for esthetic purposes, as it risks reducing the surface area for guiding plane contact.

In addition, the contour of the occlusal surface of the denture tooth will often not harmonize with the occlusal surface of the natural tooth. In order to obtain good esthetics with maximum centric contact, the denture tooth may need to be placed in hyperocclusion and then ground into a solid centric contact. When this need arises, the clinician must verify that denture teeth with the same dimensions as the natural teeth have been selected. Manufacturer-recommended molds, as taken from a mold guide, traditionally could not be used, as they were too small to allow optimum occlusal contact. Fortunately, modern, higher-end, esthetic molds now offer more realistic and accurate anatomical shapes and sizes. To that end, the choice of the posterior tooth mold should be made only on the basis of the mesiodistal and buccolingual dimensions of the opposing natural teeth. In the same manner, the choice of cusp height is based on the contours of the opposing teeth.

In most instances, a 1-mm hyperocclusion that is adjusted into contact will be satisfactory. While typically not required with modern well-positioned teeth, the occlusal surface of an adjusted tooth can be recontoured to recreate any lost occlusal anatomy. Denture teeth should be positioned and ground into suitable occlusal contact one at a time instead of arranging all the teeth into hyperocclusion at once, since some teeth will require a greater or lesser degree of hyperocclusion than others.

As the positioning of the teeth proceeds posteriorly, (or anteriorly in the case of the Class IV), the creation of small randomized diastemas will usually result in a lifelike appearance of any teeth that are visible. Likewise, if anterior teeth are included, they will need to be selected on the basis of the dimension of the edentulous area and the predicted normal anatomical dimensions of the patient's teeth. Taken together, these two pieces of information will dictate whether diastemas or crowding would be appropriate. Since anterior diastemas are unlikely to occur in one arch only, arrangements with some amount of crowding tend to be more common (Figs 8-12 and 8-13). Remember, it is very unlikely that any patient requiring anterior tooth replacement in the mandible would have perfectly straight incisors unless they are very young or have the tooth-arch discrepancy that would indicate the need for diastemas. Obviously, the patient can be expected to remember the presence of diastemas, while they may not recall the crowding. These critical esthetic decisions are best managed during the diagnostic and mouth preparation phases of therapy. As noted, the same teeth used for the diagnostic arrangement, if successful, are the ones now transferred to the partial denture. The primary areas of adjustment to the prosthetic teeth are therefore the areas of the framework that alter the available space for the arranged teeth. This is most commonly the guiding plane, clasp, and resin retention areas.

Only two situations exist where second molars would be placed in the mandibular partial denture. The first is when the opposing arch contains second molars that have the potential for continued eruption. The second is when the maxillary arch is a CD and the patient has a severe skeletal Class III maxillomandibular relationship. In the maxillary arch, the second molar should be replaced regardless, as it may be partially visible and can help prevent cheek biting.

For the RPD opposed by a CD, almost always CD/RPD, some decision on the occlusal scheme of the combined

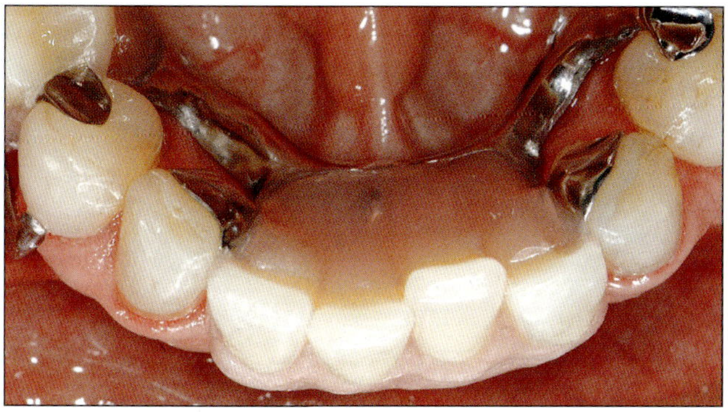

FIG 8-12 This arrangement replicates the typical crowding of mandibular incisors.

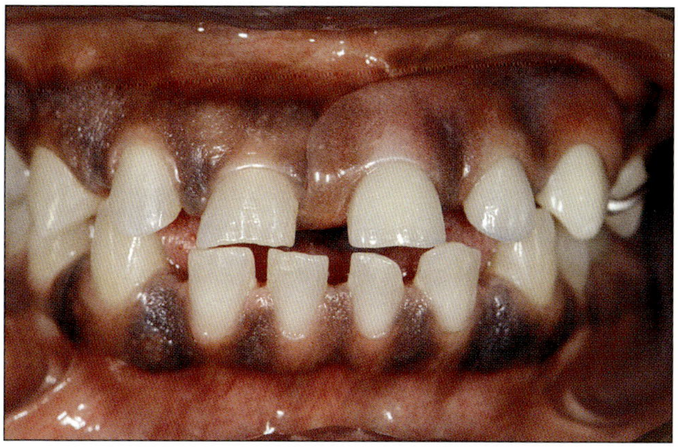

FIG 8-13 Diastemas are necessary to replicate certain occlusal and esthetic situations.

prosthesis must be made. There is no evidence that one form of occlusal arrangement is superior to any other, but for esthetic reasons, some form of cusped tooth is usually indicated because a flat tooth may be difficult to harmonize with the remaining natural teeth. Perhaps the lingualized arrangement is the most adaptable.

Final waxing for an advanced partial denture should be done prior to the final evaluation. This is critical for the clinician and patient to evaluate the contour, feel, and appearance of the prosthesis.

Unfortunately, waxing for a trial evaluation is often done in a casual manner that does not allow the clinician or the patient to fully evaluate the planned end result. The waxing must always be evaluated off the cast to ensure that adequate thickness of base material will be available after finishing and polishing. Any areas of potential sore spots, as might be found adjacent to a sharp mylohyoid ridge, should be over-waxed. These areas are then recontoured in the final resin once any pressure spots have been eliminated.

Custom staining or tinting of the partial denture flange should be completed for advanced partial dentures when gingival display is expected. Any flange area where tinting of the denture base material is planned must be waxed to exacting contours since the tinting will be superficial and easily altered by recontouring. Those flange margins that will be visible must be waxed to a very thin margin and should be slightly curved as they pass vertically since a straight line will tend to be more visible than a margin that flows with the contours of the tissues. The root surface on the facial or buccal of a prosthetic tooth can be intentionally exposed in order to mimic areas of recession for those wanting a natural esthetic result (Fig 8-14). As a final step in the waxing of the denture base, all traces of wax must be removed from the exposed denture teeth. This is normally done with a sharp carving instrument like a Walls carver. No further use of the flame is indicated, since a flash of wax will inevitably result. The object of this final waxing is to create a surface that will require no finishing, only a light polishing, since any finishing operation will remove some of the outer surface of the tooth and the tinted denture base.

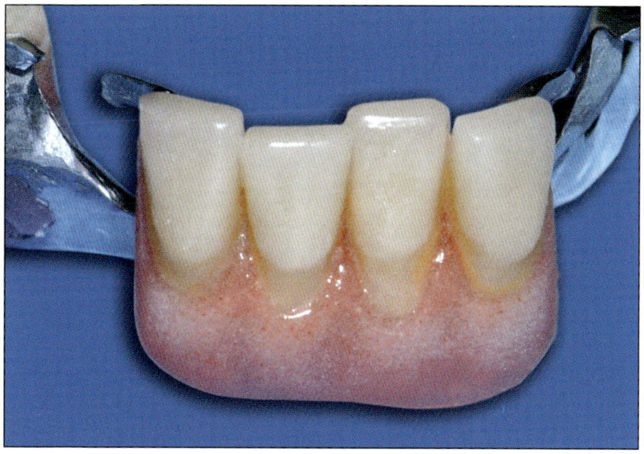

FIG 8-14 Recession waxed in for effect.

Flasking, Tinting, and Packing

The laboratory procedures of flasking and packing the RPD are more complex than those of the CD and, except for the tinting of the denture base, are not highly technique sensitive. Because there may often be many small areas of isolated base resin, a split packing of the flask is used. The technique of split packing implies that a sheet of cellophane,

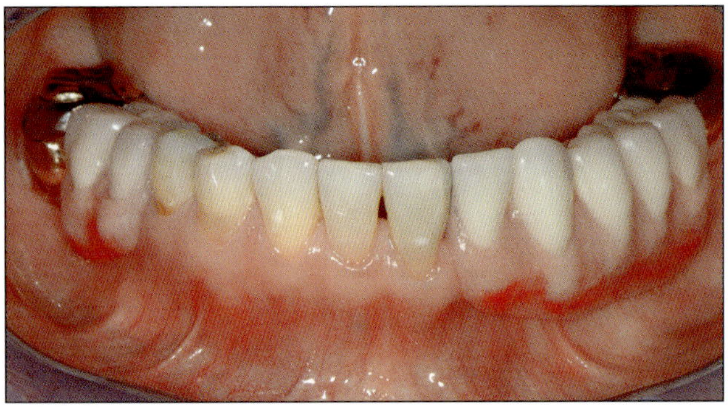

FIG 8-15 Custom staining enhanced the result.

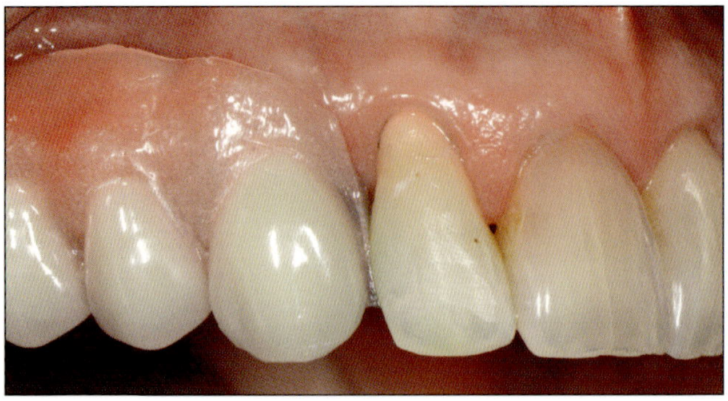

FIG 8-16 Gray show-through of guiding plane.

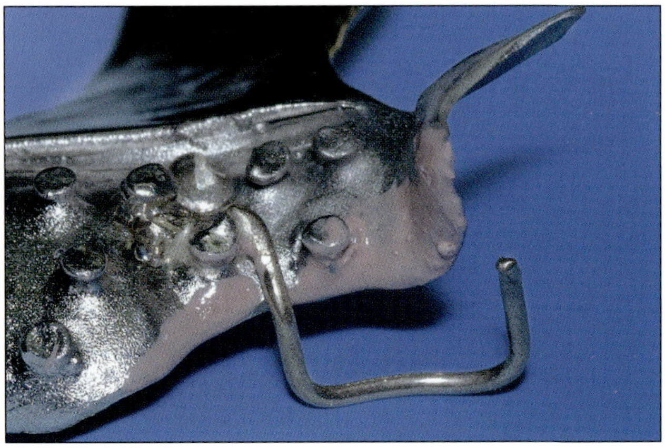

FIG 8-17 Applying an opaquer will help hide gray show-through at thin acrylic areas.

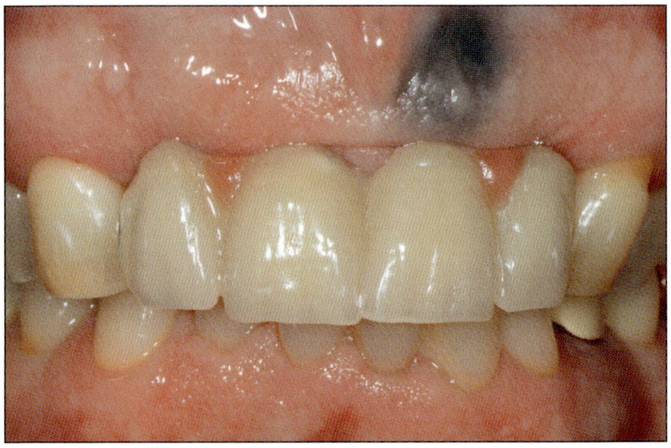

FIG 8-18 Class IV partial denture with no flange. Small areas of gingival shade composite are bonded directly to the metal base.

with resin on both sides, is kept between the halves of the flask up to the final closure of the flasks. This procedure ensures that the resin will not pull out of the interproximal areas or from around clasp arms during trial packing. At the final closure, the cellophane is removed, and the two resin surfaces are moistened with monomer to ensure a complete bond. The popularity of injection molding has reduced the necessity for trial packing or compression molding.

The custom gingival shade matching, often called *tinting*, of the flange is one of the techniques that makes the difference between a standard partial denture and a state-of-the-art prosthesis.[1-4] When skillfully done, the tinted base partial denture can be as esthetic as any prosthetic reconstruction (Fig 8-15). If these esthetic results are compared with less-than-ideal implant surgical reconstruction attempts, the benefits in saved time, cost, pain, and risks become overwhelming.

As part of the tinting of the denture base, consideration must be given to opaquing the casting in areas where the grayness of the metal may show through thin sections of the flange (Fig 8-16). Resins associated with the 4-META (4-methacryloxyethyl trimellitate anhydride) bonding agents can be used to bond on a thin layer of opaque, typically pink in color. The opaque layering must be thin so as to not interfere with the mechanical interlocking between the base resin and the bead or mesh retention (Fig 8-17). Certainly, accurate tinting to truly match the patient's gingival color is a matter of art rather than science and, unfortunately, something that cannot be done at the chair. Experimentation with coloration will be required between the clinician and technician to achieve the best results. Superficial paint-on liquid tints are available, but they are only temporary in nature. Definitive tinting requires that the tinted resins be placed in the flask and blended from the outside inward before the regular base material is added. Conventional acrylic resin tints are available from Schottlander and other companies. Composite resin coloring kits are available as well. The composite gingival shading systems are indicated in areas that are too small in volume to be conveniently packed (Fig 8-18). When used, they are layered directly to the metal base and therefore are generally not used in areas of mesh.

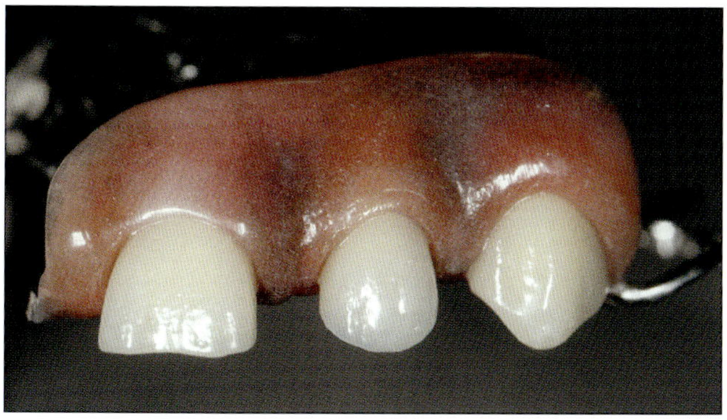

FIG 8-19 Pigmentation tinting creates a realistic end result that blends with the surrounding environment.

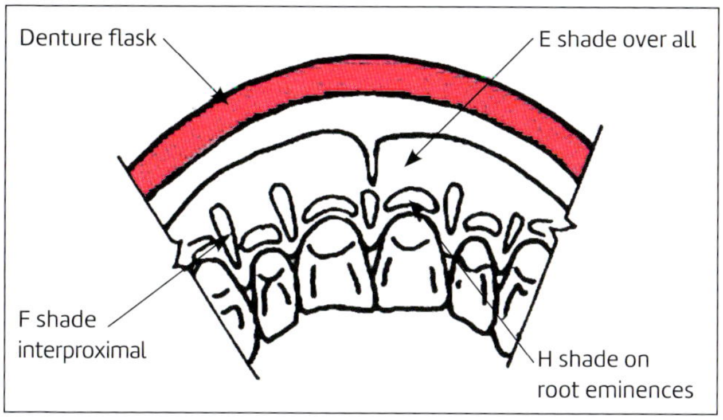

FIG 8-20 Denture base tinting guide for fair-skinned patient.

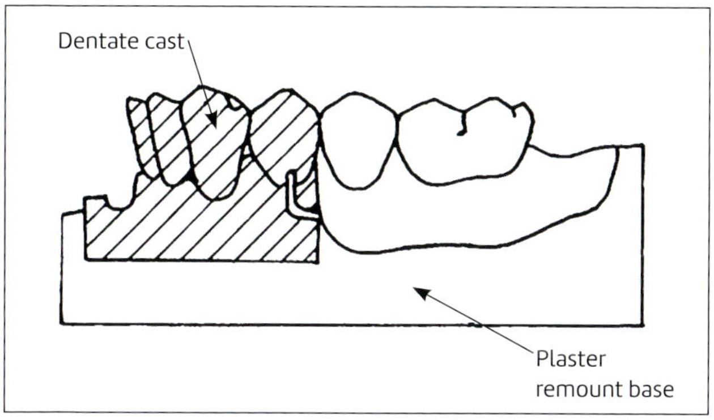

FIG 8-21 Remount cast for RPD.

The clinician interested in developing this aspect of advanced partial denture fabrication should create a series of shade tabs in conjunction with the dental laboratory that will process the resin. Kits come with various levels of detail, with more complex kits containing over 10 different shades. The vials of colored polymer will range from nearly white or very light pink, used to tint areas of firmly attached tissue over the necks of teeth, to a dark, heavily pigmented color that is compatible with patients with darker skin (Fig 8-19). The kits also contain red flocking that can be placed in the areas of unattached mucosal tissue to simulate blood vessels. The short flocking that is commonly found incorporated within denture base materials does not present a lifelike appearance; it appears awkwardly in the marginal gingival area in the random pattern that occurs with standard packing techniques. This type of flocking does, at the very least, add color to an otherwise partially translucent material. When the tints are placed on the outer surface of the base and backed up with the standard resin, the end result can be indistinguishable from natural tissue. Because a natural appearance of the visible denture base is critical to ideal esthetics, mastery of the tinting process is an essential component of an advanced level of prosthodontic care. The instructions that come with the tinting kit provide sufficient guidance for choosing the appropriate colors but do not cover the fine points of their application[1] (Fig 8-20).

Since the denture base adjacent to the prosthetic teeth has been carefully waxed to the desired contour, the final preparation of the finished base should require only the removal of the flash from the packing and the possible slight reshaping and polishing of the denture borders. Finishing and polishing of the junction of the denture tooth and the base should be kept to a minimum for the most esthetically pleasing result. Aggressive finishing tends to remove the texture and contour that provides the most lifelike appearance.

Should the partial denture be Class I or II and opposed by a CD, a remount cast must be made for the finished prosthesis. Occasionally, the dentate portion of the definitive cast can be salvaged in deflasking, but more often than not, the cast is destroyed. A second pour of the dentate portion of the final impression can be adequate for the remount cast as long as major tears did not occur upon removal of the first pour. The finished partial denture is placed on the dentate portion and a plaster base added to support the distal extensions (Fig 8-21). Any undercuts present in the denture bases must be blocked out before pouring the plaster base.

Placement

Because of the care taken to make the final impression or the altered cast impression, there should be little adjustment of the denture bases at placement. Flanges of tooth-borne segments should be short of any undercut areas. Pressure indicating paste will identify areas of possible subsequent sore spots, but it is important to remember that the correlation of a visible spot in the pressure paste and a subsequent area of soreness is far from 100%.[5] Some thought must be given before removing denture base material. When the visible mark in the pressure indicating paste is over a

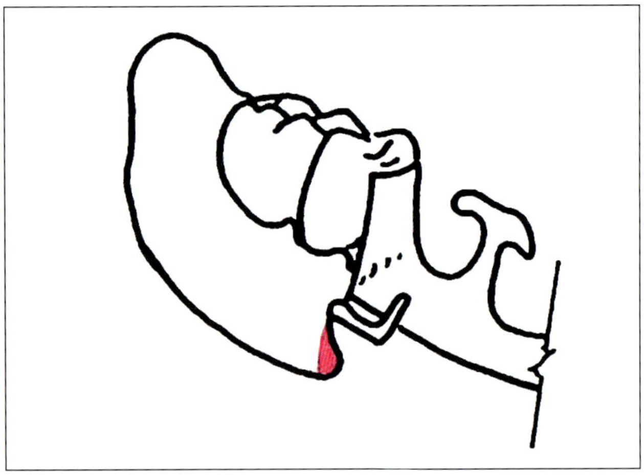

FIG 8-22 Critical undercut area generally requiring adjustment before seating the RPD.

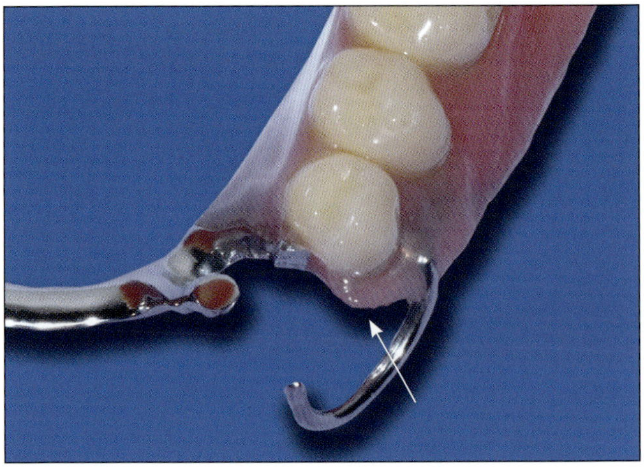

FIG 8-23 Excess acrylic *(arrow)* contacting the abutment alters guiding plane function.

thin mucosal area, such as a torus, adjustment is indicated. When the visible mark is over firm, thick, pressure-bearing areas, such as the buccal shelf or tuberosity, adjustment is likely contraindicated. The most common areas that can be expected to require adjustment are those below the height of contour of tissue undercuts. These are normally found adjacent to the terminal abutments as the ridge form transitions from dentate to edentulous anatomy (Fig 8-22). The resin in these usually minor undercuts must be relieved even if the undercuts do not initially hinder the full seating of the denture. The soft tissue in these areas is usually quite thin over the bone and tightly bound. The guiding planes will dictate the path of insertion, thus forcing these undercut areas to engage.

Another area requiring attention is the subtle wraparound of acrylic lateral to the guiding planes (Fig 8-23). This can be due to over-waxing or simply because of the sealing of the partial denture prior to investing. This is especially common with Krol-style proximal plate designs. These areas require adjustment prior to the placement appointment to restore the planned tooth-frame interface. At placement, a final clinical evaluation with marking medium is conducted in the same manner as at the framework fitting to confirm that this relationship has been maintained.[6]

In order to not traumatize the soft tissue areas, the partial denture should never be fully seated at first. Rather, pressure indicating paste is painted on the base and the partial denture seated until the first slight resistance is felt or until the patient feels pressure. The partial denture is removed and adjusted, and this careful procedure is repeated until the partial denture fully seats without the patient feeling any pressure or rubbing. The final test of this should be done by having the patient bite down or chew on bilateral cotton rolls. This simulates chewing function and can help identify areas of pressure that occur when the prosthesis is placed in function. By starting the flange of the denture base distal to the first denture tooth as was described earlier, some of these problems can be eliminated.

Retentive clasp arms might have been distorted in the deflasking process and may require adjustment at placement. Rather than trying to overadapt the clasps, the patient is better served by leaving the partial denture on the loose side with the explanation that the goal initially is to have the partial denture only minimally retentive. Because all patients will be seen for at least one postplacement visit, further adjustment of the clasps can be done at that time if the patient finds the initial retention inadequate. Most patients will understand that having the partial denture too rigidly attached to the remaining teeth is not desirable in the long run.

The altered cast procedure discussed in chapter 5 is fairly time consuming and technique sensitive. A more efficient alternative to idealize the soft tissue support is to reline distal extension areas at the placement appointment. This requires that the flange extensions achieved in the definitive impression, and therefore in the processed partial denture, are reasonably close. If the border roll is more than 3 mm short, most reline materials will not have sufficient viscosity to mold the proper contour while still flowing freely enough to not distort the soft tissue. This procedure is best considered when proper contours and extensions have been achieved, but ideal tissue-base adaptation is lacking, perhaps due to the inability to control the force of the definitive impression on the tissue. If a rebase procedure involving alterations in the flange extensions is necessary, then the resin reline material being used will need a longer working time and a thicker consistency.

Assuming the extension base in question has this minimum level of accuracy, the chairside reline lowers the risk of technical error by reducing the number of steps. Likewise, all critical steps occur in the mouth, which should ensure that the tooth-frame interface remains accurate. The primary reason why relines are not considered more frequently is the belief that the reline material is inferior to laboratory-processed acrylic resin. While generally true, this difference is not nearly as pronounced as it was in prior decades. Proper handling, use of surface sealers, and attentive framework design that keeps any acrylic material away from the marginal gingival tissue all mitigate problems with porosity and color change. It is also often ignored that the partial denture will require a reline in the future anyway, as the residual ridge resorbs. Chapter 9 discusses reline procedures in more detail, but it is mentioned here as an effective alternative for managing the challenge of combined tooth-tissue support.

Occlusal adjustments are almost always required at the placement appointment. This should be looked on as fortuitous since the absence of prematurities often means infraocclusion, which can only be corrected by the addition of new material or teeth. Under no circumstances should the patient be released if the opposing natural tooth contacts are not back in contact. A rare exception of course would be some type of onlay prosthesis that has been deliberately selected to increase the OVD. When the patient has a partial denture in both arches, the partial dentures should be adjusted one at a time to natural tooth contacts before attempting to place both partial dentures in the mouth for final adjustment. Any easily visible natural tooth contact can be chosen as a witness mark to be sure that natural tooth contact occurs, both in MIP and in excursive movements. Shim stock, ideally below a 25-μm thickness, is used to confirm that a true contact exists, while a dye-impregnated articulating paper is used for assistance in locating the areas of potential contact.

Patient Instructions and At-Home Care

As discussed in chapter 1, RPD patients require greater attention to disease risk management than other patients. Advanced treatment philosophy, based on long-term research, holds that 50% of RPD treatment success is dependent on maintenance. Specifically, RPDs will tend to succeed in the long term when disease risk is reduced and disease prevention is continued. This begins by reminding the patient of their responsibilities. As with any education, these responsibilities must be clearly and repeatedly explained. This is done both verbally and in written form. Amid the excitement and many details of the placement appointment, maintenance instructions are easily forgotten. While almost certainly not true, it is remarkable how many patients, when asked at an initial examination, will say: "My dentist never told me I should take my partial out at night." Giving the patient a written copy of instructions at the placement appointment helps to ensure that the information is retained and used (Box 8-1). It is also an efficient way to document that this education took place. After the dentist or assistant reviews the instructions with the patient, they ask them to read the written copy when they are eating dinner that night. This repetition during a quiet moment at home, after the partial denture has been used at least once, helps ensure that the recommendations are put into practice. When the patient returns for the postplacement appointment and future recalls, they are quizzed on homecare and handling of the partial denture as a further means of assuring good habits.

Along with this instruction sheet, a proper denture brush and denture cup are given to the patient. Use of the brush is demonstrated when reviewing that section of the instructions (Fig 8-24). In particular, the use of a nonabrasive soap rather than toothpaste, which will scratch the acrylic surface over time, is explained. Basic soaps provide an inexpensive and effective means of plaque removal.[7] This plaque removal is supplemented with denture cleaner solutions specifically designed for use with the various framework metals. For those patients, often elderly, who lack the dexterity to clean a complex partial denture or to accomplish effective brushing, a simple at-home ultrasonic unit can be purchased. These at-home units, less than the cost of a single cleaning, can achieve complete plaque and stain removal when used consistently.

Advanced partial dentures, especially those using the guiding plane concepts and precision attachments, are particularly stable and retentive. It is often overlooked that the patient may have a difficult time accurately seating or removing the prosthesis. The dentist must not assume that the patient will simply figure it out. Before dismissal, the patient must be able to properly seat and remove the prosthesis without any assistance whatsoever. Patients have been known to call the dentist a day after placement stating they are unable to remove the partial denture from the mouth. More concerning would be the uncontrolled forceful biting into place of a well-fitting partial denture. This has the potential to bend or break various components. Have the patient stand in front of a wall-mounted mirror after giving them some tips on placement and removal. Knowing the effort and expense just expended, a warning that biting the partial denture into place could break it is most effective when given at this moment.

Box 8-1 Typical patient instructions, given in written and verbal form, on the day of placement

INSTRUCTIONS FOR PATIENTS WITH REMOVABLE PARTIAL DENTURES

1. Placement and removal of partial dentures

- NEVER force your partial denture into place. Doing so (even by simply biting them into place) often causes them to bend and become useless. Place the partial denture down with light finger pressure using a slight "wiggle" if necessary to find the proper direction.
- You should not grab the partial denture by the clasps when removing it. These parts are the most easily bent. Instead, find and use the tooth- or gum-colored portion of the partial denture to remove it.

2. Cleaning your partial denture

- Since your remaining teeth help hold your partial denture, if you have a dirty partial denture, you will have dirty teeth. This increases the likelihood of cavities and gum disease.
- After every meal, you should:
  - Clean your remaining teeth (see Instruction 4).
  - Use a denture brush to scrub the dentures clean.
  - Apply a small amount of regular unscented hand or dish soap while brushing under warm water. This will remove debris as well as odor-causing bacteria.
  - Leave the sink basin filled with water to protect the dentures from breaking or bending if they are dropped.
- Prior to bedtime every day, you should:
  - Remove your partial denture(s).
  - Clean them as you would after every meal.
  - Soak them in plain water (replace with fresh water daily).
  - Occasionally, you may use cleansers that are specifically designed to clean partial dentures. If ever in doubt, ask your dentist first or simply soak them in water.
- Note: Bleach or abrasive cleansers such as toothpaste will destroy the dentures, so do not use them.

3. Adaptation period

- Getting used to your new dentures will take time. Do not expect results for several days or even weeks.
- During this adaptation period, you will likely experience:
  - Sore spots
  - Slight tightness around the teeth
  - Difficulty eating
  - Difficulty speaking
  - Cheek/lip biting
- These issues are almost always resolved at your first adjustment visit. If the partial denture is not used between appointments, these issues cannot be accurately corrected.

4. Cleaning your teeth

- You most likely have had an RPD made for you because you are missing multiple teeth. This means the odds of you losing more teeth are very high.
- The people who have long-lasting partial dentures are those who become very committed to doing two things well:
  - Reducing their frequency of sugar intake. The bacteria in your mouth will use that sugar to produce the acid that will cause cavities. No/less sugar = less bacterial acid.
  - Having perfect oral hygiene. Brushing the remaining teeth three times per day with fluoride toothpaste is a MUST. This will reduce the bacteria and help reinforce the teeth.
- Remember: Since the partial denture holds on to the remaining teeth, if you lose any more, you may not have enough remaining to hold a partial denture that works well.

5. Increased frequency of dental visits

- Due to your increased risk of losing teeth, a minimum of two dental cleanings per year is required.
- Often, the dentist may recommend as many as four visits a year in order to help you try and save your remaining teeth for as long as possible.

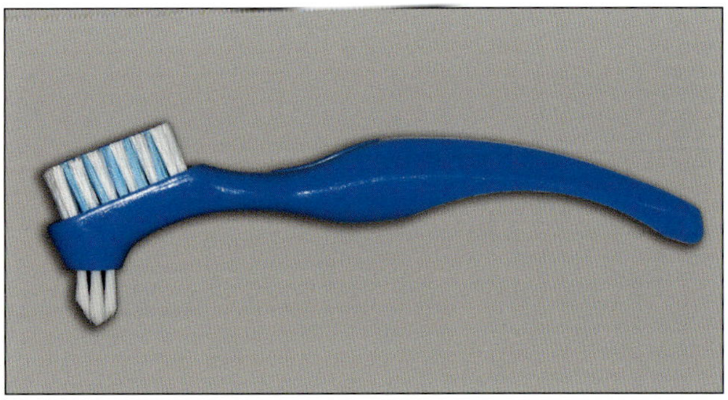

FIG 8-24 A wide-handled brush with both broad and narrow ends to access and clean all areas. The wider handle helps arthritic patients use the brush.

Then, have the patient practice placing and removing the prosthesis. Be aware, this may take 10 or 15 minutes if this is a first-time partial denture patient and it is a Class III situation. Once the patient accomplishes placement and removal, they typically have the confidence and feel to do so again, with it getting easier each time. A postplacement visit, sometime between 2 and 7 days after placement, is essential to complete the process. If all aspects of construction have been accomplished with care, there is seldom need for any additional postplacement appointments. The patient should be placed on a well-defined recall program at this point, realizing that only through regular recall and reevaluation can the full life of the partial denture be assured.

References

1. Pound E. Personalized Denture Procedures: Dentists' Manual, ed 1. Anaheim: Denar, 1973:81–87.
2. Choudhary SC, Craig JF, Suls FJ. Characterizing the denture base for non-Caucasian patients. J Prosthet Dent 1975;33:73–79.
3. Crace K. An updated guide to characterizing injected dentures. J Dent Technol 1996;13:22–27.
4. Bourke RE. Custom shade matching of gingival tissue, part 1. J Dent Technol 2003;43:24–31.
5. Yeoman LR, Beyak BL. Patient's ability to localize adjustment sites on the mandibular denture. J Prosthet Dent 1995;73:542–547.
6. Sato Y, Shimodairo O, Kitagawa N. Systematic clinical evaluation and correction procedures for support of removable partial dentures. J Prosthodont 2008:17;228–232.
7. Moore TC, Smith DE, Kenny GE. Sanitization of dentures by several denture hygiene methods. J Prosthet Dent 1984;52:158–163.

9 EXTENDING LONGEVITY

Nothing lasts forever, especially RPDs.

The ability to remove a partial denture is both a blessing and curse. By being removable, they allow the clinician to make alterations that accommodate changes in the oral condition. However, movement wears surfaces and stresses components over the many years of use. Long-term maintenance of an RPD constructed to the highest standards, as described in this book, will be minimal. It is typically limited to the occasional adjustment of retentive clasp arms and precision attachments. Resilient attachments can be expected to need replacement on an annual basis. Relines of distal extension bases and areas of recent extraction will also be required with time. So while experienced, forward-thinking treatments will minimize the effects of time, they will not eliminate it. Skill and knowledge are therefore required to manage the various issues that will arise with partial dentures as they age. The older the partial denture, the more likely it will need maintenance and repair procedures to extend its lifespan.

Long-Term Maintenance

As research continues to show, the primary factor in extending the longevity of an RPD is the dedication to disease prevention and risk reduction. Once the prosthesis has been given to the patient, many feel they are done with treatment. As the months and then years go by, old hygiene and diet habits tend to return. This is especially true for patients who return to a general dental office after having been referred elsewhere for the RPD. Some offices may lack the dedicated prevention strategies discussed in chapter 1. In these instances, when their maintenance will be overseen by a different dentist, it is the role of the RPD provider to point out the specific maintenance requirements for each individual patient.

Regular, repetitive oral and prosthesis hygiene instruction is therefore of far greater importance than the technical aspects of recall and maintenance. Referring back to previously quoted research, the life expectancy of an RPD can extend beyond 20 years if the supporting structures can be maintained. Remember, the average partial denture patient has already demonstrated some degree of inability to manage their own disease process. In the first year after insertion, high-risk patients should be seen at 3-month intervals to evaluate the response of the tissues to the partial denture and to provide oral hygiene instruction. The evaluation and critique of the patient's ability to clean, not only their remaining teeth, but the partial denture as well, is the most critical aspect of the recall appointment. This requires that the dental hygienist be given adequate time for the time-intensive, face-to-face, hands-on instruction. After asking the patient to demonstrate their brushing technique, a plaque-disclosing solution is used to stain the partial denture as well as the teeth. This will indicate those areas where plaque remains. Showing

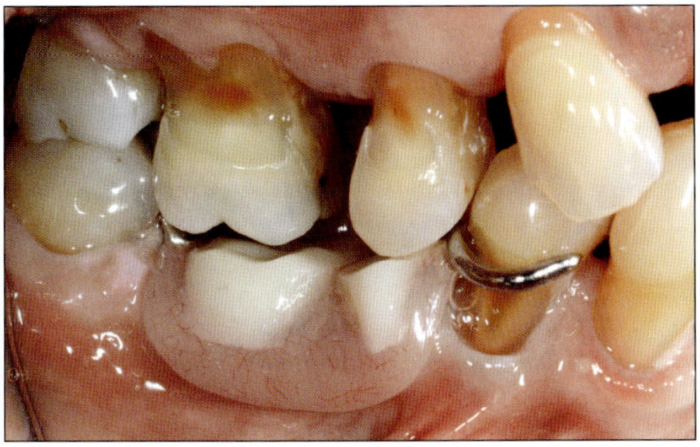

FIG 9-1 Overeruption of teeth as the RPD wore away further complicates this situation.

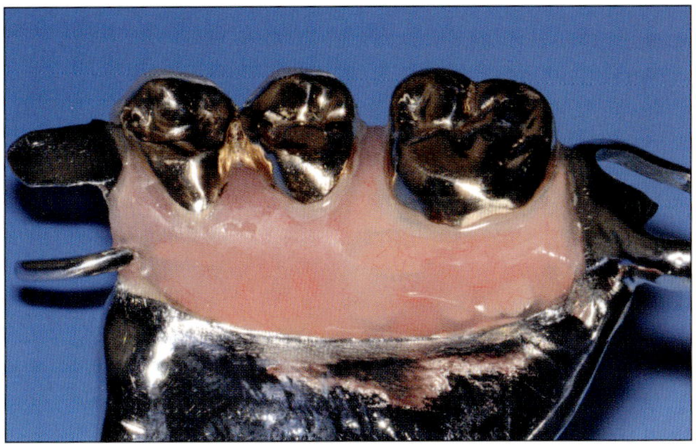

FIG 9-2 Metal occlusal surfaces were added after 3 months of use.

the patient the residual staining with a large mirror should always be done, as it will objectively and clearly demonstrate their lack of effectiveness. Often, the clinician will find that the patient has lost the denture brush that is normally given to them at the placement appointment. Cleaning the partial denture with a standard toothbrush tends to be ineffective, as toothbrushes do not have sufficient bristle length to get into all areas of the partial denture. A short brush of the kind that is used to apply pressure indicating paste has proven effective for plaque removal from the spaces formed by guide plates, rests, and clasp arms. The standard of clinical care has not been met until patients have proven their ability to keep the partial denture free from accumulations of plaque over time.

An ever-expanding number of preventive procedures and methods is found in chapter 1 and in the CAMBRA (Caries Management by Risk Assessment) protocol literature. While a twice-per-year recall may be effective for some patients, erring on the side of caution with 3- or 4-month intervals is advised, at least during the first year or two. The added frequency may be a logistical hassle for an elderly individual, but it is worthwhile to control disease. The examination completed at the recall appointment will evaluate disease control, fit of the resin denture base, and integrity of the various components. The information in this chapter discusses management of the most frequently encountered deficiencies to keep the partial denture in optimum working condition.

Metal/Porcelain Occlusal Surfaces

The use of acrylic resin denture teeth, while efficient, has resulted in the need to manage prosthetic tooth wear much more frequently than in the past. The problems created by tooth wear are twofold. First is the loss of tooth contact and, in certain situations, occlusal vertical dimension (OVD). Second, if opposing tooth contacts are against natural teeth, compensatory eruption of the antagonist tooth can create major interocclusal space issues if the eruption is left to continue for too long (Fig 9-1). When this situation is left undiagnosed or untreated, the antagonist tooth or teeth can alter the plane of occlusion so dramatically that extraction may be required.

Knowing this, it is advisable to select a material that will wear at a rate similar to existing natural teeth. While hardened composite resin layered denture teeth are an improvement over cross-linked acrylic resin denture teeth, they still tend to wear down faster than clinicians expect. The tried-and-true method of metal occlusal surfaces remains an excellent way to manage this issue (Fig 9-2). With the cost of precious metal alloys continuing to remain high, the more difficult handling characteristics and silver color of nonprecious alloys is more likely tolerated than in years past.

When the RPD is opposed by natural teeth or fixed restorations, consideration must be given to protecting the occlusal surfaces from this inevitable wear (Fig 9-3). There are many techniques for fabricating metal occlusions. Perhaps the most dependable method is to allow the patient to wear the new partial denture for a month or so to be certain that the chosen occlusal scheme is appropriate for that situation. At that point, the patient returns and the RPD is placed back on the remount cast, if one has been made. Sprue leads of 6-gauge round wax (or similar wax forms) are added to the occlusal table, one at the most posterior cusp and one at the most anterior (Fig 9-4). A silicone mold is made of the occlusal surfaces of the denture teeth to include the sprue leads. Using a resin finishing bur, the occlusal surfaces of the denture teeth are reduced by a

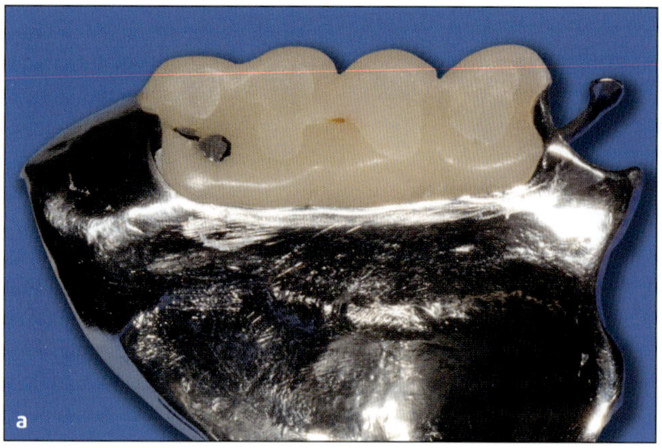

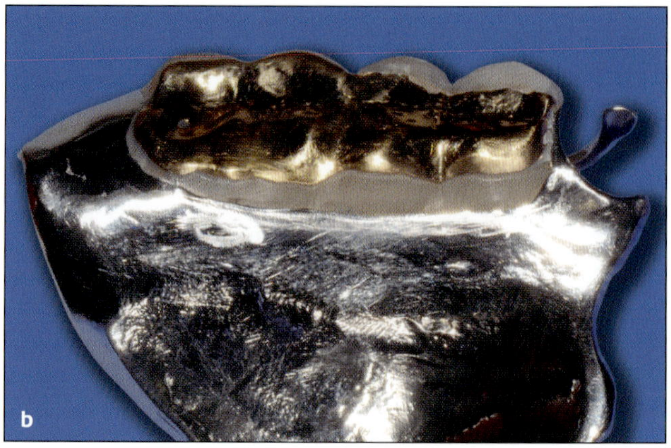

FIG 9-3 *(a)* The opposing natural dentition has contributed to extensive occlusal wear. *(b)* Metal occlusals will further extend the life of this 10-year-old partial denture.

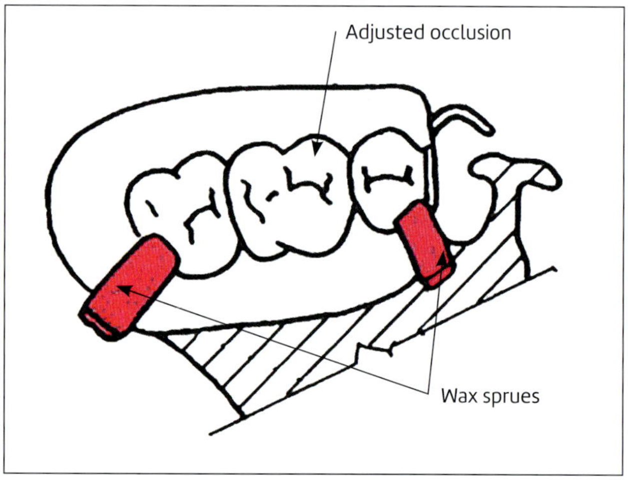

FIG 9-4 Sprue leads attached to build metal occlusal surfaces.

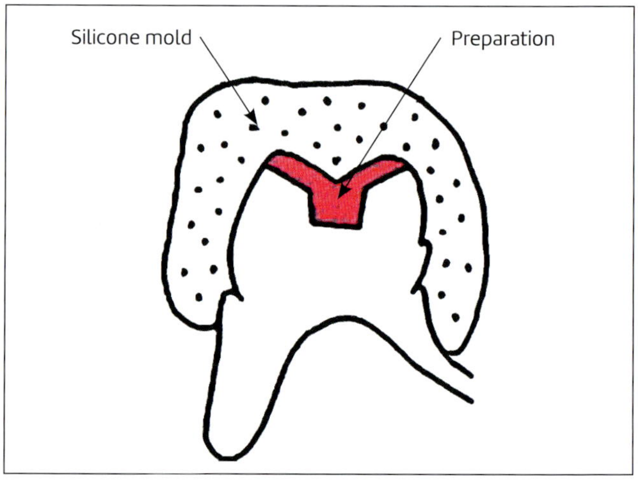

FIG 9-5 Silicone mold to duplicate occlusal surfaces.

uniform 1 mm, including the grooves. A 3-mm-deep central groove is cut into the teeth. In some instances, this groove extends into the denture base material. This groove should be wide enough to occupy one-third of the buccolingual width of the teeth (Fig 9-5). The occlusal surfaces of the denture teeth and groove are lubricated with a separating material, and the silicone mold(s) are replaced on the partial denture. Using an eye dropper, molten inlay wax is injected into one of the sprue leads until wax is seen coming out the opposite sprue. When the wax has cooled, the silicone molds are removed and any voids or defects corrected with additional wax. For those partial dentures where no remount cast was made, the wax contacts can be verified in the mouth. Once the desired occlusal contacts are obtained, the wax occlusal block is teased from the denture and sprued from the underside of the central groove with sufficient sprue leads to assure a complete casting.

Before investing the wax patterns, a retentive groove is cut into the bulk of wax that extends into the central groove (Fig 9-6). The purpose of this groove is to ensure physical retention of the casting to the cementing medium. After casting and sandblasting, a 4-META (4-methacryloxyethyl trimellitate anhydride) type bonding agent can be applied as an additional metal-acrylic retentive measure. Because it will take only a day or two to invest, cast, and finish the casting(s), the patient can leave the office with the RPD after the wax patterns are created. Despite the lack of occlusal contacts, the RPD can function reasonably well for this short duration. The alternative is to keep the RPD during the entire fabrication time frame, which may risk abutment tooth displacement.

When the castings have been finished, the patient returns, and the partial denture is placed on the remount cast (if one exists) to complete the process (Fig 9-7). Each casting is generally cemented with autopolymerizing acrylic resin to assure a bond with the denture teeth and base. This also serves to effectively fill any voids at the butt-joint margin. The viscosity of this material requires additional space that

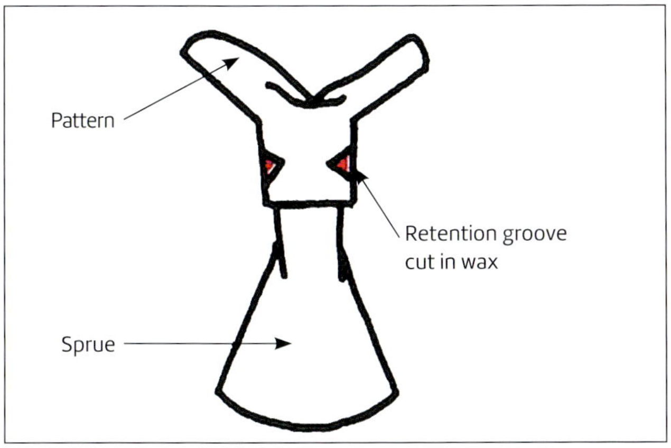

FIG 9-6 Sprued wax pattern with retention grooves.

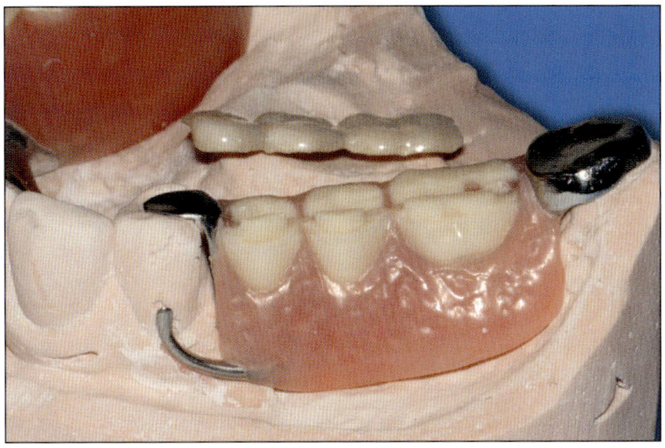

FIG 9-7 Partial denture back on remount cast and ready for cementation of zirconia occlusals.

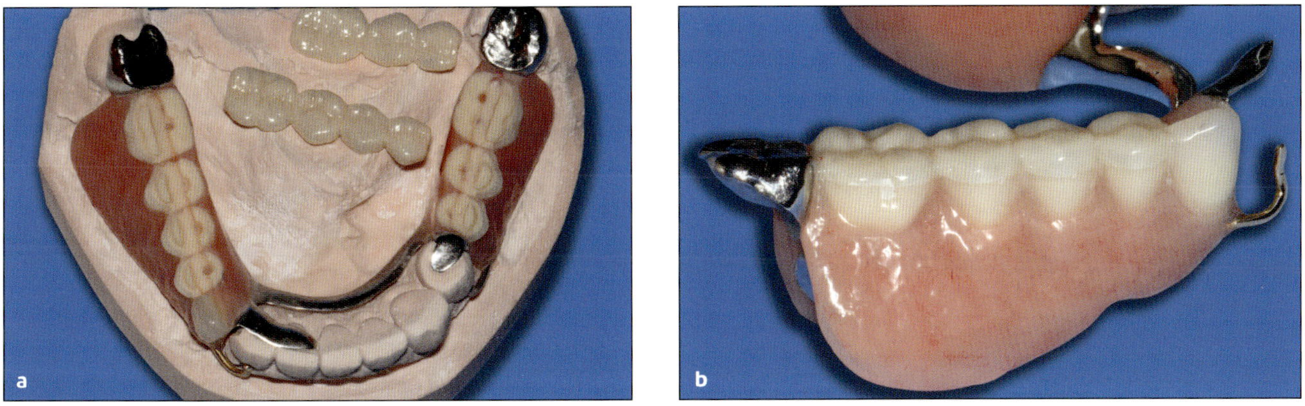

FIG 9-8 *(a)* Monolithic 3Y-TZP (3 mol% yttria-stabilized tetragonal zirconia polycrystal) zirconia occlusal surfaces prior to cementation. *(b)* Zirconia occlusal surfaces after cementation.

is created by removing a small amount from the internal surface of the prepared cavity. The casting(s) are tried on the preparation to confirm the fit. Once the occlusal contacts are satisfactory, tooth-colored acrylic resin of the appropriate shade is mixed and placed in the groove and on the other prepared surfaces. The castings, with liquid monomer painted onto the intaglio surface, are forced into place by closing the articulator to the original OVD. Excess tooth-colored resin is removed, and then a stout rubber band is placed around the articulator to hold the castings in occlusion while the articulator is placed in the pressure pot. After finishing and polishing, the metal occlusal surfaces can be expected to add considerable life to the RPD. A minor problem with this procedure is that there will be micro-leakage at the metal-resin interface that will in time leave a dark line in the resin. Using a bonding agent and minimizing the marginal gap will greatly reduce this line.

Depending on the opposing contacts, the metal need not cover the entire occlusal surface of the denture teeth. They may, in fact, take the form of large Class I restorations. When the opposing occlusion is a complete denture, the lingual cusps of its posterior teeth can be made in metal using the same technique and a lingualized occlusion created for the patient that virtually eliminates occlusal wear for the expected life of the dentures.

For those patients with high esthetic concerns, a simple solution to the wear issue is, of course, traditional porcelain denture teeth. If this is not feasible, the occlusal overlay concept can also be applied using milled ceramics, most commonly zirconia (Fig 9-8a). These would be digitally fabricated, perhaps while the patient waited. Fabricated in much the same sequence as the metal occlusals, the zirconia occlusal surfaces are more susceptible to fracture. The cost savings should theoretically be significant as the cost of material and time to fabricate can be reduced. A scan of the existing occlusal morphology is made and then integrated with a scan taken after the preparations are completed. The previous, worn-in occlusion can then replicated in the mill (Fig 9-8b). This requires that the occlusal surfaces be made before any form-altering wear has occurred.

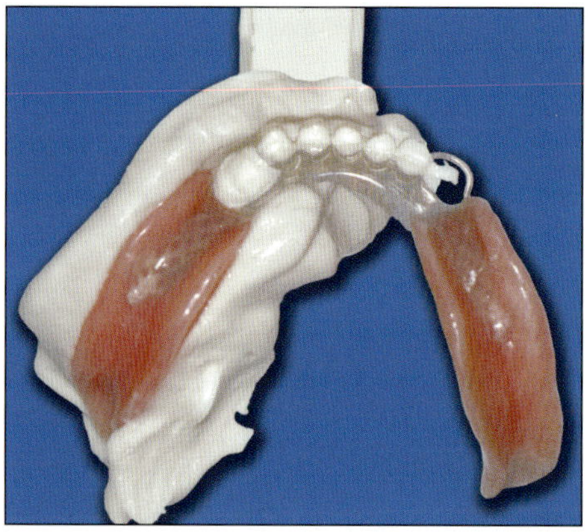

FIG 9-9 A typical sectional impression. The exposed left quadrant is held in position by the clinician while the impression is made.

Pickup Impressions for Repairs

Many of the necessary repairs and additions to an RPD will, by necessity, be made in the dental laboratory. It is incumbent on the clinician, however, to be knowledgeable in the area of framework repairs and to fully understand the clinical requirements necessary to prepare the prosthesis for a laboratory repair.

The clinician will be responsible for relating the partial denture to the mouth and for capturing this relationship in the pickup impression, regardless of the type of repair or addition. To be certain that the partial denture is fully seated during the impression, the clinician will often be required to hold the partial denture in position while the impression is being made. This requirement necessitates a sectional impression (Fig 9-9). Fortunately, repairs are almost always confined to one specific area of the denture, so a pickup impression that covers only the quadrant in question will allow the RPD to be held firmly in position. In some instances, an assistant will be required to seat the tray while the clinician maintains the relationship of the RPD. When a pickup impression (almost always made in irreversible hydrocolloid) is fully set, every attempt should be made to remove the impression and the RPD in one piece. Should the alginate separate from the RPD, the clinician must be certain that the prosthesis has been fully reseated in the impression. This will sometimes require that small amounts of impression material that may have been bent under the partial denture during reinsertion be cut from the impression before the pouring of the repair cast.

When pouring the repair cast, it must be remembered that only that portion of the arch that relates to the actual repair need be reproduced on the cast. As long as there is sufficient cast structure to ensure that the technician can remove and replace the segment(s) accurately, there is no advantage to having a larger cast. In fact, it is often easier to work with a partial cast, since seating the repair on and off the cast is facilitated and the possibility of cast fracture reduced.

Resin Repairs

The need to repair only a resin portion of the properly constructed RPD is usually related to an accident in which the RPD has been dropped by the patient and some part of the denture base fractured. When the broken part is available, it can usually be repositioned exactly based on the fracture line. It is then a simple matter to submit the denture and the fractured resin to the laboratory for repair. Occasionally, the patient will attempt to repair the fracture using cyanoacrylate (super glue). Once used on resin, accurately repositioning the two segments is usually impossible. In this instance, the cyanoacrylate is removed with an acrylic trimming bur and the remainder of the denture base prepared for a reline impression.

Approximately 1 mm of acrylic resin is removed from the entire tissue surface of the fractured denture base and the missing or broken area reformed using gray or green stick modeling compound. Once the borders of the defect have been corrected, 1 mm of compound is removed from the tissue side of the addition and a wash reline impression made in the affected denture base. The wash impression can be made with any low-viscosity impression material. The completed reline impression is submitted to the laboratory, a cast poured against the impression, and the reline and repair completed at the same time, either in a flask or a reline jig. By combining the repair with a reline, an accurate tissue surface is obtained regardless of the fracture site.

Another common repair situation is the fracture of an isolated denture tooth, almost always caused by inadequate framework design and construction. A common example would be not incorporating a supporting stud or pin to retain a lateral incisor. Because the cause of the fracture is in the framework, no successful long-term repair can be made without either remaking the specific retentive component or using one of the modern resin-to-metal bonding agents (4-META).[1] Because the cost of making and welding on a proper supporting element approaches the cost of a new casting, the bonding agents offer an inexpensive and apparently dependable method of single tooth repair. The use of these bonding agents is technique sensitive, and the manufacturer's instructions must be followed to the letter.

Metal Repairs

The most common metal repairs are associated with fractured clasp arms. For the most part, these fractured clasps can be replaced with a wrought clasp as a repair. Embrasure clasps and clasps emerging from some single-tooth edentulous spaces are the exceptions to the rule and may not be reparable. Whenever possible, a fractured cast circumferential clasp, the most commonly used clasp, should

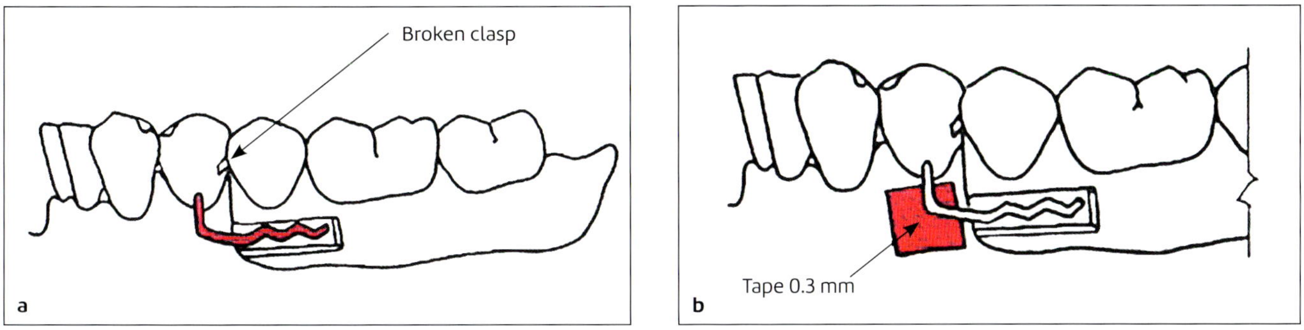

FIG 9-10 *(a)* Replacement of a circumferential clasp with a wire I-bar. *(b)* Adhesive tape square used to keep repair clasp off tissue.

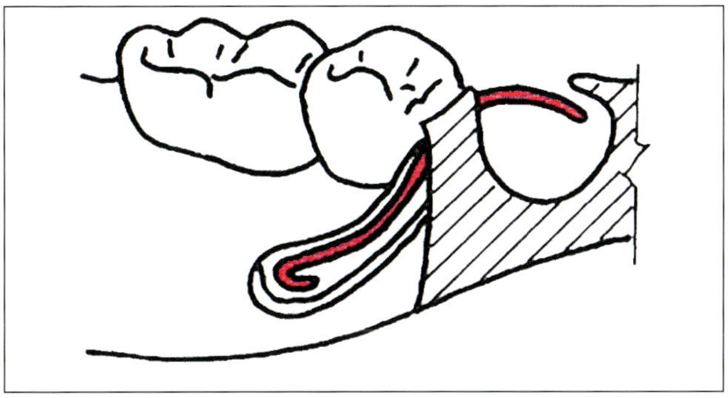

FIG 9-11 Lingual access for circumferential repair wire.

be replaced with an infrabulge wire clasp, since the replacement clasp will be contained entirely in the resin of the denture base and not involve the occlusal surfaces (Fig 9-10a). When infrabulge clasps are added as a repair, the technician must be reminded that the approach arm of the clasp must not contact the gingiva if the RPD is expected to rotate into the soft tissue, as it would if it were a Class I RPD. Instead, the clasp should be positioned so that it is slightly (0.2 to 0.3 mm) away from the soft tissue (Fig 9-10b).

Before making the pickup impression, the cause of the clasp fracture, if known, should be evaluated. It may be that the clasp was poorly designed or constructed. If this was the case, then the situation cannot be improved without additional mouth preparation, and the repaired clasp will itself fracture in the future. Most commonly, this is seen in circumferential clasps where insufficient space for the clasp was created during mouth preparation. The clasp arm or shoulder was then adjusted to allow full occlusal contact of the opposing teeth. The adjustment created a thin spot, which became a point of stress concentration and resulted in the fracture. The thickness of the metal at the fracture site can be measured, and if it is less than 1.25 mm, additional mouth preparation must be completed before the impression. For similar reasons, other tooth contours are modified to the ideal form, line angles rounded, and excessive undercuts reduced as an essential component of the repair procedure.

After all indicated mouth preparation has been done, the pickup impression is made. Again, the need to maintain the partial denture in its ideal relation to its supporting structures is essential, since the fractured clasp may eliminate the possibility that the partial denture will stay in place for a full-arch impression. Rather than send the pickup impression directly to the technician, the clinician must pour the cast and remove the denture after the stone has set so that the contours of the stone abutment tooth can be surveyed and the gauge and position of the replacement wire clasp determined and marked on the cast. The same standards of clasp construction discussed in earlier chapters apply to the repair clasp.

When the clasp in question does not have an adjacent acrylic flange of suitable proportions to allow the placement of an infrabulge clasp, the repair will require a circumferential clasp. This repair will involve the opening of the occlusal surface of the denture tooth adjacent to the repair so that the wire circumferential clasp can be brought across the occlusal surface to be embedded in the lingual resin of the denture base (Fig 9-11). As a result of the preparation of a transocclusal groove, the occlusal surface of the denture tooth will need repair as well. To ensure that the repaired partial denture will have proper occlusal contact in this area, the opposing denture or cast of the opposing teeth should be sent to the laboratory with the repair cast so that the technician can restore the occlusal surface(s) involved.

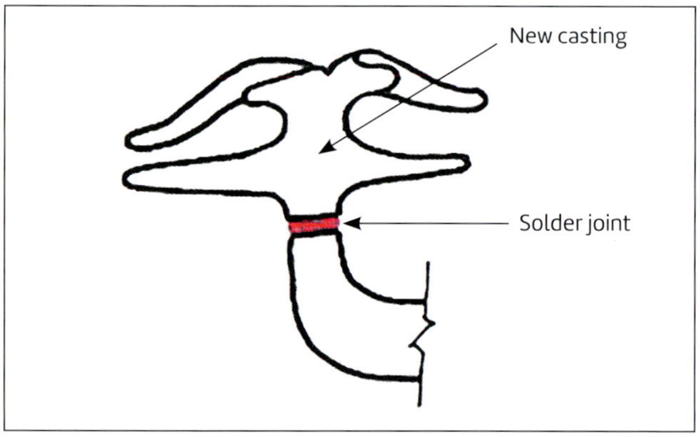

FIG 9-12 Embrasure clasp repair.

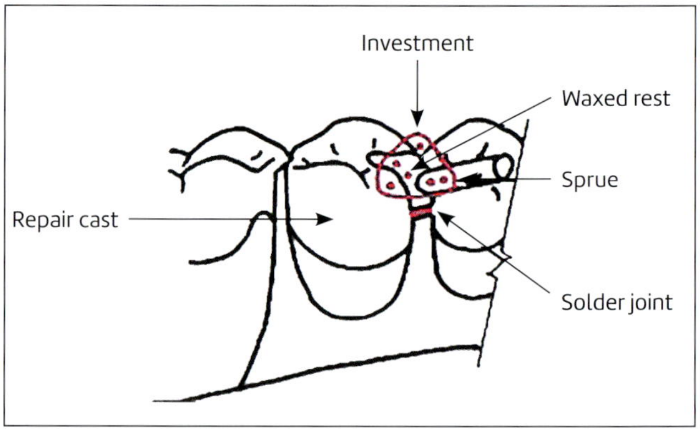

FIG 9-13 Replacement of broken occlusal rest.

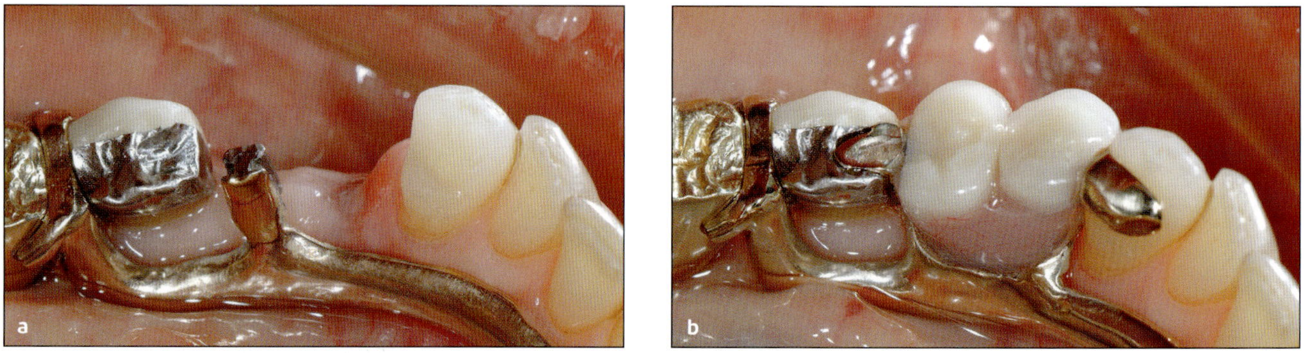

FIG 9-14 *(a)* A precision attachment RPD can still be functional if support is replaced. Note the rest preparation on the second premolar and cingulum addition on the canine. *(b)* Laser-welded addition to restore rests, guiding planes, and teeth. Note no need to replace the missing clasp.

The fractured embrasure clasp may be repaired by sectioning the lingual minor connector a few millimeters below the occlusal surface before making the pickup impression. This keeps the minor connector weld away from an area of occlusal load (Fig 9-12). The laboratory can then block out the cast, duplicate, wax, and cast a replacement embrasure clasp. This clasp, when finished and polished, can be welded to the framework to complete the repair. In most of these situations, an overlap joint is created in the new casting to maximize the strength of the laser weld rather than the classic space for soldering that is shown. Unfortunately, the cost of this type of repair is high and totally dependent on the weld for longevity. In most of these situations, it is advisable to remake the partial denture.

The same procedure of sectioning the minor connector first is used for another common repair situation, that of the fractured occlusal rest. This type of fracture can almost always be blamed on inadequate mouth preparation that leaves a marginal ridge reduction of less than the 1.25 mm mentioned before. The technician can wax the replacement rest directly on the lubricated repair cast. The rest is sprued with a small round wax sprue lead and a small amount of appropriate casting investment painted on the wax (Fig 9-13). Once the investment has set, the entire assembly can be teased from the repair cast and added to some other partial denture framework casting for final investment and casting. The finished rest addition is polished and joined to the partial denture using laser welding. The joint must meet all criteria discussed in chapter 6 for an adequately strong laser weld.[2]

The addition of a denture tooth to the partial denture to replace a natural tooth lost to caries or periodontal disease is also a common repair situation, often one that could be considered a real emergency if the tooth happens to be an anterior tooth (Fig 9-14a). The tooth can be replaced as an addition after the natural tooth has been extracted and initial healing has taken place, or—and this is often the preferred way—as an immediate replacement following the extraction. In either case, the existing framework must be capable of supporting the addition (Fig 9-14b).

As we have discussed earlier, one indication for a lingual plate is when the potential for tooth loss exists. When a lingual plate is present, the best results are obtained by drilling two small holes in the plate and welding a small

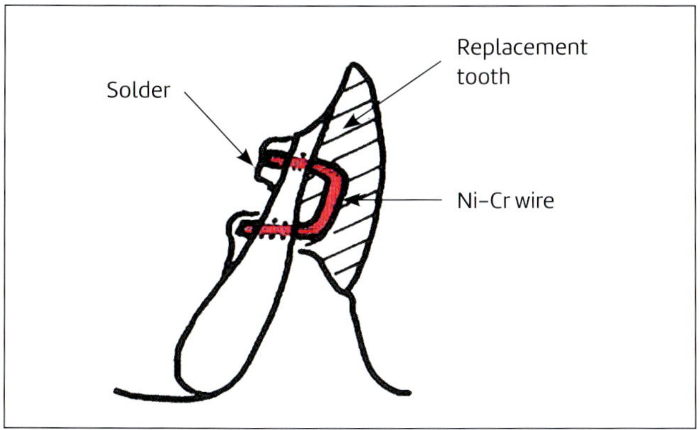

FIG 9-15 Addition of retention and denture tooth to lingual plate.

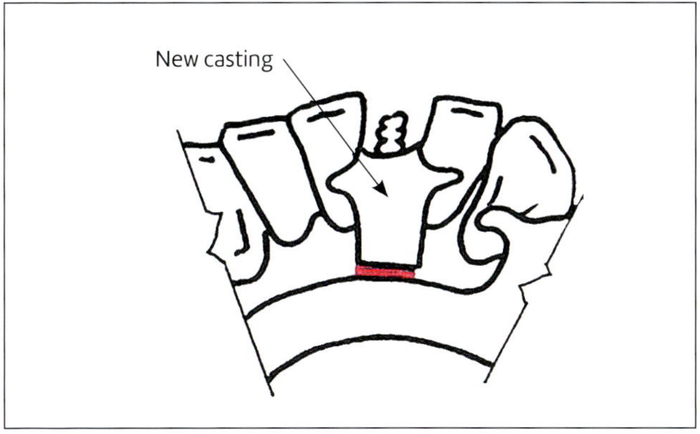

FIG 9-16 Addition of cast retention to lingual bar.

loop of wire, usually one of Ni, Cr, and Co, into the holes so that the loop is internal to the replacement denture tooth (Fig 9-15). This form of retention will be as strong as one that is part of a new partial denture framework. When no lingual plate exists and there is insufficient adjoining resin to retain a denture tooth, a cast addition, laser welded on, is indicated (Fig 9-16). As in the replacement of the broken embrasure clasp, the cost of a quality repair may approach that of a new casting. Again, and on a temporary basis, the 4-META bonding agents can be used to add a tooth to the metal framework.

Fractures of major connectors were traditionally repaired by using 800 fine solder and a resistance brazing device.[3,4] However, laser welding has completely replaced this technique. Obviously, the mandibular bar will be the easiest major connector to weld since it offers easy access over a limited distance. Maxillary major connector repairs are seldom worth the effort. The need for a major connector repair results more often from distortion rather than from outright fracture of the metal. However, there are occasionally inclusions of refractory material that collect near the sprue attachment and cause a spontaneous fracture. The patient who drops their partial denture and then steps on it can expect it to not fit well from then on. In an emergency situation, the major connector can be separated with a thin disk at the point of the perceived bend and, if both segments fit the mouth in an acceptable manner, it is worth making the pickup impression and sending the case off to the laboratory for welding. Beyond this, major connector repair is not practical.

Restorations Under Existing RPDs

It is not uncommon for abutment teeth to require some form of restoration or rerestoration during the life of the partial denture. The two- or three-surface alloy restoration that fractures at the isthmus is difficult to replace under an existing partial denture because positive contact with the rest is difficult to maintain. In these instances, if amalgam is again the material of choice, deepening and/or widening of the preparation is often required to ensure that an adequate bulk of amalgam is present. Despite the superior longevity of posterior amalgam restorations, direct composite restorations have a significant advantage when used for rest seat repairs. The partial denture can be seated over uncured composite. The composite will adapt itself to the rest seat form as the partial denture goes to place. Once cured, the result is a nearly ideal tooth-frame interface at the repair site.

Because the composite filling can be layered into the cavity, the final contact with the rest and guiding plane is best made after removal of the rubber dam and matrix. This is done after the critical dentin and enamel bonding is completed under proper isolation. After the initial restoration and rubber dam removal, the partial denture is seated to confirm that there is no contact in the area of the repair. The less space between the partial denture and the supporting surface, the more difficult the repair tends to be. Therefore, at least 1 mm of space is recommended for the second addition of composite. The partial denture is lubricated with an acceptable separating medium. Isolation protocols are followed as closely as possible to prevent contamination of the composite-to-composite bond, and uncured composite is added to the repair area. The partial denture is then seated over the uncured composite. Any large excess is removed with an explorer before curing. Light activation is usually possible in a two-stage process where the material is first activated with the partial denture in place. With fairly small rest dimensions, adequately powerful curing lights pass light laterally enough to sufficiently set the composite. This allows removal of the partial denture without distorting the restoration. The process is nonetheless typically dynamic, with the clinician lightly lifting the partial denture on and off while the assistant cures from the periphery. Once the

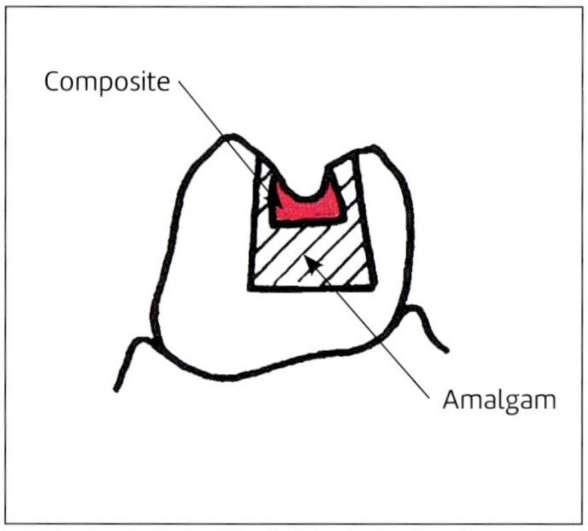

FIG 9-17 Composite and amalgam combination to retrofit a rest.

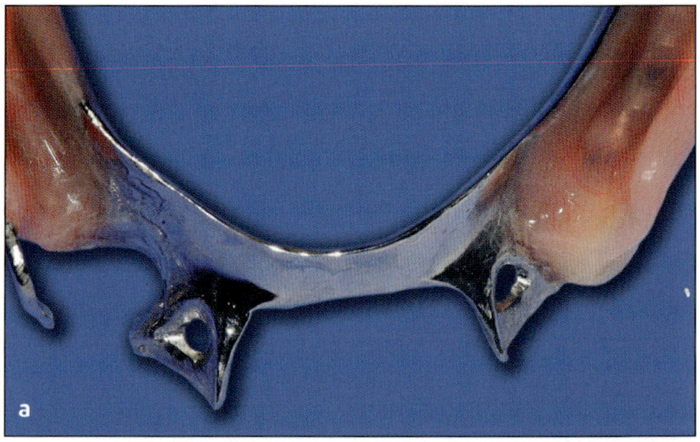

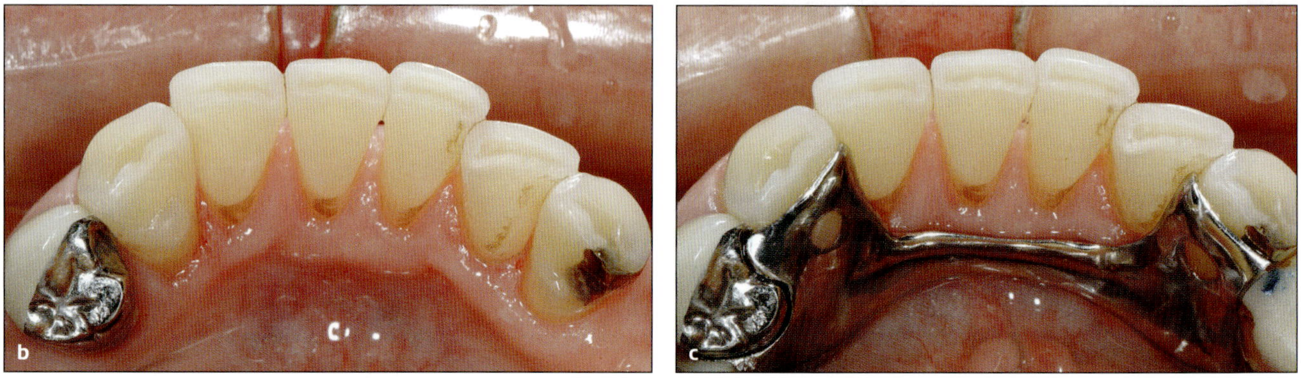

FIG 9-18 *(a)* A symptomatic 5-year-old partial denture was lacking basic support. It had lingual plates but no rests on either mandibular canine. A positive rest form was cut into the plate area at each canine. *(b)* Additive composite cingulum rest seats retrofitted to canines. *(c)* With positive support present, functional symptoms were resolved.

partial denture is completely removed, additional light curing is done directly over the uncovered restoration. Finishing of any rough margins or excess material can be completed at this time, paying close attention to leaving the now very accurate composite-frame interface unaltered.

This staged approach also facilitates the use of a combination of alloy and composite to support an occlusal rest. After the additional mouth preparation, the alloy is packed in the usual manner. Once set, a dovetailed box in the area of the rest is formed (Fig 9-17). Chemically curing composite is placed in the box and the partial denture fully seated in the mouth until completely cured. This combination of restorative materials will allow the creation of a positive rest seat contact. Some form of microfilled resin is indicated in these repair situations.

The retrofitting procedure described here results in a tooth-frame interface that is exceptionally accurate. In fact, the fit of the partial denture to these repairs is often better than the previous contact.[5] With this in mind, there are instances where this procedure can be used to improve the framework fit. One example of this situation would be a lingual plate that was designed without positive rest seats and is in need of improved stability for continued use. Cingulum rest seats can be retrofitted to these cases by first modifying the lingual plate (Fig 9-18a) and then following the additive technique just discussed (Figs 9-18b and 9-18c). Adding a solid positive rest seat often results in a noticeable improvement in performance as well as reduced mobility of teeth that the plate was displacing due to the previous inclined plane contact. Fortunately, isolation and therefore bonding is somewhat easier to accomplish in this area than for a proximal restoration in the posterior region.

Knowing the challenge of accomplishing an ideal tooth-frame interface, there are times where retrofitting a framework has been intentionally done to maximize the framework fit. This would be done by altering a definitive cast to create an ideal rest or guiding plane form (Figs 9-19a and 9-19b). The partial denture is then fabricated against this ideal form. Once completed, the abutment tooth that was modified on the definitive cast is overprepared to ensure no contact between the framework and the area of modification. Once the partial denture has been fit to all other areas, the retrofit procedure is carried out for the modified area just as if it was a composite repair (Figs 9-19c to 9-19f). In this way, it is the restoration that is being fit to the RPD rather than the RPD that is being fit to the abutment.[5] While this technically sensitive operative procedure requires a high level of skill, it is still an efficient way to achieve a nearly ideal tooth-frame interface.

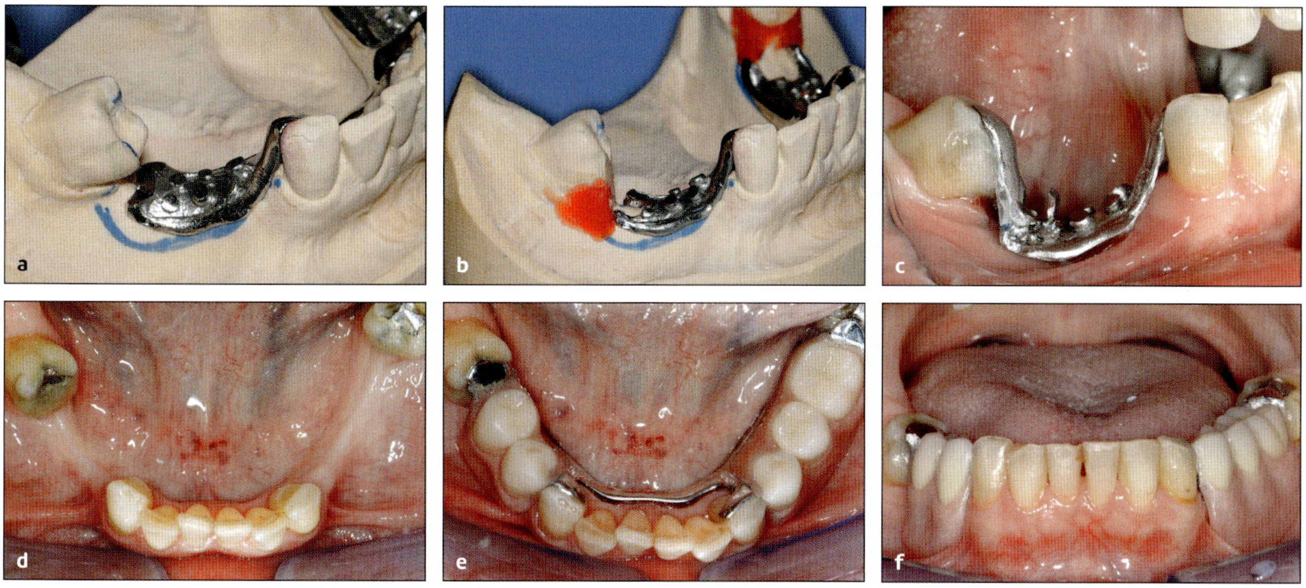

FIG 9-19 *(a)* Sectionally constructed frame with anterior segment completed. *(b)* The definitive cast is modified to create parallel guiding planes. The frame is completed to this idealized laboratory modification. *(c)* Mesial guiding planes were retrofitted to the framework at the fitting appointment. *(d)* Occlusal view of retrofitted molar abutments. Note composite bonded over amalgam. *(e)* Completed claspless RPD. *(f)* Guiding plane retention only.

Crowns under existing RPDs

In many situations, restoration of the fractured abutment with amalgam or composite will not be adequate to properly restore the tooth. Some type of crown, veneered or monolithic, will be needed. Constructing a crown under an existing partial denture is not an easy task, and if it is not done to perfection, the partial denture will not seat passively on the tooth after cementation of the crown. There are many publications discussing these issues,[6] with more recent publications highlighting the potential for improved accuracy with a completely digital method.[7,8]

ABUTMENT AND SPACING

The value of the abutment in question should once again be reviewed before the decision to crown it is made. If inadequate tooth structure remains and adjunctive procedures like surgical crown lengthening or orthodontic extrusion are necessary, then the tooth will likely not be a reliable partial denture abutment. As previously noted, endodontic treatment with post and core restorations should rarely be considered since the failure rate for this approach with partial denture abutments is high and the investment significant. This makes retrofitting a crown onto a Kennedy Class I distal abutment a rare event. It is more likely for a critical molar abutment in a Kennedy Class III situation where the tooth has sufficient structure for retention and resistance forms. Those that do not can be considered for overlaying if the partial denture would accommodate a resin-only repair to accomplish this. Overlays are discussed in detail in chapter 12.

In almost all these repair situations, the tooth will be prepared for a full crown. The clinician must verify adequate reduction to allow a minimum of 0.5 mm of metal on the axial walls and up to 2.0 mm on the occlusal surface if an occlusal rest is involved. Likewise, sufficient space for the existing clasp assembly needs to be taken into account. After preparation, the partial denture is seated in the mouth in order to visualize that space is present for all components.

IMPRESSION

As in other repair situations, the impression must be made with the partial denture in its proper relationship to the supporting abutment teeth. This requires a sectional impression with the clinician holding the partial denture in position while the assistant seats the sectional tray. The actual impression is made by removing the retraction cord and injecting the low-viscosity impression material of choice completely around the margin of the preparation. A small amount of impression material can be injected onto the remainder of the prepared tooth. An excess of material might restrict the full seating of the partial denture. The partial denture is then quickly seated in the mouth. Additional material is syringed onto the prepared tooth and into the space between the tooth and the partial denture. Once the space is filled with the low-viscosity material, the sectional tray with higher-viscosity impression material can be seated. This tray must extend on either side of the repair area so that there will be sufficient impression material to lock the partial denture into the impression. The impression and the RPD must be removed at one time since the chance of being able to accurately reposition the RPD into the impression is unlikely. The definitive cast is then poured, either by the clinician if the RPD is to be returned to the patient, or by the technician if the RPD is to be kept in the laboratory for the construction of the crown. When pouring the definitive cast, it is critical that the stone be poured directly against all parts of the partial denture with the exception of clasp arms, precision attachments, and undercuts in the resin areas. This will allow a positive seating of the casting during the construction of the repair crown.

If the patient can do without the partial denture during the repair, then the technician need only marginate the die and wax the crown to fit the framework. This is usually done by first waxing a thin coping to the margins. The partial denture is then seated on the cast, and molten wax is flowed into the space between the coping and the clasp assembly. A glass eye dropper, warmed in the flame to prevent the wax from cooling too quickly, is used to add larger volumes of wax.

CLASP

The most difficult part of the repair is the waxing of the area where the clasp will lie, if present. Not only will the wax need to contact precisely against the internal of the clasp arm, but a retentive contour will have to be built into the wax-up. The undercut formed from this contour will have to relate to the path of insertion and provide the required 0.01-inch dimension for the terminal third of the clasp arm. If the crown is to have a porcelain veneer, the task becomes even more difficult, since the porcelain must be overbuilt originally. As a result, the frame cannot be removed from the crown without fracturing off the dry porcelain.

One solution to these problems is to sacrifice the retentive clasp arm and make the facial contour to ideal dimensions. After the crown is complete, with appropriate undercut in place, a repair clasp is added to the partial denture using the techniques previously described. The resulting repair crown will have an ideal form and will often be an improvement, both functionally and esthetically, over the original abutment tooth.

MAKING A TEMPORARY RPD

Should the patient require the use of the partial denture during the repair period, the clinician will need to pour and recover the final impression and construct a temporary restoration in the shape of the original tooth form. A vacuum form made from a diagnostic cast before mouth preparation can be used to make the temporary restoration. Another technique uses a putty matrix that is made of the tooth before preparation. Missing tooth structure can be restored with soft wax before the matrix is adapted to the tooth. After preparation, the matrix is filled with tooth-colored resin and seated on the preparation. Unfortunately, some adjustment of the temporary restoration is almost always required to seat the partial denture. Areas of premature contact are best identified using the mylar-based articulating ribbon placed inside the partial denture contours when the frame is seated onto the temporary crown. Points of heavy contact show up easily and are adjusted.

The patient is allowed to wear the partial denture but is asked to return once the die has been trimmed and a wax coping dipped onto the die. The patient waits while the wax pattern is developed, using the molten wax as previously described. Because the facial surface will be shaped to ideal contours, the patient will not be needed again until the crown is completed and the repair clasp added. At this time, the crown is cemented and the partial denture seated. Occasionally, despite one's best efforts, some adjustment of either the casting or the clasp is required. Again, mylar tape is the method of choice for identifying points of premature contact. Because the clasp will be made of wire, and as often as possible in the I-bar form, the adjustment of the clasp is not difficult.

Digital fabrication methods are a possible solution to manage some of the challenges in retrofitting a crown. One efficient method is to restore the tooth form to ideal using composite. This ideal prefracture form is then scanned. Next, the tooth is prepared as previously discussed. The tooth preparation is then scanned. Most software will then allow a crown to be milled to match the prepreparation contour. These crowns, while quite accurate for experienced operators, typically require adjustment just as with the analog method. A significant disadvantage is also the fact that all-ceramic materials are more common with this workflow. However, gold and titanium alloys may be available for those situations that call for a more reliable material when esthetics are not a concern. The many variations in digital crown fabrication techniques allow for many choices on how to accomplish this difficult task.

Relines

Chairside versus laboratory

Because residual ridge resorption is chronic, progressive, and irreversible, periodic relining of the distal extension areas of the RPD is an essential component of the maintenance phase of therapy. Relines of recent extraction areas are also required. The clinician is faced with deciding between a

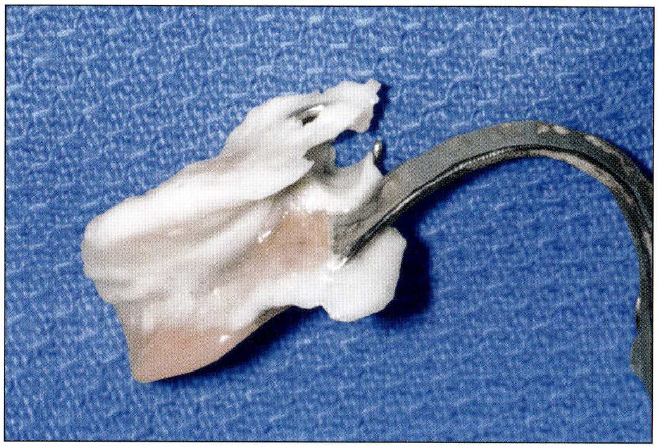

FIG 9-20 "Hot" alginate test showing buccal plate resorption and lingual contact.

laboratory reline and one done at the chair. Unlike complete dentures, where a laboratory reline is preferable in all but very temporary situations, the partial denture reline is best done in the mouth. The reason for this difference lies in the fact that the partial denture framework has a different relationship to the abutment teeth when it is being relined in a flask than when it is relined in the mouth.

When the partial denture is originally processed in a denture flask, it remains on the definitive cast so that the tooth-frame relation cannot change even if the technician fails to get the flask completely closed when packing the resin. The result of any error here would be a prematurity in the occlusion, which is easy to correct. In a laboratory reline, however, the partial denture does not stay on the cast but ends up in the other half of the flask. Now, when the technician does not get the flask completely closed, the tooth-frame relationship is destroyed and the completed reline will not seat completely onto the abutment teeth.

To avoid any chance of this disaster occurring, a resin that cures either completely or partially in the mouth is used. This allows the clinician to fully seat and maintain the casting on the abutment teeth while the resin polymerizes. The partially light-cured composite resin manufactured by Astron Dental (or similar materials) is an excellent choice for RPD relines since it is quite color-stable over time and bonds well to the resin base. In addition, it only partially cures in the mouth, which eliminates the fear of locking the partial denture in place when excess material sets around abutment teeth. Heat release, color stability, and strength of the material should all be considered.[9]

Denture base preparation

Regardless of which reline approach is chosen, the preparation of the partial denture base for the reline impression is nearly identical. In order for the reline material (either resin or impression material) to flow freely when the partial denture is seated on the teeth, the clinician must be certain that adequate space exists between the base and the supporting ridge. Just because the partial denture rocks or the patient complains of movement, it cannot be assumed that a uniform space exists under the base. To register the tissue-base relation, a thin layer of specially prepared alginate is placed in the base and the partial denture seated completely. This alginate is a mixture of one scoop of regular set alginate with two units of hot water. The resultant mix will be very low viscosity so it will not displace tissue but will set quickly because of the hot water. When the partial denture is removed from the mouth, the tissue-base relationship is easily seen and any areas of contact marked before the alginate is removed. The alginate can be torn to evaluate its thickness. More costly fast-set silicone or polyether material can work for this as well. Often there will be 1 to 2 mm of space over the ridge, especially in the mandible, but no space will exist in the lingual flange area (Fig 9-20). The clinician will need to relieve the contact areas so that 1 mm of space, at the very least, is present overall. In some instances, this will mean that the underside of the raised meshwork is completely exposed. This space is critical for the free flow of the impression material or resin.

A decision must also be made as to whether the border extensions are adequate. The free-flowing light-cured composite resins cannot be expected to create a proper border roll if the existing border is underextended more than 3 mm. If the existing borders are significantly underextended, a rebase of the partial denture should be considered. This would entail a pickup impression as described earlier. If the existing borders are properly extended, a finishing line should be cut into the resin border to provide a butt joint of the new resin with the old. This will reduce the

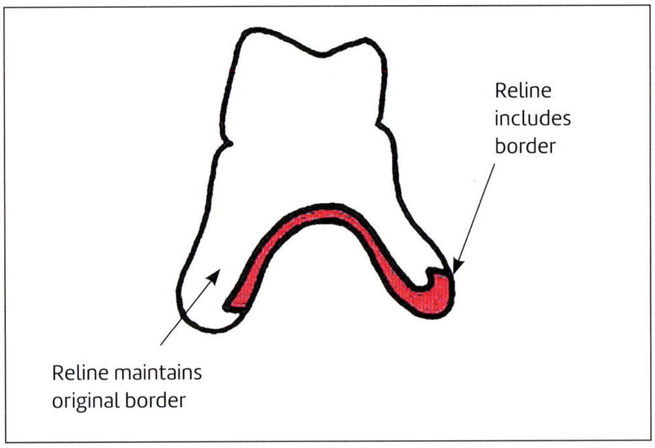

FIG 9-21 Creation of uniform relief after alginate evaluation with finishing lines.

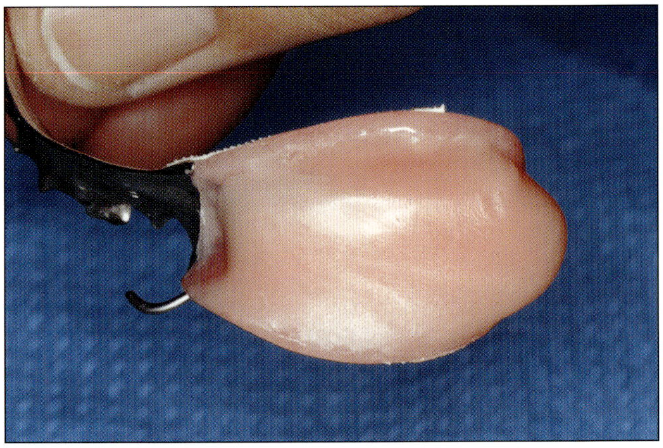

FIG 9-22 The volume of material matches that seen with the alginate test. Note that the material is not overly runny.

possibility that repair resin will peel away later, which is often the case when a very thin flash of resin exists at the border. The goal of the partial denture reline should be to add a uniform layer of new resin overall (Fig 9-21). The same finishing line should be created for an impression to be used in a laboratory reline if that option is chosen. It will give a positive line for cutting away any excess impression material before pouring the repair cast.

To reduce the incorporation of air bubbles, mixing of the reline material is best done using a vibrator. All materials have distinct handling characteristics, often with great differences in the time for the material to reach the firm but still moldable viscosity necessary for a reline. Once this point is reached, the bubble-free mix is applied to the partial denture base. Similar to a wash impression, the volume of material applied to the base for the reline should be limited (Fig 9-22). This helps prevent excess material from flowing between the tooth-frame interface and altering the partial denture orientation during placement. The hot alginate technique should have demonstrated the volume of material necessary to avoid underfilling. Seating of the partial denture must be consistent and guided completely by contacts with the abutment teeth. The clinician must avoid pressing on distal extension bases, as this will lift the framework in the anterior. Once in position, the frame must be held stable in this relationship throughout the setting of the material (Fig 9-23).

The light-cured reline material will set to a firm but resilient mass in the mouth without the generation of heat but, as with all resin materials, with a strange taste. When inserting the partial denture into the mouth for the reline, a small amount of resin can be placed in the clinician's mouth so that the initial set of the material can be evaluated. When the mass attains the consistency of bubble gum and the manufacturer's recommend time has been reached, it is safe to remove the partial denture without fear of distortion. Gross excess is trimmed away with scissors, never with a knife, to prevent peeling at the border. An oxygen barrier is then painted on the reline surface and the final set achieved in a light-curing unit (Fig 9-24). While the reline material manufacturer's own light source is ideal, a typical unit like that used to make trays is acceptable to complete the cure.

Similar preparation and reline steps are used when conventional autopolymerizing acrylic resins are used. One possible exception is the use of an acrylic bonding agent. These typically are provided as part of the kit clinicians can purchase. Likewise, there are surface sealers that can be applied to the reline material after the final polishing. While these do result in improved performance of the materials, at least initially, allergy is a common occurrence and would result in the need to repeat the reline without the surface sealer application.

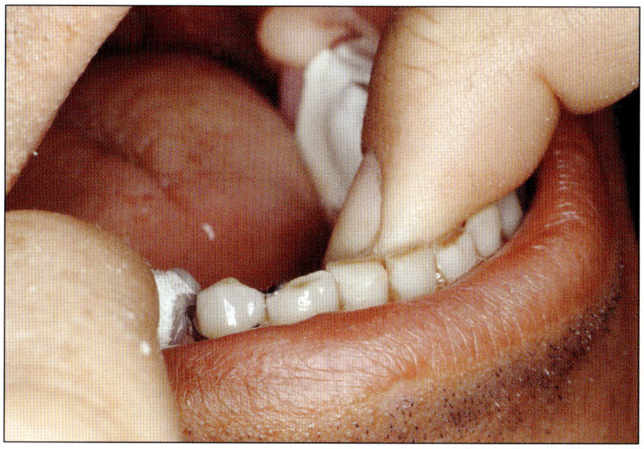

FIG 9-23 The tooth-frame relationship must be maintained with firm pressure, on the frame only, until the material has set.

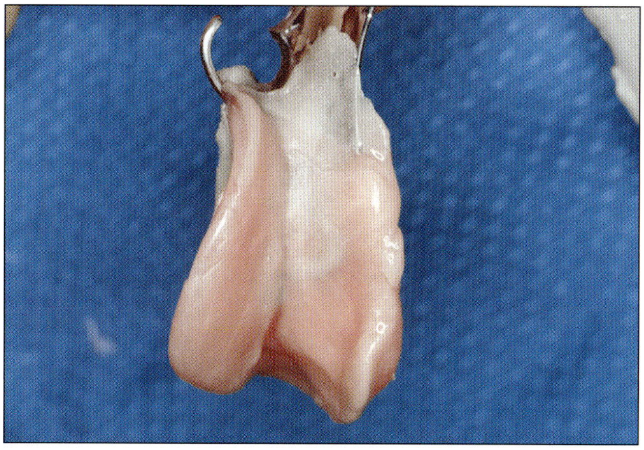

FIG 9-24 A chairside reline after removal from the mouth. Note bubble- and void-free surface.

Occlusal adjustment

To complete the reline procedure, the clinician must be prepared to adjust the occlusion. Because the loss of ridge support occurs over an extended period of time, migration of the opposing dentition or prosthesis is to be expected. This requires a clinical remount procedure if a complete denture is involved, since intraoral adjustments on unstable bases will never give the quality of occlusal contacts that can be developed on the articulator. When the opposing arch is natural dentition and significant compensatory eruption has occurred, the occlusal changes can result in overreduction of the prosthetic teeth on the partial denture. It may be necessary to equilibrate the opposing occlusal surfaces to maintain a reasonable occlusal plane. These more dramatic situations should be diagnosed prior to undertaking the reline and certainly are best prevented by attention to the need for both relining and replacement of worn prosthetic teeth.

While the base support must be evaluated as part of the annual recall examination, the actual need for a reline on a mature ridge should not occur more often than once every 4 to 6 years. When a solid tissue-base relationship exists, concern over the stress relief built into the design of the partial denture becomes purely academic. The rotation of the partial denture during function can be expected to be within the tolerance of periodontal ligaments, thus limiting any damage to the abutment teeth.

As just noted, part of the recall examination includes evaluation of the wear of the occlusal surfaces of the denture teeth. As discussed earlier, it may be appropriate to evaluate the wear of the resin teeth over a period of time, and to only convert to metal or ceramic when a total lack of contact is found. Once the need to convert to a more wear-resistant material is necessary, it is best done immediately after a reline of the base, should a reline be indicated due to resorption.

Given what is known about the need for continual maintenance of even our best efforts, the repairs, additions, and relines of all types of RPDs become a critical component of the state-of-the-art partial denture. Even though we have made every effort to design and construct the strongest possible partial dentures, we know that we will be required to perform these services, with the help of our technicians, on a routine basis, along with the ongoing efforts in combating caries and periodontal disease.

CASE STUDY:

Achieving and maintaining optimum soft tissue support

Regular maintenance is required throughout the life of an RPD. This goes beyond disease-control efforts. Residual ridge resorption will result in lost tissue-base contact. In Class I and other extreme classes, this support is critical to the function of the prosthesis. It may still become a nuisance in tooth-borne situations, as food will impact into open spaces. If mesh retention with acrylic base was selected, resorption will be relatively easy to manage with a reline procedure. This sequence demonstrates a typical chairside reline for a base that lacks ideal contact. While this is often encountered after time has elapsed, this case shows a chairside reline being used instead of an altered cast procedure. Regardless, the clinical process is the same.

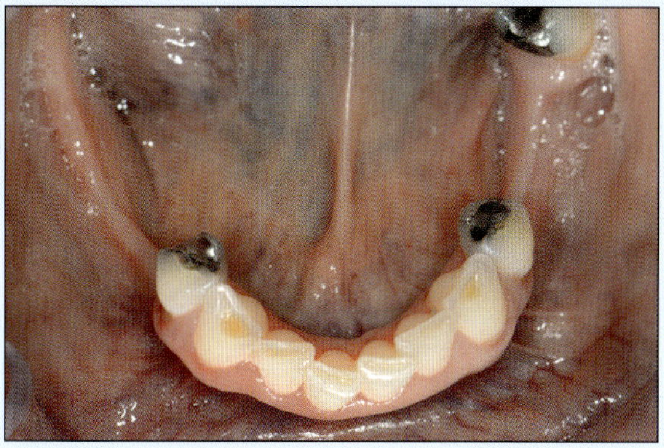

FIG 1 A 56-year-old woman was treatment planned for a maxillary immediate complete denture and a mandibular RPD. Her Cariogram score was 68% with significant improvement expected after a dedicated caries-control program. Maintaining her mandibular dentition was considered critical due to a predisposition for severe residual ridge resorption. This, along with some financial limitations, made her a poor candidate for dental implants.

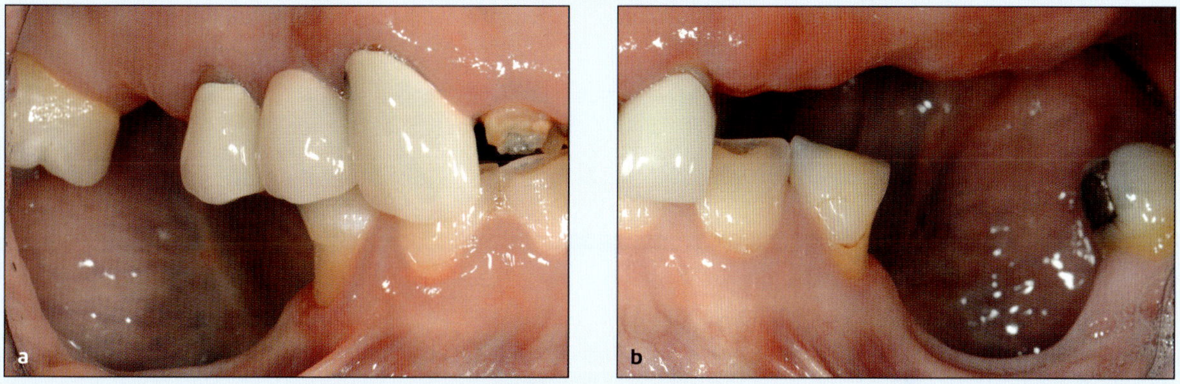

FIG 2 *(a and b)* Maximizing support and stability exclusively with rests and guiding planes would be unlikely considering the length and height of the distal extension and tooth-bound edentulous segments. Ideal tissue support was required. To accomplish this, a chairside reline was planned to be done at time of placement of the new partial denture.

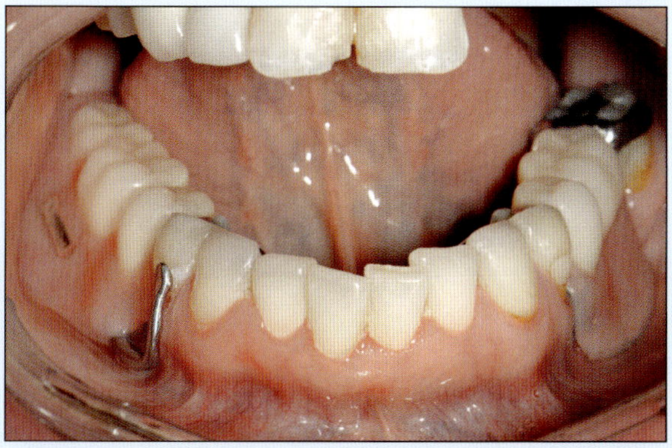

FIG 3 The Kennedy Class II Mod 1 mandibular arch offered an adequate number and position of abutment teeth. Fortunately, they required minimal restorative intervention. This resulted in a conservative and cost-effective partial denture.

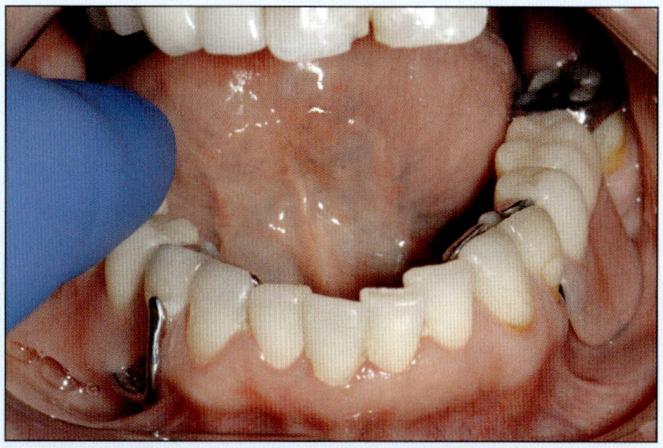

FIG 4 Lack of adequate soft tissue support was confirmed at placement. Firm pressure on the distal extension caused tipping along the fulcrum line. Note the lifting up of the rest seats on the patient's left first premolar and canine. While more ideal guiding plane contact would resist this lifting, the extent of these edentulous segments required maximum support from the soft tissue.

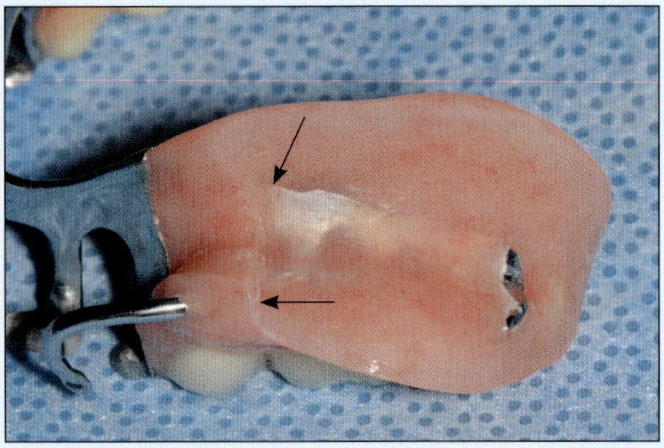

FIG 5 Proper extensions along the distal extension flanges were confirmed. The preparation of the base therefore maintained the existing length. A finish line was created along the entire periphery. This butt joint is highlighted by the *arrows*. The relief of the base is critical to ensure adequate thickness and therefore quality of reline material. The finish line ensures a secure and maintainable union between the base and reline material that is less likely to peel or leak.

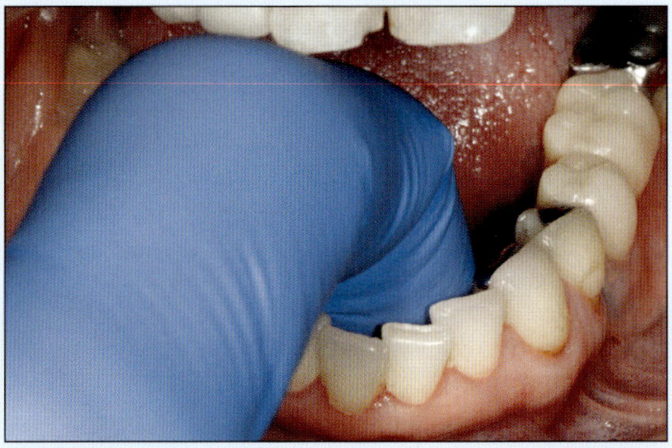

FIG 6 It is critical to maintain the tooth-frame interface during the reline procedure. Pressure is never applied to the distal extension. The frame is held in place throughout complete setting of the material. Note the slight excess material expressed on the right buccal shelf. This confirmed that an adequate volume of material was used. The rest seats are completely seated. Border molding movements can be conducted if necessary, once the material has reached a doughy consistency.

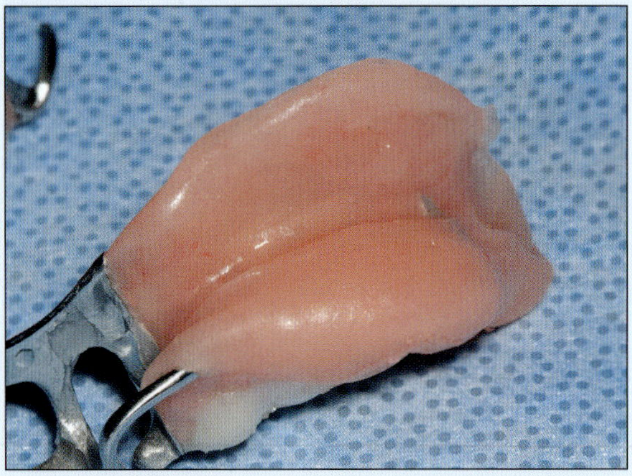

FIG 7 A high-density reline with minimal bubbles or voids was confirmed. Flexacryl Hard (Lang Dental), an autopolymerized polymethyl methacrylate, was used. The peripheral border roll appears clean, consistent, and continuous. Note how minimal material has flowed over the metal distal to the abutment tooth. This indicates close contact and that an appropriate amount of material was used.

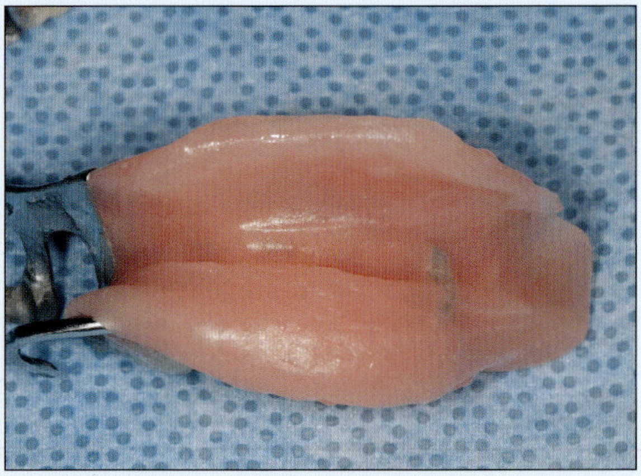

FIG 8 The material now present between the clasp arm and abutment tooth will need to be trimmed away. The efficiency of a reline was preferred to an altered cast procedure. In addition, the tooth-frame relationship could be more confidently maintained. If the patient's tongue was more powerful or difficult to control, an altered cast procedure would have been used.

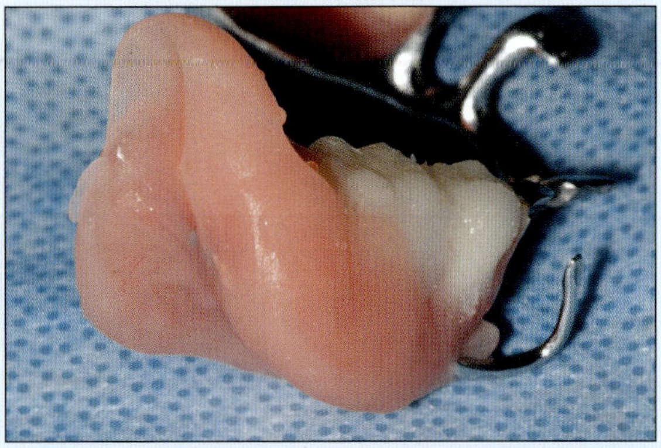

FIG 9 Material has flowed above the retromolar pad and filled the space above the buccal shelf. Activation of the buccinator muscle formed this contour. The original border can be seen showing through as the color of the reline material changes with its density. A decision is now made on whether the excess material filling this space is appropriate to manage the food bolus. In this instance, a thinner concave form was restored.

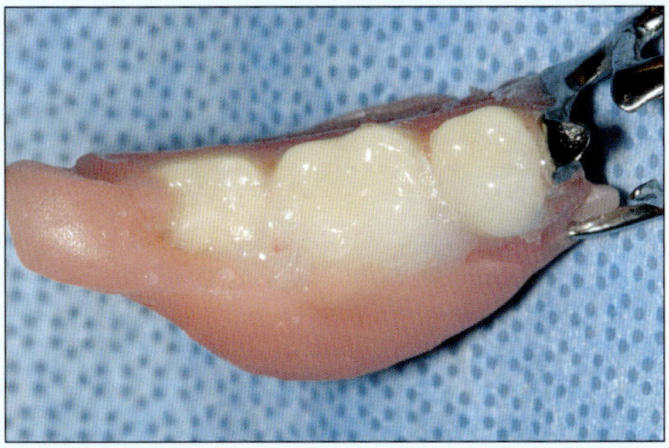

FIG 10 If excessive reline material is used, there is a risk of locking around abutment teeth. This is especially true if modification spaces are being relined. A dual-curing reline material that hardens when light-cured outside the mouth will greatly reduce the risk of binding.

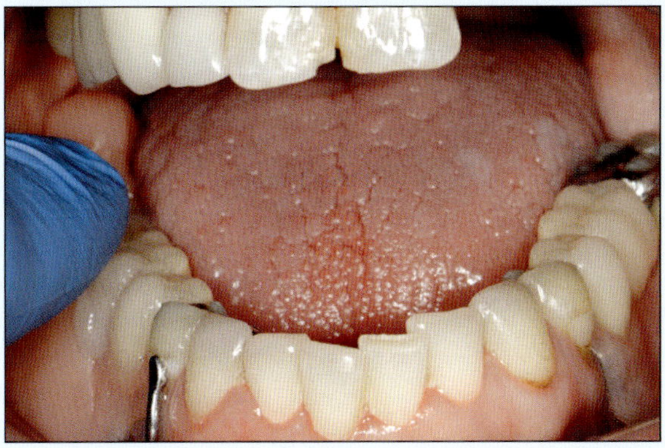

FIG 11 Effectiveness of the reline is confirmed after full curing. Firm finger pressure no longer displaces the RPD or guiding plane contact on the left first premolar. The rest seats remain in contact. Final trimming and polishing can now be completed.

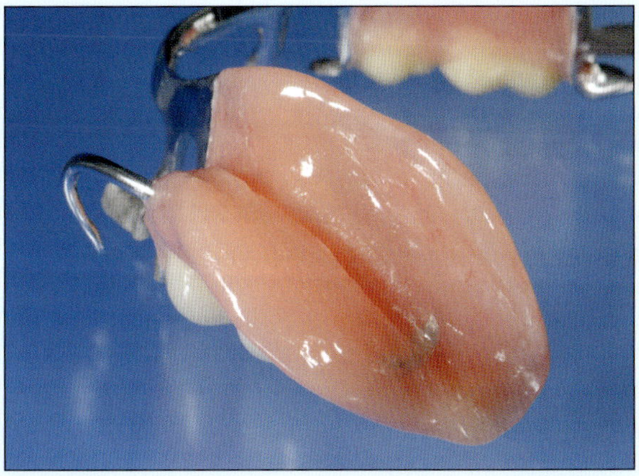

FIG 12 After trimming and polishing, a surface sealer was applied and allowed to cure. The critical buccal shelf and retromolar pad are replicated in detail. These areas must be accurately covered to provide sufficient support.

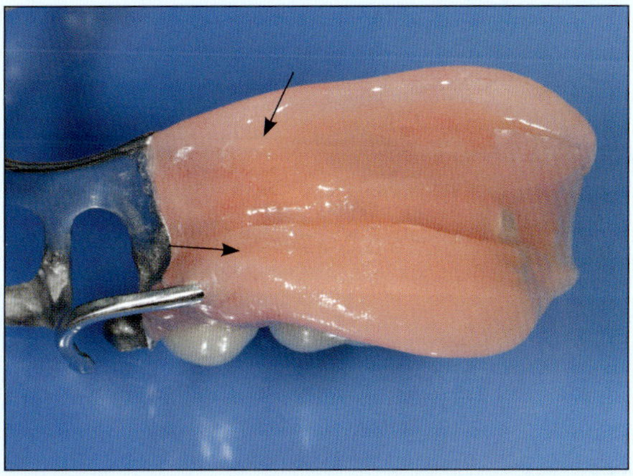

FIG 13 The *arrows* highlight the internal finish line between the reline material and the original base. An effective finish line and reline process will minimize future peeling and leakage. Note how the excess material between the clasp arm and abutment tooth has been removed and contoured.

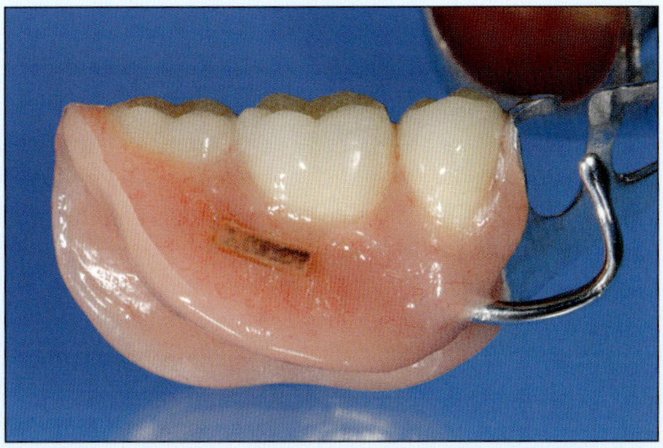

FIG 14 The color difference demonstrates the finish line between the reline material and original base. Excess length of reline material would indicate that the original flange was underextended. This process can typically be completed, start to finish, in 30 minutes.

References

1. NaBadalung DP, Powers JM, Connelly ME. Comparison of bond strengths of denture base resins to nickel-chromium-beryllium removable partial denture alloy. J Prosthet Dent 1997;78:566–573.
2. Brudvik JS, Lee S, Croshaw SN, Reimers DL. Laser welding of removable partial denture frameworks [published correction appears in Int J Prosthodont 2008;21:386. Reimers, Dave L [corrected to Reimers, Donald L]]. Int J Prosthodont 2008;21:285–291.
3. Brudvik JS, Fisher WT, Chandler HT. Repairs of metal parts of removable partial dentures. J Prosthet Dent 1972;28:205–208.
4. Brudvik JS, Nicholls JI. Soldering of removable partial dentures. J Prosthet Dent 1983;49:762–765.
5. NaBadalung DP, Nicholls JI, Brudvik JS. Frictional resistance of removable partial dentures with retrofitted resin composite guide planes. Int J Prosthodont 1997;10:116–122.
6. Tran CD, Sherraden DR, Curtis TA. A review of techniques of crown fabrication for existing removable partial dentures. J Prosthet Dent 1986;55:671–673.
7. Smith CS, Grandin H, Low K. A predictable all-digital workflow to retrofit a crown to an existing removable partial prosthesis. J Prosthet Dent 2019;121:876–878.
8. Gouveia DNM, Razzoog ME, Alfaro MF. A fully digital approach to fabricating a CAD-CAM ceramic crown to fit an existing removable partial denture. J Prosthet Dent 2019;121:571–575.
9. Bunch J, Johnson GH, Brudvik JS. Evaluation of hard direct reline resins. J Prosthet Dent 1987;57:512–519.

INTERIM RESIN-BASED PARTIAL DENTURES

10

How do we get from here to there?

The extensive prescription and use of resin-based RPDs for definitive care in general dental practice is perhaps the primary reason for the continued poor performance of partial dentures in epidemiologic research. Those reading this text—particularly graduate students lacking significant real-world exposure—may be unaware of the large degree of difference between the effort and results discussed in this text and that of a typical multi-dentist corporate or government-managed general dental clinic. With a transient patient population, frequent dentist turnover, and financial decisions often superseding clinical decisions, long-term results are rarely considered a priority. With regard to RPDs, it is no surprise then that the quickest, cheapest, and least complicated treatment modality would be provided. Outside the United States, having a metal major connector is exceedingly rare.[1–5] Within the United States, modern data from the private practice environment[6] find that the nonmetal RPD is far more common than how it is portrayed in the dental schools or in typical research.[7,8] It seems clear that financial pressures, often stemming from the inability to control the technical steps of RPD construction, quickly alter a new dentist's preference for the type of RPD they provide to patients. While not a surprise, this demonstrates yet another reason why the RPD continues to unjustly be viewed in a negative light.

The numerous significant disadvantages of the various resin and resin-like materials used for RPD frameworks are, as of yet, too great to be overcome on a consistent long-term basis. The mainstream use of polyetheretherketone (PEEK), polyamide resin (nylon), and improved polymethyl methacrylate (PMMA) resins will certainly grow.[9] However, their use for advanced RPD frameworks as discussed within this text remains limited for the foreseeable future. These materials nonetheless have worthy applications. With certain design modifications, they have improved enough that short- or perhaps even medium-term use can be considered.

An *interim prosthesis* is defined as a fixed or removable dental prosthesis designed to enhance esthetics, stabilization, and/or function for a limited period of time, after which it is to be replaced by a definitive dental prosthesis; often, such prostheses are used to assist in determination of the therapeutic effectiveness of a specific treatment plan or the form and function of the planned definitive prosthesis.

Philosophy of Use

It is rare for a patient to present in an adequate state of health and ready for fabrication of an RPD. The typical presentation, as discussed in chapter 1, is the partially edentulous patient with active dental disease. The existing prosthodontic work is usually failing, with malpositioned fixed or removable partial dentures that have lost abutments or components. Once treatment is planned for an RPD, the next most critical question becomes how to transition from this diseased, debilitated state to a healthy, reconstructed end result. Resin-based interim partial dentures are the typical answer to this question and are often required to facilitate an advanced RPD. They facilitate two distinct aspects of care. First, they provide reliable and functional prosthetics during disease management. Second, they allow immediate transition of debilitated dentitions that almost invariably present with significant malocclusions. Without this transition, there is no control over the multiple steps of the rehabilitation.

Disease management, as has been discussed, requires time. The common excuse for not properly managing dental disease before fabricating definitive prostheses is that "the patient needs something to wear." This is exacerbated by the obvious desires of patients with limited posterior teeth or missing anterior teeth. The commitment to the extensive time, cost, and effort of an advanced RPD requires that disease be fully controlled for the long term. For the patient to accept the disease-management approach, they must be provided with a capable interim prosthesis that addresses their concerns, at least in part. In this way, they can be kept engaged and motivated. For those patients ready for definitive care, mouth preparation and prosthesis fabrication will require multiple visits and time. The patient should have an interim prosthesis that is functional, comfortable, and esthetic. Ideally, it will be a prototype of the definitive prosthesis. In this way, a positive interim experience will improve the prognosis of the definitive RPD.

Whether being used strictly for disease management or to facilitate the reconstructive transition, the interim prosthesis will likely need to be modified several times over the course of treatment. Tooth and tissue contours will change with mouth preparation. What is therefore needed is a prosthesis that can be efficiently, effectively, and economically modified. PMMA resins therefore continue to be the material best suited for interim prostheses during restorative transitions. While frameworks made from PEEK and polyamide show great promise, the fact that they cannot currently be effectively and efficiently modified chairside limits their utility to interim prostheses that will require infrequent modification.

Disadvantages

The list of disadvantages with resin-based frameworks is extensive. To try and overcome the primary disadvantages, laboratories often alter design principles, creating further negative side effects. To begin with, the materials are universally weaker than metal. To reduce the risk of fracture, the major connectors are made thicker and/or wider (Fig 10-1). Small, thin components would easily break or flex, so rests and most minor connectors are typically not included (Fig 10-2). These materials are flexible when compared with metal connectors, polyamides dramatically so (Fig 10-3). This flexibility and subsequent lack of adequate hard tissue support, as provided by rests, results in a prosthesis supported by soft tissue.

Clinical experience will quickly demonstrate the consequences of relying on extensive soft tissue support. Discomfort, more rapid residual ridge resorption, recession, marginal tissue inflammation, and tissue trauma in general are all to be expected with extended time of use. The more missing teeth, the greater the reliance on the soft tissue support, and the more likely and rapid the consequences will tend to be. The detrimental effects on the limited number of remaining tooth contacts will also be exacerbated. Experienced clinicians have seen the incisal attrition, migration, and chipping that occurs once posterior contact has been lost. When a limited number of teeth are missing, for example a single incisor, a resin-based RPD tends to work well and do little harm. The remaining tooth contacts are extensive enough to limit significant functional pressure on the periodontal tissues. In essence, when a limited number of teeth are replaced, the resin-based interim prosthesis is nothing more than a cosmetic space-maintaining prosthesis.

The plaque adherence and porosity of these materials is another factor that is detrimental to periodontal health. Research on partial dentures often reflects this issue. When comparing material performance, it is important to note that the research that highlights poor periodontal response to RPDs is almost exclusively evaluating RPDs where porous resin material is present around the abutments.[10–16] In contrast to this, the research showing good or normal periodontal response to RPDs evaluated RPDs with metal frameworks that are often designed according to the philosophies in this text.[17–21] It is rare to find any clinical comparison that finds resin performance superior to metal, and the few that find no difference seem to contradict clinical experience.[22,23] This contrast in clinical results begs for comparative research. The near-total lack of head-to-head comparison of materials is something we hope changes with the arrival of the newer potentially improved resin-based or resin-like materials already mentioned.

From a biologic perspective, polyamides appear to further complicate the periodontal issues seen with other resins.[16] Similar to PMMA, plaque tends to adhere more aggressively, and porosity has not been eliminated. The ability to maintain a high-quality clinical polish on the fairly soft and easily scratched surface is difficult.[24] Special extra-soft brushes and plain nonabrasive soap are used to prevent rapid loss of surface finish. The inherent flexibility of the

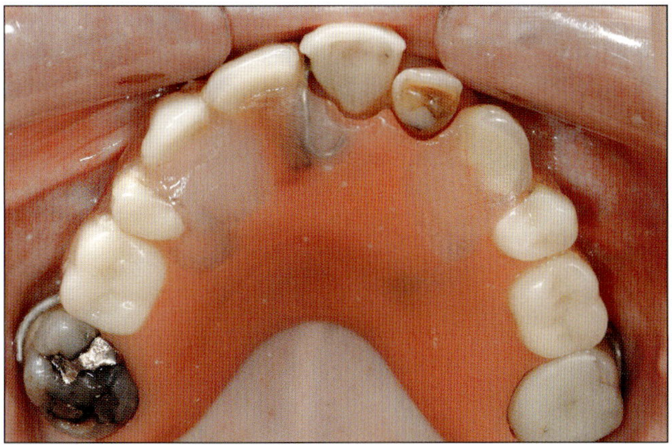

FIG 10-1 Interim resin-based RPD with excess tissue coverage and bulky major connector.

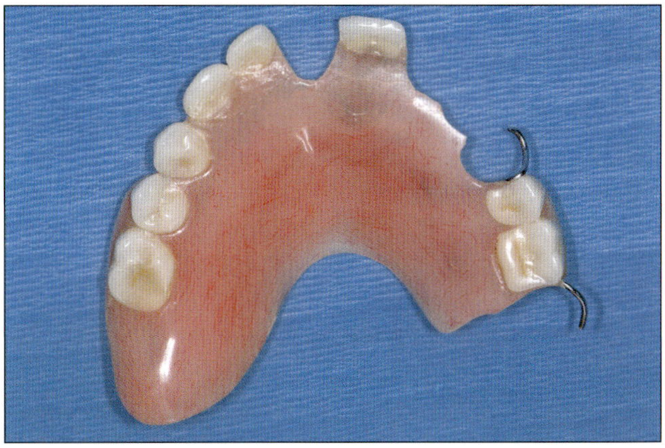

FIG 10-2 Entirely soft tissue–supported interim resin-based RPD. Note the fracture lines at the incisors due to the weak material.

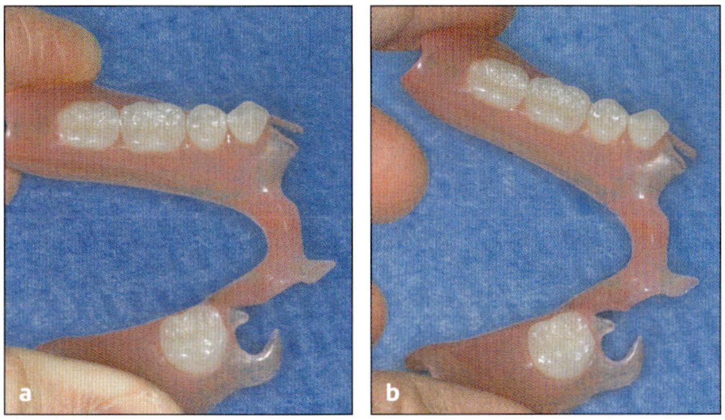

FIG 10-3 *(a and b)* A polyamide-based RPD with a lingual bar is very flexible.

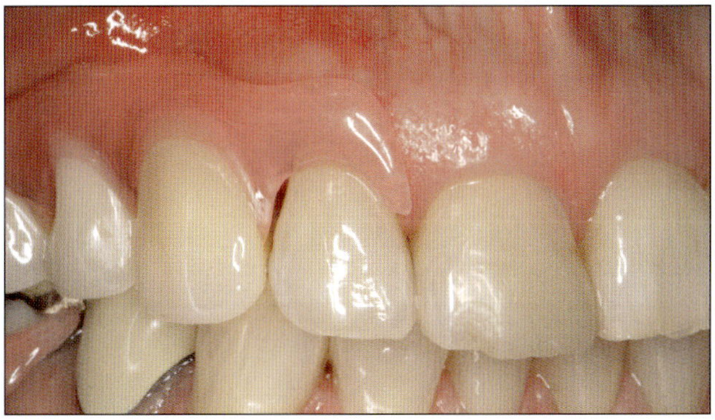

FIG 10-4 Tall and thick polyamide clasp overlaying the faciogingival of an incisor.

polyamides requires additional bulk when a certain degree of resistance to deformation is desired. This results in clasps that are significantly larger than a typical cast or wire clasp. They therefore overlay the delicate buccal gingival tissue (Fig 10-4). While the more natural color of these clasps is highlighted as a great benefit, the dramatic increase in size of these clasps tends to damage the periodontal tissue. The tissue-supported design and extensive tooth coverage is more likely to cause tissue trauma, recession, and even tooth mobility beyond that of other resin-based designs.

From a technical perspective, polyamides, and to a certain extent PEEK, lack the ease of use that clinicians have come to expect from PMMA. Take for example a simple base or contour adjustment. PMMA is smooth and reliable to cut, trim, and polish. Polyamide peels and melts when cut. Specific stones are recommended for making adjustments, but these still tend to melt the material at uncontrolled speeds, making precise adjustment difficult (Fig 10-5). The polishing process after adjustment is a similar challenge, as it is difficult to leave a truly smooth and

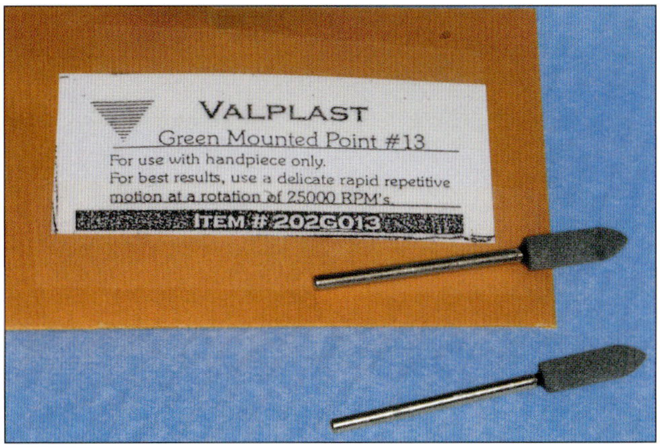

FIG 10-5 Specific stones and instructions for adjusting the polyamide surface.

polished surface. It is also not possible to make a chairside addition to these newer materials. These materials are chemically inert once cured. This means that, with the current state of the technology, bonding additional material to them is time consuming and must be laboratory based. Most laboratories would tell you it is just as easy to make an entirely new polyamide RPD as to add a tooth or base extension to an existing one. The lack of a chemically active surface also means that these materials do not bond to typical composite or acrylic denture teeth. The teeth must therefore be mechanically retained. Because the framework is flexible, these teeth are known to break off. This issue is complicated in cases where there is reduced interocclusal space or a lack of ability to completely surround the prosthetic teeth with the framework. Taken as a whole, these technical issues make it very difficult to achieve an adequate tissue-base or tooth-frame relationship. This is a major problem since the fit cannot be reliably managed. If the base cannot be accurately adjusted and efficiently modified, and if it lacks the rigidity to provide cross-arch force distribution, then the clinician has little control over the functional aspects of the prosthesis. In this context, PMMA can be made to fit both the tissue and teeth better than other resin-based or resin-like materials at this time.

It is interesting that color is used as the primary marketing scheme by the manufacturers of the newer resin-based materials. These advertisements often highlight the "ugly" clasping by metal RPDs. These statements are of course made with the typical RPD in mind and have not considered the modern advanced RPD. If they had, they would realize that the unesthetic display of clasping is not a prerequisite of a metal-framed partial denture. In fact, the bulky, eventually discolored, food-catching clasp arms of polyamide partial dentures tend to be less esthetic in practice than a well-constructed infrabulge clasp arm. Considering just the base, the polyamides are translucent and do to tend to show the underlying tissue color. However, custom staining is not an option, which once again leaves PMMA in a superior position when ideal esthetics are needed. PEEK, on the other hand, has the opposite issue as it is very opaque. Clinical reports demonstrating these materials show very opaque white clasps that do not appear much more esthetic than a small gold wire running just above a gingival margin.[25]

As these various disadvantages become clear to clinicians, the marketing and manufacturer-highlighted applications have changed. Polyamides are now being used for clasps on metal frameworks. Likewise, conventional PMMA is being used to hold the prosthetic teeth to PEEK frameworks rather than relying on the mechanical locking between the teeth and PEEK. These efforts, while well intentioned, tend to complicate the overall process of RPD fabrication by incorporating additional steps or materials. Are the savings in time and perhaps cost really worth the disadvantages that the clinician and patient will experience? When one reads the advertisements or speaks with a laboratory technician promoting these new materials, it should be clear that they are being promoted to address problems that exist for the typical general dentist–level partial denture rather than the advanced partial denture. When compared with definitive advanced partial dentures, the indications for their selection over metal frameworks are severely limited and tend to be for disease management situations only.

Expectations

When the term "interim," "temporary," or "provisional" is used, it generally lowers expectations. As noted, this has a tendency to reduce the quality of the care. Partial dentures in general—often considered temporary—suffer from lack of technical attention or effort. If interim partial dentures are created with this mindset, the less-than-optimal results will serve only to push the patient to edentulism or rash decisions with risky fixed prosthodontic options. The interim RPD, for our more advanced purposes, must therefore also be provided to higher standards.

It is expected that an interim RPD will effectively replace the missing teeth. Function, comfort, and esthetics must therefore follow, although obviously not necessarily to an ideal level. The tooth-frame and tissue-base adaptation must be controlled so that the effectiveness of the planned design, for example guiding planes, can be tested (Fig 10-6). To ignore these aspects in the interim is to lose the opportunity to resolve problems before the definitive prosthesis is created. An ineffective interim prosthesis will leave the patient wondering whether an RPD was the correct choice. Worse yet, the ineffective interim prosthesis may create periodontal complications that negatively influence surgical outcomes.

It is also expected that an interim can be accomplished efficiently. This is most notable during complicated combination case rehabilitations where fixed prosthodontics is being combined with an RPD. Efficiency in this regard comes from the ability to fabricate an interim within a limited amount of chair time. Perhaps more important is keeping the patient functional and stable throughout the course of these complex treatments (Fig 10-7). Being forced to make multiple interim RPDs as the clinical environment changes would be very inefficient. Likewise, being forced to carry out modifications or changes over multiple appointments adds to the already extensive time and effort in these cases. Working through an off-site laboratory to add a tooth or alter a base extension is terribly inefficient.

The ability to make immediate chairside alterations to an interim prosthesis is the primary reason why PMMA resins continue to be the material of choice. These modifications are most commonly needed to accommodate surgical changes such as implant placement or tooth extraction.

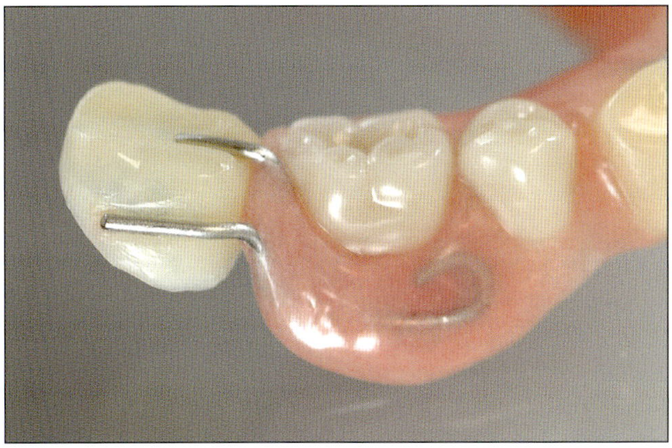

FIG 10-6 Rest seat, guiding plane, and buccal ledge incorporated into interim RPD design.

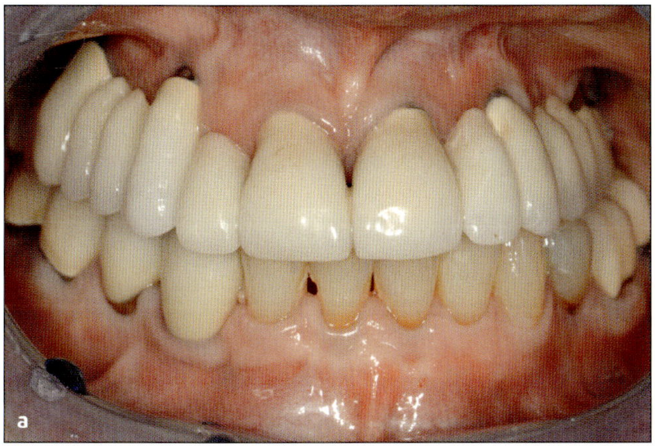

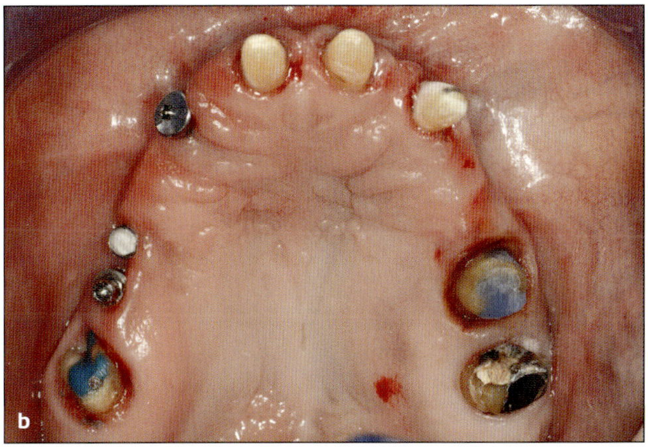

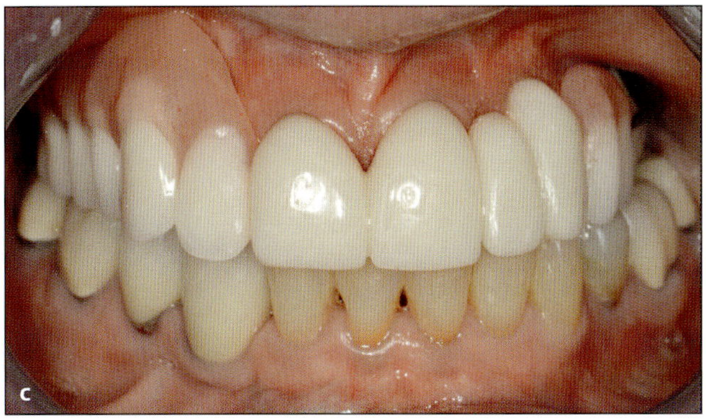

FIG 10-7 *(a)* A failing complex fixed rehabilitation in need of deconstruction. *(b)* Disassembled rehabilitation requiring immediate interim restoration. *(c)* Interim restorations allow the patient to remain stable and comfortable throughout the reconstruction.

Sectional relines are typically conducted to readapt and recontour the RPD to the surgical sites after postoperative healing (Fig 10-8). The interim RPD must also be altered when the dentist has elected to cement any new crown or bridge units prior to framework creation or when there has been a major change in the occlusal relationship due to treatment of the opposing arch. It is common for the initial form and design of the interim RPD to look much different by the time the definitive RPD will be fabricated (Fig 10-9). It should therefore be obvious how PMMA is well suited for this type of transitional prosthesis. The durability of the additions and subtractions are typically well maintained for the fairly short functional time period they are needed. These adjustments and changes occur chairside with autopolymerizing material the same day that the abutment or tissue change occurs. In this way, there is no extra visit for the patient.

The final primary expectation is that all of this occurs economically. While some charges will be necessary, in the context of the overall plan, they should be minor. The

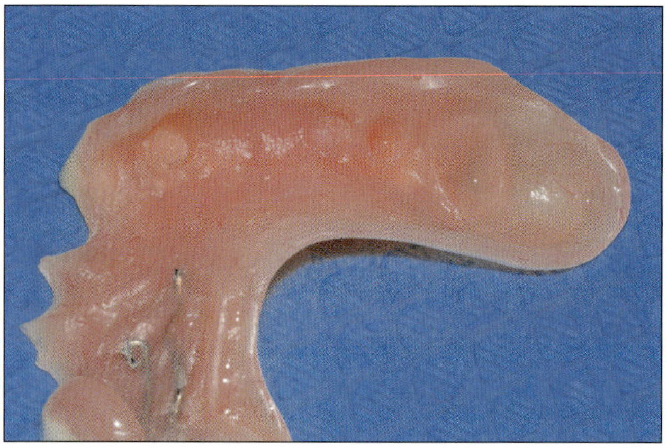

FIG 10-8 Intaglio surface relined chairside as implants have healed and teeth are restored.

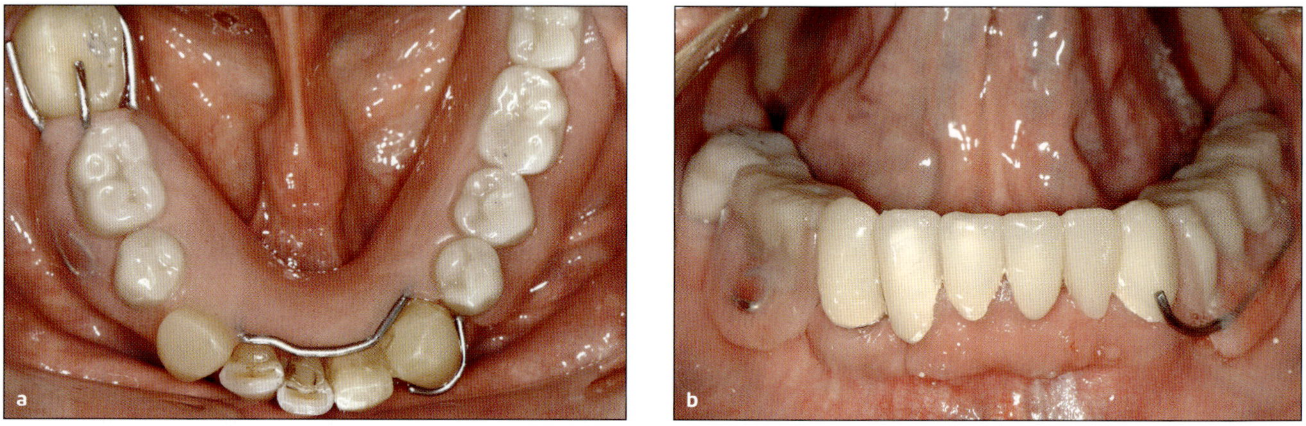

FIG 10-9 *(a)* Initial interim RPD. *(b)* Interim RPD after 18 months of service. Note the alterations to abutments, clasps, and occlusion as orthodontic, surgical, and restorative steps have been completed.

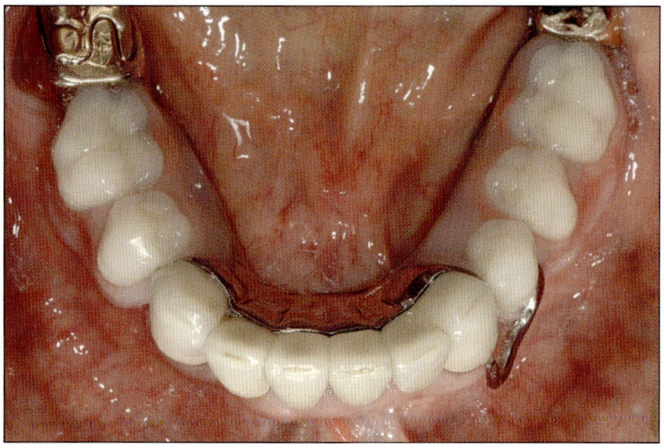

FIG 10-10 To avoid surprises, the completed RPD from Fig 10-9 is very similar to the interim in form and design.

dentist can mitigate the overall cost by using lower-grade prosthetic teeth and by maximizing the efficiencies just discussed. A successful interim prosthesis will reduce the chair time required for the rehabilitation. This is of obvious benefit to both the patient and clinician. In reality, the effort and time spent on the interim RPD will repay itself in the form of a somewhat predetermined outcome for the definitive RPD (Fig 10-10). If the interim RPD was functional, comfortable, and esthetic, the operator will have confidence that the definitive prosthesis will be the same, likely better. As an experienced clinician knows, additional appointments for small complications such as broken temporary crowns and to adjust sore areas quickly increase overhead and reduce expected profitability.

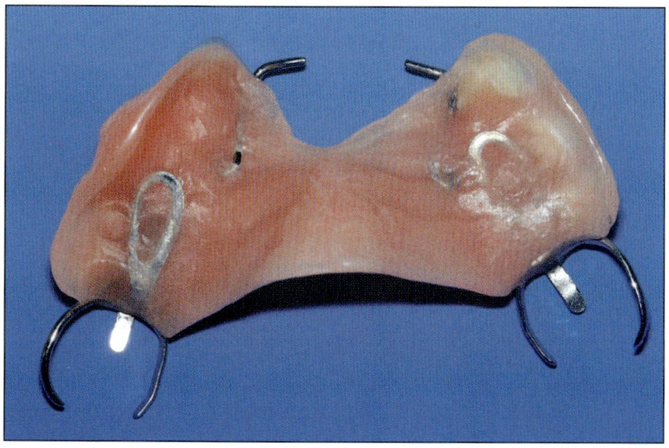

FIG 10-11 Wire rest extensions on interim RPD. Note the wide, half-round wire used on the molars.

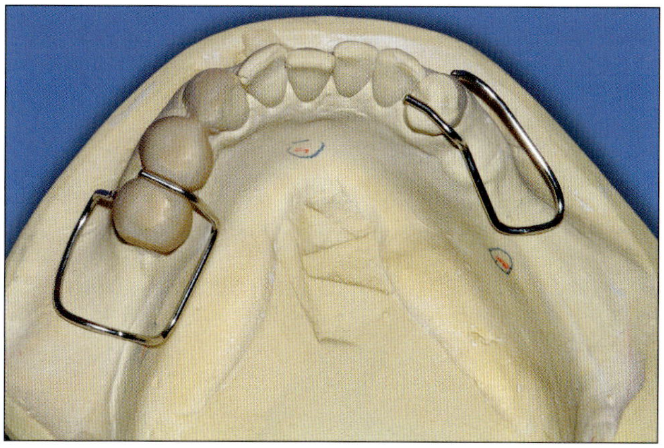

FIG 10-12 Mesial rest between premolars designed into recess within embrasure.

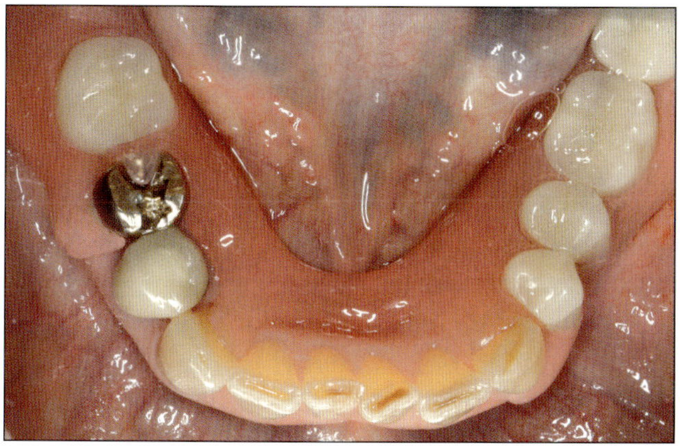

FIG 10-13 The effectiveness of the rests created on this flexible polyamide frame is questionable.

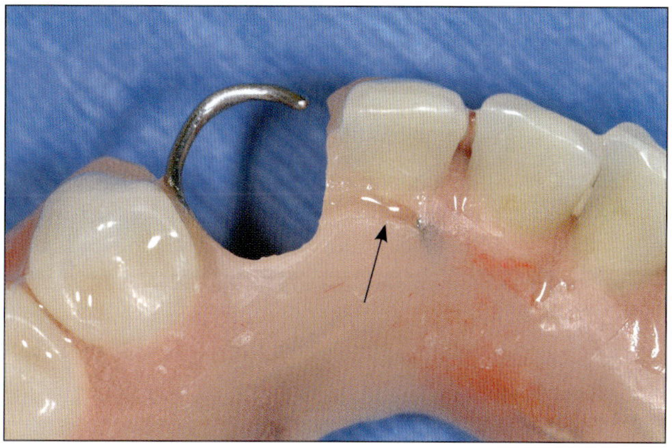

FIG 10-14 Residual recess from a failed round wire rest *(arrow)*. A larger-gauge, half-round form is advised.

Design

Several specific design considerations should be applied on a routine basis for interim resin-based partial dentures. The first and foremost among these is the addition of some form of rest[26] (Fig 10-11). The exact type and design of the rests can take many forms (Fig 10-12). The goal, of course, is vertical support. This can be accomplished with wires, acrylic extensions, ball clasps, or even castings incorporated into the major connector. The longer the interim prosthesis is expected to function, the more critical the need to have reliable vertical support. For this support to be effective, the means of resisting the vertical displacement toward the tissue must be rigid and strong. The use of thin, weak PMMA or polyamide material will not suffice (Fig 10-13). These materials will either break or flex when masticatory pressure is applied.

Wire rest extensions can be very effective and efficient but must be done with wire of adequate gauge to prevent early fatigue failure of the wrought metal (Fig 10-14). Ideally, this is done with larger-gauge half-round wire that has limited flexibility compared with round wires. These wire rests can be placed within prepared or preexisting rest seats. They can also extend over embrasures or as strut rests to ultimately function as a vertical stop (Fig 10-15). These embrasure wires can be strategically placed in areas of open occlusal contact to avoid interfering with intercuspal position. Ball clasps are also sometimes used for this purpose, as the ball end can fit nicely into either a prepared rest or an occlusal depression. Keep in mind, these balls rely on the wire diameter just adjacent to the ball itself being thick enough to resist early fatigue failure. Orthodontists are also very familiar with resin-based interim prostheses. Labial wires, as in a Hawley retainer, can be used to stabilize anterior teeth where the lack of posterior support has resulted in excessive mobility (Fig 10-16). If the mobility of these teeth can be improved by the interim prosthesis, a more definitive treatment plan can be made with more confidence.

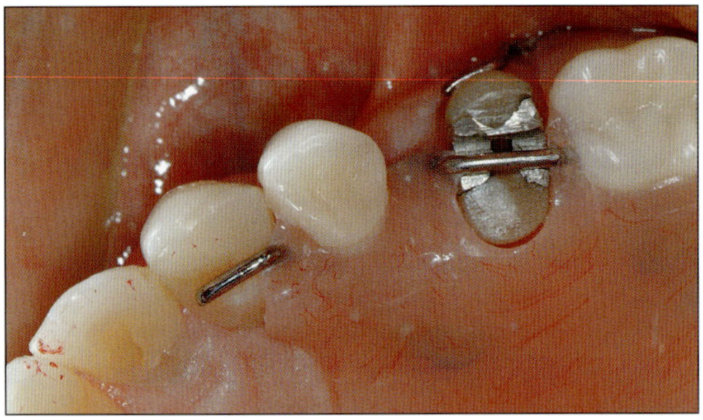

FIG 10-15 A wire strut rest used to maximize support on a lone premolar abutment.

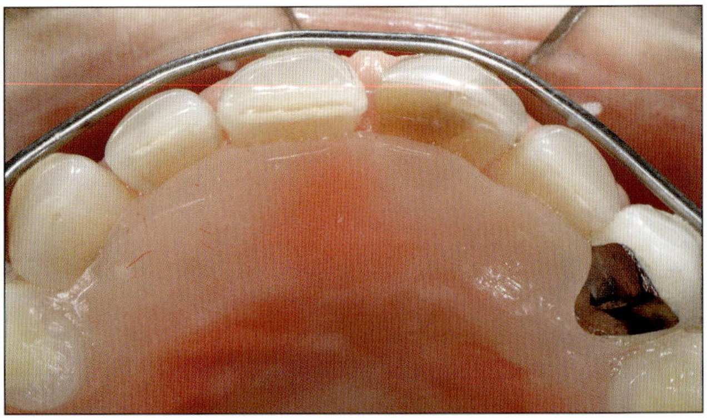

FIG 10-16 Labial wire with lingual plate to help stabilize highly mobile anterior teeth.

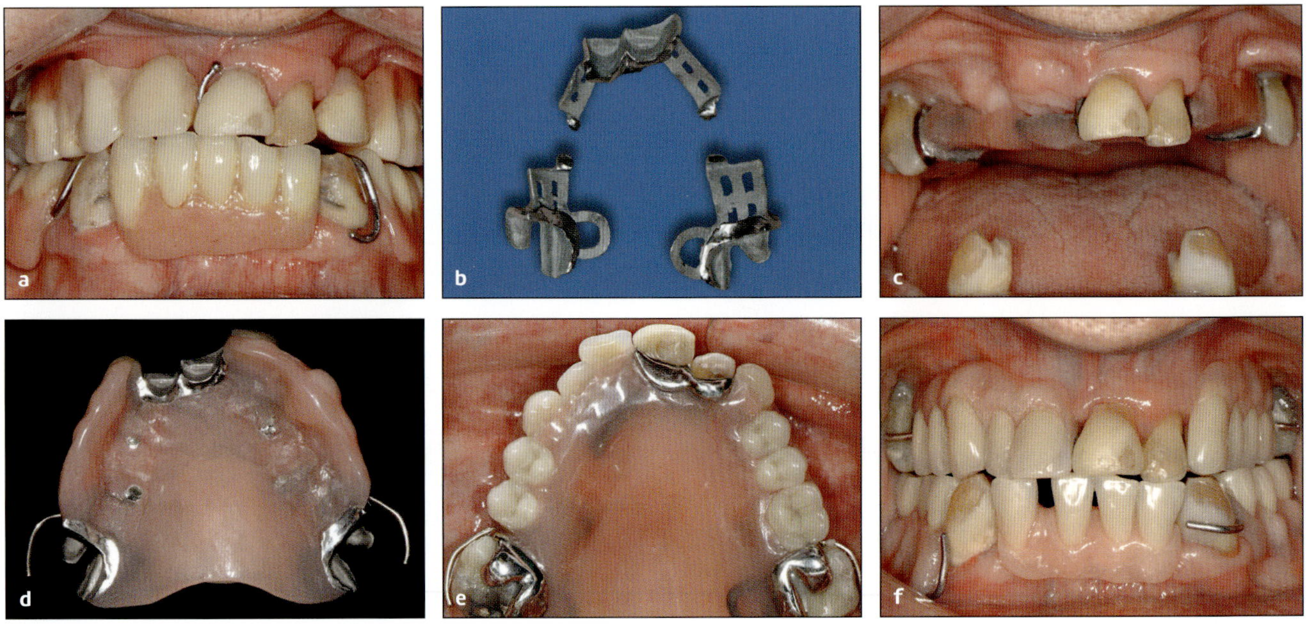

FIG 10-17 *(a)* High-risk patient wishing to avoid edentulation as long as possible. *(b)* Base metal component castings. *(c)* Optional framework evaluation. *(d)* Completed conversion prosthesis. *(e)* Resin-based major connector. *(f)* No maxillary anterior clasps.

The conversion prosthesis

More elaborate rest seat incorporation can be achieved using individual castings. Smith and Rymarz showed the use of simple clasp assembly castings that were connected by a PMMA major connector.[27] This was done to extend the longevity of interim RPDs and has proven to be quite effective. For interim RPDs that are only expected to function for several months, this is likely unnecessary effort. However, in situations where the interim's life span may need to be measured in years, this may be a critically important design addition.

Interim partial dentures are indicated for disease management situations partly due to the challenges encountered when an abutment fails and we wish to continue using the existing prosthesis. What if the existing prosthesis were designed in a way that the loss of one or more abutments did not dramatically affect its ability to continue to be used? While it is common for RPD design to accommodate individual poor-prognosis abutments, to do so in an efficient and effective manner for situations with multiple poor-prognosis abutments remains challenging[20] (see Fig 10-17a). This idea led to the development of the conversion prosthesis concept. By incorporating an interim philosophy with cast tooth-frame assemblies, the effectiveness of a definitive prosthesis can be achieved with the efficiency of a PMMA major connector.[29]

A conversion partial is an RPD whose tooth-frame assembly components are individually fabricated and then joined with an acrylic resin major connector (Fig 10-17). Cecconi et al's component partial concept, discussed in chapter 6, where the partial denture is designed and constructed in

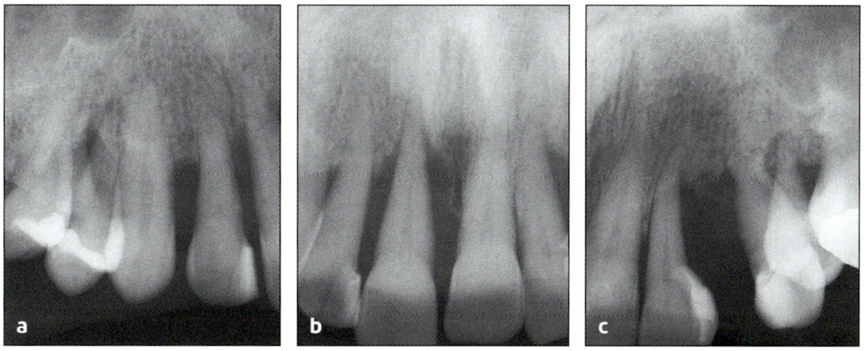

FIG 10-18 *(a to c)* A periodontally terminal dentition. Note the bone loss on all remaining teeth.

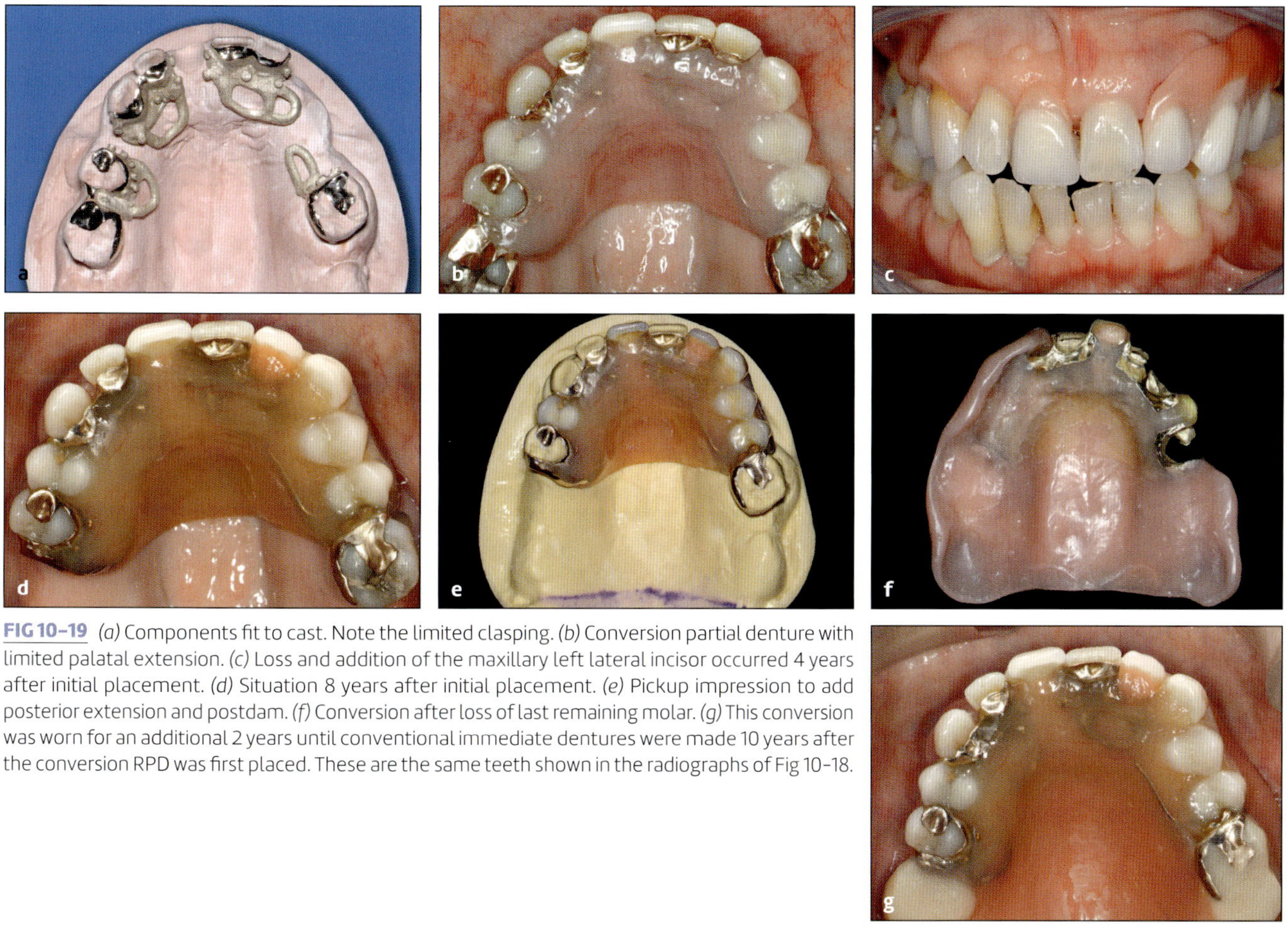

FIG 10-19 *(a)* Components fit to cast. Note the limited clasping. *(b)* Conversion partial denture with limited palatal extension. *(c)* Loss and addition of the maxillary left lateral incisor occurred 4 years after initial placement. *(d)* Situation 8 years after initial placement. *(e)* Pickup impression to add posterior extension and postdam. *(f)* Conversion after loss of last remaining molar. *(g)* This conversion was worn for an additional 2 years until conventional immediate dentures were made 10 years after the conversion RPD was first placed. These are the same teeth shown in the radiographs of Fig 10-18.

individual parts, is followed.[30] The parts are individually fitted on the definitive cast and joined during resin processing. Unlike the component system, the conversion partial does not use a metal major connector. The benefit of eliminating the metal major connector is superior convertibility. If an abutment tooth or teeth are lost, the metal component can be removed and both replaced at the same visit with minimal time and effort.

The design flexibility of the conversion partial lends itself to patients with terminal dentitions (Fig 10-18). Maximum available support, stability, and frictional retention can be maintained through the optimum passive fit achieved during fabrication. If the assembled components do not fit at framework evaluation, the dentist has a unique opportunity to correct the acrylic resin connector intraorally. The component(s) at fault can be easily sectioned from the acrylic resin frame and reconnected to the assembly using autopolymerizing acrylic resin in the mouth. However, the primary advantage is the ability to use the conversion partial as a transitional prosthesis as the remaining teeth are lost over time (Fig 10-19). If proper extensions are maintained, the conversion partial may be used as a transitional complete denture.

The conversion partial is well suited to the maxilla, where adequate rigidity may be achieved by the palatal acrylic resin. Mandibular prostheses may require a metal reinforcement to ensure adequate strength and rigidity. Also, some patients may object to the increased bulk of acrylic when compared with a metal framework.

Provisional prostheses for combination fixed-removable situations

One of the most difficult tasks faced in the construction of a partial denture is to maintain the patient with their existing partial denture throughout what may be a long treatment time. When orthodontics, implants, and perhaps even orthognathic surgery are involved, treatment time can extend to years. It is in the best interests of the clinician as well as the patient to convert an existing metal-frame partial denture to a quality resin appliance made in conjunction with any required fixed provisional restorations. While there are many possible ways of creating these provisional restorations, it is important to bear in mind the cost to the patient. The following technique creates a quality long-term provisional restoration at minimum cost to the patient. For those patients without a current prosthesis, or when the existing partial denture is of such poor quality that it cannot reasonably be converted, the provisional RPD is created new using this sequence.

The first step is to prepare the existing partial denture for a special type of pickup impression. Any component of the partial denture that contacts the remaining teeth is cut away with a large carborundum disk, leaving at least 2 to 3 mm of space between the partial denture and the teeth (Fig 10-20). This will allow the impression material full access to the teeth. A high-viscosity polyether or silicone impression material is mixed and placed on the tissue-contacting surfaces of the partial denture that have been previously coated with adhesive. The partial denture is carried to place and maintained in position while the patient is guided into MIP. If significant occlusal interferences exist, the prosthetic teeth on the partial denture should be equilibrated prior to the impression. This initial impression allows the partial denture base to be used as a record base. Unless the remaining tooth contacts are stable and accurate, the impression/record should be made in CR. This record is therefore made just prior to first contact of the natural teeth. This prevents incorporation of existing occlusal interferences. Before removing the partial denture, a second impression (alginate this time) in a stock dentate tray, preferably sectional, is made over the partial denture and the remainder of the denture-bearing area. Special care is taken to ensure that alginate is wiped onto all remaining teeth and into the space created between the partial denture and the teeth when the framework was sectioned.

The two impressions are hopefully removed together and poured in buff stone. When the alginate portion of the impression is removed from the cast, the elastomeric impression inside the old partial denture is left in place until the cast has been articulated with the opposing cast. Once articulated, the partial denture is carefully removed from the cast, leaving the impression material in the partial denture. At this time, any diagnostic waxing for the fixed provisional component is done according to standard techniques. Rest preparations and guiding planes are prepared, and undercuts ideal for infrabulge I-bar clasps are created. Once the waxing is complete, that cast is duplicated and the partial denture is now placed on the duplicate cast. Space between the partial denture and the new abutment tooth form must be verified to ensure accurate relation to the duplicate cast. Flanges are also cut away from the partial denture to create space for the retentive wire bar clasps. These Ni-Cr-Co wire clasps are adapted and waxed into place on the cast. Additional wax is added to complete the desired form of the provisional partial denture. Because the resin provisional will need to be thicker than the old framework, at least one thickness of baseplate wax must be added to all areas of bare metal framework. The outline of the provisional RPD will necessarily cover a greater portion of the mouth than did the old metal-based RPD (Fig 10-21). For the mandibular provisional, special care must be taken to wax the lingual plate area of the major connector to provide for adequate strength in the resin. Because the pickup impression was made in coordination with an accurate occlusal record and final adjustments to the abutment tooth contour were made prior to duplication of the articulated cast, there is no need to articulate this processing cast.

The completed waxed partial denture is placed in the first half of the processing flask in a normal manner. The second half of the flasking is the key to making this technique possible. The exposed denture with its added wax contours is covered with a stiff elastomeric silicone mold release material such as Flexistone (Detax). Immediately after placing this material, usually with the finger to ensure that no voids are created, the second half of the flasking is completed using the normal mix of dental stone. This immediate pouring of the stone onto the as-yet not-set silicone is essential to keep them from separating during the boil-out and opening of the flask. Once set, the flask is boiled out in the normal manner. When the flask is opened, the old partial denture is easily removed from the mold. After completing the boil-out, the cast is painted with separator. A small amount of autopolymerizing resin is added to the tang of the bar clasps to stabilize them during packing. The reason for selecting the infrabulge clasps for this provisional denture should now be apparent. Had a normal circumferential clasp been used, it would have had to cross

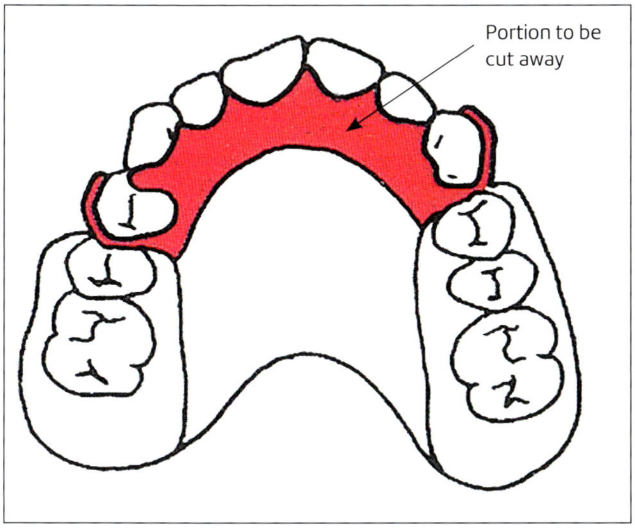

FIG 10-20 Preparation of an old RPD for conversion to a resin-based provisional RPD.

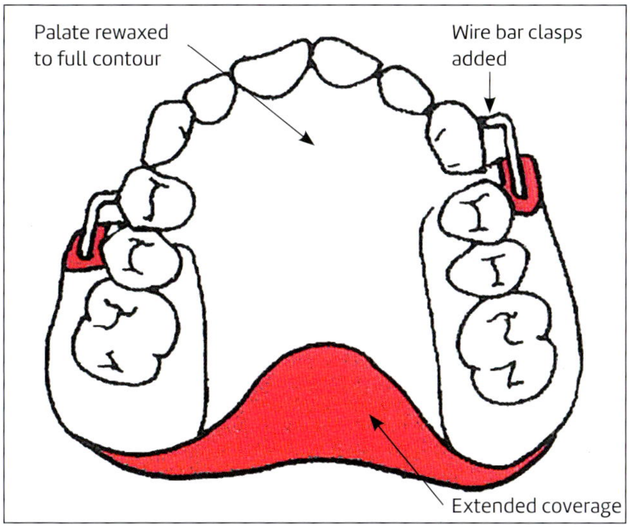

FIG 10-21 Final waxing of converted cast partial denture.

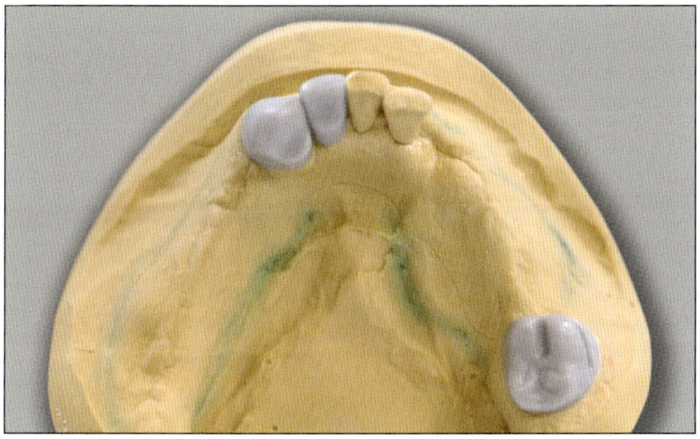

FIG 10-22 Waxed provisional contours ready for shell creation.

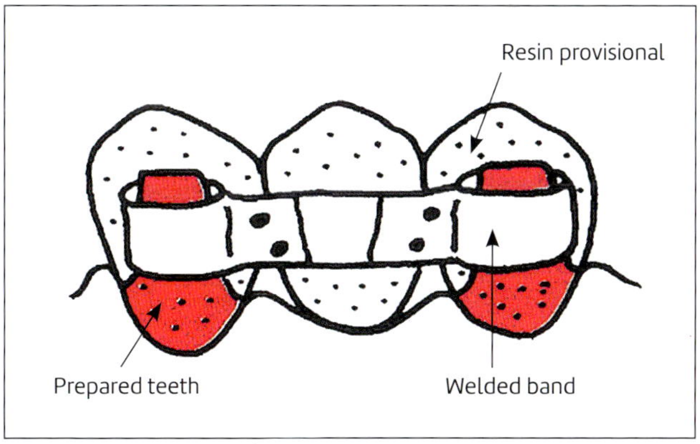

FIG 10-23 Fixed provisional reinforced with welded orthodontic band material.[31]

the occlusal surface of the RPD, which might have made removing the old RPD from the flask difficult.

The technician then has the option of either cutting the resin teeth and their associated resin from the old partial denture in block form and placing them back in the mold or pouring tooth-colored resin into the tooth negatives in the elastomeric material. If they choose to pour new resin into the negative, the flask would then be placed in a pressure pot for the cure of the new denture teeth. This segment of teeth will have to be removed from the mold and the excess resin removed before placing them back into the mold for final processing. In either case, the provisional partial denture is packed in a high-impact heat-cured resin and processed and finished in the normal manner.

The original definitive cast, with its waxed fixed provisional contours, is now used to create an eggshell fixed provisional for relining in the mouth (Fig 10-22). Additional wax is added to the marginal one-third of the teeth receiving provisionals to ensure there is adequate resin at the margin, and a putty mold of the wax-up is made. Tooth-colored resin of the appropriate shade is painted into the putty, usually with both incisal and body resin, and the mold placed in the pressure pot. Because the fixed provisional restoration will be required to support the removable provisional restoration, the stresses placed on the temporary cement seal will be great, especially if the provisional RPD is a Class I and can rotate in function. Any washout of cement and resultant caries will create a disaster that can be at least partially overcome by reinforcing the provisional with orthodontic band material.[31] The band material is loosely adapted to the preparation and spot welded in the interproximal areas as well as in the edentulous pontic areas. When completely adapted, the band is placed in the mouth and the fixed provisional shell relined in normal fashion, resulting in a metal-reinforced provisional fixed unit that has an increased resistance to flexure and cement seal failure[32] (Fig 10-23). In some

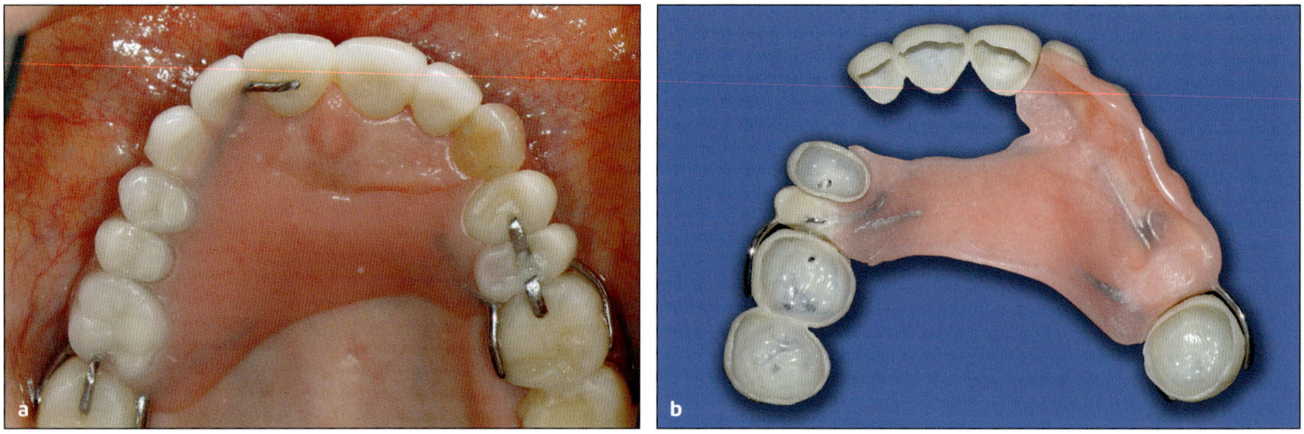

FIG 10-24 *(a)* Accurate interfacing between the fixed components and the partial denture. *(b)* Fixed components with limited frame contact can be sticky waxed into position to stabilize them during relining.

instances, a cast reinforcement for the fixed provisional is advisable. The fixed portion can also be easily milled from monolithic PMMA. The digital form would come from a scan of the wax-up. Milling of a provisional must still result in a shell to be relined. The clinical performance of these milled shells is superior to autopolymerized acrylic shells due to the improved strength, density, and color stability of premanufactured monolithic material.

Because the fixed provisionals and the provisional RPD were made from the same cast, they will fit together with minimal adjustment (Fig 10-24a). In fact, it is in this state that the relining of the fixed provisionals onto the prepared teeth will occur. When multiple separate shells are present, it may be helpful to sticky wax less stable single units to the RPD in order to manage the entire assembly with confidence (Fig 10-24b). To reline the fixed provisionals without regard to the RPD will almost guarantee that their relationship will change and that unnecessary adjustments to the resin partial denture will be required. Rather than completely fill the fixed provisional restorations with resin to reline them, only a small amount of resin should be placed in the eggshell. Then, the entire provisional assembly, fixed and removable, is seated and directed to place using the occlusion with the opposing dentition and the contact of the partial denture against the supporting soft tissue as the guides for proper placement. The small addition of resin will imprint the occlusal/incisal portion of the prepared teeth and positively relate the provisional. It is also advisable to coat the resin-based partial denture with separator in case any acrylic leaks in between the tooth-frame interface. The removable provisional is then separated from the fixed units and the relining of the fixed provisionals completed without interference.

Once the fixed provisional is completed, the fit of the provisional RPD is adjusted to reduce often excessive frictional retention due to this technique. AccuFilm (Parkell) or Fit Checker (GC America) is used as if the final frame was being evaluated. The amount of movement allowed is generally greater than if this were a definitive prosthesis to help avoid problematic technical failure of the weaker acrylic. The result of all this will be a combined fixed and removable provisional restoration that can be adjusted and added to as needed while other forms of mouth preparation are made. The only chair time expended will be that needed to make the double impression pickup impression and the clinical fitting procedures, so the cost to the patient and clinician will be low. If the patient's current prosthesis cannot be used in this manner, a trial base will need to be fabricated to facilitate the initial articulation. The only downside of this provisional combination will be the added bulk of the resin-based removable portion when compared to the old metal partial denture. Patients generally tolerate this bulk since they know that it will only be temporary.

Immediate provisional resin-based partial dentures

Many of the patients whose ultimate treatment will be some form of a precision attachment partial denture with associated fixed prosthesis enter our practices with failing restorations, some fixed and some removable. They are in immediate need of a provisional restoration to carry them through the initial phases of treatment. Often, a failing fixed partial denture will present with the loss of retention of one abutment, leaving the bridge supported by only one abutment, and the patient is well aware that the bridge is

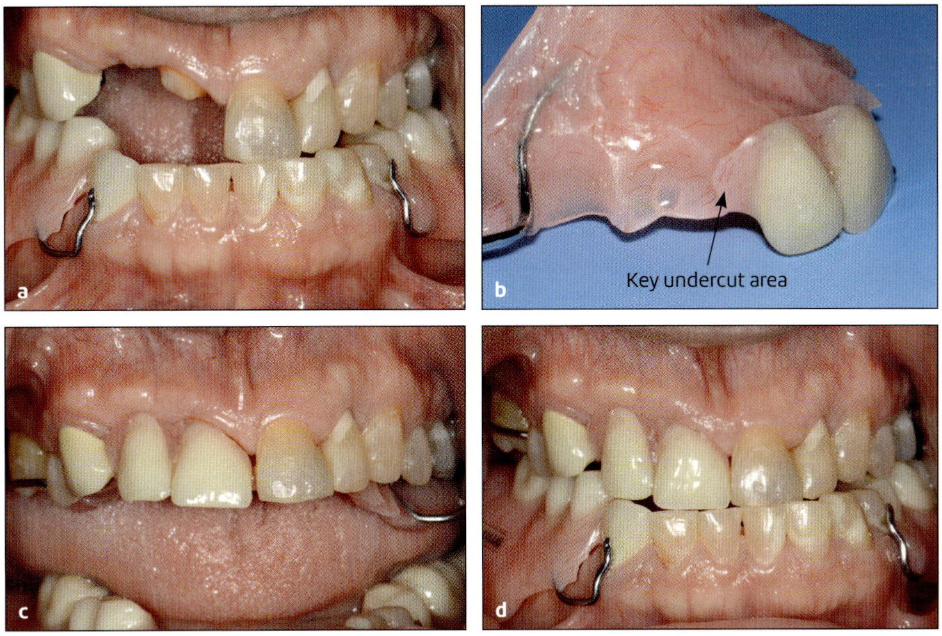

FIG 10-25 *(a)* Skeletal Class III malocclusion, partially edentulous, and high caries risk. *(b)* Mesial undercut on the first premolar is not modified in the mouth or blocked out on the cast. *(c)* Interim RPD laterally rotating into position. Note that the embrasure wire clasp on the patient's left is yet to engage. *(d)* Completely seated prosthesis. The rotational path eliminated the need for an anterior clasp and reduces tissue

loose. The first step in treating this type of patient must always be to obtain the very best possible initial impression of the affected arch. Any attempt to remove the defective fixed partial denture without a usable initial cast of the arch will require a more traditional technique with additional appointments and increased cost if the defective restoration is completely undermined with decay, and it is not possible to maintain it in place for a later impression. The patient is without the bridge or a conventional provisional partial denture, especially if a large number of teeth are involved, many days away from completion.

A very quick solution to the problem that will provide an almost instant replacement can be made using a combination of autopolymerizing tooth-colored resin, orthodontic resin, and nonprecious I-bar wire clasps. When the original alginate impression is removed from the cast, those teeth that will need replacing are poured immediately in the appropriate tooth-colored resin, and the alginate is placed in the pressure pot. The block of teeth is removed and trimmed, and the stone teeth are removed from the cast. Wire clasps, again preferably in the I-bar form, are adapted and sticky waxed to place. The new resin tooth segment is substituted for the stone teeth and the ridge trimmed as for any immediate denture situation. Any obvious undercuts on the lingual surfaces of the teeth to be contacted with the denture base are blocked out with baseplate wax to roughly 90 degrees. After coating the cast with a separating medium, the bulk of the partial denture is formed in the fine-grained orthodontic resin, either pink or clear, and the entire project is placed in the pressure pot.

The resulting partial denture can be expected to closely approximate the defective restoration in tooth position and arrangement. If the patient requires the extraction of nonrestorable teeth, the teeth are removed and the provisional partial denture is seated and adjusted as needed. A piece of clear thin plastic, normally used in trial packing of dentures, is then placed over the sockets, and tissue conditioner is added to the partial denture before it is inserted. The tissue conditioner will act as a soft bandage for the initial healing. The purpose of the plastic sheet is to prevent the conditioner from being forced up into the socket. Once the tissue conditioner begins its initial set, the partial denture can be removed from the mouth and the plastic easily peeled away.

Most immediate provisional partial dentures need only one clasp arm per side. As I-bars, these clasps are much easier to adapt initially and are readily adjusted to the abutment teeth if necessary. Any areas of this quickly made provisional prosthesis that do not fit satisfactorily can be easily readapted with any autopolymerizing reline resin.

The basic sequence and philosophy for temporization of fixed-removable partial denture situations is such that almost any definitive design feature can be utilized. The following examples demonstrate this fact. A rotational path design (discussed in detail in chapter 12) can be utilized with a resin-based interim partial denture (Fig 10-25).

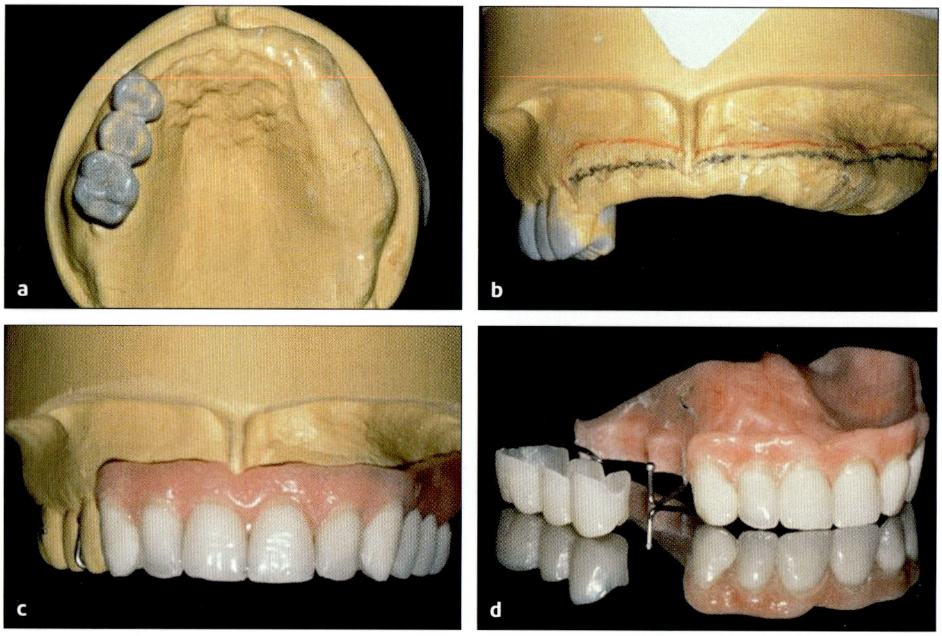

FIG 10-26 *(a)* An extreme Class II arch will result after extraction of the maxillary left sextant. An immediate provisional RPD is needed. *(b)* Height of contour *(black line)* surveyed in relation to the abutment tooth design. The *red line* is the planned extent of the flange. *(c)* The denture base of the immediate RPD extends just beyond that height of contour, resulting in a short flange. *(d)* Shell ready to reline. The removable component will serve as a guide while relining the fixed component.

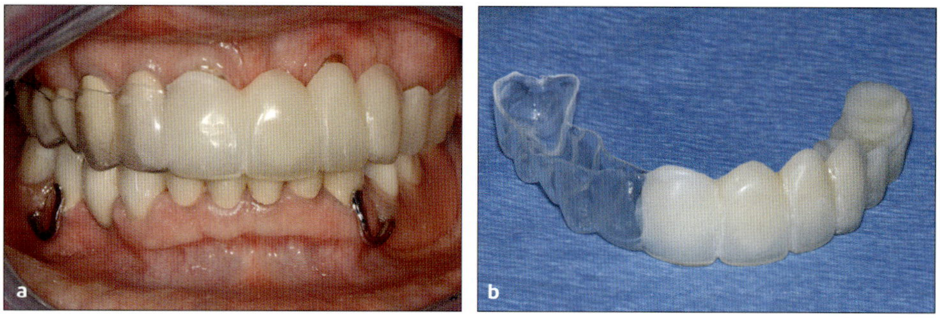

FIG 10-27 *(a and b)* Intraoral and extraoral views of an Essix retainer.

Space and strength are, as usual, typical limitations. The functional undercut is typically on teeth, but it can be on soft tissue. This can be effective when managing a fixed-removable provisional for extreme Class II situations, especially when implants are planned for the edentulous segment (Fig 10-26a). The rotational path allows the resin base to engage the soft tissue undercut on the edentulous side. The base will extend just beyond the height of contour on the edentulous side in an area that would be parallel to the lingual surfaces of the remaining teeth (Fig 10-26b). Engaging this undercut area prevents rotation of the base away from the ridge, which should result in retention of the edentulous side of the prosthesis (Figs 10-26c and 10-26d). If the patient's soft tissue in that area cannot tolerate the rotational pressure, then that resin extension will have to be removed and denture adhesive used to gain retention.

Lingual clasping is also possible with provisional resin-based prostheses. As with definitive prostheses, this is typically a simple matter of managing the height of contour of the fixed portion of the reconstruction so that a lingual clasp arm becomes a retentive element. However, this concept can also be applied to situations that will ultimately be completely fixed. Long-span quadrant reconstructions with implants typically require removable interim prostheses. Essix retainers can be used effectively in these situations but often break down in a short time and are typically not as functional or esthetic as a resin-based RPD (Fig 10-27). However, the resin-based interim prosthesis can be complicated by the fact that the abutments are only to be used temporarily until the implant prosthesis is fabricated. Therefore, abutment modifications are generally not advised. In this situation, the interim prosthesis can suffer from exaggerated clasp positions that can be unesthetic and therefore unacceptable to particular patients.

These scenarios can benefit from lingual clasping. A resin-based interim partial denture is made in the usual fashion with the exception of the anterior abutment. Here, when the occlusion allows, lingual modification with composite

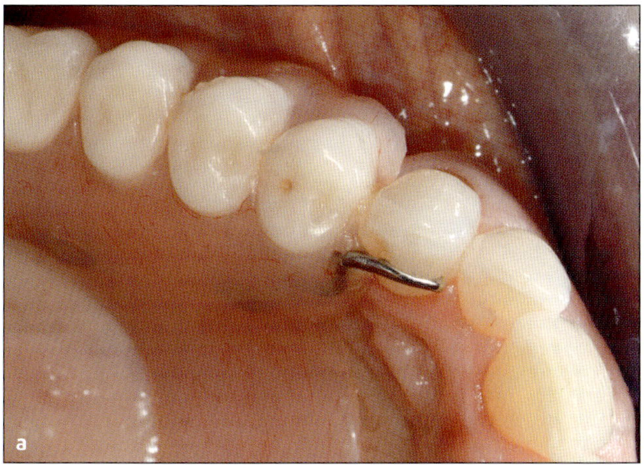

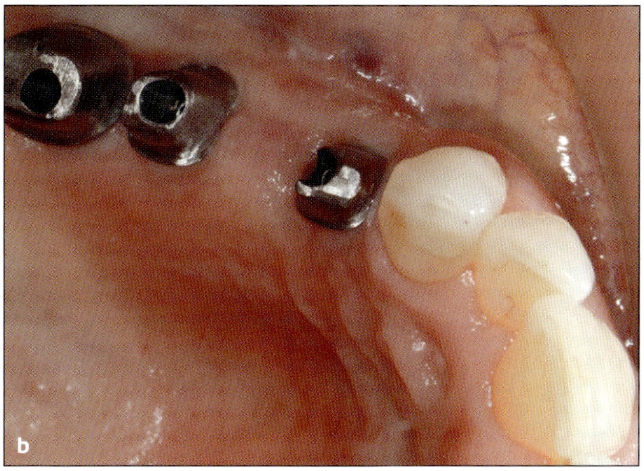

FIG 10-28 *(a)* A lingual retentive clasp engages a temporary composite undercut. *(b)* The composite is removed once the implant restoration is complete.

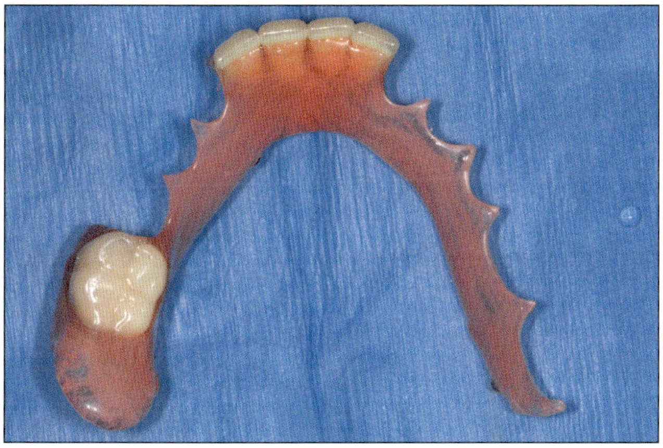

FIG 10-29 Flexibility of the connector allows engagement of lingual undercuts. This provides adequate stability when replacing few teeth.

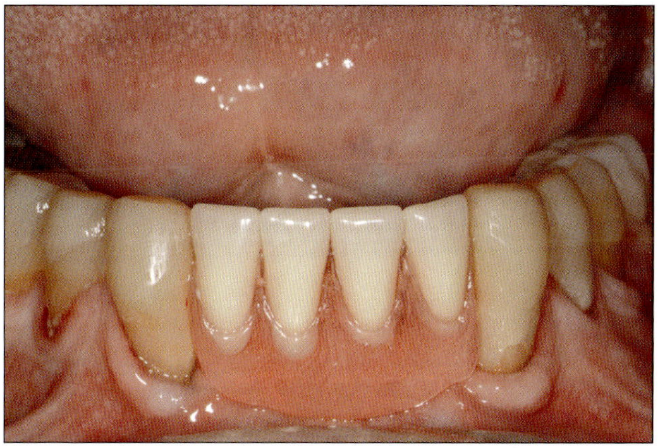

FIG 10-30 Lingually engaged polyamide interims are indicated to replace mandibular incisors. Note the lack of buccal components.

resin can create a small undercut. A short wire is then used to engage this small undercut (Fig 10-28a). When the abutment is a canine, this wire can often also act as a rest. While the composite will wear with time, the prosthesis is typically not required beyond 8 months. Clinical experience has shown that the composite undercut, if not overused, tends to last at least this long. For ease of fabrication, the lingual wire can be designed and incorporated as if it is simply a rest seat. Once the partial denture is fit, the composite is added directly to the tooth with the partial denture completely seated. After curing of the composite, the wire can be flexed lingually with an instrument to ensure disengagement prior to removal of the partial denture. From there, minor adjustments to the composite addition are done to customize the retentive force. This ensures that the wire remains passive and will prevent unwanted abutment tooth displacement. Once the implant restoration is completed, the composite modification is removed and the enamel repolished (Fig 10-28b).

The flexibility of a polyamide interim RPD is another opportunity to utilize lingual undercuts. A simple lingual plate design with no buccal wires or extensions can in fact be quite retentive by engaging a portion of the lingual undercuts on the mandibular posterior teeth (Fig 10-29). These teeth tend to be lingually inclined. In fact, it is easy to engage these undercuts to the extent that the partial denture is not able to be removed, even with great effort. For this reason, the definitive cast must be blocked out appropriately prior to duplication. This is a procedure often ignored by laboratories making polyamide partial dentures out of efficiency rather than for accuracy. When controlled, this engagement will result in more than adequate stability and retention for the replacement of lost mandibular incisors. When these are the only teeth missing and a disease management plan is required, this material-specific design is indicated despite its periodontal and hygiene disadvantages (Fig 10-30).

The case for interim RPDs to facilitate advanced RPDs is clear. What is worthy of further debate is whether the newer materials and simplistic techniques most often associated with resin-based RPDs should be considered for definitive prostheses. The answer, as usual, is that it depends. The majority of everyday general dentists in the United States will continue to prescribe these materials as "definitive" partial dentures as long as they lack the technical understanding or willingness to devote clinical time to RPDs. Their fallback position, if ever pressed on the issue, is the phrase, "It works for my patients." There are certainly low-risk patients who can tolerate the biologic, technical, and esthetic disadvantages of these materials without major consequence. In fact, we have all seen decades-old "flippers" that appear to be doing no harm. The challenge for the clinician of course is to identify these patients. Even when identified as low risk, are clinicians willing to offer a weaker, less functional, and less hygienic prosthesis to a patient who is seeking a higher level of care? To that end, the medium- and long-term use of resin-based RPDs is certainly possible. However, if the goal remains the advanced partial denture, a metal framework will continue to be the ideal for the vast majority of disease-controlled situations until there is a comparable alternative.

References

1. Lewandowska A, Speichowicz E, Öwall BE. Removable partial denture treatment in Poland. Quintessence Int 1989;20:353–358.
2. Thean HP, Payne JA, Jeganathan S. The use of removable partial dentures amongst private dental practitioners in Singapore. Singapore Dent J 1996;21:26–30.
3. Radhi A, Lynch CD, Hanningan A. Quality of written communication and master impressions for fabrication of removable partial prostheses in the Kingdom of Bahrain. J Oral Rehabil 2007;34:153–157.
4. Schwarz W, Barsby M. A survey of the practice of partial denture prosthetics in the United Kingdom. J Dent 1980;8:95–101.
5. Lynch CD, Allen PF. The teaching of removable partial dentures in Ireland and the United Kingdom. Br Dent J 2007;203:1–5.
6. Pun DK, Waliszewski MP, Waliszewski KJ, Berzins D. Survey of partial removable dental prosthesis (partial RDP) types in a distinct patient population. J Prosthet Dent 2011;106:48–56.
7. Curtis DA, Curtis TA, Wagnild GW, Finzen FC. Incidence of various classes of removable partial dentures. J Prosthet Dent 1992;67:664–667.
8. Öwall BE, Taylor RL. A survey of dentitions and removable partial dentures constructed for patients in North America. J Prosthet Dent 1989;61:465–470.
9. Campbell SD, Cooper L, Craddock H, et al. Removable partial denture: The clinical need for innovation. J Prosthet Dent 2017;118:273–280.
10. Carlsson GE, Hedegård B, Koivumaa KK. Studies in partial dental prosthesis III. A longitudinal study of mandibular partial dentures with double extension saddles. Acta Odontol Scand 1962;20:95–119.
11. Carlsson GE, Hedegård B, Koivumaa KK Studies in partial dental prosthesis. IV. Final results of a 4-year longitudinal investigation of dentogingivally supported partial dentures. Acta Odont Scand 1965;23:443–472.
12. Carlsson GE, Hedegård B, Koivumaa KK. Late results of treatment with partial dentures. An investigation by questionnaire and clinical examination 13 years after treatment. J Oral Rehabil 1976;3:267–272.
13. Tuominen R, Ranta K, Paunio I. Wearing of removable partial dentures in relation to periodontal pockets. J Oral Rehabil 1989;16:119–126.
14. Yusof Z, Isa Z. Periodontal status of teeth in contact with denture in removable partial denture wearers. J Oral Rehabil 1994;21:77–86.
15. Zlatarić DK, Čelebić A, Valentić-Peruzović M. The effect of removable partial dentures on periodontal health of abutment and non-abutment teeth. J Periodontol 2002;73:137–144.
16. Manzon L, Fratto G, Poli O, Infusino E. Patient and clinical evaluation of traditional metal and polyamide removable partial dentures in an elderly cohort. J Prosthodont 2019;28:868–875.
17. Bergman B, Hugoson A, Olsson CO. Caries, periodontal and prosthetic findings in patients with removable partial dentures: A ten-year longitudinal study. J Prosthet Dent 1982;48:506–514.
18. Bergman B, Hugoson A, Olsson CO. A 25 year longitudinal study of patients treated with removable partial dentures. J Oral Rehabil 1995;22:595–599.
19. Schwalm CA, Smith DE, Erickson JD. A clinical study of patients 1 to 2 years after placement of removable partial dentures. J Prosthet Dent 1977;38:380–391.
20. Chandler JA, Brudvik JS. Clinical evaluation of patients eight to nine years after placement of removable partial dentures. J Prosthet Dent 1984;51:736–743.
21. Kapur KK. Veterans Administration cooperative dental implant study—Comparisons between fixed partial dentures supported by blade-vent implants and removable partial dentures. Part II: Comparisons of success rates and periodontal health between two treatment modalities. J Prosthet Dent 1989;62:685–703.
22. Wright PS, Hellyer PH. Gingival recession related to removable partial dentures in older patients. J Prosthet Dent 1995;74:602–607.
23. Meinig DA. Removable partial dentures without rests. J Prosthet Dent 1994;71:350–358.
24. Ucar Y, Akova T, Aysan I. Mechanical properties of polyamide versus different PMMA denture base materials. J Prosthodont 2012;21:173–176.
25. Zoidis P, Papathanasiou I, Polyzois G. The use of a modified poly-ether-ether-ketone (PEEK) as an alternative framework material for removable dental prostheses. A clinical report. J Prosthodont 2016;25:580–584.
26. McCartney JW, Fiks S. The all-acrylic resin mandibular removable partial denture: Design considerations. J Prosthet Dent 1997;77:638.
27. Smith RA, Rymarz FP. Cast clasp transitional removable partial dentures. J Prosthet Dent 1969;22:381–385.
28. Hansen CA, Clear KE, La Mar SD. Removable partial denture design considerations where periodontally compromised teeth exist. Int J Periodontics Restorative Dent 1997;17:89–93.
29. Waliszewski MP, Brudvik JS. The conversion partial denture: A clinical report. J Prosthet Dent 2004;91:306–309.
30. Cecconi BT, Campagni WV, Cecconi ML. The component partial. A new RPD construction system. J Calif Dent Assoc 1997;25:371–376.
31. Hazelton LR, Brudvik JS. A new procedure to reinforce fixed provisional restorations. J Prosthet Dent 1995;74:110–113.
32. Hazelton LR, Nicholls JI, Brudvik JS, Daly CH. Influence of reinforcement design on the loss of marginal seal of provisional fixed partial dentures. Int J Prosthodont 1995;8:572–579.

PRECISION ATTACHMENTS

11

Attachment brands come and go; the principles remain.

The precision attachment denture has long been considered the highest form of partial denture therapy. It combines fixed and removable prosthodontics in such a way as to create the most esthetic partial denture possible. It also has the reputation of lasting far longer than the conventional partial denture despite evidence to the contrary.[1,2] What possible biologic reason could exist to support this reputation? It has long been our belief that the reason this prosthesis is generally so successful is that the clinician and the laboratory simply must take greater pains in every aspect of construction just to get the precision attachment partial into the mouth. Because the cost of this particular therapy is apt to be far greater than for a conventional partial denture, there is a greater likelihood of long-term follow-up care and high-quality maintenance by the patient. If the more conventional partial denture, one that is clasp-retained, is constructed as described in this text, then there is no inherent reason that the attachment-retained partial should be superior.

The precision attachment partial denture should differ only in the means of its retention when compared with the clasp-retained partial denture. The only reason for utilizing this mechanical device is to replace the visible clasp arm. All other functions of the partial denture can be performed by conventional means if they are understood and the partial denture is constructed to the highest standards.

Traditionally, the use of a precision attachment required the construction of one or more crowns as part of the treatment. With the advent of milled guiding plane surfaces, resin-bonded components, and lingual clasping, a whole new era has opened for the attachment-retained partial. An era, in fact, where attachments may often be unnecessary. The now inherent demand for ideal or supernormal esthetics has made many of our patients unwilling to accept visible clasping. This results in an increasing need to be able to offer this type of prosthesis. The combination of these two seemingly unrelated statements should result in a more sophisticated partial denture, one in which tooth structure will not have to be sacrificed to allow maximum esthetics.

Because the construction of the precision attachment partial denture is technically demanding, the need for the clinician to fully understand the implications for the dental laboratory is critical for success. It is to that end that the subject is presented in some detail in this chapter. The sheer number of attachments on the market makes a truly comprehensive evaluation next to impossible. A solid understanding of the use of the basic categories of attachments will provide the clinician with tools to evaluate other systems as they come on the market and to choose those that offer the greatest potential for long-term success.

Box 11-1 Common precision attachment manufacturers and distributors

Sterngold Dental, LLC
23 Frank Mossberg Drive
Attleboro, MA 02703
1-800-243-9942
www.sterngold.com

Preat Corporation
2625 Skyway Drive, Suite B
Santa Maria, CA 93455
1-800-232-7732
www.preat.com

XPdent Corporation (Bredent)
12145 SW 131st Avenue
Miami, FL 33186
1-877-328-3965
www.xpdent.com
www.bredent.com

Zest Anchors, LLC
2875 Loker Avenue East
Carlsbad, CA 92010
1-800-262-2310
www.zestdent.com

Cendrest Métaux (MedTech)
Biel, Switzerland
www.cmsa.ch/en/medtech/prostheticline
Available in the United States through Sterngold Dental, LLC

Rhein83
Via E. Zago, 10/ABC
40128, Bologna, Italy
United States office:
1-877-778-8383
www.rhein83usa.com

Common Clinical Procedures

A number of clinical procedures common to the use of any attachment system must be mastered before a real level of confidence can be achieved. Many of these steps have been presented briefly in the preceding chapters but are discussed here in more detail. Of particular note are the details regarding surveyed crowns discussed in chapter 4.

Diagnostic procedures

Because space will almost always be a major consideration and a problem for precision attachment selection and use, a diagnostic wax-up and setup is essential for every case. As noted in chapter 1, there is no point in even considering the design portion of treatment until all diagnostic steps are completed. This is even more critical when considering precision attachments. Regardless of what is found in the opposing arch, a diagnostic tooth arrangement must be verified intraorally so that tooth position can be evaluated by both the clinician and the patient. The final position of all teeth and the denture base must be known to ensure that the space requirements of the attachment system under consideration can be met. When insufficient space is available, either the system selected or the oral environment must change, through surgeries, orthodontics or tooth modification, or—in very special situations—an increase in the occlusal vertical dimension (OVD). The clinician will need an up-to-date comprehensive catalog of attachment systems that indicates all dimensions of each unit. In choosing an attachment system, the laboratory must be a willing collaborator, since it must have experience with the chosen system or be willing to learn along with the clinician. Recent consolidation has resulted in several traditional attachment companies combining or closing. Most catalogs can be found online and are a required resource for planning the dimensions required (Box 11-1). The catalogs and websites also typically give valuable technical guidance and precise descriptions of the various systems.

The pickup impression

The process of accurately relating the partial denture framework to the precision attachment components is an essential step in the clinical procedure sequence required to construct a precision attachment partial denture. The clinician must utilize a technique for making a final impression for the RPD framework that includes picking up the completed fixed components from the mouth in such a way that the position of the units remains accurately related to the remainder of the mouth. Having the actual crowns on the definitive cast allows precise positioning of the attachment components, a task that may not be possible when working on a stone replica of the crown, due to the probable fracturing of thin projections of stone. It also allows the definitive cast to be used as a milling cast to provide a stable platform for milling metal surfaces of the fixed components. The pickup technique was discussed in terms of conventional surveyed crowns in chapter 4 (see Figs 4-29 to 4-31). This procedure will require a custom impression tray and an impression made with a relatively rigid material, usually a silicone or a polyether. The fixed units will have to be either completely stable on the tooth because of the inherent fit of the casting or, if there is a potential for movement during the pickup impression, they will have to be temporarily cemented to keep them from moving. The cementing medium for this procedure must be one that will allow the unit to be removed from the mouth with the impression, since replacing a unit in an elastic material runs the risk of creating an inaccurate relationship. A small bead of Fit Checker (GC America), placed just internal to the margin, will usually maintain the casting-tooth relationship. An equally small bead of Temp-Bond (Kerr Dental) with petroleum jelly (eg, Vaseline, Unilever) can also be used.

When the impression is removed from the mouth and is found to be acceptable, resin dies that have been made previously are placed into each fixed unit and the impression boxed and poured. These dies are made with an autopolymerizing resin, like GC Pattern Resin (GC America), with a retentive wire projection to lock them into the dental stone of the definitive cast (Fig 11-1). The completed crown is first lubricated, and then resin is added up to the margin. A wire that has been serrated is inserted into the resin mass, and the resin is allowed to set. The portion of the wire that protrudes from the crown is bent into some retentive form to retain it in the stone. When seated into a crown that has been picked up, the resin die must be very stable. With the die in position, the margin of the crown must typically be protected with a thin layer of wax. This facilitates easier removal from the set stone cast and will protect delicate porcelain butt margins. The definitive cast must always be poured in improved die stone to gain maximum resistance to fracture and abrasion.

A very real potential exists for fracturing any porcelain butt margins that may be present when the impression is removed from the definitive cast. In addition, tall thin stone teeth are apt to break when more rigid impression materials are used. These same rigid impression materials will not allow easy removal of a tray from a picked up bar. Any of these events would be time consuming to remedy. For this reason, the impression tray is best made of acrylic resin. Unlike light-activated composite tray material, they can be heated with an alcohol torch and softened enough to peel the tray off the cast without fear of damaging the underlying stone teeth or fixed components. Stock metal trays, perfectly adequate for most framework impressions, obviously do not offer this option and should not be used. Once the tray is removed, the impression material can be easily separated from the cast.

Pickup of attachment components

Each attachment system will require slightly different pickup techniques, requiring some level of experience to routinely join them to the casting without introducing error. The clinician must be aware of the techniques for joining attachment components to the framework directly in the mouth as well as on the cast. In many instances, it may be appropriate to join the attachment to the framework out on the bench, since it is generally easier to make a quality bond on the bench and then take it back to the mouth to verify the accuracy of the relationship. Verification steps are essential to success with precision attachments. Some attachments, such as clips for bar-clip attachments, will be picked up using a laboratory autopolymerizing resin of the same color as the denture base.

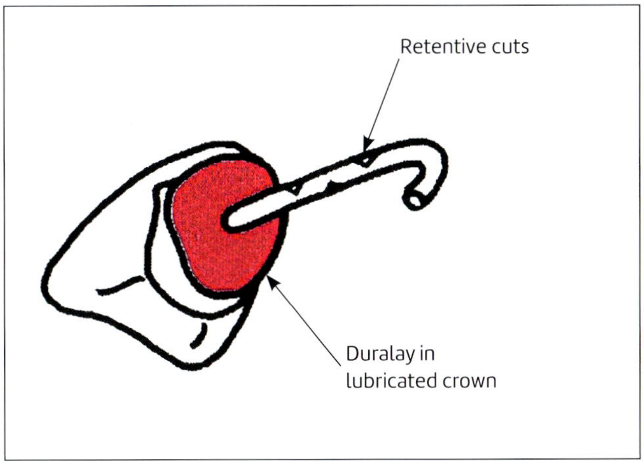

FIG 11-1 Pickup die with wire retention.

Many systems require that some portion of the unit, either the matrix or patrix, be joined to the RPD casting in the mouth. These chairside techniques are best done with the aid of the chairside assistant. The same approach used for certain types of repair impressions will be needed. In other words, the clinician must relate the components while an auxiliary places the resin and cures the mass. As with the repair, either an autopolymerizing resin like GC Pattern Resin or a light-cured composite resin can be used. The light-cured resin is more expensive but quicker to use. The chairside method is often selected as a means to control the positional relationship of the components. Laboratory environments, no matter how detailed, may not be able to replicate variable tissue resiliency or tooth mobility. These movement issues are managed by having the clinician maintain the appropriate position of the various components while the assistant places and cures the resin. The positional relationship is thereby maintained throughout the process.

The quality of chairside resin connections can be improved with preparation of the housing, if one exists. The housing is sandblasted and coated with an appropriate metal bonding agent. Prior to the appointment, a thin layer of the connection material of choice is added. Applying a precured layer of resin in a controlled laboratory environment ensures that the weak link between metal and resin is maximized. The more forgiving resin-to-resin connection is then completed in the mouth. The layer of resin must be thin so as not to interfere with the already limited amount of available connection space.

Joining attachment components to a framework is most often done with resin. This is primarily for convenience and retrievability. Attachment systems can also be soldered or laser welded to the framework. This choice depends primarily on the amount of available space and the ability to create an accessible framework-component joint. When space is at a premium, the soldering/welding option is definitely the technique of choice. If future component replacement or retrieval will be necessary, this stronger, more permanent connection is contraindicated.

In addition to these specific techniques, altered cast impressions and precise maxillomandibular relationship records must be available for the construction of the precision attachment partial denture. Timing and management of the tissue-base relationship is dependent on the resiliency and design features of the framework. In most instances, the altered cast impression or functional reline will be made after the attachment system has been joined to the framework since the object of the altered cast is to record the support of the soft tissue in relation to the abutment teeth through the fit of the casting. However, when there is extensive redundant soft tissue or maxillofacial defects, it can be beneficial to have a more stable base and thereby framework while making the attachment connection. In these situations, the partial denture is more or less completed when the attachment is finally connected to the frame or base. The management of resiliency during the connection process is also dependent on the system and case classification. Bars and many stud attachments have the option of including a spacer. The idea of the spacer is to create a buffer for tissue compression during function. This is a moot point in Kennedy Class III situations but may have significant influence in an extreme Class II unilateral situation. If a spacer is not used, the attachment will act as a vertical stop, which must be accounted for within the overall design.

Crown preparation for intracoronal attachments

When intracoronal attachments are to be used as a part of an abutment crown, the preparation design for the abutment tooth will have to be modified from that of a standard full veneer crown preparation. In order to create a crown that has a normal emergence profile and dimension, some form of box preparation that will relate to the dimensions of the chosen attachment must be made. If the chosen attachment will not fit within the normal contours of the abutment in question, a slight overcontouring of the crown is acceptable only if the gingival one-third of the contour is maintained as normal. A review of pulpal anatomy is essential to preclude overpreparation of the abutment tooth. This may require the preparation on the bench of extracted teeth with dimensions similar to those of the actual abutment tooth. The presence of secondary dentin and the determination of its depth become critical issues. When considering the preparation depth, the minimum thickness of the alloy, usually around 0.5 mm, must be added to the dimensions of the attachment matrix. If this reduction places the tooth at risk for overpreparation, the choice of attachment system must be reevaluated. The choice of an extracoronal attachment instead of an intracoronal is an obvious solution to the problem. Intracoronal attachments are better utilized when placed into pontics where there will be no possibility of affecting abutment strength. After years of experience reevaluating abutment fractures, due most often to the excessive reduction of tooth structure, intracoronal attachments can no longer be recommended over the new generation of extracoronal attachments. We therefore now reserve their use to pontics only.

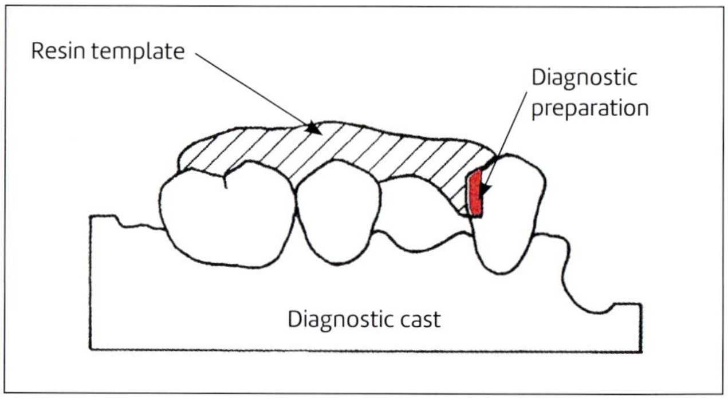

FIG 11-2 Preparation guide for intracoronal attachment.

The stone tooth representing the abutment on the diagnostic cast must be prepared to accept the matrix plus the minimum space necessary for the metal of the crown. The matrix can be tried in place on the prepared stone tooth using the holding device that fits into the dental surveyor. Once adequate space has been created, a template can be quickly constructed to transfer the preparation form to the mouth. The prepared stone tooth and the occlusal surfaces of adjacent teeth are painted with a separating agent and an autopolymerizing resin placed into the cavity and onto the occlusal surfaces of the adjacent teeth (Fig 11-2). When set, the template can be trimmed of excess resin and taken to the mouth to verify the dimensions of the matrix cavity by placing it onto the adjacent teeth and modifying the preparation

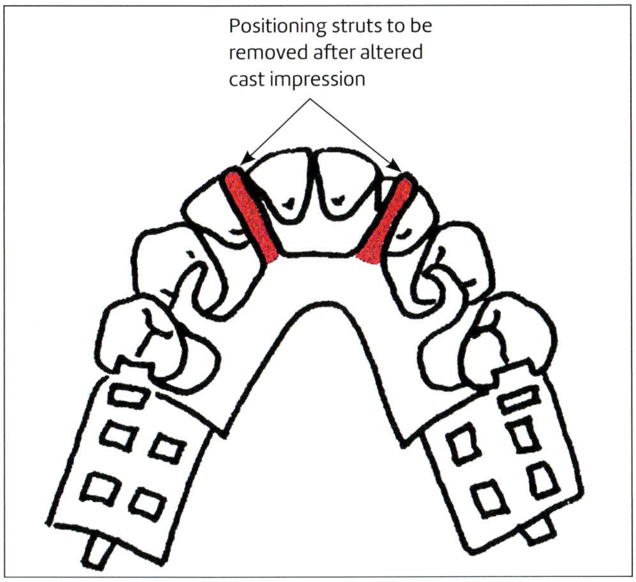

FIG 11-3 Casting modification for precision attachments.

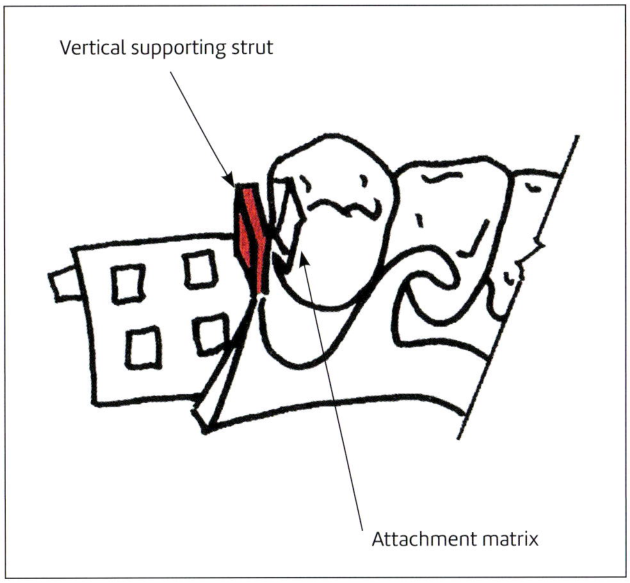

FIG 11-4 Casting modification to support an intracoronal attachment.

until it accepts the form. The use of this simple preparation guide reduces, but does not eliminate, the risk of overpreparation of the tooth at the same time that it guarantees that there has been enough reduction to allow the matrix to be placed within the normal contours of the abutment tooth.

Modifications of the framework design

At times, there may not be sufficient contact areas between the framework and the remaining teeth to ensure positive orientation during the pickup operations described earlier. This will be true most often when attachments are used that will also bear some of the vertical support of the partial denture. In these cases, additional struts are added to the major connector and extend to the occlusal or incisal surface of at least two widely separated teeth (Fig 11-3). The strut is waxed directly on the refractory cast and has the dimensions of a normal minor connector. The struts provide a very positive position of the framework in the mouth while attachments are joined to the casting and while altered cast impressions are being made. After these two operations are completed, and the fit of the attachments verified, the struts are cut from the major connector, and the surface is returned to a normal contour and finish.

Many partial denture frameworks will need a strut added to the retentive mesh area in order to have something to which the patrix can be either soldered or attached with resin (Fig 11-4). The exact shape of this strut will be dependent on the attachment system used, but since it is such a critical element, its design must be reviewed with the laboratory. This is best done after diagnostic cast preparations that result in visualization of the attachment-strut interface.

Custom housings

Perhaps the most difficult of the problems associated with attachments is the lack of vertical space. The large number of parts that must fit within such small dimensions is almost invariably a challenge; the matrix, the patrix, a housing, resin retention, and a denture tooth all must have minimum dimensions to function without failure. Unless there has been some loss of supporting proximal bone, it is unlikely that sufficient space will be found adjacent to the terminal abutment in Class I situations, especially if that abutment happens to be a premolar. With space at a premium, the thin overlying denture tooth typically fractures in short order, with debonding of the prefabricated housing often occurring a short time later. This is no doubt among the most frustrating, yet preventable, course of events with precision attachment partials after so much time and effort has been spent. A custom housing that is stronger and often more esthetic than a typical resin overlay is an invaluable means to improve the longevity and appeal of the precision attachment partial.

Custom housings that are laser welded to the RPD framework combine the housing, resin retention, and denture tooth into a single component and thereby reduce the space required. Made out of cast metal, the housings can be made exceptionally thin while maintaining strength.

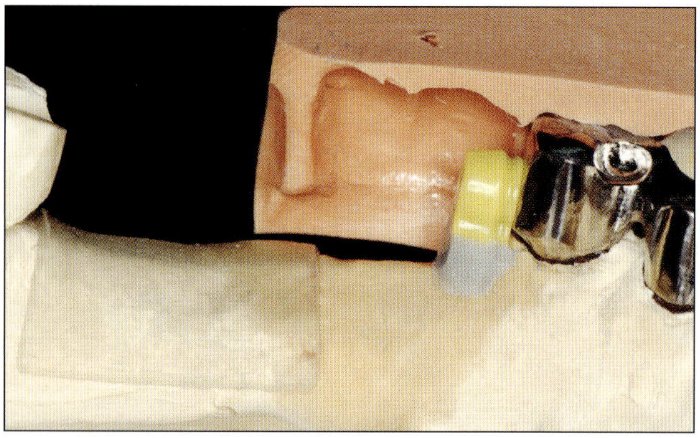

FIG 11-5 Putty matrix indicates space available for custom housing. Note the relief pad and blocked-out matrix in position prior to impression for refractory cast.

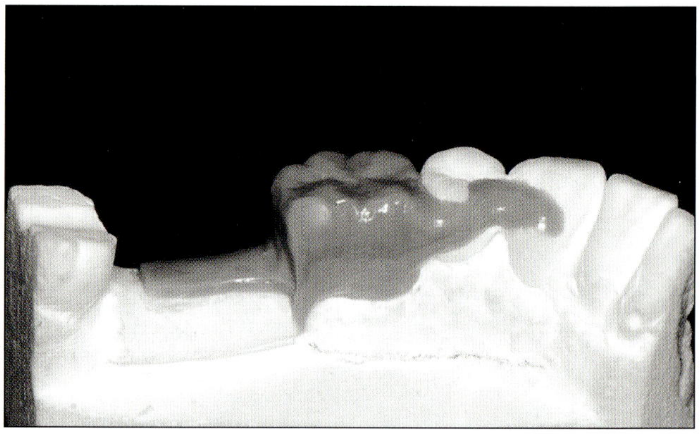

FIG 11-6 Full-form wax-up of custom housing on refractory cast before cutback for porcelain. After cutback, the wax-up will be invested directly on this refractory cast.

Additionally, porcelain fused to the proper cast alloy allows more ideal control of esthetics when thin resin would otherwise show the dark color of underlying components. When made, they must still allow for efficient replacement of the worn inserts that they retain and protect. These features are called housings since they house or protect the attachment apparatus, be it the matrix, patrix, or both. In many instances, these need be nothing more than metal occlusal surfaces that prevent occlusal wear and thereby prevent exposure of the underlying manufactured housing. In other more limited space situations, these protective overlays can replace the prosthetic tooth component entirely while still remaining separate from the manufactured housing. However, in many instances it is most efficient to create the housing in a way that replaces the housing and prosthetic tooth portion of the area in its entirety.

The fabrication of a custom housing for a resilient extracoronal attachment is explained here since it lends itself to the creation of a housing that will contain the resilient matrix, thus taking the place of the separate housing.[3] This same concept can be used for other attachment housings in a very similar fashion. Constructing the custom housing is always a space management challenge. It is an absolute necessity that a clinically derived diagnostic wax-up and trial arrangement be completed to perfection prior to purchasing components and beginning the fabrication process. The diagnostic cast must be as accurate as any final impression, especially at the marginal gingiva of the potential abutments, since this is where the critical occlusal-gingival measurement will be made. As discussed, this total dimension allows proper selection of an attachment system that will fit within the given space. Once selected, a matrix/patrix set is ordered and placed within this space. With the attachment system held in position with a small amount of wax, a measurement is made from the top of the overlying component, in this example the matrix, to the opposing tooth. This measurement will determine the type of custom housing, whether it will be all metal or metal and porcelain/composite, and crestal bone must be removed to lower the placement of the patrix. A putty matrix, made from the diagnostic setup, indicates the amount of vertical height available for the housing and can be repeatedly referenced as fabrication progresses. In Fig 11-5, it is in position on the definitive pickup cast prior to housing fabrication.

The housings are likely to be so thin vertically that they cannot be waxed, sprued, and removed from the definitive cast without distortion. This requires creation of a separate and special refractory cast so they can be cast as individual units (Fig 11-6). Once cast, they are confirmed, veneered, and picked up to be laser welded to the frame. Fortunately, the laser weld can be brought very close to the veneer without harming it (within 0.5 to 1.0 mm). Remember that laser welding allows dissimilar metals to be joined. Chrome-based framework alloys can therefore continue to be used while a metal-ceramic alloy of choice can be used for porcelain veneered custom housings.

The custom housing is typically in an area that requires additional RPD components. Most common among these is a rest, as resilient extracoronal attachment systems are not to be used as a means of support. These rests are best incorporated into the custom housing casting. When they are, this becomes an opportunity to incorporate the sectional construction method for framework fabrication. As described in chapter 6, by eliminating the influence of casting shrinkage, an RPD that is fabricated in sections prior to being joined together has the potential for an ideal framework fit. This is perhaps one of the reasons why precision attachment partials experience good results in the hands of careful operators. The use of machined parts for attachment systems forces dentists to utilize sectional construction,

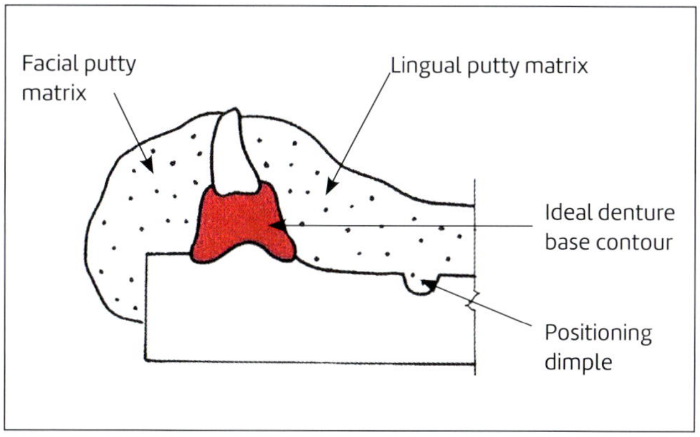

FIG 11-7 Putty matrix over patient-approved arrangement and wax-up.

which in turn results in frameworks that fit and therefore function as they are intended. Several examples with exact step-by-step fabrication details can be found within the literature on this topic.[3,4]

Bar-Clip Attachments

The bar-clip attachment has its origins in turn-of-the-century dentistry when the Gilmore clip system was made available to the profession. It was commonly used with copings or crowns over vital teeth and later with endodontically treated teeth in which a post coping system supported a solid bar about 8 gauge in diameter. The attachment mechanism was a plate-gold U-shaped clip of various lengths, retained in the resin of the prosthesis or soldered to some internal framework. Bar-clip systems are widely used with implant-supported overdentures of many different designs and are available from a variety of manufacturers. In cross section, the bars can be round, pear-shaped, U-shaped, or rectangular. The round and the pear-shaped forms are intended to allow some rotation of the attachment device perpendicular to the long axis of the bar. Among the most popular are the Hader bar, Dolder bar, CM rider bar, and Ackermann clip and bar.

Advances in organic chemistry have resulted in the creation of resilient clips made of thermoplastic materials that are very inexpensive and can be rapidly replaced by the clinician. They have the disadvantage of wearing more quickly than the gold plate clips. These plastic clips are offered with a thin metal retainer housing, with retentive contours on the inner surface to retain the clip. They are, in turn, held in the resin of the denture with retentive contours on their outer surface.

Attaching the bar

When used as an attachment for an RPD, the bars, either in the form of a castable plastic pattern or as a wrought precious metal bar that is intended to be soldered, are attached to elements of the fixed prosthodontic component. It is again essential that diagnostic wax-ups and trial arrangements are created to relate the position of the denture teeth to the position of the bar in order to ensure that adequate space exists—not only for the bar, the clip, and the clip retainer, but for the teeth and associated resin that will usually be placed directly over the bar-clip assembly. When space is limited, the use of a protective metal covering over any thin resin areas is indicated. This will often take the form of a cast-metal occlusal surface for a posterior tooth since the expected wear of a resin denture tooth in function can result in breakage over the clip assembly.

Once the diagnostic wax-up is complete and the teeth to be replaced on the partial denture have been tried in the mouth and verified esthetically, a putty matrix of the teeth is made with a positive seat on the cast to allow both the clinician and the technician to find the ideal position for the bar relative to the denture teeth (Fig 11-7). As part of this decision, the vertical position of the bar relative to the soft tissue will have to be selected. If the bar is placed on the tissue of the ridge, or even slightly above it, experience has shown that the tissue will, in time, hypertrophy and will not only come into contact with the underside of the bar but extend up along the sides of the bar into any space not occupied with the clip. Perhaps the best position of the bar in relation to the tissue is just high enough off the tissue to allow the tip of a mini proxy brush to pass under the bar. The patient must assume responsibility for daily stimulation of the tissue as well as keeping the undersurface free from plaque. The contours of the bar where it connects to the

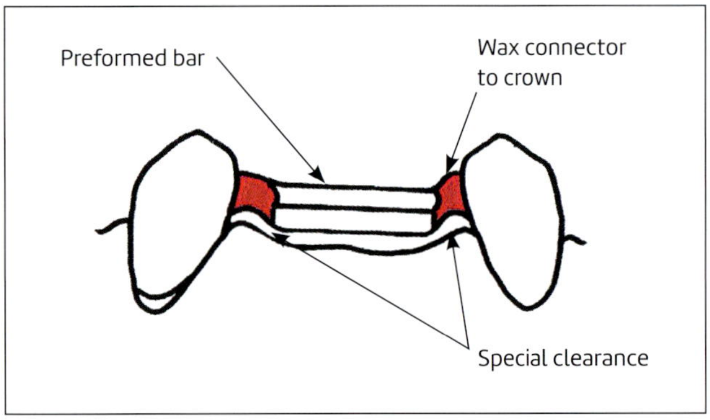

FIG 11-8 Relationship of plastic bar pattern to gingiva.

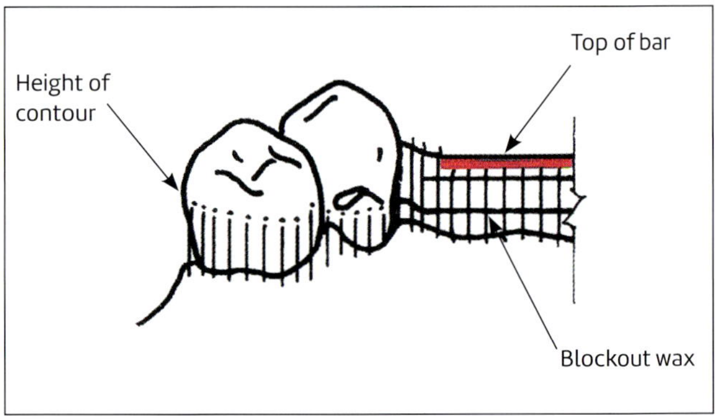

FIG 11-9 Blockout of bar and abutment crowns.

crowns or copings must also be carefully evaluated, as the clearance required for the marginal gingival tissue is even more critical than for the bar as a whole (Fig 11-8). The level of the bar in these areas will, almost without exception, need to be raised. In practical terms, this means that the bar must be cut short of the connector area, maintaining sufficient length for the clip, and then waxed into contact with the crown, usually in a curved segment. As this connector is closer to the incisal/occlusal plane, space may become a problem, even if adequate clearance exists over the length of the bar.

Usually the plastic bar pattern is cast to one side of the fixed component and soldered to the other side after relating the segments in the mouth or from the definitive cast. The preformed bar is connected in a similar fashion, most commonly by laser welding, after any ceramic component has been completed. The solder or weld joints must always be larger in circumference than the bar itself. In the finishing and polishing of the bar, care must be taken not to touch the section of the bar that will receive the clip since any change in dimension will reduce the retentive effect of the clip. Other areas of the bar—solder joints and tissue surface, for example—will receive the same degree of finish as the fixed units. When the fixed components, including the bar, have been completely assembled and finished, they are picked up in the final impression for the removable framework as described earlier so that they are available to the laboratory technician during the subsequent construction phases.

Attaching the clip

It is not essential to use the clip with the bar. In fact, in instances where space is at a real premium, the bar makes an ideal anterior rest for the partial denture. Conventional clasping or other attachment systems elsewhere in the mouth will then provide the necessary retention. This approach also serves as a less expensive alternative to fixed pontics in many situations, most commonly when mandibular incisors are missing and the option is either to include them with the fixed component as pontics or to replace them with the partial denture. As a result of adding the bar in the anterior region, the two sides are more effectively splinted and an ideal rest created. A disadvantage to this use of the bar is that the patient is forced to wear the partial denture at all times for esthetic reasons.

Whether the clip will be used or not, the bar is to be blocked out along with the other components of the remaining dental arch. The superior surface of the bar is left free of blockout wax so that the partial denture casting will contact the bar along that surface up to the solder joint area where a slight amount of relief is appropriate (Fig 11-9). This blockout of the bar presupposes that the bar and associated fixed components have been picked up from the mouth in their finished state and are a part of the definitive cast submitted to the laboratory for construction of the framework. If a clip is to be used, it, along with its housing, must be in place on the bar at the time of blockout so that a refractory replica the exact size of the housing will be created (Fig 11-10).

The clip must be placed in such a way as to ensure that its midline is parallel to the path of insertion, as indicated by the prepared guiding planes on the abutment teeth, permitting both wings of the clip to be flexed the same amount when the clip is activated during insertion and removal. The clip will be reproduced in the refractory cast to create an opening in the casting exactly where the clip is to be positioned. The outer surface of the casting adjacent to the opening will require retentive beads or loops to retain the attaching resin (Fig 11-11). The tooth replacement retention in the area of any bar-clip attachment or the bar alone is to be metal with beads or other mechanical projections. This will always be superior to having that area only in resin since the limited space will require the

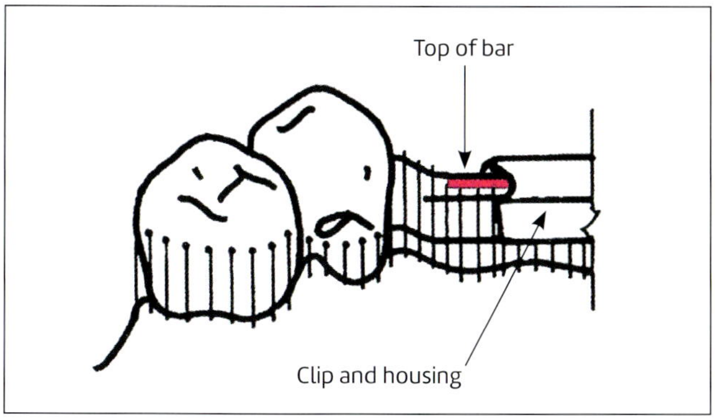

FIG 11-10 Blockout of bar and clip.

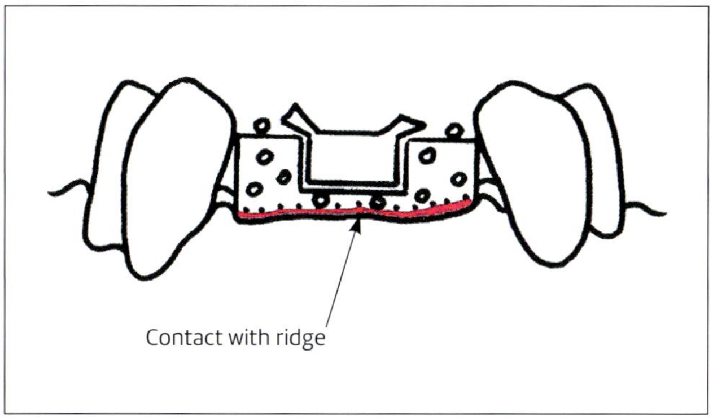

FIG 11-11 RPD casting-clip relationship before pickup.

strength of the full metal coverage. The metal coverage must extend to the crest of the remaining ridge just anterior to the bar with the remainder of the denture base in resin of the appropriate color. When that resin is thin, it will be necessary to have the laboratory opaque the facial aspect of the metal so that it will not be seen through the partially translucent denture base.

When the casting is returned from the laboratory, all components are seated in the mouth if some natural teeth are present or on the definitive cast if all contacts are on fixed units, and its fit corrected as required. If the casting contacts only the fixed components present on the definitive cast, then the clip, or the clip housing, depending on the system in use, should be attached to the frame on the definitive cast with a small amount of autopolymerizing resin, either pink or tooth-colored, depending on the area of attachment. When uncrowned abutment teeth are part of the design in addition to the fixed restorations present on the definitive cast, then the clip should be attached to the frame in the mouth, with all fixed restorations completely seated. Only after the clip is attached to the framework is the altered cast impression made (where indicated) and maxillomandibular relationship records completed. The object is to have the framework and associated abutments in their final relationship before any support of the soft tissue is obtained. This will ensure that no misalignment occurs during processing of the denture bases.

Before the flasking of the denture bases, the fixed components are removed from the definitive cast so they will not be subjected to the high pressures of trial packing. The metal housing in the area of the clip is filled with a silicone mold release material or a putty to protect the clip and housing. The fully waxed denture is seated on the definitive cast, and the borders are sealed. The first half of the flasking will cover the resin cores that once supported the fixed components in addition to any exposed areas of the framework in the standard fashion. The silicone will make the cleanup of the clip area very easy since no stone will be present.

Clip replacement

The clips, either metal or plastic, will eventually wear and will need replacement. In general, the plastic clips will wear much faster than the metal clips, but since they are now in a metal housing, they can be replaced in seconds with minimal effort. Their life expectancy can be improved in two very important ways. First, if the remaining teeth and fixed units are milled at 90 degrees to the path of insertion/removal, the wings of the clip will flex equally and minimally as the clip is activated. Second, if the patient can be made to take some responsibility for the method of insertion of the precision attachment partial (eg, to never bite the partial to place but use only finger pressure), the load on the clip will be controlled. These two suggestions are applicable to all partial dentures but are especially pertinent to the precision attachment partial with a resilient component.

In replacing the plastic clip, any dental hand instrument that can fit inside the metal housing can be used to slide the old clip out of the housing. The new clip is placed on the insertion tool that is specific to that clip and snapped into place. Replacement of the metal clip will require that the old clip be ground out of the partial denture by making an access hole over the clip, usually just lingual to the replacement teeth. The hole must be large enough to allow access to the entire clip and its retentive extensions. These retentive extensions on the new clip are covered with a thin coat of autopolymerizing resin of the appropriate color that is allowed to cure under pressure outside of the mouth. The new clip is placed on the bar, making sure that it is aligned with the path of insertion, and the partial denture is seated over the clip. By completely covering the retentive elements of the clip with resin outside the mouth, the clinician will

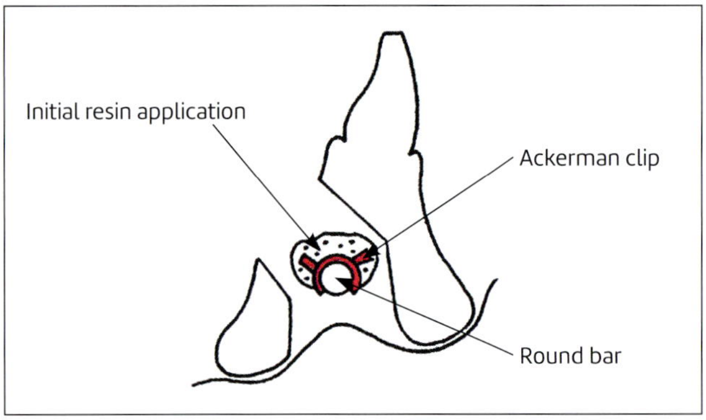

FIG 11-12 Cross section of mandibular overdenture showing replacement of Ackerman clip (gold).

ensure that no voids are created and an optimal resin-clip connection exists when the clip is actually connected to the partial denture in the mouth. Only enough additional resin need be added by picking up polymer with a wetted brush and placing it through the access hole to create a solid joint (Fig 11-12). The patient is typically instructed to close lightly into maximal intercuspal position to verify the proper base-clip relationship and then open the mouth slightly while the clinician holds the denture in place. Once the resin has completely cured in the mouth, the partial denture is carefully removed and the remainder of the required resin added to fill the internal contour to its prerepair condition. The exterior hole is filled to excess, after which the partial denture is placed in the pressure pot for the entire curing time. By filling to excess and then finishing away the top layer, the density of the added resin will be maximized.

The bar-clip combination offers a relatively inexpensive attachment system that has been used successfully for a few generations. It is adaptable to many situations and is easy to maintain. Its only real disadvantage is that it does require a good deal of space, both vertically and horizontally, and so cannot be used universally.

Intracoronal Precision Attachments

The intracoronal attachment that is classified as precision comes from the manufacturer as two components: a matrix and a patrix. These are often accompanied by a paralleling guide that fits into the dental surveyor as well as devices to activate the attachment after fabrication. The matrix is waxed into the crown or bonded into a preparation in the tooth. The patrix is attached to the framework in some fashion, usually by laser welding. In many instances, the patrix will have some retentive component that can be activated and readjusted as wear occurs.

These attachments, being machined to close tolerances (0.001 inch on average), cannot be expected to allow for controlled freedom in rotation of a denture base, and as a result, they are used in all tooth- or tooth/implant-supported partial dentures. There are a number of intracoronal attachments that have an integral hinged component intended to offer stress relief to a distal extension base. The use of this hinged attachment does not, in the author's opinion, fulfill the need to distribute the maximum load to the selected abutments. Instead, it places an uncontrolled amount of force on the tissue least likely to withstand the load: the edentulous ridge. Because we know that resorption of the edentulous ridge is an ongoing, irreversible process, the use of any hinged device places an additional maintenance requirement on the clinician. The distal extension base must be kept in ideal contact with the underlying tissues through relines to minimize soft tissue impingement and stripping of tissue. Due to its poor clinical performance, this type of attachment has all but disappeared from use in the modern partial denture.

Dimensions and space requirements

The standard intracoronal attachments that contain no moving parts do, however, offer excellent retention and esthetics for the tooth-borne partial denture. Because these attachment systems become a part of the crown or pontic, they must be contained within the normal contours of these restorations. The average dimension of the intracoronal attachment is just over 1.5 mm, and allowing for a minimum of 0.5 mm of metal in the crown internal to the matrix, it can be easily seen that a minimum of 2 mm of reduction in the area of the attachment is essential to keep the final unit within normal contours. It may be that bonding the patrix into a prepared cavity in the tooth would require less axial reduction than for a casting, but this treatment modality is in its infancy without longitudinal studies to support its use.

There is general agreement that, in addition to the axial space requirements, the tooth must have sufficient clinical crown height to accept a matrix with a minimum vertical height of 3.5 mm. The height of most matrices as received from the manufacturer is 6 mm, but it is not common to find a crown capable of accepting the total length. Obviously, the greater the vertical height of the attachment complex, the greater the potential retention and stability that can be expected. There are a number of split attachments that have some form of latch, such as the Stern Latch (Sterngold). These can be effective in shorter heights, since the actual retentive mechanism is a split casting with a ridge at its most gingival portion (Fig 11-13). Because of the split casting, the ridge can compress on itself and snap into a recess in the matrix.

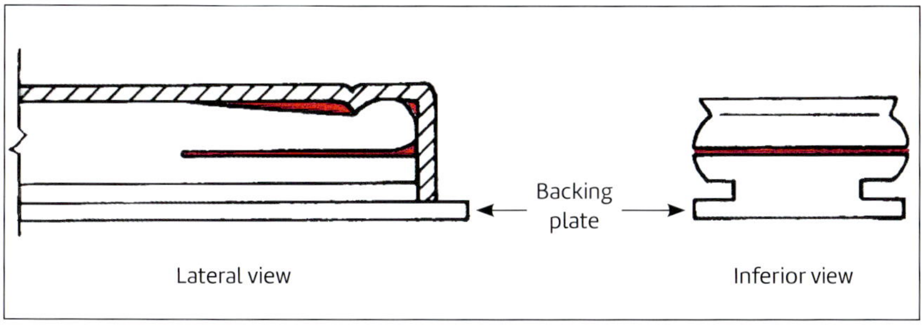

FIG 11-13 Intracoronal attachment (Sterngold, gingival latch). *Red* denotes space within the attachment latch area.

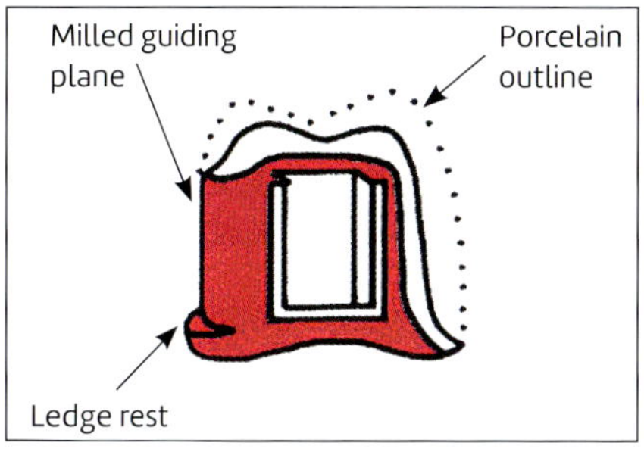

FIG 11-14 Veneer outline for intracoronal attachment. *Red* denotes exterior polished metal.

These space requirements must be taken into careful consideration during the diagnostic waxing and positioning of the denture teeth. In the younger patient, where large pulp chambers and a lack of secondary dentin are found, it may not be possible to use an intracoronal attachment; extracoronal attachments will be necessary for these patients. The width of the matrix in a buccolingual direction will be in the range of 3 mm, a dimension that can be accommodated in most abutment teeth. For example, the width of the patrix for the Stern Latch is 2.3 mm.

Before mouth preparation on the actual abutment teeth, all guiding plane preparations on the remaining teeth that will not be treated with crowns or other castings must be made and verified. It is far more practical to make the attachments and any guiding planes on their crowns to match the path of insertion/removal as it exists on the other prepared teeth than to make the attachment containing crowns first and then try to parallel guiding planes to match the path. Because these attachments are very precise, it is nearly impossible to match their path after they are in place. The same system of diagnostic mouth preparation as suggested for the conventional partial denture must be employed with a careful verification of the check cast before beginning the actual preparation of the teeth to be crowned. As with conventional surveyed crowns, the definitive cast must include all other teeth involved with the partial denture and transfer the desired path of insertion/removal to the technician through tripod marks or similar surveyor-based references.

Laboratory construction of intracoronal precision attachment crown and pontic units is not difficult, although some experience is necessary to use the surveyor and special tools to position the matrices perfectly parallel to the indicated path of insertion. Some discussion with the technician is needed as to the extent of the porcelain coverage on the abutment crowns since the matrix will require a small amount (0.4 mm minimum) of metal around it that is free of porcelain (Fig 11-14). These abutments will often also require milled guiding planes and appropriate contours to accept rests, all of which will influence the cutback of the metal for veneering.

The intracoronal attachment will not normally be indicated on the mesial surface of anterior teeth since the alteration of contour will most likely prove to be unacceptable (the canines being the only possible exception). Generally speaking, anterior edentulous spaces are better restored with fixed pontics than with components of the RPD.

Taking the impression

When the crowns have been completed and have been found to be acceptable for esthetics and occlusion, the final impression for the removable framework is made. A firm-setting elastomeric impression material, either silicone or polyether, is used in a custom tray with ample retention (holes and adhesive) to ensure that the impression material does not separate from the tray during removal of the impression from the mouth. These materials are not intended to impress large undercuts as may be found on unprepared natural teeth. Because the goal of the final impression is to relate the fixed components to the remainder of the arch and to allow the pickup of these components without distorting the final impression, it is often necessary to block out large undercuts, furcations, undersurfaces of pontics, and any other area where the resistance to removal is apt to be so high as to threaten the integrity of the final impression. Any number of materials can be used for the blockout of these areas. Wax, alginate, or a dedicated blockout material such as OraSeal putty (Ultradent) are examples that should be considered.

Ideally, the crowns and other fixed components should remain in the impression because repositioning them into the impression reduces accuracy. As discussed earlier, resin dies should be available to insert in the crowns prior to pouring the definitive pickup cast. The modern impression materials used in these situations can be comfortably

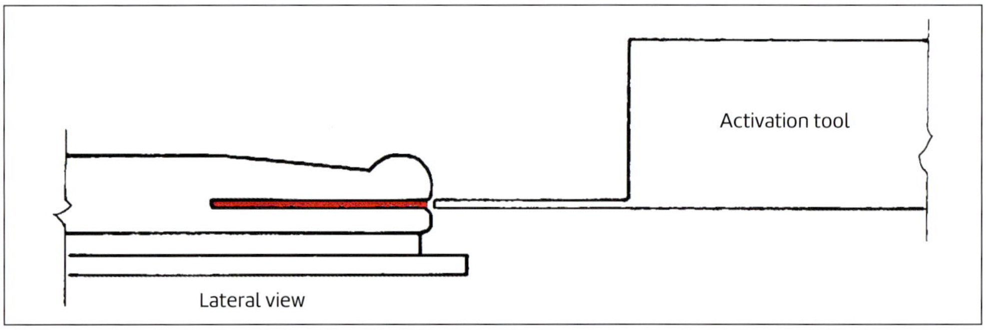

FIG 11-15 Reactivation of Stern Latch attachment.

transported to the dental laboratory without fear of distortion, and the construction of the definitive cast left to the technician. A diagnostic cast must accompany the final impression to inform the technician of the prescribed design of the framework. It is much easier to convey specific requirements via a diagnostic cast with a neat and careful drawing of the outline of the framework than to try to describe the desired outcome over the phone or on the work authorization form.

Verifying fit

The same requirements of design and construction as described for the conventional partial denture must be adhered to for the precision attachment framework. When the frame and definitive cast are returned to the clinician, the fit of the frame in the mouth and to the crowns must be verified before the patrices are picked up in resin, either in the mouth or on the definitive pickup cast. The decision as to where to best join the attachments to the framework is dependent on many factors, and there is no one correct way. It must be remembered, however, that in every instance, the frame/attachment relationship must be identical from the mouth to the definitive cast before the construction can continue. Most intracoronal attachments will be joined to the framework by soldering or laser welding since space is likely to be a critical limiting factor.

The fit of the framework must be reverified after the laser welding operation in every instance. Only when the tooth-frame relation meets the highest standards can other procedures be undertaken. The completion of the case, once the frame fit is established, is relatively standard as far as records, positioning of the denture teeth, and processing of the base are concerned. An area of special consideration is the protection of the patrix connection when the amount of resin over or around this area is minimal (less than 2 mm of tooth or base resin). In these instances, metal occlusal surfaces are to be constructed, usually in type IV gold, and added to the denture teeth to ensure that subsequent wear will not break through to the patrix.

At insertion of the intracoronal attachment partial denture, any undercuts to the path of insertion/removal where resin has extended will have to be carefully identified and recontoured to fully seat the partial denture. Because the path of insertion will be so precise, the finished partial denture must never be forced to place on initial seating until all possible undercuts in resin have been identified and adjusted. The soft tissues of the mouth occlusal to areas of slight undercut may compress and allow the full seating of the partial denture but will not allow the partial denture to be removed without pain or discomfort to the patient. If pressure indicating paste is placed on all resin areas and the partial denture inserted with light pressure until resistance is felt, either by the clinician or by the patient, areas of difficulty can be identified without fear of tissue irritation.

There remains only the activation of the attachment, in those attachment systems where this possibility exists. In general, the patient should be informed of the intention to use only the lightest activation that will satisfy the patient's needs for retention, since the lower the level of activation, the better the chance to reduce distortion and the need for repeated adjustments. Activation is accomplished with the use of specific tools provided by the manufacturer that distort the patrix by increasing the opening of the split areas of the metal (Fig 11-15). The tools are carefully calibrated to ensure that overactivation does not occur, a frightening situation where the partial denture cannot be removed from the mouth without excessive force. For this reason, it is not wise to allow the patient to reactivate their attachments by themselves. Assuming that every aspect of construction of the intracoronal precision attachment partial has been done to the highest standards, the attachments should only need periodic reactivation, undertaken as a part of normal recall activities. Systematic recall for these patients is perhaps as critical as high standards of construction for the long-term success of the entire treatment. Certainly, these two components of treatment are far more important than variations in design of the partial denture.

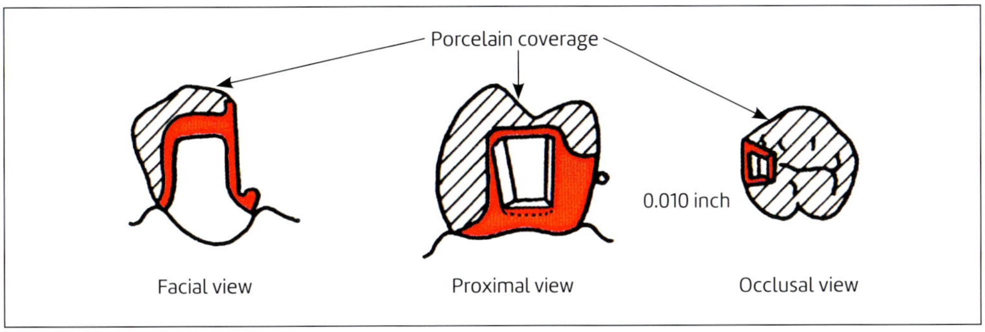

FIG 11-16 Cross sections of Thompson dowel rest semiprecision intracoronal attachment.

A wide assortment of intracoronal attachments is available to the clinician, all based on the same general principles described here. Dental technicians will have their favorites, depending on their experience; however, their experience is based upon fabrication issues and not on clinical evaluation. Therefore, while one attachment system may be easier to construct, it does not follow that the system will work as well as some other type over the expected lifespan of 20 years. The sheer number of attachments precludes that any one clinician or technician will have had sufficient experience working with all attachments to define the selection in any scientific manner.

Intracoronal Semiprecision Attachments

Because of the very low tolerances of the precision attachment, little stress relief is possible when it is used on Class I partial dentures, especially in the mandible. When only a few compromised mandibular anterior teeth are available as abutments, as is so often the case, many clinicians elect to relieve the stress of mastication to the abutments by splinting all remaining teeth and transferring some of the load to the edentulous ridge. While it is theoretically possible to do that with precision attachments that utilize a hinge component in the patrix, as stated earlier, that is not advisable. There is a type of attachment, usually referred to as a *semiprecision attachment*, that utilizes an intracoronal box and a resilient lingual clasp arm, preferably wrought, for the actual retention. The bottom of the box in the crown has a slight lip and a rounded base that allows the patrix rest to rotate slightly in function but that will not, because of the lip, slip distally and unseat (Fig 11-16). To disengage, the entire partial denture must move vertically the distance of the raised lip before the patrix is free of the matrix. The esthetic effect of a semiprecision attachment is the same as for a precision intracoronal attachment with no evidence of the RPD visible on the facial aspect of the abutments.

The semiprecision attachment, as defined by the *Glossary of Prosthodontic Terms*, 9th edition,[5] is laboratory fabricated rather than made from prefabricated parts. Despite this, the term is occasionally applied to attachments using prefabricated plastic components. The Thompson dowel attachment is the best known of this type of laboratory-fabricated device. It is made by waxing the matrix within the abutment crown to a homemade former and then creating the patrix rest pattern in resin directly in the finished casting of the abutment. Similar attachment forms are made by some commercial manufacturers. Because the space they require in the crown will be the same as the precision attachment, without the retentive effect found in most precision patrices, the use of this design is not as easy to defend. If a posterior isolated abutment on a tooth-borne side of the partial denture is less than ideal and unlikely to survive the projected lifespan of the partial denture, the Thompson dowel attachment is indicated for the more anterior abutment tooth (usually a premolar). When the distal abutment tooth is lost, the partial denture can be quickly converted to a distal extension without having to be concerned about the stress relief of the attachment system.

A matrix former can be easily handmade in wax and attached to a straight resin sprue of sufficient length and dimensions to allow it to be placed in the vertical arm of the surveyor after casting in any alloy (usually a nonprecious partial denture alloy). It is finished and polished and then machined using the side of a large, flat disk to ensure that the walls of the matrix will have no undercut areas. The original Thompson dowel attachment had both a right and a left matrix former, the lingual walls of which were set at right angles to the internal wall. The buccal walls diverged slightly to allow ease of rotation while still providing a guiding plane surface parallel to the path of insertion/removal. The buccal divergence also allows easier positioning of the attachment for insertion by the patient. The metal former is lubricated with a silicone spray, and wax is added in excess to create the matrix. The wax pattern is removed from the matrix former and reduced to have walls approximately 0.3 mm thick. The crown pattern is cut away on the distal aspect to a thickness of 0.3 mm, and the matrix pattern is added to the crown using the surveyor to carry the wax matrix to place. Once the matrix has been fully tacked into

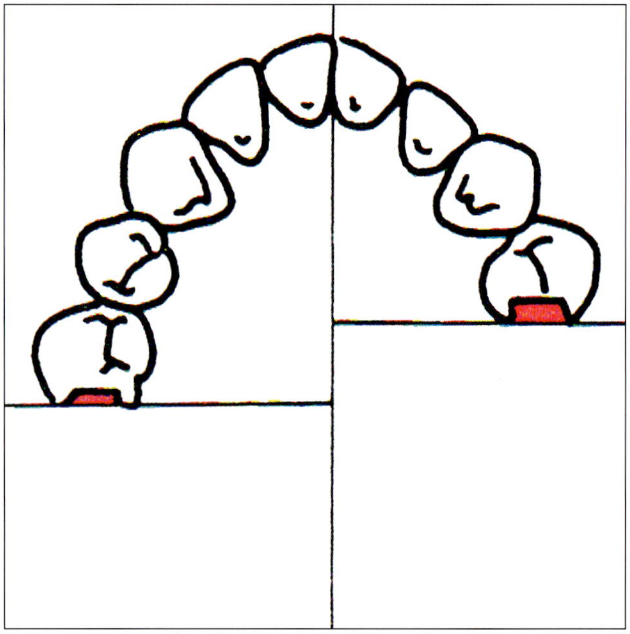

FIG 11-17 Parallel placement of Thompson dowel rests.

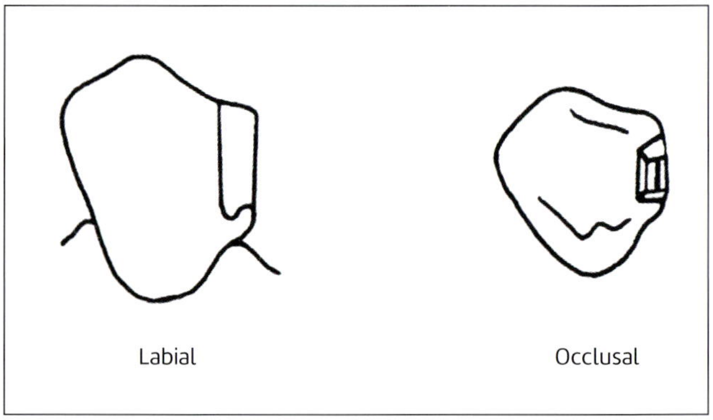

FIG 11-18 Alteration of contour of a canine to accommodate the precision attachment.

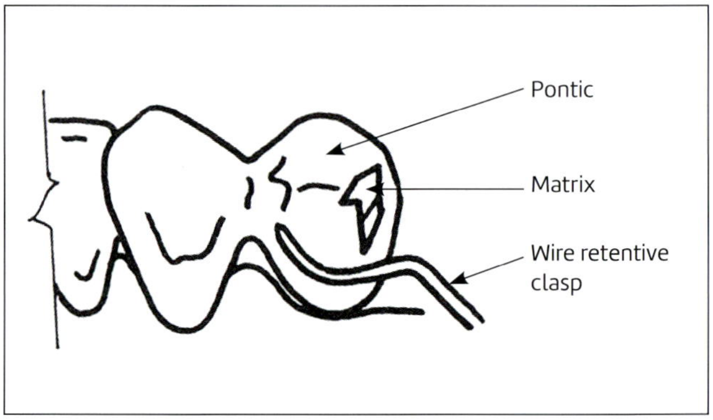

FIG 11-19 Cantilevered first premolar to contain attachment (Thompson dowel).

place and the contours reestablished, the former is removed from the wax pattern.

Because this attachment is semiprecision, it can be completely hand waxed without the use of the matrix former. Parallel or tapered burs are used on the wax pattern to create the walls to the desired dimensions and angles. A round bur can be used to create the depression for the rotational ridge. Surveyor-type milling machines with wax-cutting burs, and typically speed control, make the shaping of a matrix—and guiding planes for that matter—a relatively simple procedure.

It should be obvious that the matrix form must be parallel to the path of insertion/removal as dictated by the guiding planes prepared on any unrestored teeth present in the arch that will be used as abutments. When this attachment is used for a Class I partial denture, the internal walls of the matrix must be set parallel to each other and at right angles to the midsagittal plane of the arch (Fig 11-17). This positioning of the matrices is essential to allow rotation of the bilateral distal extension bases. When the terminal abutment is a canine, it is often necessary to shape the distal half of the tooth like a premolar to place the distal surface parallel to the distal surface on the opposite side of the arch (Fig 11-18). When the remaining teeth are to be splinted, as they often are in these cases, a premolar can be cantilevered off the terminal canine to contain the attachment. Because the actual retention of the partial denture will be created using a lingual wire circumferential clasp, the use of a premolar pontic will allow a longer clasp arm than would be possible on the canine, with a more natural approach to a mesiolingual undercut area (Fig 11-19). If the abutment teeth are not to be splinted across the arch, double abutting must be considered, with additional rests and guiding planes prepared on the nonsplinted teeth. The use of this attachment in a nonsplinted mandibular first premolar, for example, would be contraindicated due to the load that could be placed on the tooth if the distal extension base were not kept in full contact through subsequent relines.

The lingual surface of the waxed crown(s) is prepared to accept the terminal third of a light wire (20 gauge) circumferential clasp running to the mesiolingual. The entire lingual surface can be shaped to allow the clasp arm to lie in a depression in the metal, with the final one-third passing

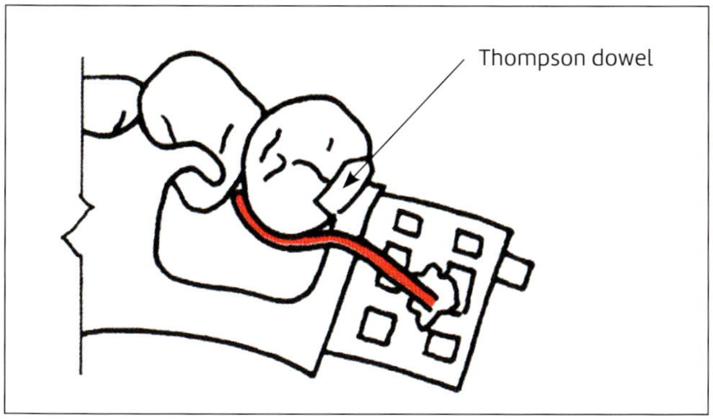

FIG 11-20 Lingual retentive wire with full extension into embrasure.

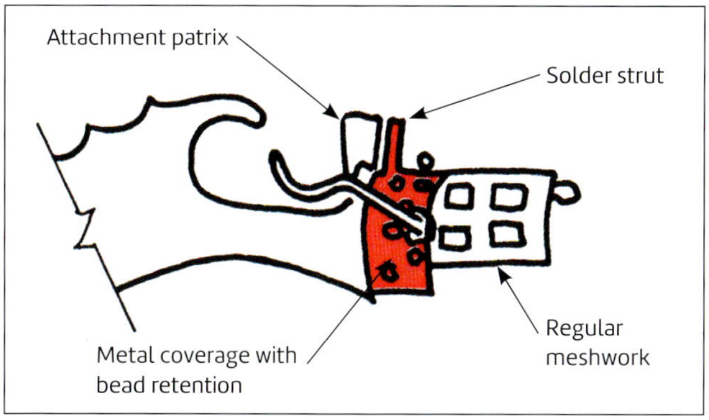

FIG 11-21 Metal coverage of ridge under attachment to be laser welded/soldered.

into a 0.01-inch undercut relative to the path of insertion/removal of the matrix and the remainder of the guiding planes in the mouth. The clasp arm is to be extended as far to the mesial as the embrasure contour will allow to create the longest possible retentive arm (Fig 11-20). The height of contour must be planned to leave a 1-mm space between the gingival border of the clasp and the gingival tissue.

Once the castings have been completed and veneered, they are picked up from the mouth in the final impression for the partial denture. The patrices are now formed in resin and their tangs in either resin or wax. At this time, a decision on the method of attachment of the patrices to the framework will have to be made. If the patrices are to be laser welded to the framework, the area of attachment should be all in metal with the internal finishing line distal to the weld area (Fig 11-21). This requires that the relief wax begins distal to the weld area. In addition, a strong support strut should extend vertically as if it were a guiding plane; this facilitates welding from at least three different directions. If the intent is to attach the patrices to the frame with resin and keep them in resin, then an evaluation of the available space occlusal to the meshwork must be made. Remember, when space is at a premium, the welding method is preferred. With adequate space, there is an advantage to keeping the connection in resin so that the attachment component can be replaced with minimum destruction to the partial denture.

When the shape of the tang is established, the wax and resin pattern is invested and cast in the same alloy or one slightly softer than was used for the crown. This is done so any wear with time will occur on the patrices, which are relatively easy to replace, rather than the matrices. Type III gold will probably be slightly softer than the ceramic alloy chosen for the crowns. The definitive cast, with the patrices in place, is now ready for blockout and duplication. The waxing of the framework will depend on the manner in which the patrices are to be attached. Once again, the framework is protected from any internal finishing by the technician, and only after a quality fit is verified in the mouth will the patrices be attached to the frame, either on the cast or in the mouth. Care must be taken to ensure that the patrices are fully contacting the internal wall of the matrix when they are added to the frame, since it is in this relationship that the tissue base relationship will be confirmed. Even though the clasp arms have not yet been added to the casting, an altered cast impression would be made if indicated. Only after the altered cast with its maxillomandibular relationship record is returned to the laboratory will the wire clasp arms be added and the case finished.

Because there is no buccal clasp arm on this type of partial denture, a Class V cavity is cut into the most anterior denture tooth to serve as a ledge where the patient can place a fingernail to remove the partial denture. The Thompson dowel attachment offers freedom to rotate for the Class I partial denture, with ease of adjustment of the wire retentive clasp. As is typical for intracoronal attachments, the main disadvantage is the bulk of the matrix and the need for 3.5 mm of vertical height. When reviewing the overall design of a Thompson dowel case, one finds it is remarkably similar to the advanced designs in this textbook utilizing lingual clasping. This makes it difficult to defend these dowels as superior to the similar functional and esthetic results achieved with proper rest, guiding plane, and lingual clasp designs described previously.

Extracoronal Rigid Attachments

There are a variety of extracoronal attachments available to the clinician. Some of these are rigid; that is, they do not allow any rotation of the partial denture in function. Others are hinged, offering a stress-breaking action to the distal

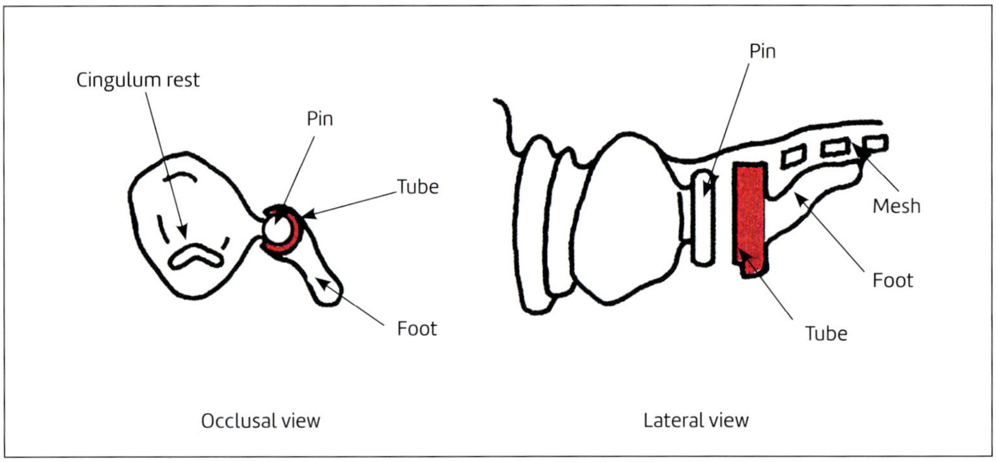

FIG 11-22 Pin-tube attachment.

extension base. As was noted, there seems to be little advantage to placing greater load on the extension base through the use of hinged attachments. These hinged attachments are therefore not considered justifiable and will not be discussed further. However, a number of resilient extracoronal attachments that permit a limited amount of movement of the denture base for the Class I partial denture situation are available. Both the rigid and the resilient have a distinct place in the tooth and tissue–borne partial denture.

The great advantage of the extracoronal attachment is that it does not alter the normal contour of the abutment crown, being entirely outside of these contours, and therefore does not require additional tooth reduction. An additional advantage of the rigid attachment is that the entire length of the attachment, from the gingival tissue to the occlusal plane, can be used for frictional retention. This makes it invaluable in situations with short abutment teeth.

A simple rigid extracoronal attachment is one commonly referred to as the *pin-tube attachment* (Fig 11-22). For most of these, the pin (patrix) is added to the fixed unit and the matrix (tube) to the partial denture. The attachments can be easily made by hand. They are also available from attachment manufacturers (eg, Preci-Vertix from Preat Corporation, Interlock and Tube Lock from Sterngold). Some intracoronal pin and tube attachments can be used as extracoronal attachments by reversing the patrix and matrix so that, instead of having the matrix in the crown, it becomes part of the partial denture. Resilient retentive sleeves have been added to the matrices of pin-tube attachments. The most commonly used of this special form is the vertical Hader bar. A similar form is the Preci-Vertix, which, according to the manufacturer, can be used either as a rigid attachment or, when the coronal portion of the patrix is reduced by 0.3 to 0.5 mm, as a resilient attachment.

All of these simple attachments can be constructed using the same principles with little expected variation. They differ from older systems in that the matrix is lined with the aforementioned resilient sleeve that can be easily and inexpensively replaced as needed for retention. The matrices come with a precisely machined metal cover that has retentive contours on its outer surface to which resin can adhere. The metal matrix covers are intended to stay in the partial denture for its normal life, allowing the resilient inner matrices to be replaced.

The milled abutment as a precision attachment

Extracoronal rigid attachments, like their intracoronal counterparts, are indicated in Class III situations where minimal to no flexure of the partial denture bases is expected. The effect of these specific attachment systems is that they significantly restrict the path of placement and removal of the partial denture. The vertical slots or keyways, whether in metal or resilient material, act as very precise machine milled surfaces that dramatically increase the stability of the prosthesis. Looking back at the definition of a guiding plane, it is clear that these types of rigid attachments are often nothing more than machined guiding planes. Obviously, some have added "tricks" like the Stern latch, but the functional result of increased stability comes from the effect of the milled parallel surfaces.

The realization that truly parallel milled surfaces of abutment teeth, and especially abutment crowns, combined with ideally fitted frameworks are in fact precision attachments has been a revelation.[6,7] With the modern techniques described in this text, the fit of this type of RPD can now be so precise that, especially on mandibular

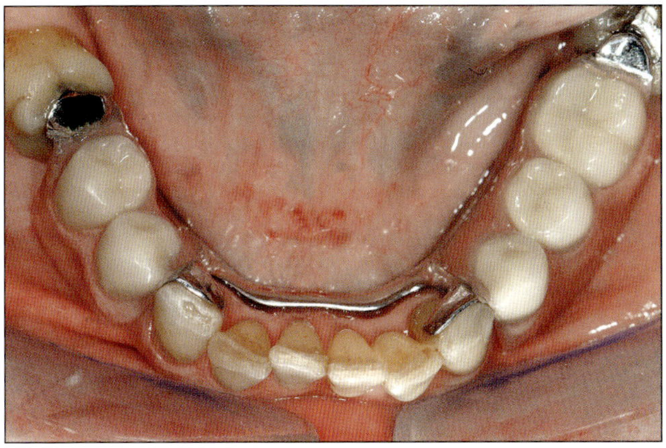

FIG 11-23 The milled surface can in fact function as a "precision attachment partial." This is a Class III RPD stabilized and retained only by rests and guiding planes.

Class III situations, no other means of retention may be required (Fig 11-23). The philosophies prescribed in this textbook now come to fruition. This kind of precision fit, once achievable only with machined precision attachment components, reduces conventional clasping to one clasp per side or less. If that clasp assembly is in the posterior of the mouth or if the clasp is on the lingual surface, then no visible clasp needs ever again be seen. In the minds of those who utilize these concepts, precision attachments become unnecessary. The additional steps, expenses, and maintenance of these complicated systems are eliminated in favor of the milled guiding plane.

While the entirety of this text highlights the specific details of advanced RPD design, it is hoped that at this point the inherent simplicity of the philosophy is becoming apparent. Eliminating clasps, reduced need for attachments, minimizing minor connectors, limited tissue coverage, and abutment selection all point to frameworks that are easier to fit, more comfortable, and more stable.[6] For example, a Class III partial denture using the milled surface concept would typically have lingual circlet clasps on the molars, a lingual or dental lingual bar major connector that does not cover any lingual marginal gingiva, and abutment teeth easily accessible for hygiene whether the partial denture is in or out of the mouth. The minimized presence of the partial denture when in the mouth is greatly appreciated by any patient who has ever had to wear a "conventional RPD." This is also appreciated by the dentist, who should have less to repair, replace, or maintain over time. The techniques required to create this type of RPD have been presented throughout this textbook.

Extracoronal Resilient Attachments

Despite dentist attempts to avoid distal extension situations, they remain common in clinical practice. As has been noted, this requires management of shared tooth-tissue support. Resilient attachments are an attempt to avoid putting too much stress on RPD abutments. They allow some degree of movement of a distal extension base so that some amount of pressure can be shared by the residual ridge. The *Glossary of Prosthodontic Terms*, 9th edition,[5] defines a resilient attachment as the following:

> **Resilient attachment (1998):** An attachment designed to give a tooth-, soft tissue–, or implant-borne removable dental prosthesis sufficient mechanical flexion to withstand the variations in seating of the prosthesis as a result of deformations of the mucosa and underlying tissues to avoid placing excessive stress on the abutments.

Attachment systems vary in the amount of resiliency they can or will provide. This brief discussion of resilient attachments moves from less resilient to more resilient but should not be taken as absolute. With ever-evolving changes in designs and materials, the clinician must be conscious of the need to reevaluate the specifics of preferred systems over time.

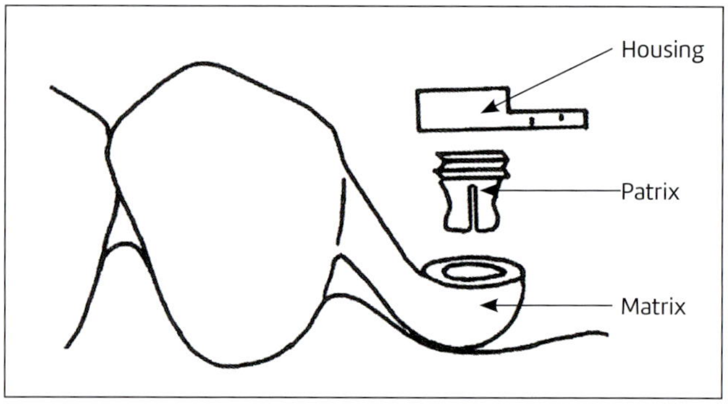

FIG 11-24 Ceka Revax attachment.

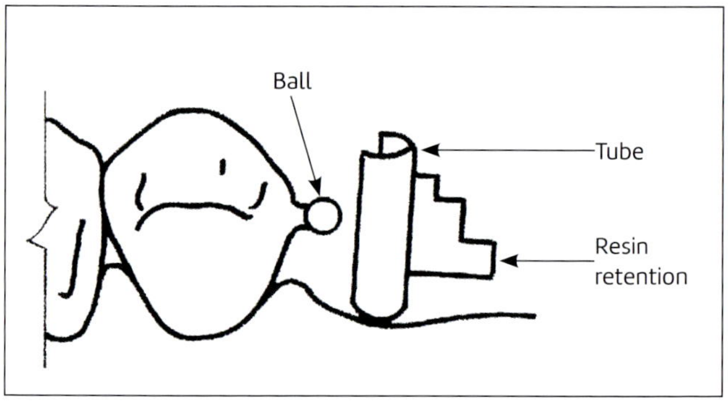

FIG 11-25 Roach attachment (ball and tube).

Ceka attachment

A well-known and long-used system is the Ceka attachment (Preat Corporation). This attachment differs from the others in that the patrix is a split metal post that is adjustable and snaps into a metal matrix attached to the proximal surface of the abutment crown. This system has many modifications for use in a variety of situations. The patrix post is threaded so that it can be screwed into the holding device and easily replaced if damaged or worn. A spacer ring is used to allow the possibility of stress relief, creating a vertical space of 0.3 mm when the spacer has been removed after construction. This space allows a small amount of rotation of the partial denture, which will place some of the load on the tissues of the denture base. An innovation from the 1980s called the Ceka Revax attachment places the matrix in contact with the gingival tissues in a way that allows easy access for hygiene, both under the matrix and between the matrix and the axial surface of the abutment crown so that the gingival tissues are never compromised (Fig 11-24).

Roach attachment

A very old system that has been in use since the 1920s is the Roach attachment. The patrix of this attachment is a partially split, adjustable round ball that extends out from the axial surface of the abutment crown. The ball comes as a finished casting that can be soldered or cast to the axial surface of a crown. The matrix of this system is a tube, in much the same form as discussed earlier. In its earliest form, the tube was made from plate gold and was attached to the partial denture by means of a metal tang that had been soldered to the tube. The modern edition has a tube with one form to be used if the attachment is to be soldered to the framework, another if the matrix is to be attached with resin (Fig 11-25).

Because the patrix is a ball, the contact with the matrix is only at the circumference. This allows for more rotation than any of the other systems. The increased stress relief available with this system is indicated for use in compromised dentitions where a conscious decision has been made to transfer load from the abutments to the supporting tissues of the denture bases. The exact amount of rotation allowed with the Roach attachment is a factor of the space between the tube and the axial wall since the tube can only allow rotation to the point where it comes in contact with the crown. In all the systems that allow rotation, the amount of movement that is desired is slight, since regular maintenance will keep the amount of space between the base and the tissues to a minimum. If the precision attachment partial denture is ignored for long periods of time, no attachment system will permit control of the rotational forces.

VKS attachment

The modern equivalent of the Roach is the VKS-SG by Bredent (XPdent), and it is this attachment that is currently found to be the most practical, inexpensive, and easy to use of all the extracoronals. The VKS consists of a castable pattern of a ball extending from a flat plate, as does the Roach, and uses a resilient matrix (Fig 11-26a). The ball is added to the abutment crown adjacent to the edentulous area using a dental surveyor and is parallel to all milled surfaces.

The matrix for this attachment is a thermoplastic "snap" that is contained in a housing that is either preformed in resin and therefore castable, or in metal for use when the matrix is to be attached to the framework with resin. The matrix has an indentation on both sides, which serves to retain it within the housing until it requires replacement (Fig 11-26b). As discussed, a custom housing can be created in metal-ceramic and veneered with porcelain or in a nonprecious metal and veneered with composite. Either can then be laser welded to the framework. This is essential

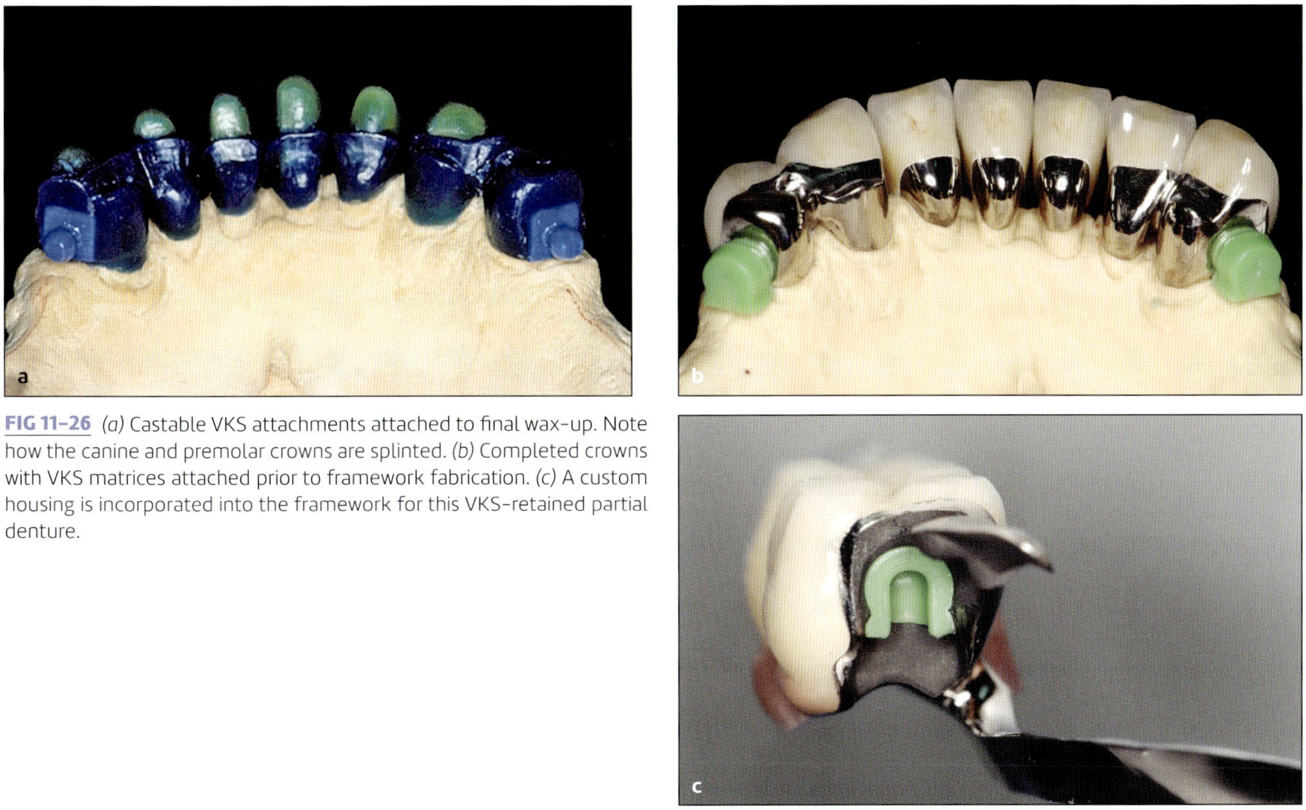

FIG 11-26 *(a)* Castable VKS attachments attached to final wax-up. Note how the canine and premolar crowns are splinted. *(b)* Completed crowns with VKS matrices attached prior to framework fabrication. *(c)* A custom housing is incorporated into the framework for this VKS-retained partial denture.

for situations with minimal vertical space (Fig 11-26c). The VKS comes in two sizes, a 1.7-mm and a 2.2-mm ball along with appropriate snaps and housings. The 1.7-mm matrix seems to provide more than enough retention for any RPD on the mandible when combined with appropriate milled surfaces. The "snaps" are easy to replace and can last from 3 months to over a year. This typically depends on the volume of milled surfaces available to restrict the path of insertion and removal. This attachment, like the Roach, does allow some rotational movement before binding.

Attaching the patrix

After all fixed units have been waxed to full contour and milled for maximum guiding plane surface area, the patrices of whatever system that has been chosen are added to the axial surfaces of the abutment crowns using the special alignment tools provided by the manufacturer. The patrices are generally patterns made in some form of hard resin that is amenable to burnout and casting in standard metal-ceramic alloys. The alignment tool is placed in the dental surveyor at the same tilt of definitive cast as was used for the wax milling of the guiding plane surfaces. It is critical that the path of insertion/removal to be used takes into account the height of contour of the edentulous soft tissues as well as the remaining teeth.

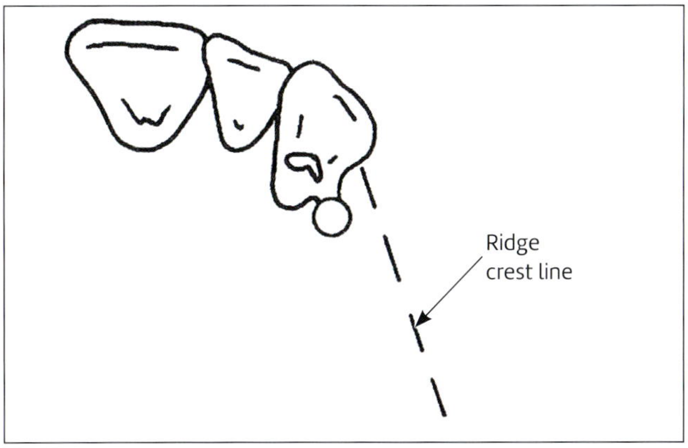

FIG 11-27 Extracoronal attachment placed lingual to the center of the proximal surface.

The plastic pattern, or preformed metal patrix, is to be placed somewhat to the lingual of the center of the proximal surface (Fig 11-27). This step ensures that the bulk of the matrix will not interfere with the esthetics of the buccal cusp of the replacement denture tooth. The average patient can tolerate a slight excess of contour to the lingual since esthetics are not involved. The patrix (in the pin systems) is to extend from a contact with the edentulous ridge to the occlusal plane. This length can be maintained in systems that utilize an open tube. If the system requires a capped

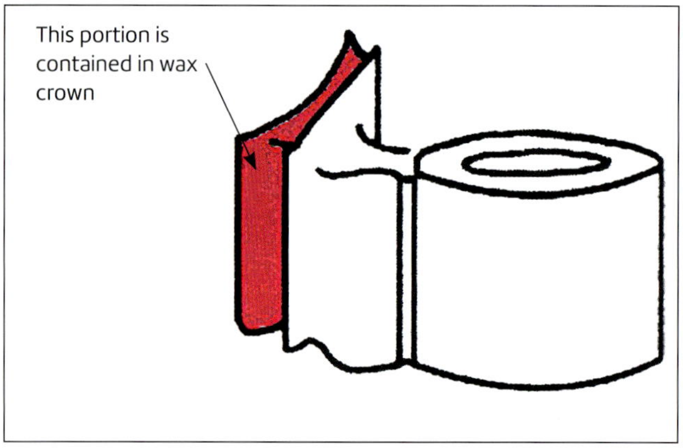

FIG 11-28 ERA patrix (Sterngold), castable plastic.

housing, the patrix will have to be shortened to accommodate the housing. The decision of which type of system to employ often hinges on the amount of vertical space available. The patrix pin must extend far enough out from the abutment tooth that floss can be passed under the pin and up to the marginal gingiva. Most plastic patterns come with a self-limiting platform that, when waxed into the normal contour of the abutment tooth, automatically controls the extension into the edentulous area (Fig 11-28).

When the teeth bearing the extracoronal attachments are to be veneered with porcelain, the extension of the cutback for the veneer is critical. The veneering material must not be allowed to contact the matrix portion of the attachment. In most cases, this requirement will cause the margin of metal to extend further to the facial and lingual surfaces than it would in a veneered crown not involved with the attachment. This extension beyond the normal cutback is generally in the area of 1.0 to 1.5 mm and does not usually create an esthetic problem since the attachment is most often found on the distal proximal surface of the abutment tooth.

Final steps

After casting, the technician is careful to leave the patrices untouched; any finishing and polishing will decrease the retention of the system. The fixed units are finished and veneered and are then included on the definitive pickup cast for the partial denture framework as described earlier. This step is essential for the extracoronal attachment since the patrices are so small that they would not stand up if impressed and poured in stone. By having the actual casting on the definitive cast, the technician creating the partial denture can wax out the contours and prepare the refractory cast so that the attachment of the matrices is precise and accurate. When all the remaining teeth in the arch are part of the fixed component, the matrices are best picked up on the definitive cast and verified in the mouth. When some of the abutments are natural teeth not associated with the fixed units, the task of picking up the attachments becomes slightly more complex since the stone replicas of these abutments may be damaged during the process. In this situation, it is best to place all the fixed components in the mouth, fit the frame, and then attach the matrices with autopolymerizing or light-activated resin. The complete assembly must then of course be returned to the definitive pickup cast for verification. Tolerances for the relationship of components in the precision attachment partial denture are much finer than for the conventional partial denture, so the use of magnification whenever possible is essential.

Most of the extracoronal attachment systems are self-aligning when it comes to joining the matrices to the patrices. The components need only be fully seated on each other and the resin applied. Some systems, the Roach for example, have aligning tools for the matrices that are to be used with the dental surveyor. These systems must be attached on the bench. As noted with intracoronal attachments, for each of these systems, the decision whether to solder the matrices to the framework or to attach them with resin must be made on an individual basis with space requirements as the biggest factor. Both means work well and, with care, will not cause problems.

When an altered cast impression is indicated, for any or all of these systems, it can only be made after the attachments have been joined to the framework. A separate appointment will often be required to obtain this impression and the subsequent maxillomandibular relationship records since the addition of resin to the matrices/patrices requires access to the retentive meshwork in the same areas as would be used to join the altered cast trays. For these situations, it is recommended that the attachment component be soldered/welded rather than attached with resin since the resin of the altered cast tray may attach to the attachment, making removal of the tray a real problem. With the attachments fully seated, the altered cast impression can be made with confidence since the support of both the hard and soft tissue has been optimized.

The trial arrangement and wax-up of the partial denture containing extracoronal attachments is generally not complicated except for placing the denture tooth that sits over the attachment assembly. Often, this first tooth will need to be hollowed out to a mere shell. In order to not have the denture base resin show through the tooth, it may be necessary to pack a small amount of tooth-colored resin, preferably heat-curing, under the tooth before the remainder of the denture base is packed. When space is at a premium, the previously discussed metal occlusals or custom

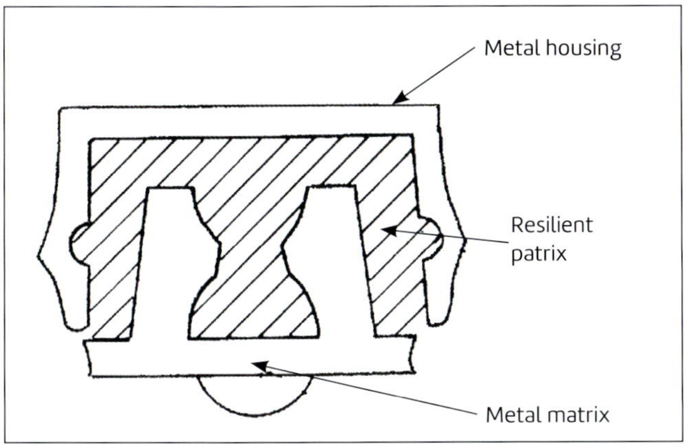

FIG 11-29 ERA cross section, overdenture matrix, with no space created (processing patrix in position).

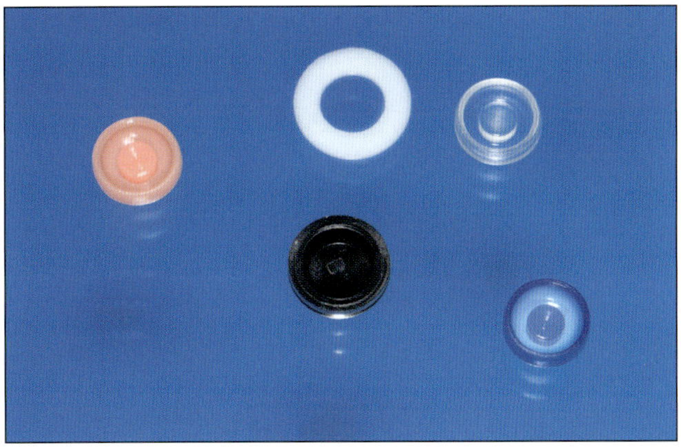

FIG 11-30 Standard Locator inserts along with white spacer ring and housing with black processing insert.

housings are needed to prevent rapid wear and associated destruction of the attachment assembly. The cost of adding a small onlay or three-quarters crown form to the partial denture is minimal compared to the cost of repairing the attachment partial denture down the road.

Additional extracoronal attachments

A final group of extracoronal attachments remains to be discussed. While several resilient attachments like the Bredent VKS have been discussed, the term is more apt to be applied to the developments best illustrated by the ERA (Sterngold), OSO, and Locator attachment systems. These systems were developed to allow for stress relief and for simple and rapid replacement of the resilient components. These systems often wear out quickly but are so easily replaced that some patients can do the job themselves.

The ERA system is similar to the Ceka attachment already described, the difference being that the patrix in the ERA is a plastic material that snaps into a matrix ring attached to the crown (Fig 11-29). The ring comes as a castable plastic pattern or a machined stainless steel cast to component (see Fig 11-28). For the smallest version, called Micro-ERA, a minimum of 3.0 mm vertical distance is recommended. Four different levels of retention are available with four slightly different plastic patrices. A metal housing with internal retentive grooves for the plastic inserts and external ridges for resin retention is included with the attachment system. The patrices are color-coded, with the white unit being the most flexible and progressing through orange to blue to gray as the most rigid. Sterngold now makes yellow and red "oversized" patrices that are designed for use when the matrix wears out, leaving a "wider" interface. Studies have indicated that after a short time, there is no clinical difference between the retention of the four colored units.[8] Most situations will need only the white patrix, as the amount of retention it gives is more than adequate when combined with other frictional retentive components of the partial denture. A trephine bur is provided that allows rapid removal of the worn patrix. An insertion tool is provided that carries the new patrix into the partial denture and forces it to place in the housing. The entire operation takes less than a minute. A processing patrix is also a part of the system. It is slightly longer than the colored units that are installed after processing and thereby creates some space for movement of the patrix within the housing. This built-in spacer is the source of the stress relief described by the manufacturer. The ERA has been popular due to its ease of replacement and the slight amount of flexibility it allows. The Locator system, in both its original and new R-TX forms, also has variable retention level inserts (Fig 11-30).

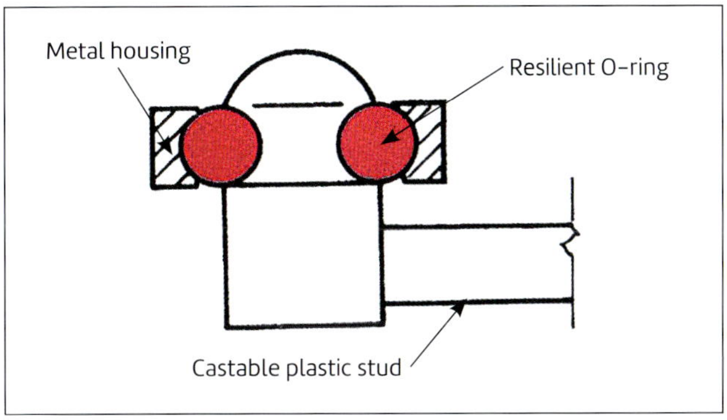

FIG 11-31 Resilient stud attachment (OSO), extracoronal, in cross section.

The OSO attachment is actually classified as a stud attachment, with a patrix looking somewhat like a doorknob and with a rubber O-ring matrix. The O-ring comes, in its most recent form, with a metal housing not unlike that used with other systems (Fig 11-31). The system also uses

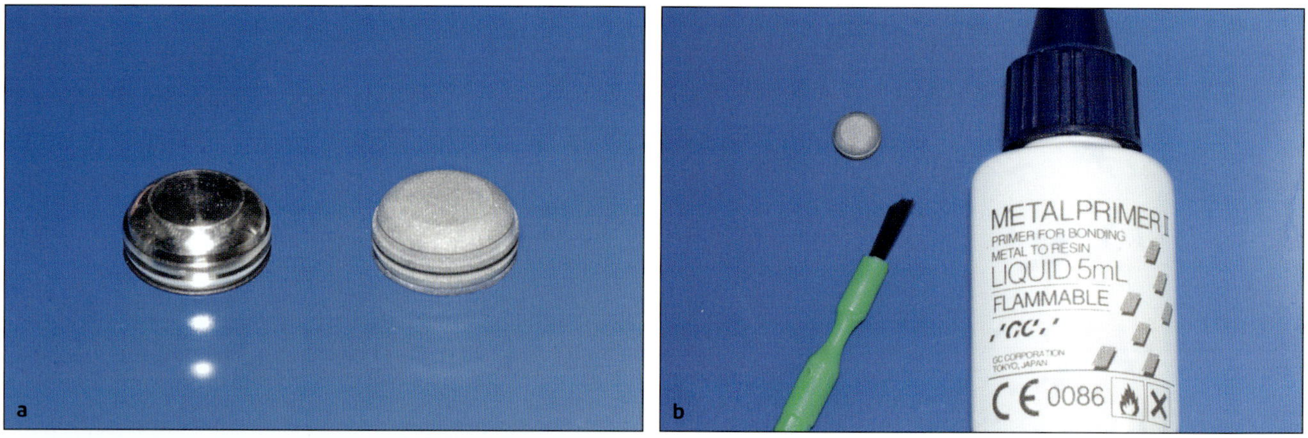

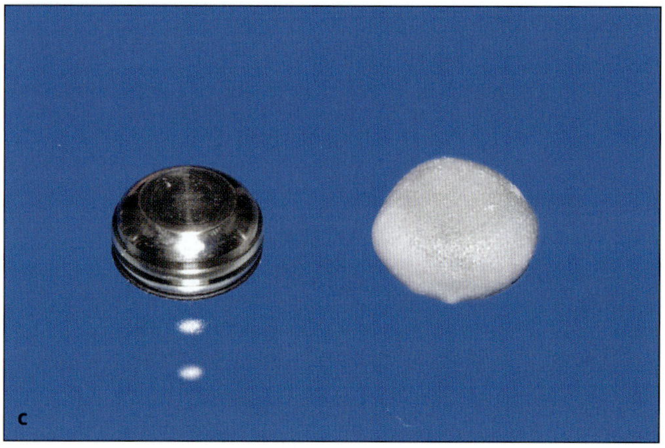

FIG 11-32 *(a)* A smooth, machined housing *(left)*. The sandblasted housing *(right)* will be more effectively retained. *(b)* A metal bonding agent is applied to the housing after sandblasting. *(c)* A layer of autopolymerizing resin is applied in the laboratory and cured in a pressure pot. This ensures an optimum metal-resin bond prior to pickup of the housing in the wet oral environment.

a processing ring that is replaced by a soft rubber ring before being placed in the patient's mouth. Because the ring is quite soft, it wears down quickly. Fortunately, it is easily replaced since the old ring can be picked out with an explorer or small tweezers and the new ring pushed into place with any small blunt-ended instrument. The patrix comes as a castable plastic pattern that can be attached as an extracoronal attachment or, in a slightly different form, as an overdenture stud. It is the most flexible of all the attachment systems and is therefore of greatest value in situations where tooth support is minimal.[9] This system has a special advantage over all the other current systems, especially when used as a "stop attachment" placed in the edentulous areas of a Class I, II, or IV partial denture. Here, the top of the ball of the metal patrix serves as a vertical stop that is independent of the retentive component. This is far superior to a system where the resilient component bears the load as a stop.

For the most part, the metal housings for the patrices of the ERA, Locator, and other resilient attachment systems will be attached to the framework of the RPD with resin, not soldered. These patrices can be related either in the mouth or on the cast. Laboratory preparation of the housings is made necessary by the fine retentive grooves and smooth machined surface on the external of the housing. This is inadequate for a maximum-strength metal-resin bond. Sandblasting (Fig 11-32a), use of a metal bonding agent (Fig 11-32b), and laboratory application of a thin layer of autopolymerizing resin (Fig 11-32c) are required as previously discussed. After connection, any bulk of the resin can be thinned appropriately to fit within the confines of the partial denture without damaging the interface. Autopolymerizing tooth-colored resin can also be used to reduce show-through of the metal housing for those situations in which space is limited and esthetic demands are great. All internal traces of resin must be removed, preferably under magnification, after the processing patrix is removed from the housing and before the retentive patrix is snapped into place.

The resilient attachment systems work best when their path of insertion/removal is restricted by the guiding planes prepared on the abutments and the well-fitting guide plates of the modern framework. When a restricted path of insertion exists, the patients cannot jam the attachment to place from a variety of directions. They are limited to the path dictated by the planes. They must be advised that if they wish to minimize the wear and replacement of the resilient elements, they must place the attachment partial denture with their fingers only, never biting it to place. When the resilient component is forced to function only along its intended axis, the wear is greatly reduced. The manufacturers often show these attachments as being the only connection between the partial denture and the abutment teeth, implying that they function as an adequate rest system in addition to providing retention. It is apparent that this approach ignores the modern principles of support and stability and should therefore not be copied.

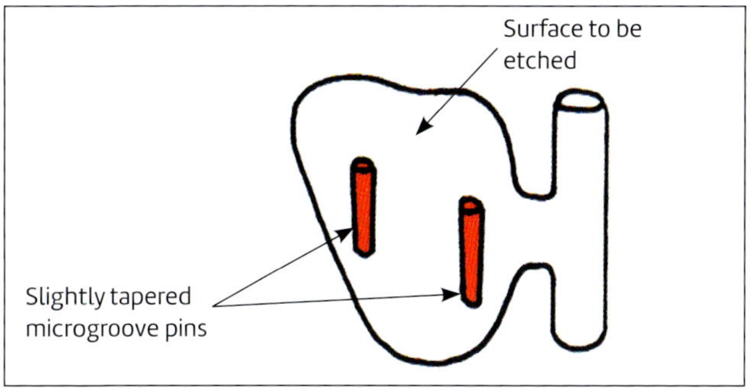

FIG 11-33 Internal view of resin-bonded pin attachment with microgrooves.

Attachment retention

It has been implied that all extracoronal attachments are cast as a part of abutment crowns. This is not strictly true, as a high level of success has been demonstrated with the use of resin-bonded extracoronal attachments. While it may not appear that an etched and bonded restoration would have sufficient retention to the tooth to resist the additional stress of an attachment, when microgroove preparation on the abutments is combined with careful patient selection, the bonded attachment is a successful and conservative means of obtaining the benefits of an attachment system (Fig 11-33). A review of articles by Taylor et al and Marinello et al will acquaint the reader with the parameters of this therapy.[10,11] In these cases especially, the attachments should only have retentive responsibilities. Support and stability must come from the other components as dictated clearly within this text. For example, additional abutments with positive rest preparations will reduce any load on the bonded attachment and should increase its length of service. All the extracoronal attachments discussed in this chapter are amenable to bonded restoration and have been used successfully over the years.

There are a variety of stud attachments that can be used for retention of the RPD, even though they are generally intended to be used in the overdenture. The stud attachments placed either in the endodontically prepared tooth, or onto an implant, create potential problems for the precision attachment partial denture since their angulation is limited by the long axis of either abutment. They are to be placed first and the remainder of the guiding plane/attachment surfaces aligned with their long axis. If their alignment causes the other components to be aligned beyond a rational limit, the use of the root or implant for retention should be redesigned and used as an occlusal stop only. When multiple teeth or implants pose this angulation problem, a bar is typically the means by which reangulation can occur.

A mastery of these few attachment systems will cover the needs of most prosthodontists as well as provide a basis for the understanding of those systems to come. While the actual attachments can be expected to change and improve with time, the techniques for their use are standard and must be a part of the technical background of clinician and technician alike. Fortunately for both clinician and technician, the manufacturers of attachments provide excellent instructional material, generally at no cost. Because systems are constantly being redesigned, the inclusion of great technical detail in any text is apt to be a waste of time. The precision attachment, in combination with the other aspects of advanced partial denture construction, offers us the possibility of making retentive, strong, and problem-free prostheses that are esthetically undetectable by the patient while also not interfering with their oral health.

References

1. Studer SP, Mader C, Stahel W, Scharer P. A retrospective study of combined fixed-removable reconstructions with their analysis of failures. J Oral Rehabil 1998;25:513–526.
2. Owall B, Jonsson L. Precision attachment-retained removable partial dentures. Part 3. General practitioner results up to 2 years. Int J Prosthodont 1998;11:574–579.
3. Goto Y, Brudvik JS. Custom precision attachment housings for removable partial dentures. J Prosthet Dent 2002;88:100–102.
4. Domagala D, Waliszewski MP. A maxillary laser-welded component removable partial denture—A clinical report. J Prosthet Dent 2009;101:1–6.
5. The Glossary of Prosthodontic Terms: Ninth Edition. J Prosthet Dent 2017;117(5S):e1–e105.
6. Chaiyabutr Y, Brudvik JS. Removable partial denture design using milled abutment surfaces and minimal soft tissue coverage for periodontally compromised teeth: A clinical report. J Prosthet Dent 2008;99:263–266.
7. Brudvik JS, Shor A. The milled surface as a precision attachment. Dent Clin North Am 2004;48:685–708.
8. Gamborena JI, Hazelton LR, NaBadalung D, Brudvik J. Retention of ERA direct overdenture attachments before and after fatigue loading. Int J Prosthodont 1997;10:123–130.
9. Chen IC, Brudvik JS, Mancl LA, Rubenstein JE, Chitswe K, Raigrodski AJ. Freedom of rotation of selected overdenture attachments: An in vitro study. J Prosthet Dent 2011;106:78–86.
10. Taylor TD, Gerrow JD, Brudvik JS. Resin-bonded components for maxillofacial prosthesis construction: A clinical trial. J Prosthet Dent 1988;59:334–339.
11. Marinello CP, Scharer P, Meyenberg K. Resin-bonded etched castings with extracoronal attachments for removable partial dentures. J Prosthet Dent 1991;66:52–55.

12 SPECIAL PROSTHESES

Nontraditional RPD designs are preferred in specific situations.

Several special design modifications for advanced RPDs are different enough to merit a special chapter. As has been noted, the variability of the partially edentulous environment creates unique situations. Standard RPD design philosophy cannot be expected to apply in all of these specific situations. It is here where the ingenuity of numerous dentists over time has resulted in specific methods to manage what would otherwise be significant compromises for traditional design. No other chapter better demonstrates how the RPD can be an effective solution where other treatments would be impractical or irrational.

Splinting with the RPD

The use of the RPD to support multiple teeth with mobility has long been questioned. Certainly, fixed prostheses offer a more dependable means of joining loose teeth into a single unit. There will be situations, however, when the RPD will be called upon to offer maximum support to the remaining teeth, either for financial reasons or because of the number and position of missing teeth in the arch. The best treatment for these situations is obviously some combination of fixed and removable prostheses where ideal contours (ie, guiding planes and rest preparations) can be created on all remaining teeth. Careful, well-planned mouth preparation of multiple teeth, coupled with ideal casting control, can offer excellent support to weakened dentitions and has been shown to actually reduce mobility over time.[1]

Perhaps the most effective means to achieve these results is by the use of a "strut" or continuous occlusal rest preparation as shown by Kratochvil.[2] Instead of a series of multiple regular occlusal rests, this continuous rest runs from tooth to tooth as a channel in the center of the occlusal surface of the remaining teeth and is joined to a proximal guide plate at either end of the segment of contacted teeth (Fig 12-1a). The channel needs to have a width of 3 mm and an absolute minimum depth of 1.25 mm in order to have adequate strength (Fig 12-1b).

The splinting effect comes from the rigid guide plates at the proximal ends of the continuous rest. Keep in mind that these are typically very tall posttreatment periodontally involved teeth. The additional available height of these teeth should result in extensive surface area on which to create the frictional contact that results in rigid lateral stability. The buccal and lingual sides of the intracoronal preparation must be slightly tapered with rounded internal angles to facilitate a complete seating of the RPD. These surfaces *must* draw with the prepared guiding plane surfaces and therefore must be reevaluated during the surveying of the check cast before final impressions. Any undercuts within the strut preparation must be removed. When an extension of this rest is placed on the last tooth in the arch, normally a second molar, the recommended minimum dimensions should guarantee rigid rest despite the cantilever from a more anterior tooth.

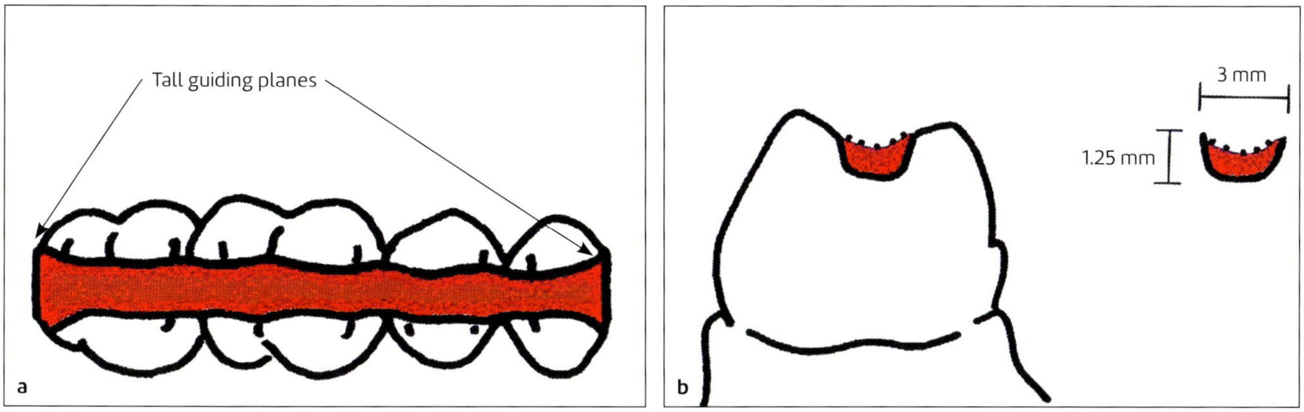

FIG 12-1 *(a)* Strut rest, occlusal view. *(b)* Strut rest in cross section.

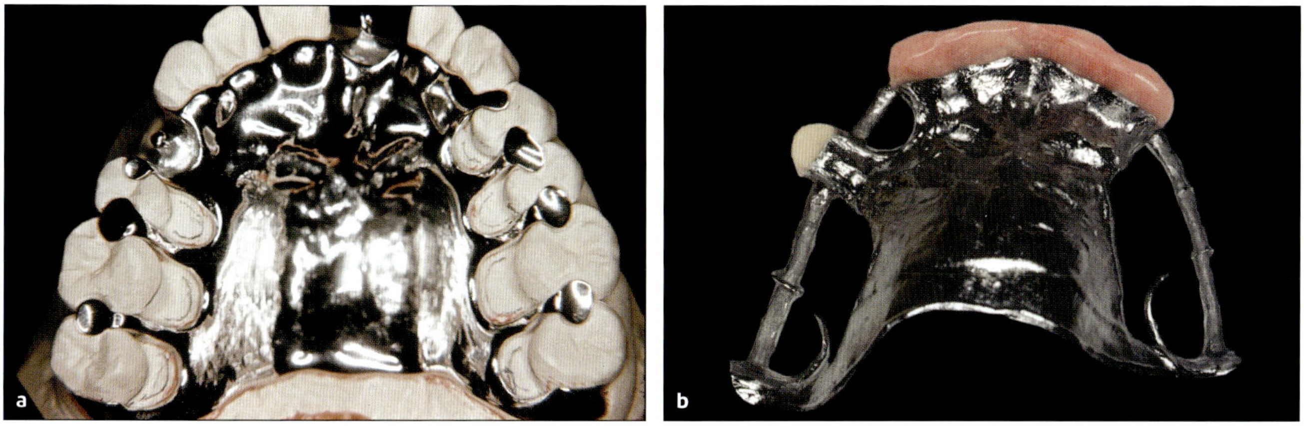

FIG 12-2 *(a)* Traditional rest designs are less effective and less hygienic for splinting. Note the number of minor connectors. *(b)* Strut rests more effectively and hygienically splint teeth together.[3] Note the absence of ancillary minor connectors.

Because the rest will be in occlusion with the opposing arch along its total length, some modification of the waxing technique is required to minimize the amount of occlusal adjustment on this very hard alloy. The laboratory can either articulate the refractory cast and wax directly to the opposing occlusion, or the rest can be waxed on an articulated definitive cast and transferred to the refractory during the final waxing of the partial denture. The advantage of the latter technique is that it allows the clinician to create the desired occlusion on the definitive cast rather than try to describe it to the technician. When waxing the occlusal strut to be transferred, a hard wax should be used to reduce distortion during removal from the lubricated cast and placement on the refractory. Modern milled waxes, being very tough and often acrylic-like, are very useful in this scenario. After finishing, the surface of this special rest should be sandblasted so that any eccentric interference to disclusion can be easily identified during the first few days of wear. After the adjustment period, the final polish can be easily restored with rubber points and a rag wheel with polishing compound.

When this special rest is properly constructed, it will stabilize loose teeth both in centric occlusion and in eccentric movements. With the partial denture fully seated and with ideal tooth-frame contact, the teeth cannot move independently from the partial denture. Specifically, each individual tooth will be supported vertically as well as laterally. This is accomplished without excess extracoronal components that would complicate peripheral hygiene efforts (Fig 12-2).[3] While this rest may not be "esthetic," it normally appears as a series of occlusal amalgams to the eye of the patient. Anterior teeth involved with this type of splinting require positive rests, either cingulum or incisal, to maintain the tooth-frame relationship during loading. Simply plating the lingual surfaces will not "splint" mobile teeth. The strut rest is therefore much more common for posterior teeth.

This type of framework is far more complex than the standard RPD, and misfits can be expected. The surface area of tooth-frame contact is greatly increased by the continuous rest form. When a misfit is encountered, cutting and laser welding the misfit components provides a relatively simple solution.[3] However, knowing the challenge, sectional construction is

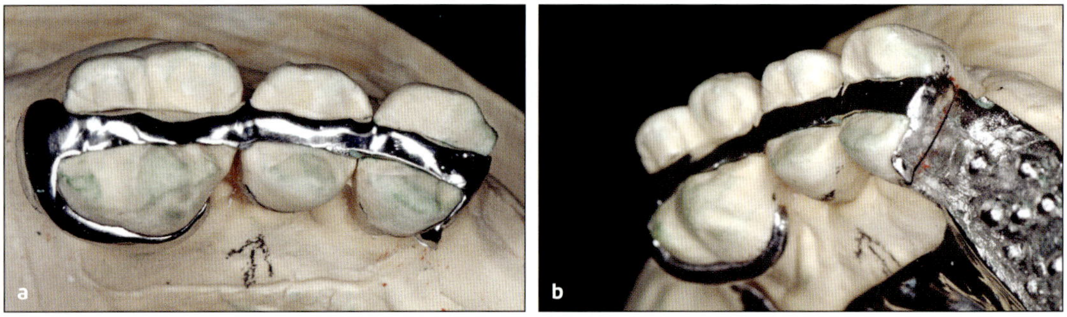

FIG 12-3 *(a)* This strut rest segment is ideally fit to the cast. Sectional construction is often preferred for these more complex castings.[3] *(b)* These components are closely related and ready for indexing. Minimizing the gap results in a strong weld.[3]

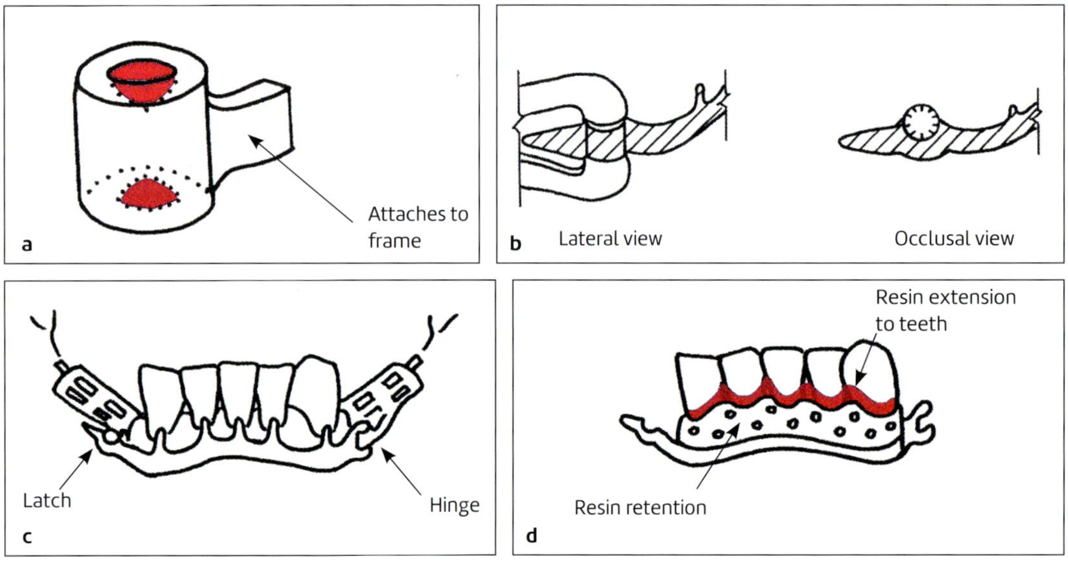

FIG 12-4 *(a)* Design of hinge. *(b)* Design of latch. *(c)* Frontal view of hinged major connector. The bar uses only pins in this design. *(d)* Frontal view of hinged major connector. In this design, the bar is made as a plate that can be veneered for improved esthetics.

indicated from the start. The strut rests and the occlusal portion of the anterior and posterior guide plates that connect the rest to the basic frame can be made as a second casting (Fig 12-3a). The basic frame is cast, finished, and fitted, and if acceptable, it is returned to the definitive cast to be "reduplicated" in refractory material so that the strut component is waxed and cast to the prepared contour of the basic frame with an overlap for the laser weld. As noted in chapter 6, this approach results in the strongest weld since there will be no need for a filler material (Fig 12-3b). When the parts are related together at the time of the resin pickup, either in the mouth or on the cast, there will be a positive metal-to-metal contact.

Hinged Major Connectors (Swinglock)

The hinged major connector is another special prosthesis that offers excellent splinting capabilities as well as a means of retention when normal tooth contours are not available for any reason. First introduced by Dr Joe Simmons in 1963, the "swinglock" design was, at that time, a patented technique for hinged major connectors.[4] A barrel-shaped hinge with retaining dimples is attached to the major connector with a minor connector that will, in most instances, exit from an edentulous area (Fig 12-4a). On the opposite side of the arch, a retaining latch of some sort extends in a similar fashion via a minor connector (Fig 12-4b). Connecting these two terminals is a bar with projections to the gingival enamel of the enclosed teeth that swings from the hinge and snaps into the latch. When the prosthesis is in the closed and latched position, all the enclosed teeth are locked together (Fig 12-4c). The bar of this partial denture can usually be placed in the vestibule, so it is seldom visible. Because the bar swings into its final position, it will normally be in a soft tissue undercut without damage to these tissues. The bar portion can take many forms, one of the popular options being a plate that runs from the vestibule to just incisal to the dentinoenamel junction. The outer surface of the plate has a gingival finishing line and micro bead retention for a thin resin veneer (Fig 12-4d). When the plate is opaqued and suitably custom stained, this gingival apron can blend in as natural gingiva (Fig 12-5).

The laboratory has two options for constructing the hinge/latch combination. The most common technique uses the patented components, hinge and latch, which are

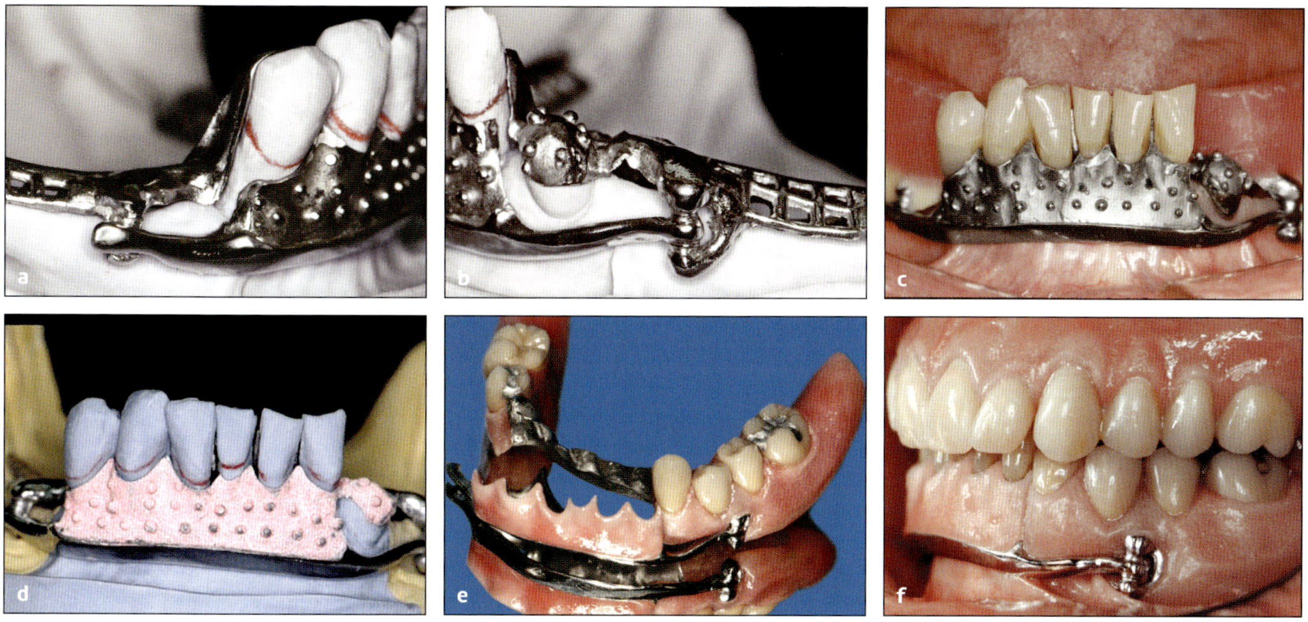

FIG 12-5 *(a)* Latch is on the patient's right. *(b)* Hinge is on the patient's left. *(c)* Labial plate design can improve strength, comfort, and esthetics. *(d)* Labial plate and bead retention are opaqued to hide the gray of the metal. Note that an altered cast impression was necessary. *(e)* Completed swinglock RPD. *(f)* The hinge is closed and latched on the patient's right side.

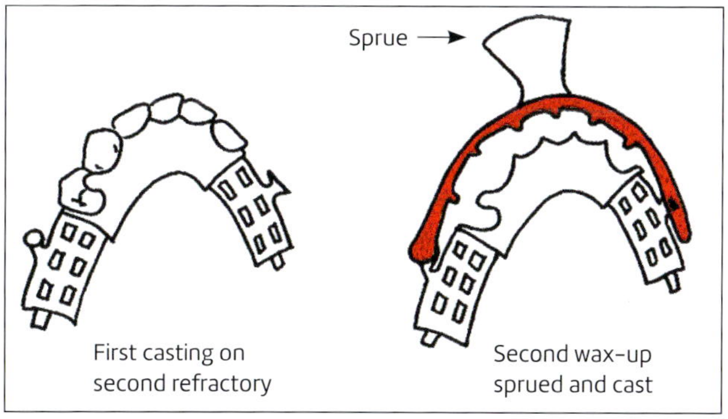

FIG 12-6 Double casting for hinged connector.

added to the wax-up of the partial denture and retained in the casting by means of retentive contours in the metal. A more sophisticated and potentially more precise approach involves two castings. The first casting contains the basic structures of the partial denture and the hinge and latch. After this section has been cast and finished, it is returned to the definitive cast and reduplicated; the casting remains in the duplicating agar, and the refractory material is poured against it. On this second refractory, the bar component is waxed to the hinge and latch (Fig 12-6). It is invested and cast to the first casting. A very precise hinge and latch results since the freedom of movement is created by the thickness of the oxide layer that forms on the first casting when it is placed in the furnace to burn out the second (bar segment) refractory. Using this technique, it is possible to make smaller and more precise joints than one can achieve with commercial components.

The swinglock concept was originally presented as a technique requiring no mouth preparation of any kind. Subsequent clinical usage has demonstrated that rest preparations are needed to ensure that the entire assembly does not slip gingivally on the teeth.[5] Because the hinged gate effectively holds all the teeth it touches in contact with the main casting, mesial migration of these teeth will not occur. A single, positive rest form of any type on each side of the casting will keep it from settling. The hinged prosthesis has the same requirements for the management of any distal extension base (especially on the mandible). Because these castings are far more complex than the standard partial denture framework, the clinician can expect to be charged a fee 75% to 100% higher than for a routine partial denture casting. This additional expense and the predictability of mandibular implant overdentures combine to minimize their frequency in actual practice.

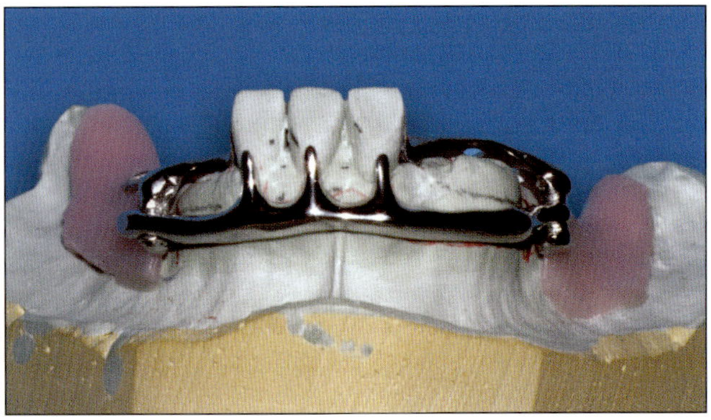

FIG 12-7 A common indication, lack of adequate abutments for a Kennedy Class I.

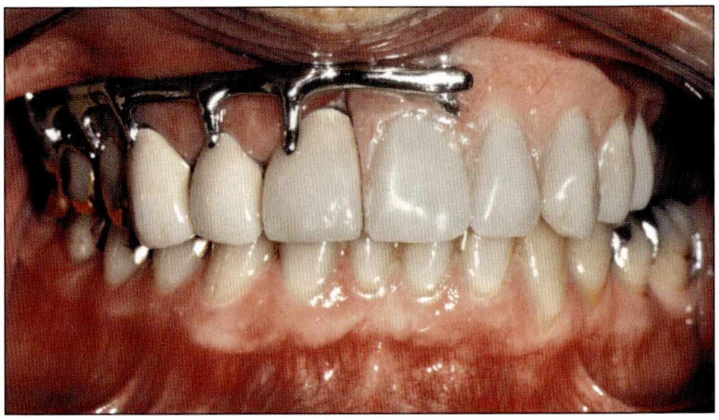

FIG 12-8 Unilateral maxillary situations require additional support.

The hinged appliance has two major indications. The most common use is in compromised mandibular situations where only a few anterior teeth remain (Fig 12-7). When one or both of the mandibular canines is missing, it is often next to impossible to obtain adequate retention by clasping a lateral incisor. In these situations, the remaining teeth are often compromised periodontally, which makes splinting them into one multirooted abutment advisable.[6] It is critical, however, to provide a positive rest seat on the terminal abutment on either side to eliminate the possibility of settling. The other, and less often indicated use, is for maxillary situations where the remaining teeth are all on the same side of the arch, often in a more or less straight line (Fig 12-8). These are the extreme Kennedy Class I or II situations mentioned in chapter 3. This situation is often found in maxillofacial patients where a maxillary tumor has caused the loss of half of the maxilla. The splinting effect of joining all the remaining teeth is often the only means of supporting and maintaining the prosthesis in these obturator situations.

Special problems exist for the hinged appliances that are not found in the routine partial denture situation.[7,8] There must be enough of a buccal vestibule remaining for the labial bar. When this space is minimal, the bar may have to be changed to a veneered plate in order to have sufficient strength (see Fig 12-5c). The labial bar is sometimes very objectionable to the patient because of the bulk in the lip. The only alternatives to the use of the hinged appliance for these compromised situations are either splinted, full-coverage restorations of all remaining teeth with attachments, the use of implants, or some combination of the two. Some patients, such as elderly patients or those compromised by arthritic changes in their hands, will have trouble opening and closing the lock mechanism and will require both training and patience to be able to utilize this design. Some of these patients benefit from a tool or "key" that helps open the gate.

Rotational Path of Insertion

The rotational path of insertion partial denture is a special prosthesis normally used in maxillary Class IV situations where anterior visible clasping is objectionable. This special design utilizes rigid projections into mesial proximal undercuts on the prime abutments (those adjacent to the anterior edentulous space) to retain the anterior part of the RPD (Fig 12-9a). Because these projections are not clasps, in that they do not flex, they must be placed into the undercuts by inserting the partial denture first in the anterior area and then rotating the posterior section of the casting to place. The rigid projections act as the rotational points, hence the name "rotational partial denture"[9] (Fig 12-9b). Because the posterior part of the casting must be rotated to place, any projections that might interfere with the rotation must be eliminated from the design. This usually implies that there be no modification spaces in the posterior segments and that the major connector be open from the rest in the anterior all the way to the minor connector for the posterior clasp (Fig 12-9c). If a modification space was present, then the additional properly utilized guiding plane surfaces would make anterior clasping unnecessary, and the rotational design would not be required.

The prime abutment teeth must have well-defined, positive rest preparations. Any movement of these teeth over time may result in loss of the retention of the RPD or its ability to completely seat onto the abutment teeth. This design provides anterior retention since the anterior segment cannot rotate down and out of the mouth when the partial denture is fully seated. While seated, the rigid projections remain in the anterior undercuts. The posterior part of the casting is held in place by embrasure clasps on either the first or second molar, bilaterally (Fig 12-10a). The positive rests on the prime abutments provide a solid stop against movement toward the tissue. The result is a retentive partial denture that replaces anterior teeth without visible clasps in the front of the mouth (Fig 12-10b).

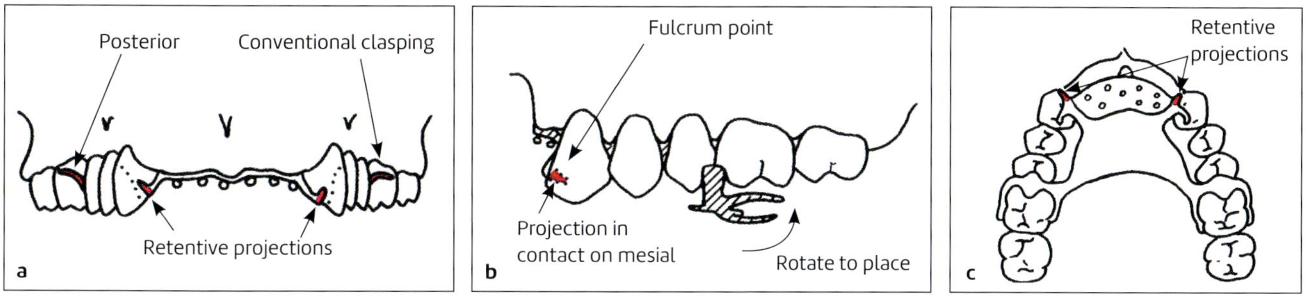

FIG 12-9 *(a)* Rotational path RPD casting fully seated. *(b)* Anterior component seated, before rotation. *(c)* Class IV rotational partial denture, occlusal view.

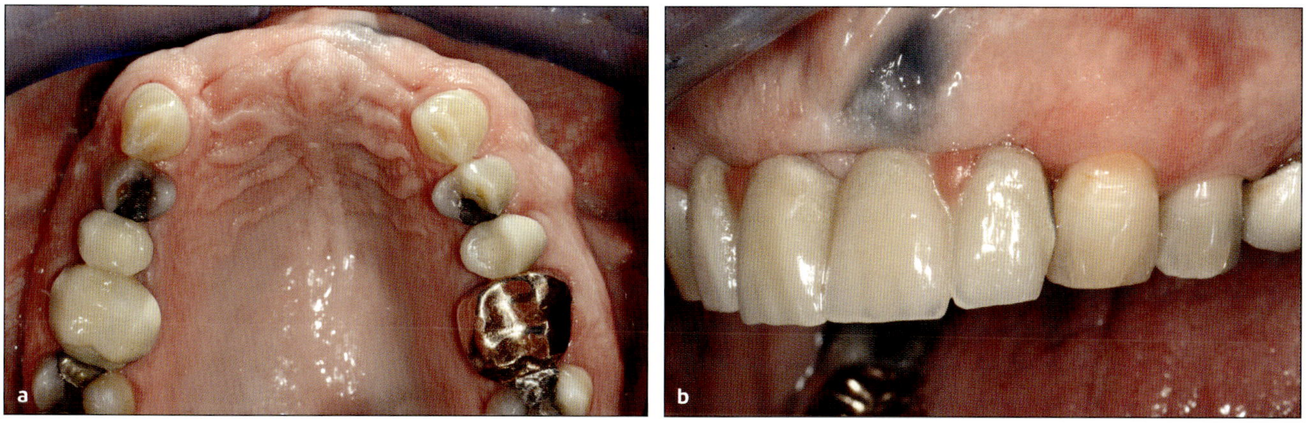

FIG 12-10 *(a)* Rotational path is indicated with a Class IV maxillary arch. Note the embrasure clasp preparations between the molars. *(b)* A lateral view of retentive projections into the mesial undercuts for this rotational path partial denture. Note that the flange was completely eliminated in this situation.

The projection into the proximal undercut can take the form of a clasp-like arm if the tooth involved is an anterior tooth, or a part of the minor connector if the prime abutment is a premolar (Fig 12-11). Very special care must be taken in the laboratory to ensure that this projection is in no way altered, either in the blockout (of which there should be none under the projection), or in the electrolytic stripping and finishing of the metal. This projection must contact the tooth in order for the retention of the anterior segment to be acceptable; therefore, the casting must be fitted first to the mouth and then placed on the cast without regard to possibly scraping the cast. The clinician can expect to find interferences to the rotation of the casting. These must be identified and adjusted intraorally using some form of disclosing material. This is one instance where adjustments of interferences may best be made on the teeth themselves rather than on the casting. For example, lingual heights of contour of nonabutment teeth that are interfering with the rotation of the major connector can be adjusted instead of altering the major connector itself. Care must be taken when adjusting the rigid projections since, as opposed to a clasp, they will be too short and rigid to bring into tooth contact by bending with pliers.

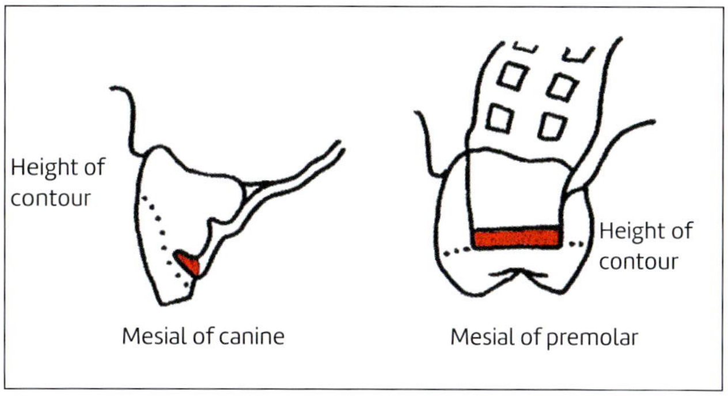

FIG 12-11 Rotational elements, no blockout.

Because the anterior segment must be rotated into place, the anterior flange can only extend to the height of contour of the edentulous ridge and must be tapered to a very thin margin to avoid creating a ledge that will accumulate food (Fig 12-12). When a major anterior ridge defect exists, for example with a cleft lip and palate, there may be no anterior undercut whatsoever (Fig 12-13). In these situations, the flange is fully extended to provide lip support, and the resin retention of choice is likely raised retentive mesh. As

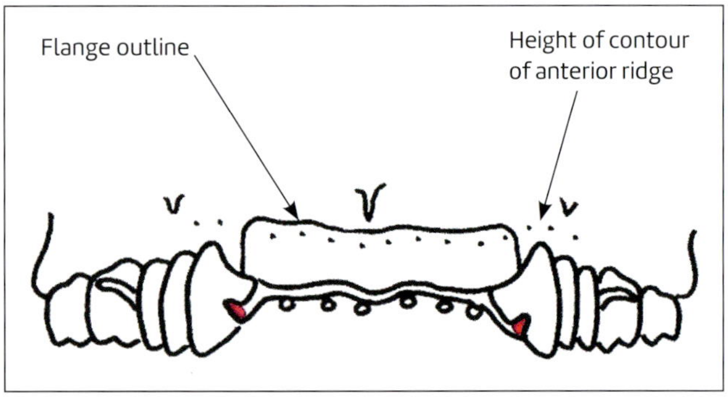

FIG 12-12 Flange extension for Class IV rotational partial denture showing height of contour limitation.

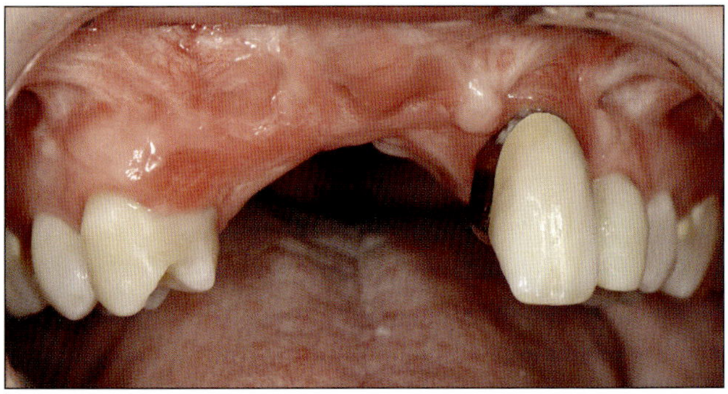

FIG 12-13 Cleft lip and palate situations often lend themselves to the rotational design.

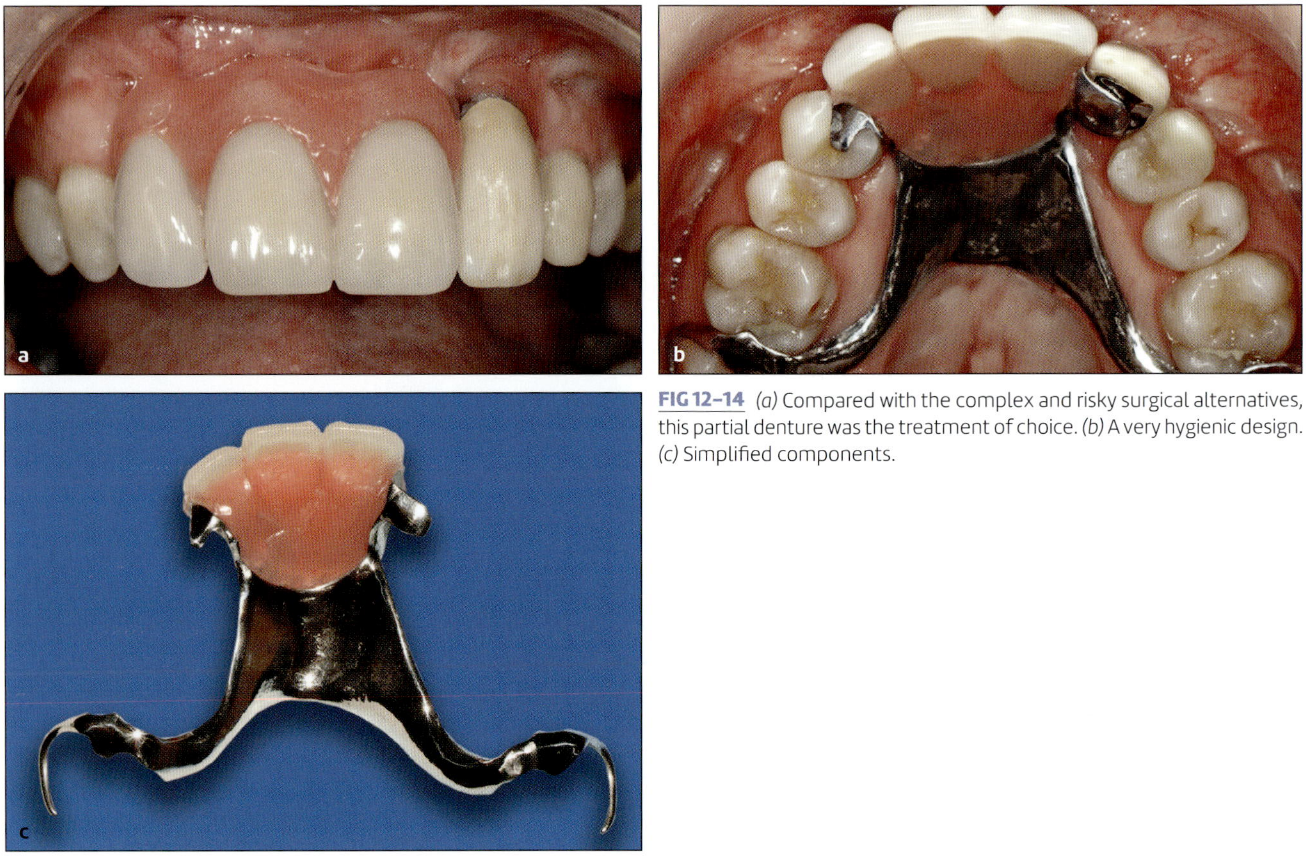

FIG 12-14 *(a)* Compared with the complex and risky surgical alternatives, this partial denture was the treatment of choice. *(b)* A very hygienic design. *(c)* Simplified components.

previously noted, a large soft tissue defect can be expected to eventually need a reline. In mature ridges without loss of contour, the metal base with suitable retentive devices for the denture teeth is preferred.

Custom staining of the flange is especially important in these cases as it complements the effect of the hidden "clasp." When skillfully done, the clinical results are often more esthetically pleasing than the complex and risky surgical reconstructions that such large defects require (Fig 12-14a). With the limited numbers of components and ability to remove the prosthesis, the soft tissue response and patient comfort tend to be very good as well (Figs 12-14b and 12-14c). Depending on where the metal of the casting ends on the facial gingiva, the casting may need to be opaque to ensure accurate tinting of the denture base. Because the resin in the labial flange will almost always be on the thin side, some experimentation with the tinting will be required. There will not be the normal depth of denture base resin to back up the tints, and as a result, the colors will not appear as one would expect from the tinting of a standard denture base.

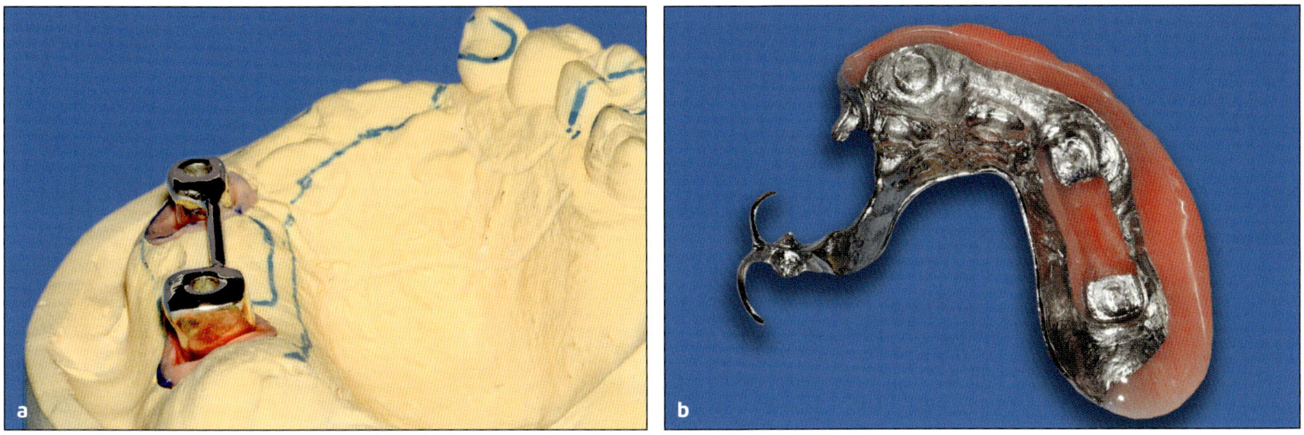

FIG 12-15 *(a)* An implant bar designed with buccal undercuts and proximal guiding planes to manage an extreme Class II arch. *(b)* Using a lateral rotational path, this partial denture engages the buccal undercuts shown in part *a* and is retentive without a clip.

It is also possible to reverse the rotation direction by placing the rotation points in the posterior area of the mouth. This design has been advocated in the literature for Class III mandibular partial dentures where the posterior abutments have tipped mesially, leaving large proximal undercuts. Rigid, cast metal is extended into these mesial undercut areas, and the partial denture is rotated to place on that axis. No guiding plane is possible on the distal aspect of the anterior abutments, so retentive clasping is required on these teeth. There is no disadvantage, either functional or esthetic, to posterior clasping, so there appears to be few situations where this design is preferred.

There are also rare instances where a lateral rotational path can be beneficial. Again, the idea is that clasp assemblies can be eliminated in favor of rotational elements locking into undercuts. Conventional guiding plane support and retention requires abutment teeth to be reasonably vertical. Debilitated partially edentulous malocclusions can present with otherwise healthy teeth that are significantly canted or tipped. If orthodontics and additive modifications are not feasible, it is possible to utilize a rotational design to manage these flared teeth. This would be specifically for a sizeable Class III situation with no modification spaces on the contralateral side. A pair of tipped abutments can be maintained and preserved from overreduction by rotationally engaging the lateral portion of the undercut created by the flaring of the teeth. An embrasure clasp then engages on the contralateral side. In this scenario, a cingulum rest is often not possible and instead must be replaced by an incisal rest due to the rotational positioning. Other lateral rotational path uses include unilateral implant-assisted partial dentures (Fig 12-15) and interim acrylic partial dentures that use a tissue undercut.

The patient will often require some extra time and instruction in the placement and removal of the rotational path RPD. While some loss of retention over time can be expected, the amount of actual wear from the friction of rotation is really minimal so that the partial denture should be serviceable for a normal period of time.

Overlays and Onlays

As noted in chapter 2, in the world of RPDs, an overlay is really nothing more than a large and very effective occlusal rest. In all instances, they serve as definite and reliable vertical support. They are indicated when the structural condition or positional relationship of an individual abutment tooth is poor.[10] Structurally compromised teeth can be overlaid to maintain their value as vertical support and to eliminate the high-risk lateral forces that tend to lead to coronal fracture. Teeth that have tipped out of the plane of occlusion yet are otherwise healthy can be "leveled" simply by creating an onlay rest for the occlusal surface. Both of these scenarios eliminate the need for and risks of extensive restorative dentistry, namely surveyed crowns.

When treatment planning, it is common to encounter root canal–treated and structurally compromised teeth (Fig 12-16a). Expending significant resources on rehabilitating these teeth with sophisticated cores and surveyed crowns is typically required but rarely indicated. These abutment teeth tend to fail due to functional overload and are often better maintained as overpartial abutments. Benefits include reducing the risks of tooth fracture, improving the crown-to-root ratio of the abutment, reducing additional treatment costs, simplifying the design, and of course maintaining vertical support from a tooth that would otherwise be extracted (Fig 12-16b). This is of particular importance when done

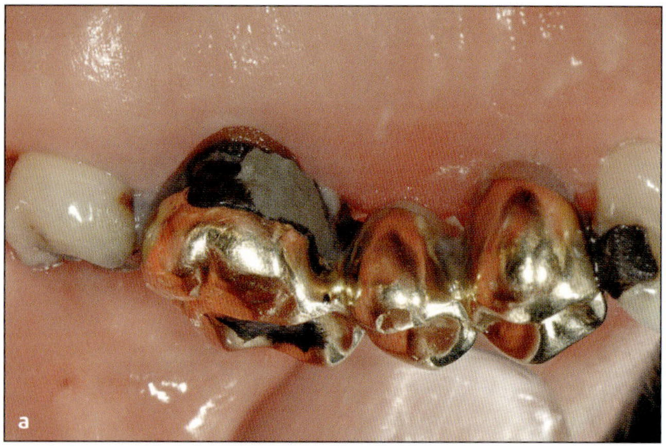
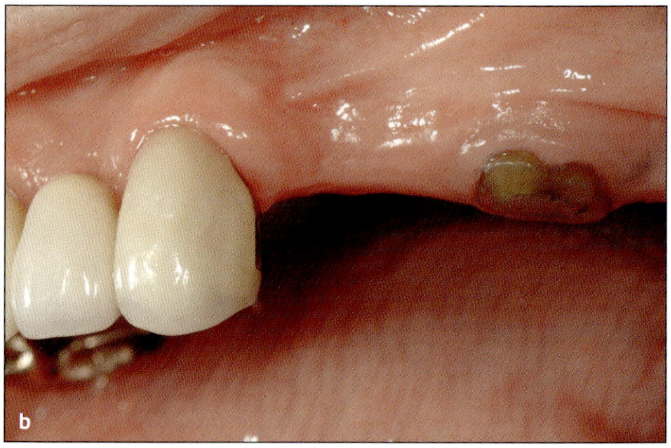
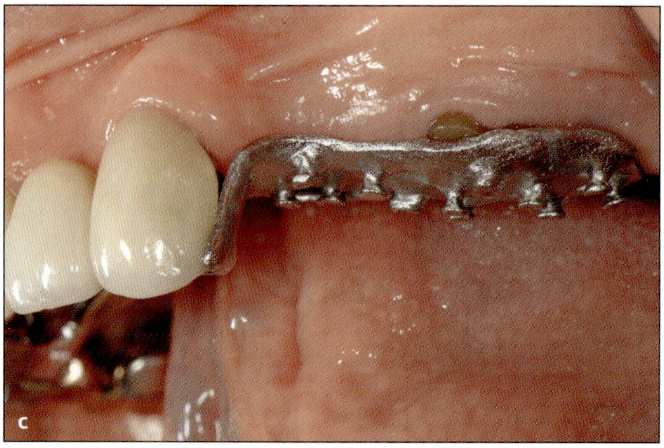

FIG 12-16 *(a)* Lingual view of a typical debilitated maxillary left first molar that previously received root canal therapy but has limited remaining tooth structure to support a surveyed crown. *(b)* The same first molar after it has been reduced and sealed with amalgam. *(c)* By overlaying the first molar, a distal extension is avoided.

to maintain distal abutment support since it reduces the complications common to distal extensions (Fig 12-16c).

Disadvantages of the overdenture concept are primarily related to the increased caries risk associated with the anaerobic environment that is created. Fortunately, if the patient's overall caries risk has been managed as discussed in chapter 1, good results can be achieved with daily topical fluoride application. This is best done by having the patient apply a drop of fluoride gel to the overlay prior to seating it after their morning oral hygiene routine. It must be noted that if overpartial abutments do need to be removed in the future for any reason, it generally does not appreciably alter the design of the partial denture. This is in contrast to needing to redesign a partial denture after the loss of a surveyed crown that accepted a clasp assembly. With this in mind, what may be considered a hopeless tooth as far as crown and bridge dentistry is concerned may in fact be valuable as vertical support for an RPD even though it may serve as such for only a few years.

To maintain a root as an overdenture abutment, the remaining coronal portion of the tooth is cut away (Fig 12-17a). Prior to completing the coronectomy, a rubber dam is applied, and the root canal space is obturated to a subgingival depth of at least 4 mm with glass ionomer or amalgam. This is to maintain a dentinal seal and leave room for future adjustment or attrition over time. The coronal "cap" is generally left 1 to 2 mm supragingival and in the shape of a dome. This is to maintain gingival health and to make it easy to fit the framework over the root (Fig 12-17b). This dome will allow the partial denture to be designed to rest on top of the retained root without the difficulty of replicating sharp line-angles. The portion of the partial denture that overlays this root should be in metal, not in mesh, to maximize hygiene and vertical space (Fig 12-18). Once overlaid, the buccal flange is typically minimized or eliminated as the ridge contour has been maintained along with the root. Strategically, it does not make sense to overlay a single premolar when the adjacent teeth are present. Overlays are generally done for strategic maintenance of support and therefore tend to be within larger edentulous spans. However, there are rare situations where an entire arch is overlaid. These situations tend to be extreme open occlusions or worn dentitions where a conventional fixed reconstruction is not indicated or feasible[11,12] (see case study in this chapter).

The need for an overlay to correct occlusal plane issues is most often found when there is an isolated mandibular

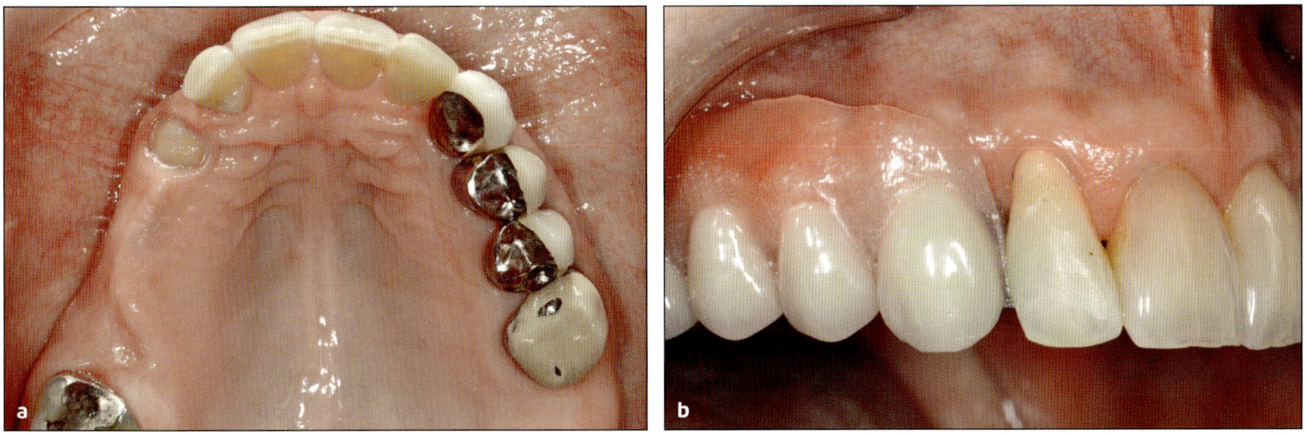

FIG 12-17 *(a)* A failed maxillary right canine is maintained to lend support to the weak lateral incisor in a Class V arch. *(b)* Overlaid canine. Note the guiding plane contact on the lateral incisor and the short flange.

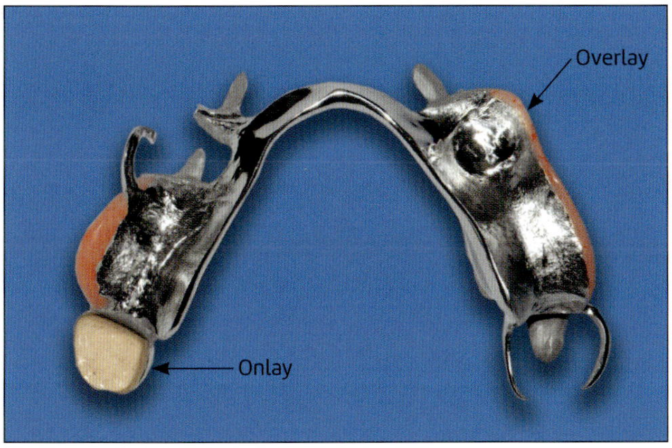

FIG 12-18 Overlaid weak mandibular left first premolar with short flange and metal base. The right second molar also has an onlay.

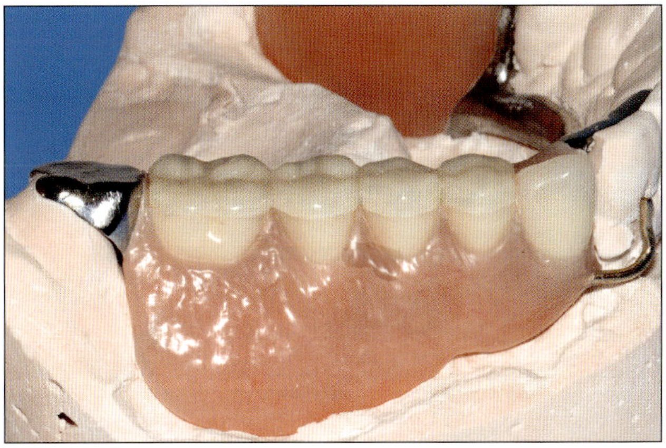

FIG 12-19 An onlay is used to restore the occlusal plane and ensure vertical support.

molar (second or third) with an opposing complete denture. The isolated molar has likely tilted mesial and lingual to the point where the mesial is below the desired plane of occlusion. This leaves the tooth unable to provide occlusal stability for the opposing arch (Fig 12-19). In some instances, such as with a mesially tipped mandibular third molar, one need only overlay that portion of the tooth that is outside the plane of occlusion. This technique can also serve as a means to judiciously "shoe" smaller or weakened cusps that would otherwise be at risk of fracture with normally recommended occlusal rest preparations.

Overlays used to correct occlusal issues are simply onlays that are a component of the RPD. The design of the "onlay prep" modification must not be as detailed as with cemented restorations. Instead, a generally flat surface with rounded line-angles and a smooth transition into the guiding plane surface are the key goals beyond the already discussed abutment modification principles. When fabricating the RPD itself, there are two ways of managing this situation; the time-honored one is to wax the onlay on the articulated and lubricated definitive cast and then transfer the wax pattern onto the refractory. There it is joined with wax to the waxed frame rather than attempting to articulate the refractory.

The second technique involves sectional construction. Here the onlay is made as a separate casting, perhaps of a different alloy (gold in some form), and then laser welded to the completed framework. The onlay should contact whatever guiding plane can safely be prepared. This guide plate minor connector will be extended to form a tang that fits into a recess in the resin retentive metal of the edentulous area (see Fig 6-29). A retentive bead or two, when placed on the external of the plate, will provide additional resin retention above the weld. A gold onlay, while more costly,

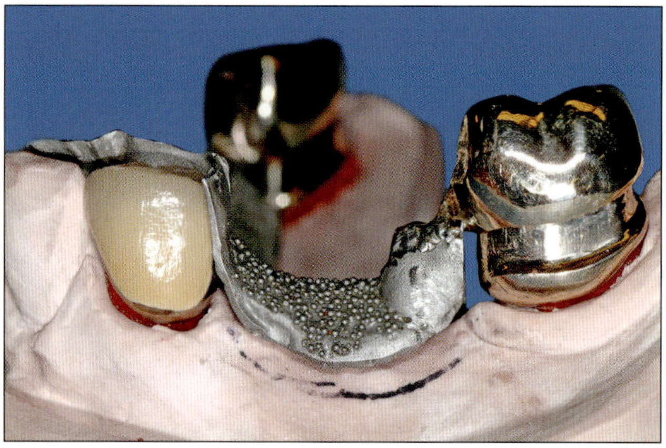

FIG 12-20 A coping on the mandibular left second molar supports an overcrown attached to the framework.

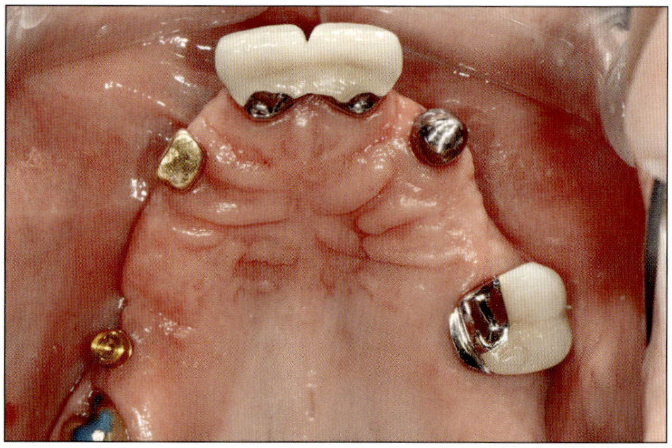

FIG 12-21 Copings on the implant at the maxillary right canine site and the natural left canine allow the necessary reangulation. Note the overlay on the right second molar and residual implant at the right first molar site used for retention. (See Fig 12-29 for the RPD.)

will be much easier to adjust and polish when compared to a stellate alloy. As discussed in chapter 6, sectional construction eliminates the distortion inherent in full-arch castings. The intraoral pickup and laser weld results in the best possible fit of the partial denture.

Copings

Copings are discussed here as they are a natural progression of overdenture designs and can be a prosthesis philosophy in and of themselves. They are the most basic precision attachment system. A thin-walled coping cemented in place on the abutment tooth permits an overcoping or crown, attached to the RPD, to fit over it (Fig 12-20). This overcoping is therefore part of the RPD framework. As with any overlay, a coping will, in every instance, act as a vertical stop for the partial denture. In most cases, it can also provide frictional retention. This allows a coping to be very effective when used in combination with other attachment systems that provide direct retention or with conventional clasping in other areas of the mouth (Fig 12-21). Perhaps the most significant additional benefit of a coping design over conventional mouth preparations is the ability to provide excellent lateral stability. They have been used for many years for extensive splinted fixed restorations, commonly referred to as *perio-prostheses*, with great success. Some attributed this to the fact that the entire superstructure could be removed by the patient for total hygiene access. Moreover, should a coping abutment be lost for any reason, the tooth can be removed and that area of the framework filled with resin to become a pontic. In many cases, these large restorations could be used even after the loss of multiple abutments. Great success in using this approach for complete overdentures has also been well documented in the literature.

These copings are usually milled to the planned path of insertion/removal or with a slight taper, around 2 to 5 degrees. The taller the height of the coping, the greater the tendency to taper it. The height of the coping varies with the crown-to-root ratio and the integrity of the remaining tooth structure. When very little tooth structure remains, a short dome-shaped coping can be made to maintain the structural integrity of the maintained root. While mechanically holding the root together with a ferrule, copings also protect the exposed tooth structure of the root from erosion and/or attrition. This type of coping is designed the same as an overlay since they will not accept lateral forces that are detrimental to the structurally weak teeth they cover.

Any posterior tooth or root can be considered for a coping restoration. Often, one root of an otherwise periodontally involved molar will have sufficient bone remaining to justify its retention in the mouth. When this root is maintained, an effective tooth-borne partial denture can be constructed in a situation that would otherwise result in a distal extension base. The decision to utilize a coping instead of a simple overlay is predicated on the tooth in question being structurally adequate for use in crown-and-bridge dentistry. The same structural parameters that determine whether a tooth can serve as a bridge abutment are considered. If the tooth is not deemed worthy, it is either overlaid or considered ancillary to the overall design.

In today's world of digital and implant-focused dentistry, teeth that can still be used in this manner are often

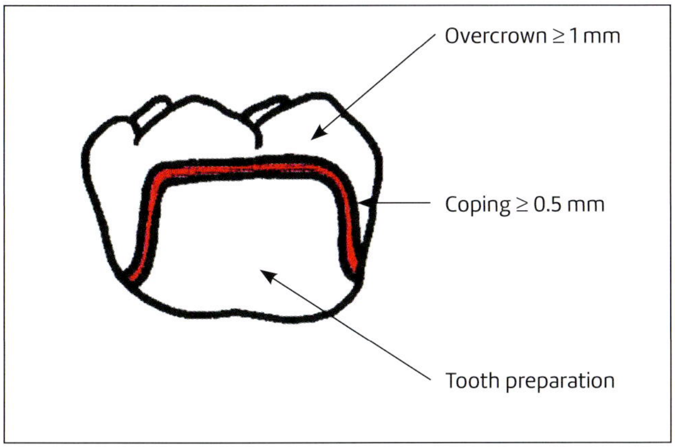

FIG 12-22 Vital tooth coping with minimal overcrown (thickness).

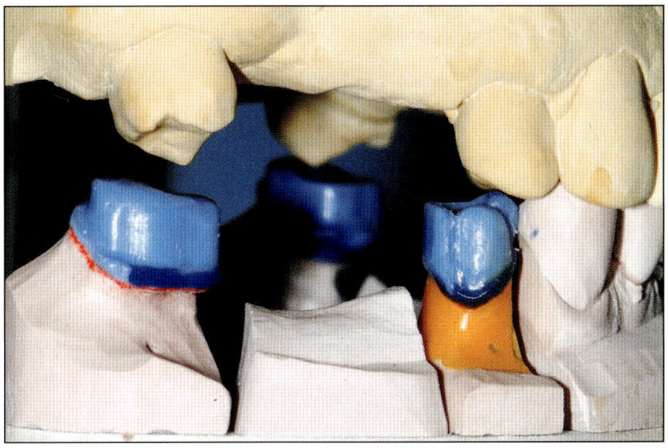

FIG 12-23 Extensive interocclusal space lends itself to a coping with an overcrown.

extracted. Few clinicians spend the time to properly disinfect and reconstruct debilitated teeth. This is an invaluable skill for creating advanced RPDs, as the ability to rehabilitate critical teeth is often all that stands between the patient being happy with a Class III partial denture as opposed to a complete denture. A critical element in the restoration of badly broken-down teeth for copings is the need to obtain a minimum 2-mm ferrule on solid tooth structure. More is obviously better, and the ferrule that does exist should be nearly parallel to provide maximum resistance form. When endodontically treated teeth are used, this ferrule will reduce the possibility of root fracture. In many instances, it will be necessary to perform crown-lengthening procedures to gain sufficient tooth structure supragingivally since the coping margin should be placed at the gingival margin. Again, this level of investment is often an indication to use the tooth as an overlay as opposed to a coping.

Space is one of the primary contraindications to fabricating copings. Vital coping abutments may be challenged to allow sufficient occlusal reduction without pulpal consequences. Significant space is required to allow both the coping and the overcrown to have sufficient thickness to withstand occlusal wear. At least 1.5 mm must be available, with the coping needing 0.5 mm and the crown taking up the remaining space (Fig 12-22). For this reason, the occlusal surface of the crown should be in metal since porcelain would require at least 2.5 mm reduction. The need for a facial veneer in the overcrown is a more common requirement. Slightly less than the 2.5 mm space can be used, and it will still hold shade and contour. Nonvital abutments are obviously more adaptable to the use of a ceramic overcrown. Because of these space requirements, situations where there is excessive interocclusal space are well suited to a coping design (Fig 12-23).

The construction of a milled coping starts with a diagnostic wax-up and trial arrangement that will include the opposing arch, be it a complete denture or a partially edentulous restoration. The design of the partial denture is determined and drawn on the diagnostic cast with indications for subtractive mouth preparation. The stone teeth that represent the abutments are prepared for either additive or subtractive mouth preparation to a chosen path of insertion/removal, and the vital abutments that will be used for copings are prepared to the appropriate dimensions and angulations. This diagnostic cast becomes the blueprint for the actual mouth preparation. Endodontically treated abutment teeth usually do not require the same level of diagnostic preparation since there is much more freedom in creating the desired milled contours. After the cast is used as a guide for mouth preparation, it can be used as a prescription for additive mouth preparation to the technician. The stone coping teeth are prepared, waxed, and milled on a surveyor using a blade attached to the vertical arm of the surveyor. The diagnostic cast will then represent all the desired contours in such a way as to ensure that the technician will be able to reproduce them in the final restorations.

The actual preparation of the coping abutments occurs only after all the subtractive mouth preparation has been completed. In this way, the prepared guiding planes can serve as vertical indicators of the final path of insertion/removal during the preparation of the abutments that will receive copings.

The definitive impression must involve all the teeth in the arch as well as all edentulous landmarks that will be

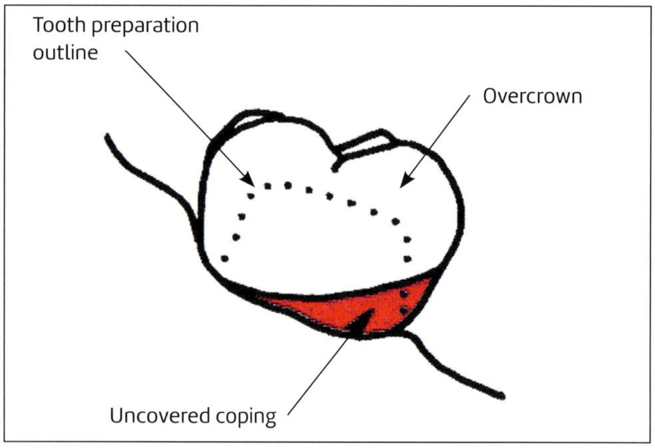

FIG 12-24 Overcrown margin options. Note the reangulation of the tipped molar.

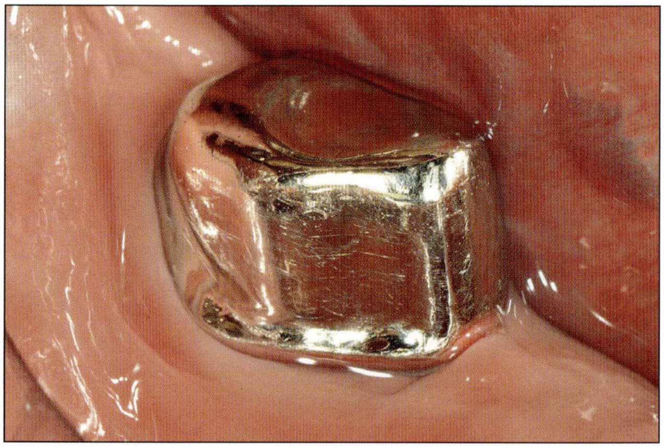

FIG 12-25 Coping with margin placed just above the gingiva.

required for the construction of the final partial denture framework, even though the casting will never be made from this cast. Once the dies have been trimmed and the casts articulated, the copings can be rough waxed by first dipping the prepared dies in molten wax to establish a thickness of at least 1 mm and then milled to the desired taper using the dental surveyor or with wax burs in the parallel milling machine that must be available in the dental laboratory chosen to support the treatment (see Figs 4-24 and 4-25). Copings can also be formed from thin vacuum-formed plastic sheets that are cut short of the margins to allow for full margination using wax. The use of the resin coping results in a more uniform coping thickness.

When the milling is complete, the waxed copings are marginated to allow for a coping margin of at least 1 mm. The placement of this margin will determine the margin of the overcrown. Because of the angulation of an isolated tooth relative to the path of insertion/removal that the partial denture must take, it may not be possible to mill all sides of the coping to that path for the full length of the coping. In these situations, the margin of the overcrown or overcoping will rise or fall according to the milled surface (Fig 12-24). This ability allows all but the most severely tipped teeth to be utilized as a coping abutment. The more surfaces that can be paralleled, however, the more the frictional retention of the partial denture can be increased.

The coping is then invested and cast in a type IV gold to reduce long-term wear (Fig 12-25). After finishing, it is returned to the definitive cast. The coping should never be thinner than 0.5 mm in any portion. The copings can now be milled to bring them to ideal contour and parallelism. Great care must be taken in thin areas, obviously, but this should not be a problem in the hands of an experienced technician. The metal is best left in a sandblasted or matte surface finish since there is no advantage to a high polish, except at the margin with the tooth.

The decision between an overcoping that will have no occlusal anatomy and an overcrown with normal occlusal contours is based on the position of the tooth in the arch and the available interarch space. In general, overcopings are used if occlusal contact with the opposing arch is not essential, such as with an unopposed mandibular third molar. When a controlled occlusal contact form is needed, then the overcrown is indicated. The overcrown is then waxed, cast, finished, and veneered if indicated. Both the coping and the overcrown are returned to the mouth so the final impression for the partial denture casting can be made. This impression must pick up the overcasting(s) as it would any surveyed crown, since they must all appear on the definitive cast. In certain situations, such as with sectional construction, it may be more reliable to do the pickup impression of the copings prior to fabrication of the overcrown. This typically allows more precise control of the occlusal form and contact, but more importantly, it allows for ideal designing of the joint between the overcasting and partial denture framework. When the copings are being picked up, it is often helpful to leave the sprue or a cast extension attached (Fig 12-26). This extension will ensure a more stable pickup of typically small smooth copings that are devoid of undercuts.

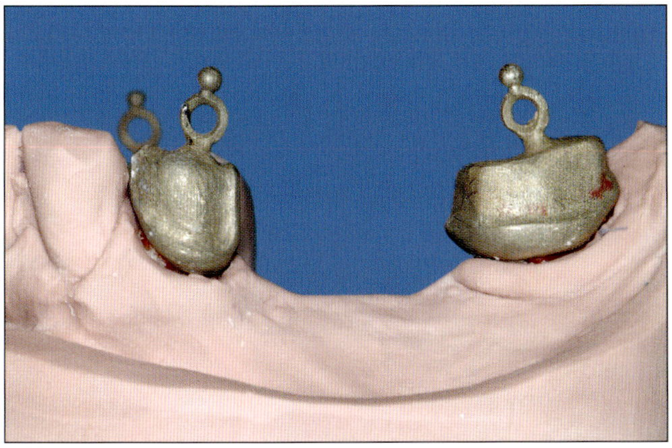

FIG 12-26 Extensions that stabilized the copings during the pickup impression will now be cut off since the pickup cast is set.

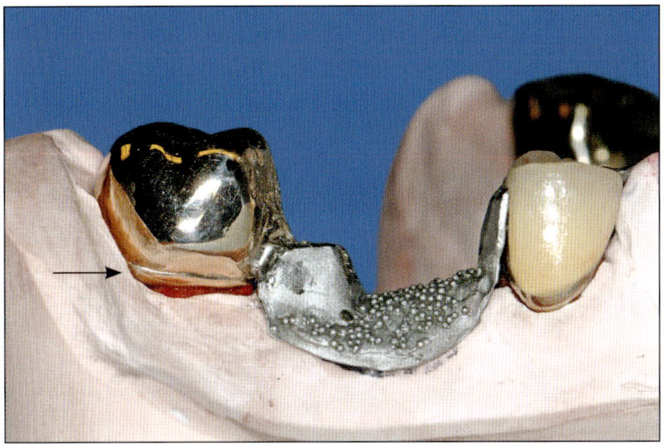

FIG 12-27 Overcrown laser welded to partial denture framework with fit confirmed on the pickup cast.

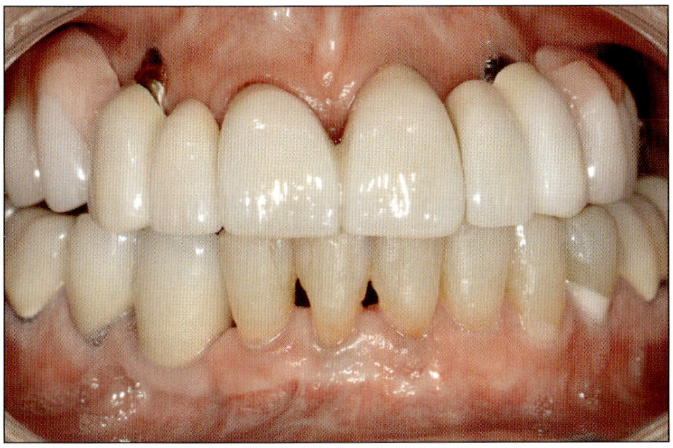

FIG 12-28 Porcelain-fused-to-metal overcrowns for the maxillary canines allow better shade matching and reangulation.

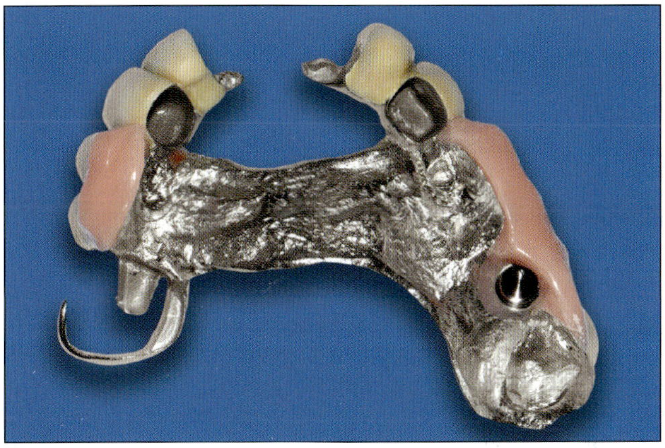

FIG 12-29 Sectionally constructed laser-welded coping partial denture. (See Fig 12-21 for the associated clinical image.)

The coping attachment, whether an overcoping or overcrown, will be laser welded to the framework in most situations (Fig 12-27). It is possible to attach retentive loops or beads to the overcoping and retain that unit in the resin base, but the need for this approach is limited to retrofitting situations. While these coping-crown situations are most often found in the posterior part of the mouth where a display of metal is acceptable, they can certainly be veneered if they are used in an esthetic area. In these instances, the use of a high noble or noble metal alloy will allow porcelain veneering for optimum shade matching and wear resistance (Figs 12-28 and 12-29). The difference in alloy composition will not appreciably interfere with laser welding the components together. Therefore, one need not rely on composite or acrylic veneering with its relatively quick deterioration and staining.

These special RPD designs provide options to maximize support and stability in situations that often present with poor prognoses. This ability to stabilize teeth, specifically where periodontal destruction has taken place, positions RPD therapy among the most cost-effective and adaptable prosthodontic treatments available. It is hoped that these special designs are not forgotten, as their effectiveness in disease-controlled situations has been clearly demonstrated.[13]

CASE STUDY:
Managing an unusual malocclusion

The ability of RPDs to conservatively manage unique partially edentulous situations is unmatched. In this example, a partially edentulous elderly patient with a malocclusion present since her youth was left with few reasonable options. Had her problems been more aggressively managed at a younger age, it is likely the situation would not be as complex. The surgical procedures needed to correct these types of malocclusions and simultaneously replace missing teeth are costly and risky. The overlay RPD selected here, despite still requiring localized surgical mouth modification, was far more appropriate than the alternatives. Here we demonstrate how this type of prosthesis cosmetically replaced her missing anterior teeth, stabilized the remaining abutments, modified her severe malocclusion, and did so in an economical way.

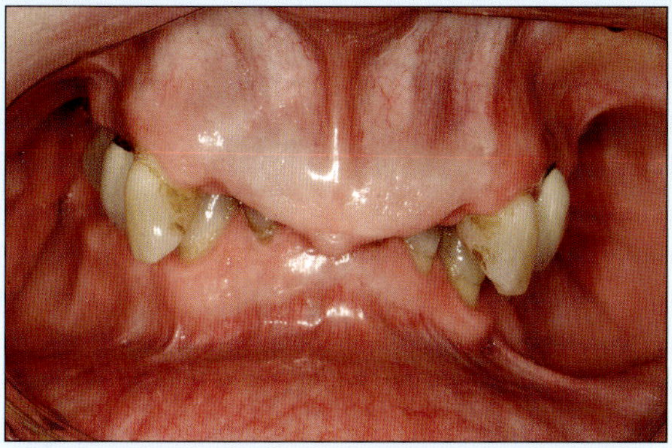

FIG 1 A 78-year-old woman recently had both maxillary lateral incisors removed. The coronal portion of both abutments fractured off along with the four-unit fixed partial denture they were supporting. While this patient presented with a low disease risk, she was a high functional risk due to limited abutments and a severe skeletal Class II malocclusion.

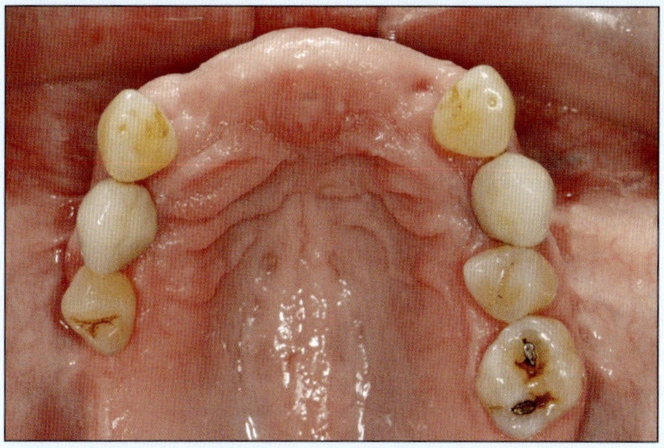

FIG 2 Over the decades, this patient adapted to her unusual malocclusion. Dentists accommodated this tolerant patient with locally focused treatment planning decisions. Her primary maxillary left second molar remains, and nonanatomical crowns exist on malpositioned dental implants at the first premolar locations.

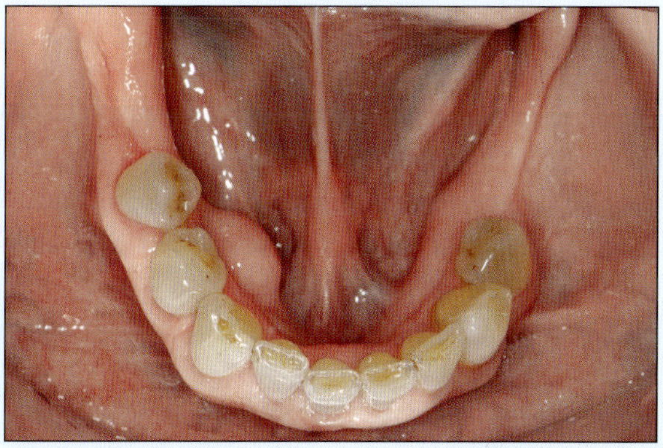

FIG 3 Likewise, her mandibular arch lacks molars, and has for decades. The Kennedy Class I mandibular arch lacks space on the posterior right due to hyperplastic gingival tissue along the ridge crest. The mandibular left first premolar is infraoccluded and well below the plane of occlusion.

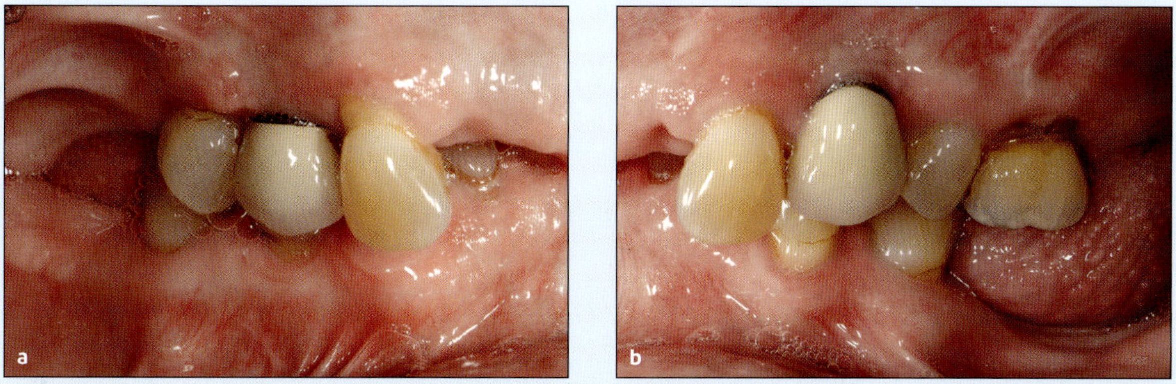

FIG 4 *(a and b)* Lack of interocclusal space is evident at all areas. Lack of adequate abutments precluded reliable crown and bridge options. The patient declined dental implant–supported reconstructions due to the complexity and cost. An overlay RPD option was offered as a means to restore her maxillary anterior teeth and to test a more normal occlusal scheme.

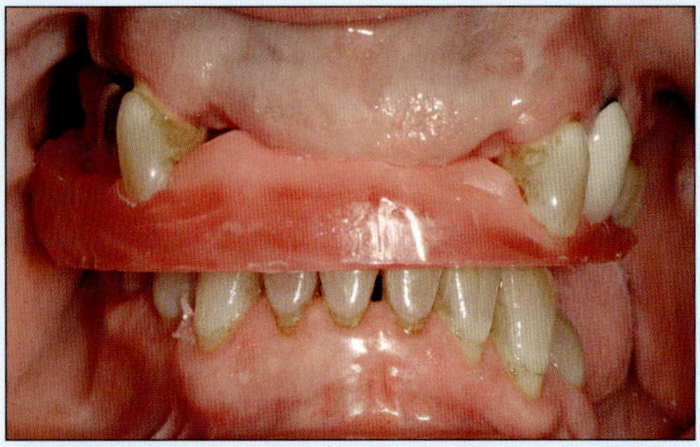

FIG 5 In order to create sufficient restorative space and to restore facial form, a significant increase in the occlusal vertical dimension (OVD) was planned. An overlay trial base with wax occlusion rim was used to evaluate and transfer the new position.

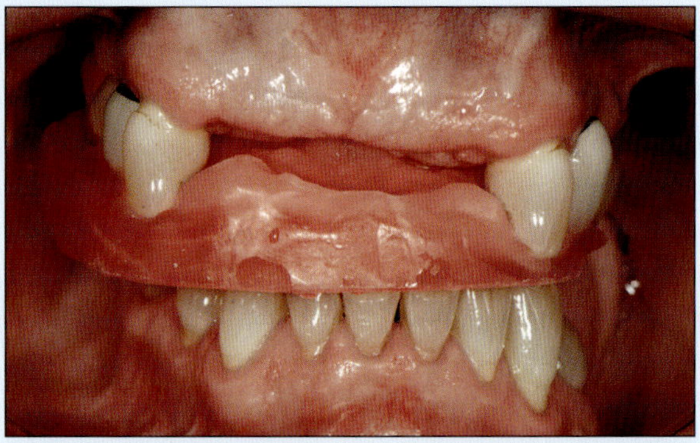

FIG 6 As discussed in chapter 4, mouth preparation is completed prior to RPD fabrication. Here, the results of localized alveoloplasty of the maxillary anterior residual ridge are confirmed by reinserting the previous trial base and wax rim. Adequate restorative space is now present for both the RPD framework and prosthetic teeth.

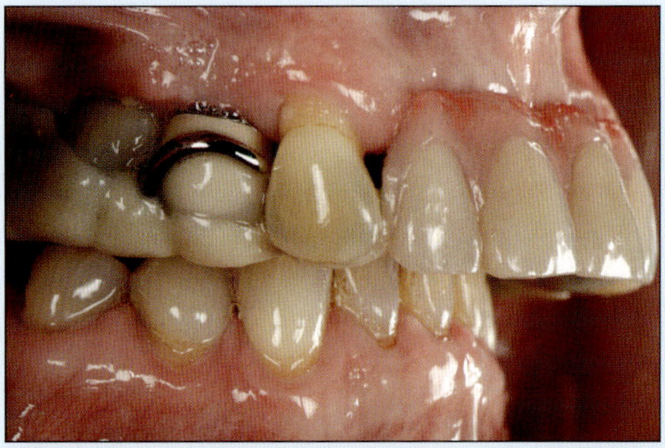

FIG 7 The patient in maximal intercuspal position after RPD completion. Note the increased OVD, now held completely by occlusal contacts on the RPD itself. The creation of these complicated and detailed occlusal contacts requires either transferring wax patterns from the articulated definitive cast or articulation of the refractory cast itself. Regardless, additional time to equilibrate the contacts will be necessary once the framework fit is confirmed.

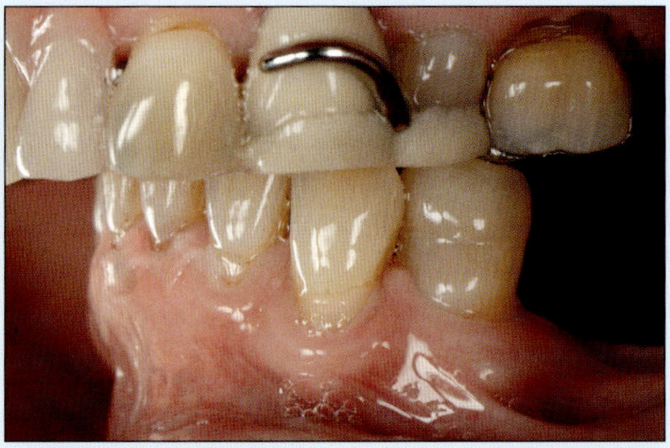

FIG 8 Embrasure style clasping is typically used where the cast framework comes over the occlusal surfaces of the teeth. In this instance, guiding planes were available and prepared on several surfaces where overreduction of the abutment was not a risk. Note the bonded porcelain onlay for the mandibular left first premolar, placed to level the occlusal plane.

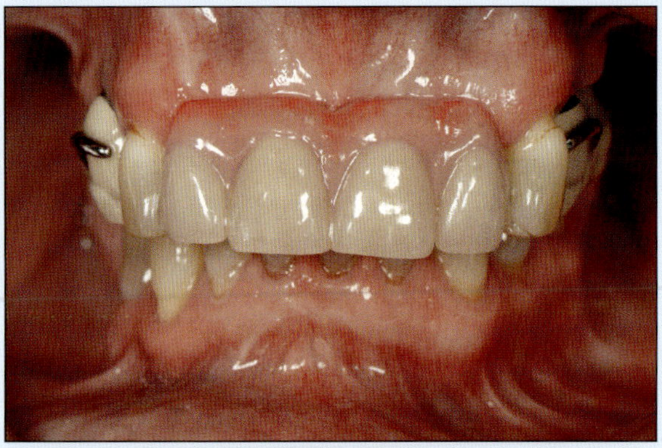

FIG 9 While the skeletal malocclusion remains, this was an economical and efficient improvement for this patient. Functionally, these designs are especially dependent on framework fit. The extensive tooth-frame contact surface area requires skill in casting and fitting procedures to achieve stability. Without this stability, retention can be a challenge. Additional clasping is therefore commonly employed with these designs.

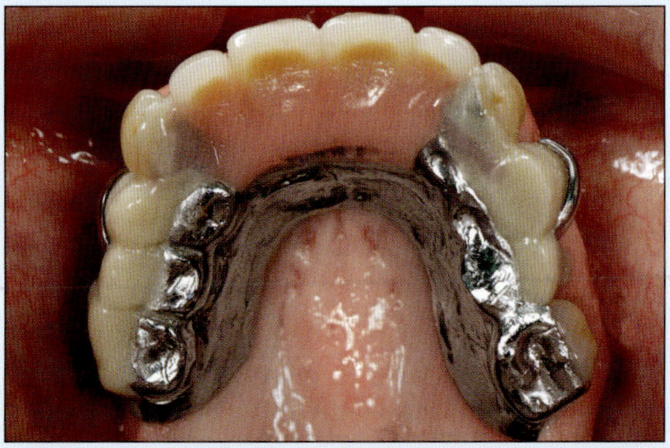

FIG 10 This overlay RPD covers all occlusal surfaces. In so doing, all opposing occlusal contacts are on the RPD itself. Note the slight indentations present in the metal occlusal portion of the overlay framework. The mandibular incisors nearly contact the acrylic of the anterior portion of the RPD. The areas of overlaid processed tooth-colored acrylic resin are supported by the framework and retained by beads in the casting. Over time, these areas tend to chip and wear away.

References

1. Rudd KD, O'Leary TJ. Stabilizing periodontally weakened teeth by using guide plane RPDs. J Prosthet Dent 1966;16:721–727.
2. Kratochvil FJ. Maintaining supporting structures with a removable partial prosthesis. J Prosthet Dent 1971;25:167–174.
3. Ma PS, Brudvik JS. Managing the maxillary partially edentulous patient with extensive anterior tooth loss and advanced periodontal disease using a removable partial denture: A clinical report. J Prosthet Dent 2008;100:259–263.
4. Simmons JJ. Swinglock stabilization and retention. Texas Dent J 1963;81:10–12.
5. Schulte JK, Smith DE. Clinical evaluation of swinglock removable partial dentures. J Prosthet Dent 1980;44:595–603.
6. Bolender CL, Becker CM. Swinglock removable partial dentures: Where and when. J Prosthet Dent 1981;45:4–10.
7. Becker CM, Bolender CL. Designing swinglock partial dentures. J Prosthet Dent 1981;46:126–131.
8. Chan MF, Adams D, Brudvik JS. The swinglock removable partial denture in clinical practice. Dent Update 1998;25:80–84.
9. Jacobson TE. Rotational path partial denture design: A 10-year clinical follow-up—Part II. J Prosthet Dent 1994;71:278–282.
10. Brewer AA, Fenton AH. The overdenture: Removable partial dentures. Dent Clin North Am 1973;17:732–746.
11. Farmer JB, Connelly ME. Treatment of open occlusions with onlay and overlay removable partial dentures. J Prosthet Dent 1984;51:300–303.
12. Winchy AM, Morris JC. An alternative treatment with the overlay removable partial denture: A clinical report. J Prosthet Dent 1998;79;249–253.
13. Becker CM, Kaldahl WB. Using removable partial dentures to stabilize teeth with secondary occlusal traumatism. J Prosthet Dent 1982;47:587–594.

13 IMPLANTS WITH PARTIAL DENTURES

Support where it is needed most.

Dental implants have proven so successful that most partially edentulous patients at least consider them as an option. This has allowed patients to realize long-term positive results with fixed prosthodontics where it was previously impossible. However, with time and experience, dental implants appear to have complication rates very similar to those of natural teeth. The idea of replacing every missing tooth with a dental implant is fraught with challenges and complications. This realization is exponentially critical in the context of partially edentulous patients. Recall the lesson from chapter 1 that these patients have demonstrated the ability to lose teeth. Uncontrolled disease is an absolute contraindication for partially edentulous dental implant therapy (Fig 13-1a). When these high-risk patients are treated with short-sighted, quadrant-focused dental implant replacements, the results are predictably unfortunate (Fig 13-1b). To make matters worse, when the remaining teeth are eventually lost, the integrated implants limit and often complicate effective full-arch prosthodontics (Fig 13-2). It typically would have been better for these implants to never have been placed in the first place. Some hesitancy is therefore necessary when implants are being considered for an RPD situation.

Treatment Planning Context

Any discussion of implants with RPDs begins, once again, with a risk analysis. The disease- and time-dependent assessments of chapter 1 form a philosophical baseline to determine whether a partial denture should be considered and then whether strategic implant placement would be appropriate. Due to the expense and frequent technical challenges with implant therapy, there must be a higher level of confidence in long-term risk assessment when considering them for a partial denture situation. One reason for this is that a partial denture, when well designed, can be fairly easily modified when additional teeth are lost. This is not necessarily the case when dental implants are among the abutments. In addition, dental implant therapy may increase the financial investment in an RPD to the point where longer-term options can be completed at a comparable cost.

When limited numbers of abutments remain, it is tempting to see value in using one or more strategic implants to help support or retain a partial denture. Unfortunately, the fact that there are limited numbers of remaining teeth means the implants that would be added would generally be the primary available support. It is often more appropriate in these situations to sacrifice the remaining one or two quality individual teeth so that more ideal implant positioning can occur for an implant-retained tissue-supported complete overdenture. This isn't really a sacrifice so much as a strategic use of remaining resources. A poorly positioned implant that complicates future care is the same cost as an ideally positioned implant. What is the real cost, function, and effort difference between a two-implant-retained tissue-supported overdenture and a partial denture that uses a dental implant

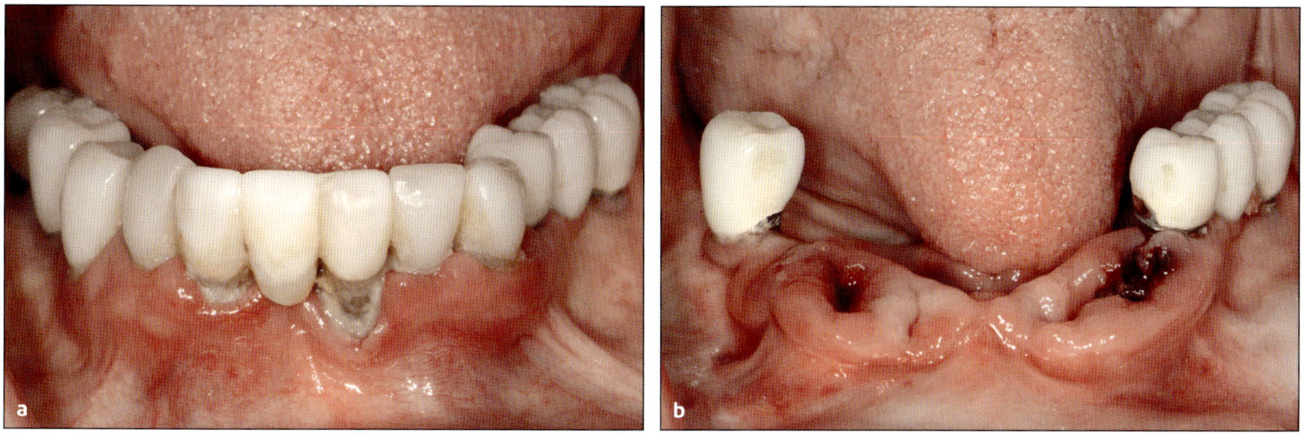

FIG 13-1 *(a)* Implants were used to replace the posterior teeth in a paitent with high risk of periodontal disease. The disease predictably returned. *(b)* After the remaining teeth are lost, the patient is left with poorly spaced implants, and previous work must be redone.

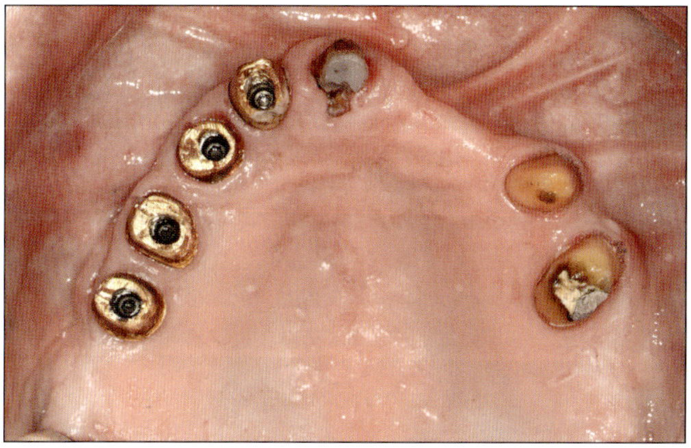

FIG 13-2 A failed fixed reconstruction immediately after disassembly. The unilateral and shallow implant positions will complicate the next reconstruction.

to replace a mandibular canine when only the contralateral canine and four incisors remain? Add to this the fact that the remaining teeth are rarely in ideal condition and will continue to be at high risk for further disease.

For those inexperienced in treatment planning, the idea of strategic extraction can, without a doubt, be abused. This partly explains the continued trend toward implants and away from conventional prosthodontics. In fact, the current implant-centric treatment planning is a driving factor behind the recommendation to base decisions on risk factor analysis rather than strictly technical issues. For the purposes of our further discussion, implants must only be considered for patients when the disease risk is low and when it can continue to be adequately controlled. When this limiting factor is strictly adhered to, dental implants facilitate results with advanced partial dentures that were previously unattainable.

The suggested ninth "rule" for application of the Kennedy classification is to consider an integrated dental implant equivalent to a potential natural abutment tooth. When present, an implant can be used in a multitude of ways. Regardless of how it will be utilized, it has the potential to provide support. Rule 9 is therefore a tool to be used during the treatment planning phase. When designing a partial denture, it should now be standard practice to evaluate how a dental implant would alter the Kennedy classification. Because we know that the use of—and satisfaction with—Class I partial dentures is lower than Class III situations, changing a Class I or II to a Class III has the potential to directly and significantly improve the expected outcome of the case. This ability to safely and predictably alter the Kennedy classification ultimately gives the dentist control over the chronic problems associated with the loading of the edentulous ridge.

The ideal use of one or more implants for the RPD is to eliminate the distal extension base, especially in the mandible[1] (Fig 13-3). The second indication, similar to the first, is to add support to an extensive modification space, for example an extreme Class II or IV arch. A third and more complex indication is to replace a critical abutment tooth or teeth.[2] Understanding of the numerous possibilities is best begun by looking closely at the various options for the implant-RPD interface.

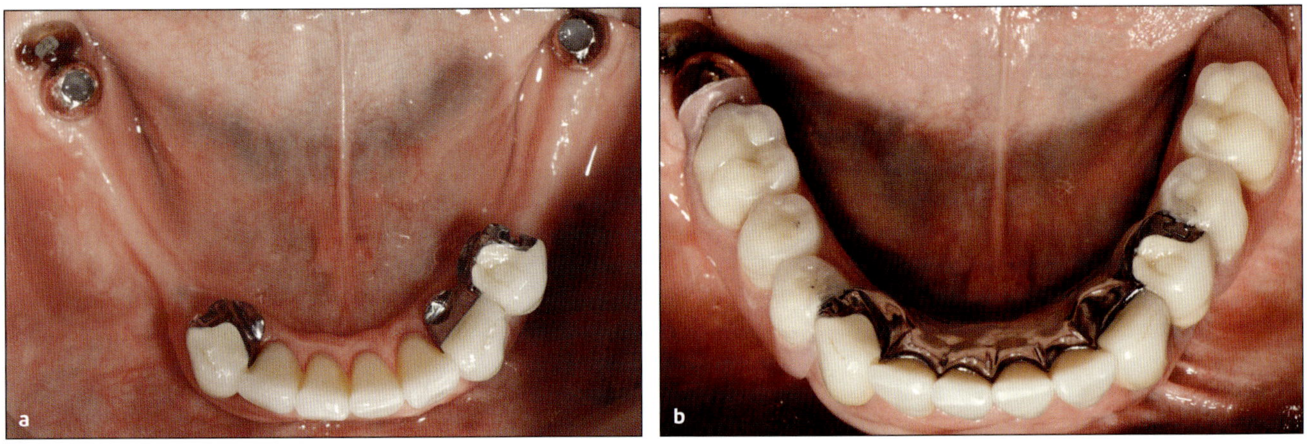

FIG 13-3 *(a)* Distal stop case. The abutments were custom-made for the patient, and the distal root of the right second molar was temporarily maintained. *(b)* Completed RPD. Posterior support allows the use of precision attachments.

Table 13-1 Summary of dental implant RPD abutment designs

ABUTMENT DESIGN	ABUTMENT TYPE	CONNECTION STYLE	USES
Prefabricated abutments	Prefabricated	Overlay	Support
Prefabricated attachment abutments	Prefabricated	Attachment	Support, retention
Custom attachment abutments	Custom	Attachment	Support, stability, retention
Custom abutments	Custom	Coping	Support, stability
Full crown form	Crown	Clasp assembly	Support, stability, retention

Implant Abutment Design

The design of the abutment that will attach to the implant body can take many forms. This is fortunate considering the nearly unlimited variety of partial denture situations. Abutment types can be generalized into five basic categories (Table 13-1).

Each category has the potential to provide specific types of force transmission, as defined in chapter 2. There is also a typical connection style that the associated partial denture will utilize to interface with the specific abutment type. Once the treatment planning has determined the best location for a strategic implant, there must be a clear understanding of what this implant abutment is going to be asked to accomplish in terms of the RPD function. Only after this is determined can the type of abutment be selected. It would not be logical to select a type of abutment and then ask that it provide functions beyond its capacity. The form must follow the function. The uninitiated will tend to select prefabricated attachment abutments knowing they are simple and inexpensive and provide retention. However, they may be completely inappropriate if the case has not been specifically designed to coordinate with the attachment design.

Prefabricated abutments

Prefabricated abutments come in many shapes and sizes. They can be easily modified, reshaped, and repolished. The simplicity of using a healing abutment for support, whether in its original shape or customized, is a major advantage (Fig 13-4). A potential problem arises from the fact that the healing abutments tend not to hold the necessary preload when torqued to place. While not as significant an issue as it once was, experience has shown that screw loosening of the healing abutment can occur with time.[3] As long as the patient is aware of this possibility and the healing abutment

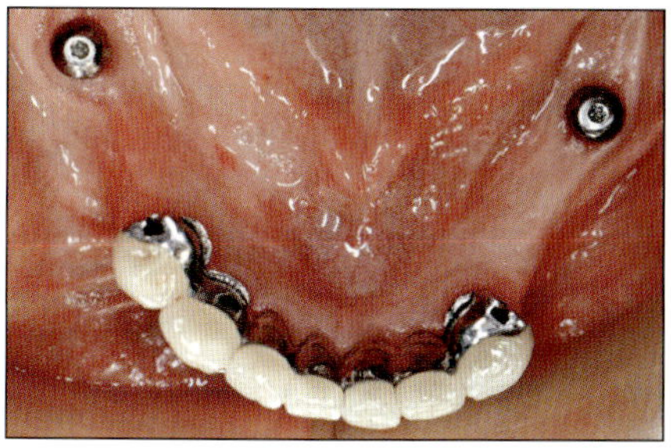

FIG 13-4 Modified healing abutments are used as distal stops to make this a Class III arch. Stress relief is no longer necessary.

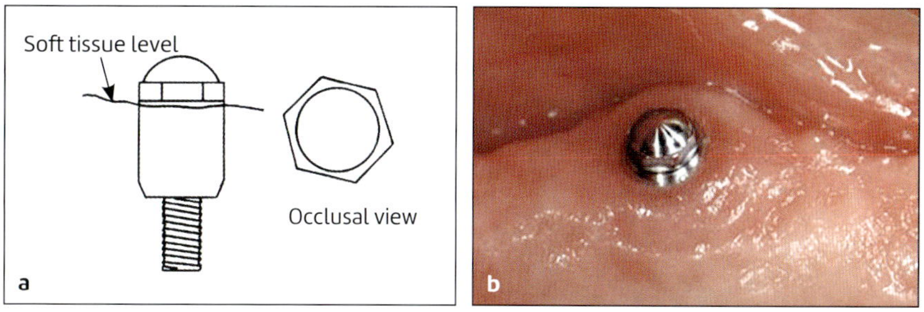

FIG 13-5 *(a)* Support-only abutment design without a center hex. *(b)* Dr Brudvik prototype abutment, with undisturbed dome shape, in clinical use.

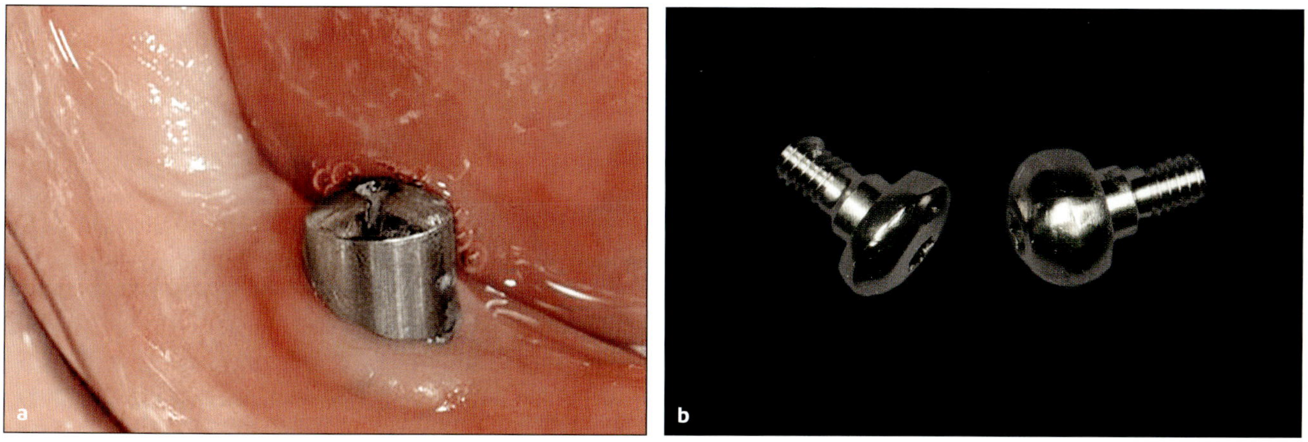

FIG 13-6 *(a)* Unmodified healing abutment with lengthy vertically parallel surfaces. *(b)* Healing abutments with dome shape, after lateral surface modifications.

is periodically inspected at recall appointments, no damage is apt to occur should it loosen. The modification of abutments that can receive greater torque has solved this problem for most situations.

With time, the top of these abutments will wear, even when contacted by acrylic resin. Should this be allowed to continue, there is potential for the hex to become distorted, or in severe cases, worn away. Having the hex at the top of the abutment, right at the point of contact, makes this difficult to avoid. An alternative design for a prefabricated abutment was created by Dr Brudvik and used in prototype form on several patients at the University of Washington (Fig 13-5). This abutment maintained the contoured form of the occlusal stop while moving the driver hex to the gingival portion of the abutment. This leaves the supporting area undisturbed and will maintain ideal retrievability. As will be discussed shortly, this is how the majority of ball attachment type abutments are designed. Dr Brudvik's design was never manufactured in any significant volume due to low demand; however, with the ability to copy-mill nearly any design, this shape can be manufactured with modern CAD/CAM technology.

These designs all strive to cap the implant with a rounded abutment that would provide point contact on its most superior surface. There should be no lateral contacts at all in order to only load the implant with vertical stress. Because healing abutments typically have vertically parallel lateral surfaces, they will need to be modified to create the desired dome shape (Fig 13-6). This is preferred to simply blocking out around the abutment, as this would leave either lateral surface contact, or if relieved, excessive space for plaque accumulation. The point contact between the abutment and the partial denture is designed to allow a slight movement, or slide. This slight amount of movement allows for the

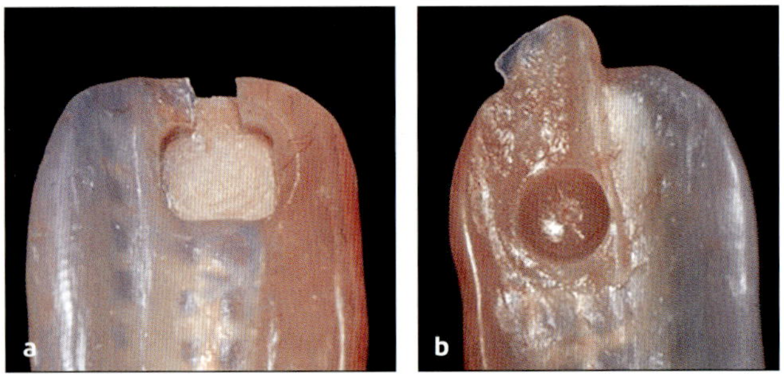

FIG 13-7 Before *(a)* and after *(b)* reline procedure to create contact with abutment.

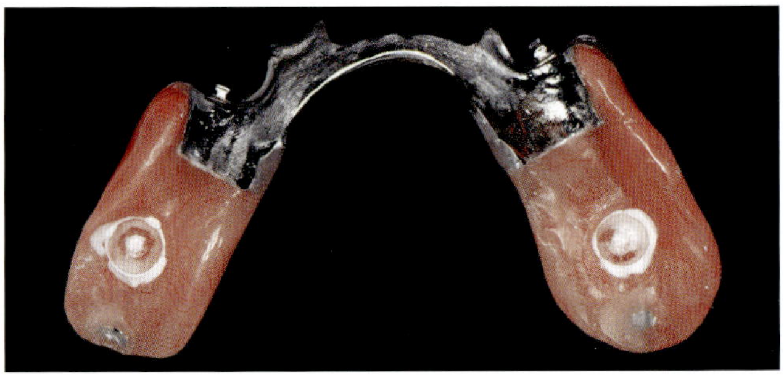

FIG 13-8 Fit Checker (GC America) being used to evaluate and modify abutment contact.

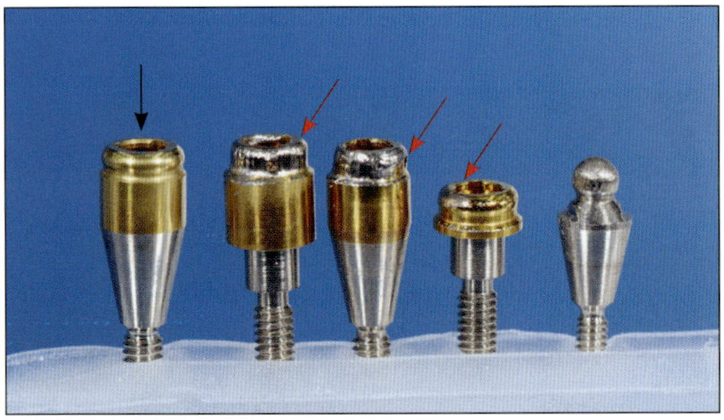

FIG 13-9 Various Locator abutments with ball abutment on right. The abutment to the left *(black arrow)* is a new abutment; the three in the middle are worn abutments *(red arrows)*.

expansion and contraction of the mandible during opening and closing as well as the slight physiologic movement of the remaining natural abutment teeth. By allowing this slight movement and ensuring no lateral contact, these prefabricated abutments serve exclusively as support to resist the vertically directed forces of mastication.

The connection for these designs is perhaps best achieved by a sectional reline using an autopolymerized acrylic resin at the placement appointment as part of the final adjustment procedures (Fig 13-7). To maintain this contact throughout the life of the partial denture, periodic evaluation of the wear to both surfaces and consideration to relines or replacement of the prefabricated abutment is required (Fig 13-8). These relines tend to be localized to the site of the abutment since the tissue is no longer being loaded to any significant degree.

Prefabricated attachment abutments

Prefabricated attachment abutments are available in various sizes and designs (Fig 13-9). Similar to healing abutments, they are very economical. These abutments are considered when a retentive element is desired. The top of these abutments is most commonly either a ball or a ring design. The various attachment manufacturers have contracted with implant part manufacturers to produce Locator, ERA, OSO, and other attachment designs for the ever-increasing variety of dental implants. When planned and executed properly, these will provide excellent retention. In providing this retention, there is some semblance of lateral stability created. This is because basically all implant attachment designs engage vertically, rather than horizontally, like a tube and plug.

Despite its presence, this is not a feature that should be relied on. When these resilient attachments are asked to act as primary stabilizers, they will tend to distort, wear, let loose, and not function appropriately (see Fig 13-9). For the purposes of this book, when in prefabricated form, these abutments are only asked to provide retention and support. By default, the attachment abutment connection with the partial denture will, in most instances, provide vertical support. While it is possible to use spacers to initially prevent the partial denture from resting on the attachment, this typically is not enough space to prevent contact as a distal extension base is depressed during function. The space, while present initially, is also lost, as residual ridge resorption occurs.

When the implant has been positioned within a tooth-bound space, supported on either end by natural abutment teeth, the retentive element is not asked to provide support.

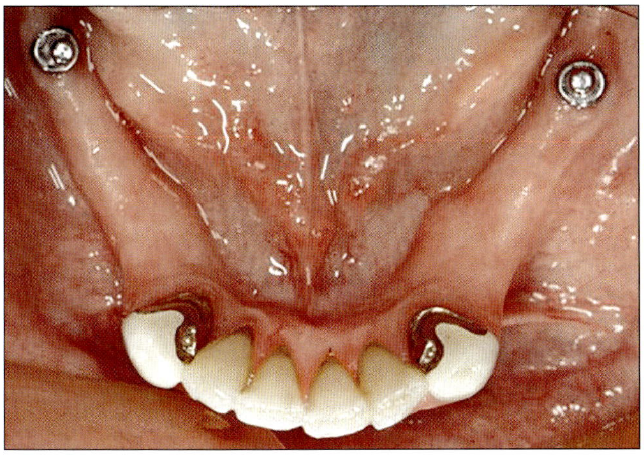

FIG 13-10 Distal prefabricated attachment abutments must also serve as support.

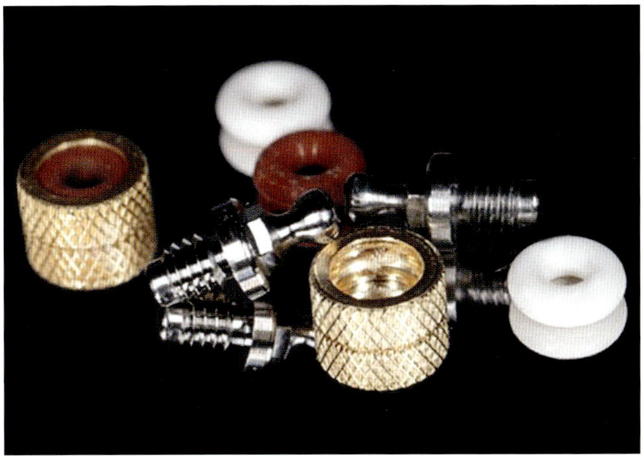

FIG 13-11 Classic OSO abutments with open housings and retentive rings.

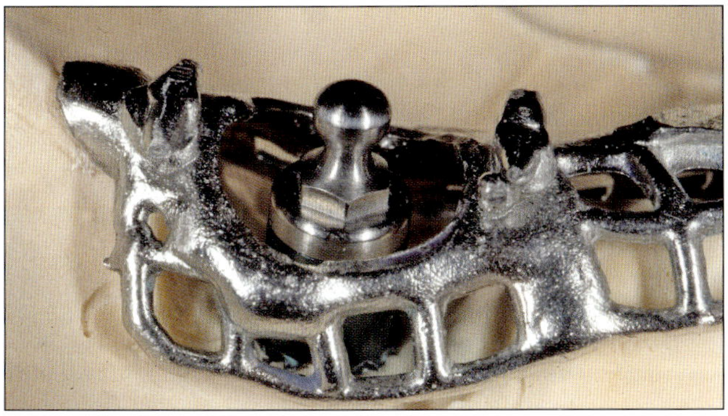

FIG 13-12 The hex and retentive area are below the supporting contact at the top of the OSO.

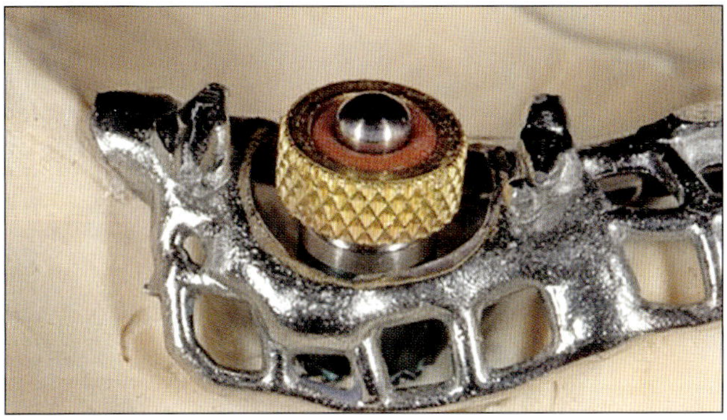

FIG 13-13 An open housing leaves the top of the abutment available to provide a vertical stop.

This assumes the abutment teeth are stable with normal physiologic mobility. When designed to only provide retention in these tooth-bound situations, the attachment abutments do very well, with a greatly extended time before replacement of the retentive inserts is necessary. This is no doubt due to the limited amount of movement and stress the attachment is required to resist.

When the abutment will be asked to provide support, the partial denture connection is designed to control the point of supporting contact (Fig 13-10). A common first choice is a ball attachment such as the OSO or Sphero Flex (Rhein 83). As noted in chapter 11, these designs are the most flexible of all the attachment systems and are therefore of greatest value in situations where movement is expected[4] (Fig 13-11). When used as support, the top of the ball of the metal patrix serves as a vertical stop that is independent of the retentive component (Fig 13-12). This is far superior to a system where the resilient component bears the load as a stop. In reality then, these abutments are treated like healing abutments that have had a circumferential undercut created below the occlusal point of contact. A rubber or metal O-ring or cap seats over this height of contour to engage the undercut.

Currently, the vast majority of attachment designs come with metal housings. This ensures a reliable means of retaining the resilient matrix within the prosthesis and also facilitates efficient replacement of the worn insert. When used in partial denture applications, it must be remembered that these housings are typically designed with complete overdentures, and therefore maximum resiliency in mind. If the goal is to also provide support, the presence of a spacer or gap within the manufacturing parameters of the housing must be known. For example, housings for the OSO attachment come in closed and open forms. The closed form is designed to preserve a space above the ball. This preserves resiliency and therefore does not provide vertical support, at least until further significant resorption of the ridge. The open form leaves the top of the ball exposed and in so doing leaves the option of providing a vertical stop (Fig 13-13).

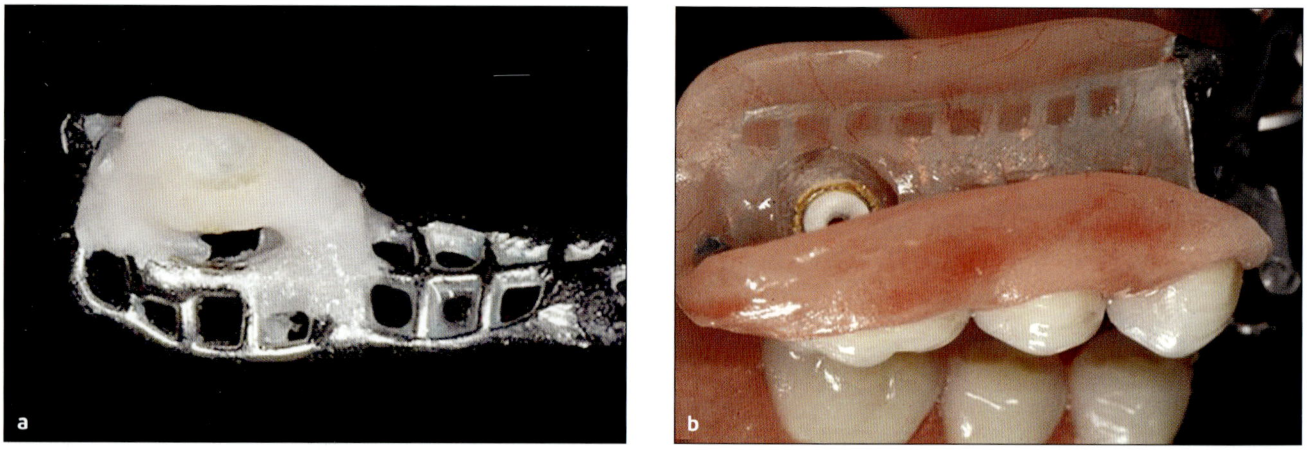

FIG 13-14 *(a)* Open housing after intraoral pickup. The vertical stop is in acrylic resin. *(b)* Housing within the base after tinting and processing.

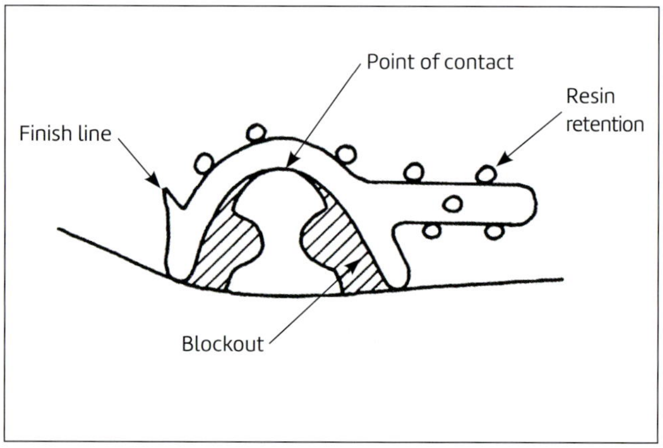

FIG 13-15 Design of protective custom housing for implant stud attachment.

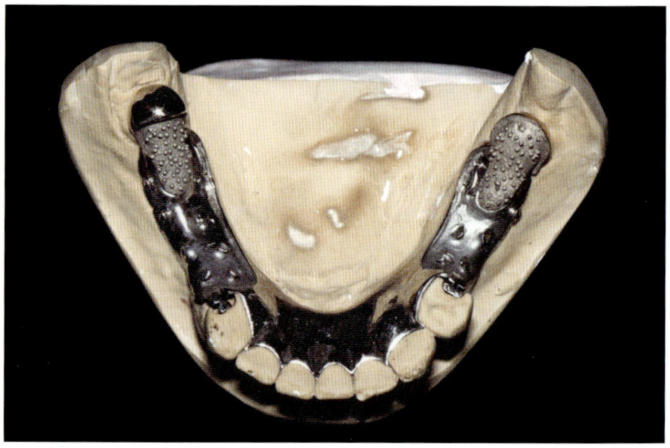

FIG 13-16 Custom housings for distal implants, ready for connection to framework.

If support is desired, the clinician must choose between allowing that contact to be in the resin of the denture base, or making a custom metal casting to ride on the ball (rounded occlusal stop). If the contact is only in the resin of the denture base, then contact can be added at processing of the base or at the time of housing connection (Fig 13-14). Either way, it occurs after the framework fitting is complete. As discussed in chapter 11, when and how this connection process occurs is determined by several factors. The less movement of the base, the longer the abutment-resin contact should be expected to last. In certain high-movement situations, such as mobile anterior abutment teeth, wear of the abutment-resin contact should be expected in a relatively short period of time.

If the clinician decides to make a custom housing, fixture analogs must be present on the definitive cast for the partial denture casting. Before metal housings were available, the patrix or ball was blocked out so that only the center of the ball surface would contact (Fig 13-15). Nowadays, for the OSO design, the open metal housing is placed and the blockout provided only below the housing. This unit is then duplicated in refractory. If the overcasting is to be retained with resin alone, it is waxed with retentive beads or loops to lock into the denture base. A tang extension, running to the retentive meshwork, is often required so that the casting or housing can be picked up from the mouth after framework fitting. In situations where space is reduced, the tang extensions are welded to the retentive meshwork of the partial denture casting (Fig 13-16). This process should seem very familiar to the custom housings described in chapter 11. The presence of the metal-to-metal vertical stop contact is generally maintained indefinitely. In fact, since the nonprecious alloy tends to wear the titanium alloy of the abutment, the ball attachment is what may require replacement after multiple years of use. This is the primary reason why it is preferred to have the driver hex below the ball, rather than at the top where contact will occur. While the ball attachment designs are preferred, they also require the most vertical space. The ring designs, like Locator, require significantly less.

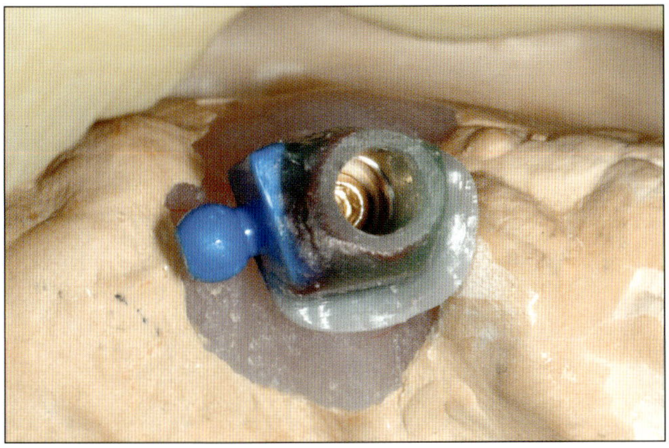

FIG 13-17 The abutment will provide support with the ledge, stability with guiding planes, and retention with the attachment.

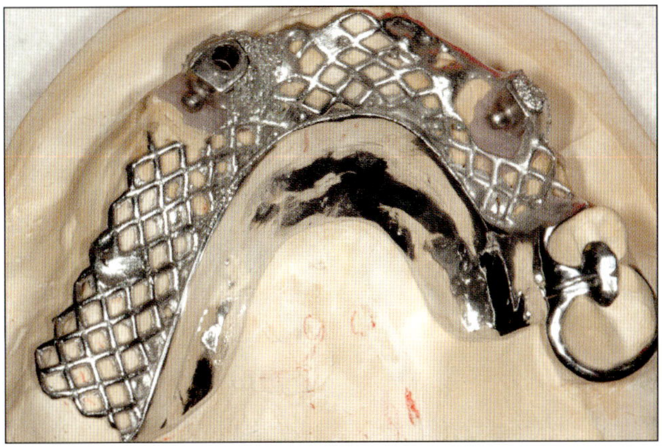

FIG 13-18 The framework interfaces with rests and guiding planes on the custom abutments to support and stabilize the prosthesis.

Custom attachment abutments

The prefabricated abutment options work very well when the implant angulations are manageable. For many reasons, this is not always the case. Despite modern computer-guided surgery and planning, it is difficult to guarantee precise implant angulation. One must also take into account that RPD options generally need to be more cost effective. The available complex surgical treatments, especially guided surgery, tend to be significantly expensive. In addition, a number of RPD reconstructions are previously failed fixed reconstructions, many with dental implants in locations planned with other goals in mind and with angulations well outside of ideal.

Custom abutments, both with and without attachments, are necessary to best manage complicated implant positions. The implant position inaccuracy can be in angulation, depth, mesiodistal position, or a combination of all three of these. Not only will a customized abutment allow the best chance of adequately managing these positional issues, but it facilitates incorporation of support and stability as well as retention. In this way, the abutment can function in a way similar to primary natural tooth abutments.

The process for planning and creating the abutment and its interface with the partial denture is basically identical to that described in chapter 11. In those situations for which an attachment component is intended, space is usually at a premium, especially if the implant is placed quite posteriorly. A measurement taken from the occlusal surface of the opposing tooth or matrix of the diagnostic arrangement must show that space exists. The abutment, the attachment components, sufficient resin to pick up the attachment, and the denture tooth will all require significant thickness. As in any attachment situation where space is minimal, the occlusal surfaces of the denture tooth over the implant are protected with metal occlusals. Where space is severely limited, a custom housing with the potential for veneering for an adequate esthetic result is often required.

The custom attachment abutment can be used for the isolated single implant at any position in the mouth. These abutments, traditionally castings, should be designed with a vertical stop as well as the attachment (Fig 13-17). Implant angulation becomes nearly irrelevant since this casting is made to be parallel with the path of insertion determined by the other RPD abutments. The logical progression of this alignment is to include a milled guiding plane along the surfaces not involved with the attachment. The end result is a partial denture framework that will rest solidly on the vertical stop, a simple flat plane contact that is easy to verify and fit. It will also contact along the vertically parallel guiding plane surfaces, assuming the fabrication and fitting procedures previously highlighted are followed (Fig 13-18). Once fit, the attachment is left to provide the retention. By segmenting these functions, they can each be verified independently. More importantly, the function of the attachment is protected from damage and wear both during placement and removal as well as during function.

This degree of customization is often necessary when the esthetic replacement of the missing tooth is a priority. Customizing the abutment will often preserve enough interocclusal space that the framework and acrylic teeth can be overlaid as desired. The cost of the abutment then could potentially save the effort and expense of a custom housing. When the space is too tight, even for this to occur, the abutment optimizes the existing space for the housing. Much of the frustration encountered with implant-supported partial dentures comes from the failure to manage the available space or the various forces. The cost and effort to correct the repeated fracture, overcontouring, misfit, and debonding

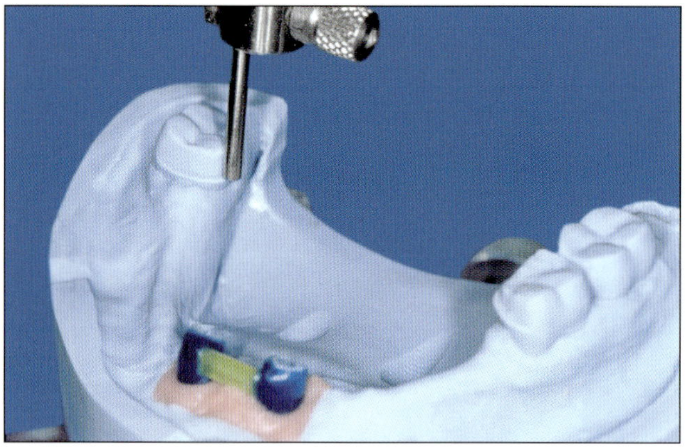

FIG 13-19 Bar being designed according to the path of insertion as determined by the teeth.

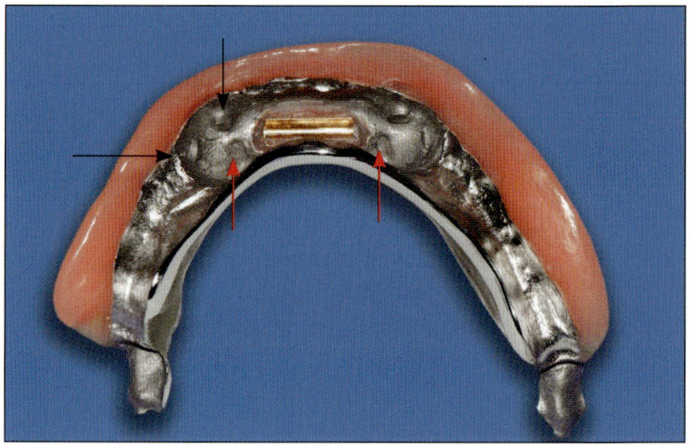

FIG 13-20 The *red arrows* indicate support contact on top of the customized bar, while the *black arrows* indicate lateral surface contact.

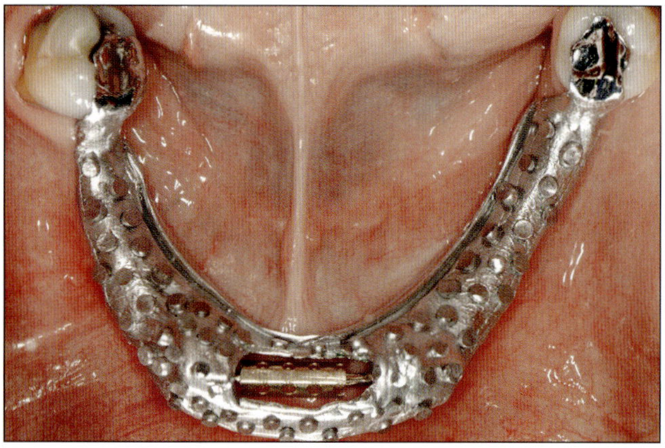

FIG 13-21 Extreme Class IV arch modified by two implants and a bar to be Class III. The frame-abutment contacts protect the clip.

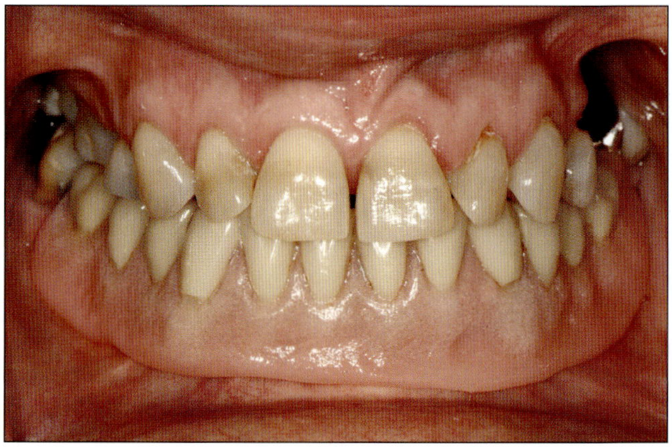

FIG 13-22 The customized bar supports the RPD against natural teeth. This RPD easily converts to an overdenture if molars are lost.

that results when implant attachments are connected without control of the space quickly exceeds the cost or effort of making the customized parts to begin with.

When more than one implant is to be used, a bar is often the ideal customized design. Bars have been effectively used to manage misaligned implants in overdenture situations since the earliest dental implant days and have proven exceptionally reliable. As will be discussed in detail in chapter 14, misalignment can be managed and retention achieved more reliably than when individual resilient attachments are used. The shape of the abutment in the area of the implants is customized to match the path of insertion of the RPD while the retentive bar element is positioned accordingly (Fig 13-19). Customization of the abutment area, by way of a flat occlusal surface, results in solid vertical support for the RPD (Fig 13-20). The vertical load, achieved by contact of the framework on the platformed abutment area or the bar itself, is directed to the implants without relying on any plastic retentive element or clip (Fig 13-21). As is shown in chapter 14, the lateral surfaces of the customized abutment portions of the bar are milled to be parallel to the path of insertion. This creates lateral support by means of guiding plane surfaces. Anteroposterior rotation can be created, if necessary, by blocking out the lingual area of the abutments. The bar, when used in nonround form, needs to be parallel with the path of insertion. The implants can have nearly any alignment. When a completely round form of bar, like the Ackermann, is used, even this relationship of the bar is irrelevant.

The bar option facilitates more extensive reconstructions (Fig 13-22). The splinting of what are often shorter and/or narrower implants will improve the distribution of force to the bone, and perhaps more importantly from the standpoint of reducing complications, the prosthetic connection. The more extensive the bar, the greater the need and opportunity to incorporate milling of lateral surfaces. In doing so, the stability of the partial denture can be greatly increased. In reality, the guiding plane concepts highlighted throughout this book are applied to the bar. Custom implant abutments, of any design, are therefore created with the same technical RPD concepts in mind as if they are natural tooth abutments.

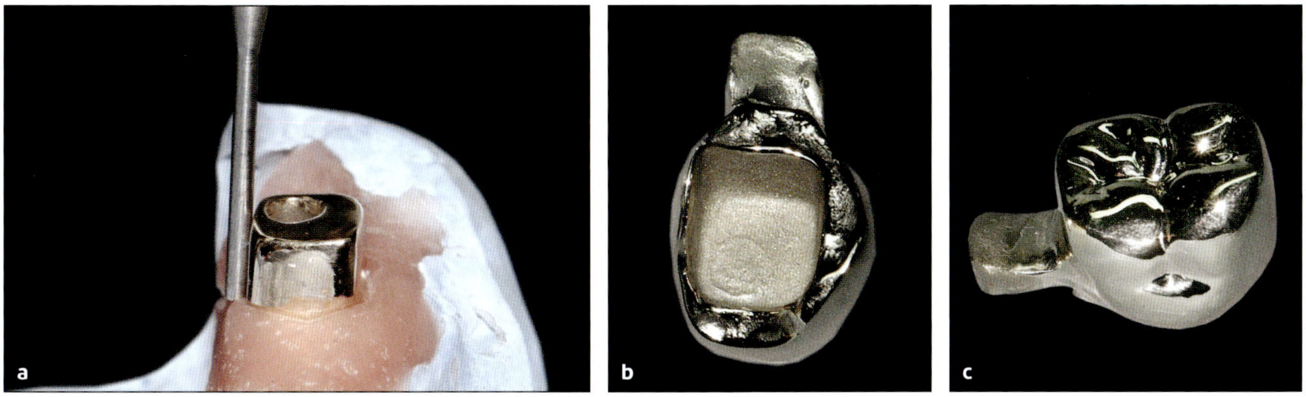

FIG 13-23 *(a)* The box form facilitates a large increase in guiding plane surface, while the flat occlusal surface is ideal support. *(b and c)* Cast full-form coping with extension for laser welding. The intaglio surface will fit over the abutment.

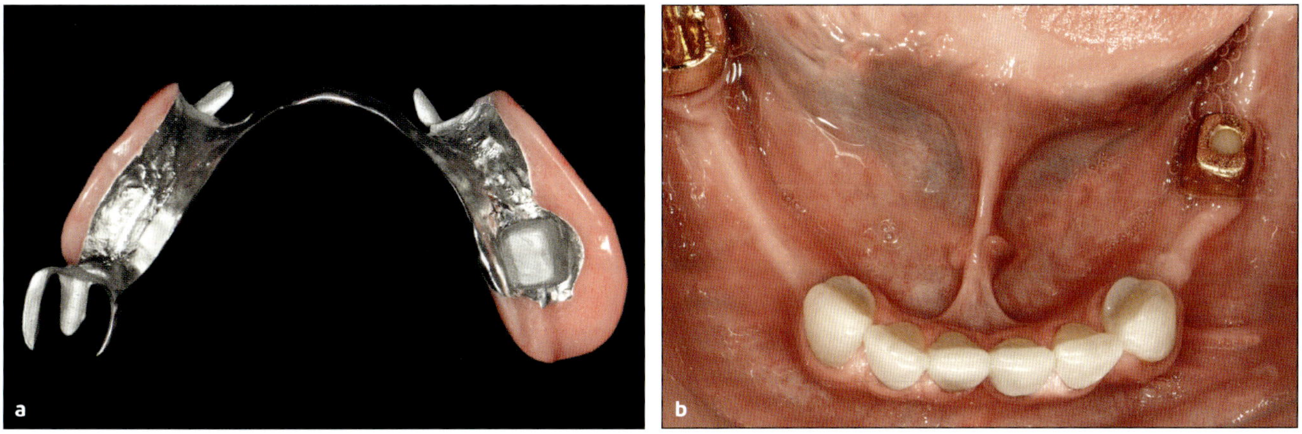

FIG 13-24 *(a)* Now a Class III arch, greater guiding plane volume results in the need for a single retentive clasp at the mandibular right second molar. *(b)* A box form custom abutment at the mandibular left first molar site, milled to the path of insertion.

Custom abutments

Designing and incorporating support, stability, and retention with an implant abutment is fairly complex. Perhaps it is not necessary to go to these lengths? Recall for a moment that optimized volume and accuracy of frictional guiding plane contact will result in a retentive prosthesis. In most instances, the volume of guiding plane surface that can be created with a custom implant abutment is far greater than on a natural tooth (Fig 13-23a). If the guiding plane surface area is increased to this degree, and the other four criteria for frictional guiding plane retention discussed in chapter 2 are met, the result should be a prosthesis with much less need—perhaps no need—for additional retentive features.

If this is the goal, the abutment-frame interface occurs best in the form of a coping (Figs 13-23b and 13-23c). Discussed in detail in chapter 12, this coping design can be a fairly straightforward way to incorporate a key implant abutment while still maximizing its benefit beyond support alone (Fig 13-24a). The simplicity is due to the ease of design and elimination of additional retentive elements. These custom abutments are usually made to the fixture level and are designed more or less in a box shape, with the subgingival form being contoured with a gradual taper toward the diameter of the platform. The box shape is milled according to the path of insertion with a flat occlusal surface and rounded edges to eliminate any sharp line angles (Fig 13-24b). The taper of the walls of the box can vary based on the amount of frictional retention desired and the expected challenge of fitting the coping over the abutment. When used in the common distal abutment situation, for example a second molar site, the mesial and lingual of the box is milled to 0 degrees. The distal of the box, often shorter in functional height due to the contour of the residual ridge, is tapered to around 4 degrees. This leaves the buccal to have a slight taper, usually 2 degrees, in order to facilitate fitting of the framework. Traditionally cast to machined interfaces, these abutments are also available through CAD/CAM processes. Custom angulated and tapered titanium alloy abutments are available from Atlantis, a division of dental manufacturing giant

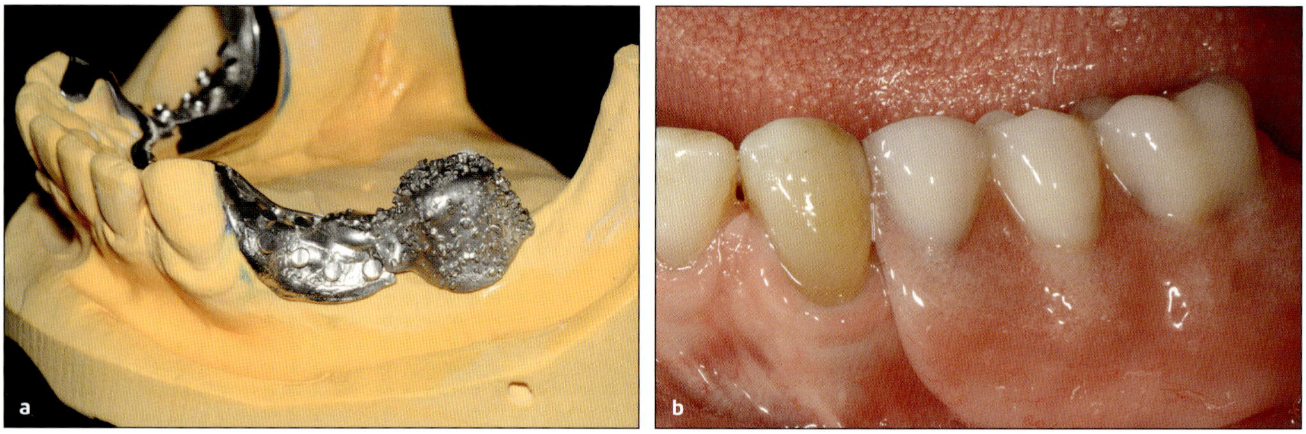

FIG 13-25 *(a)* Coping designed to be veneered by acrylic resin. Note the laser-welded connection. *(b)* Extensive interocclusal space for veneering of frame.

Dentsply Sirona. Marketed for full-arch prostheses called Conus (Dentsply Sirona), these abutments are designed to support a coping, as discussed here.

The overlay coping itself is designed to contact the surfaces of the abutment as milled, while the exterior surface can take two basic forms. When extensive space is present, it is generally prudent to plan to overlay the coping with acrylic and a prosthetic denture tooth. The exterior surface is designed with bead retention and perhaps an external finish line, if the ideal contour places the flange extension near the abutment (Fig 13-25). Due to the additional forces placed on the coping, an extension running to the retentive meshwork is required so that the casting can be more rigidly retained by acrylic or better still by laser welding to the major connector. This process is no different than that of a custom housing.

The second form, used in situations where space is limited, is to overlay the abutment with a coping that takes the full form of a tooth (Fig 13-26a). This requires that the implant be located fairly accurately within the residual ridge (Fig 13-26b). When the coping is a full-form tooth, there is no need for a flange of any sort around the abutment (Fig 13-26c). This tends to optimize the gingival health around these implants. This is often the design of choice when the opposing arch is natural dentition. The coping, made of metal, can be fit into the limited space of second molar sites without risk of fracture. This will also virtually eliminate occlusal wear over the implant. Because there is no resilient attachment insert to change, maintenance is further reduced (Fig 13-26d). Some disadvantages may be the increased cost, if a precious alloy is used, of the significant amount of metal and the need for attention to detail with the coping process. For the maker of advanced partial dentures, these advantages appear to outweigh the negatives.

Full crown form

From the standpoint of complexity, the various custom abutment options all share a disadvantage. The RPD is designed to overlay the abutment, be it an attachment, bar, or custom abutment. Not only is this a somewhat unfamiliar procedure for many dentists, but it adds an additional layer of decision-making and therefore complexity. If, as Rule 9 implies, the implant is thought of as a natural tooth abutment, why isn't it used in the same manner as a natural tooth? Put another way, why not put an ideally shaped, contoured, and shaded abutment tooth on the implant? The obvious first benefit of this is that the partial denture design can be managed in a more conventional manner with rest seats, guiding planes, and clasp assemblies if indicated (Fig 13-27a). Another advantage is that the patient retains the occlusal contact and esthetics of the tooth when the partial denture is out of the mouth (Fig 13-27b). When the cost of a custom abutment for a crown and the crown itself is considered, this may not in fact be any more costly from a laboratory perspective than the cost of a custom attachment abutment, custom housing, and associated management of the partial denture framework.

Nearly the full scope of design possibilities exists when using a full-form crown as an RPD abutment. This is because there is less concern about overpreparation of the supporting core. In other words, there is no pulp to be concerned with, and the metal of the abutment is stronger than if it was residual dentin. Depending on the implant position, intracoronal precision attachments and lingual clasping may both be possible due to greater leeway with contours. This may facilitate their use and improve hygiene where extracoronal precision attachment designs are normally recommended.

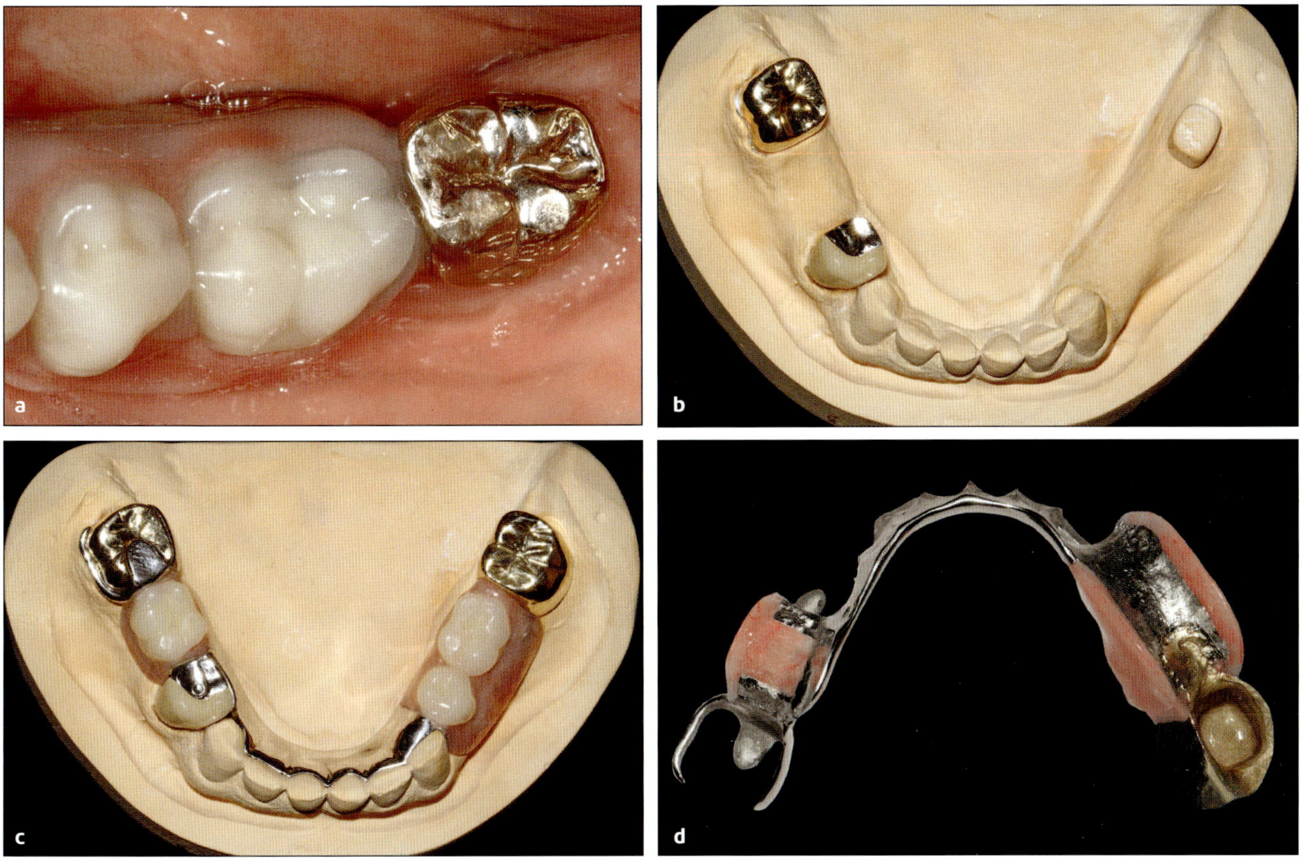

FIG 13-26 *(a)* Full-form coping over custom abutment; no flange is necessary. *(b)* Class III situation with custom abutment at mandibular left second molar site. *(c)* Full-form coping on the second molar implant aids support and stability so that a single clasp is all that is required for retention. *(d)* Uncomplicated RPD design with its many benefits. Note the laser-weld joint. No attachment means less maintenance.

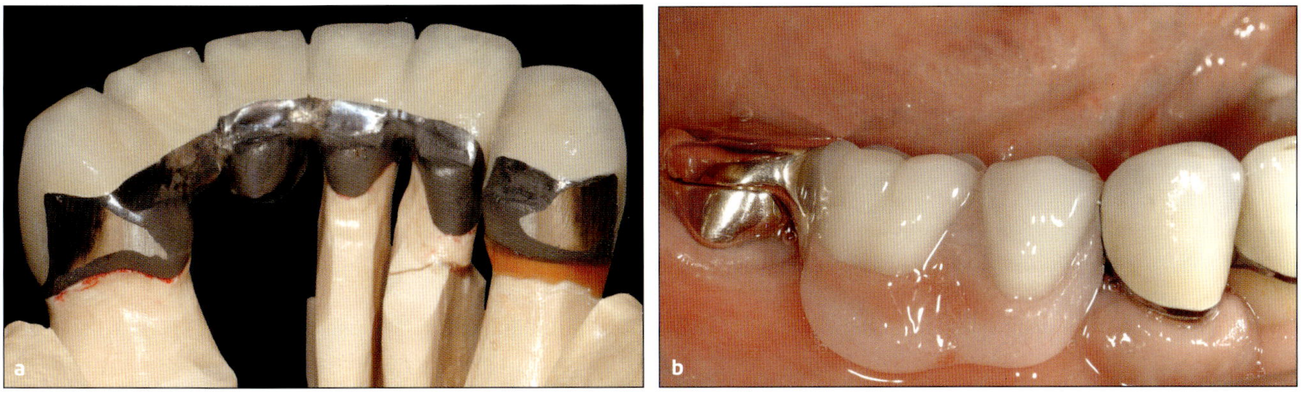

FIG 13-27 *(a)* Full-form surveyed crown for mandibular right canine implant after initial milling. Note the rest seat. *(b)* The canine implant-supported surveyed crown at placement. Note the distal guiding plane.

The sequence for fabrication of the full contour crown abutment should follow that of surveyed crowns (see Fig 4-29). The natural tooth abutments must set the path of insertion first so that the implant crown is fabricated to align accordingly. One possible disadvantage of concern is the physiologic difference between an osseointegrated implant abutment and a natural tooth abutment with a periodontal ligament. This issue continues to be debated within fixed prosthodontics, with opening of the proximal contacts with natural teeth being a common complication.[5]

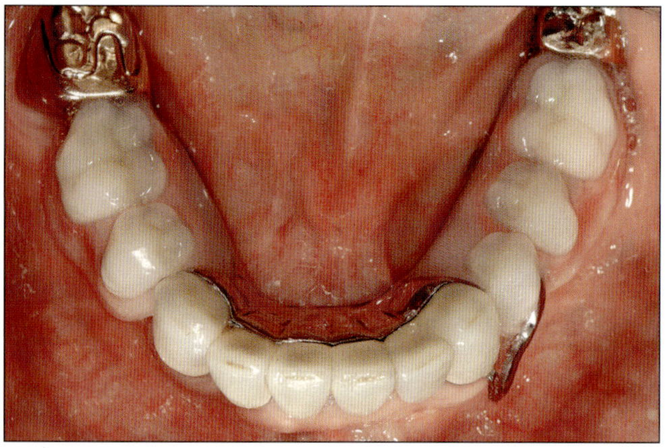

FIG 13-28 The canine implant crown receives minimal torque in this Class III arch.

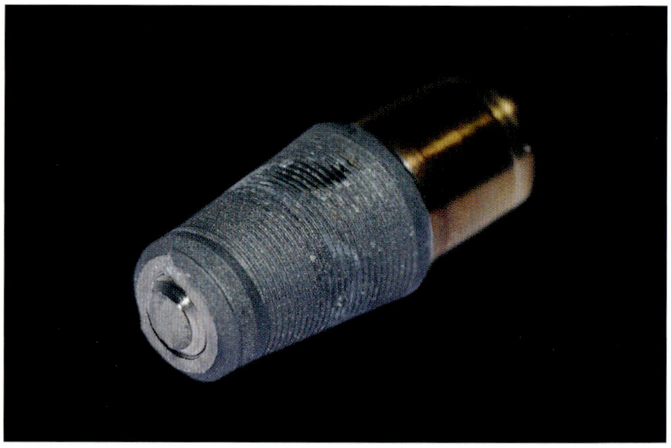

FIG 13-29 Fractured implant body. Note the screw fracture and thin periphery of metal.

The hypothesized risk for a partial denture is one where the natural tooth abutments migrate away from the framework or where the implant abutment, without a ligament, receives the vast majority of the occlusal load. These are difficult risks to quantify because RPD frameworks are less rigid in function than their cemented fixed partial denture counterparts. The issue may therefore be most legitimate for Class III situations where support and stability are maximized. Would a natural tooth migrate away from the framework due to its difference with one or two implant abutments? This has not been our experience, probably because of a focus on positive rest design and framework fit. Nonetheless, issues such as continued facial growth and the frequent opening of proximal contacts between natural teeth and implant crowns is evidence that the difference between implants and natural teeth must be respected and considered if long-term results are to be expected.[5] Unfortunately, there is only clinical experience to guide us at this time.

Another possible risk to be mentioned is one of overloading an implant or its abutment. The level of risk for fracture is no doubt directly related to the strength of the structural components and the patient (Fig 13-28). Larger, more robust implants and implant components can be relied on to handle loads better than narrow, weaker, implant designs. This type of treatment planning is no different than when considering the strength of a debilitated abutment tooth. If a narrow-diameter implant is present at the canine position of a distal extension, it would not seem wise to use a rigid design, like a coping, to make the connection. Implants and screws are at risk of fracture just like natural teeth (Fig 13-29). In light of this fact, the treatment planning decisions are quite similar, from a risk analysis standpoint, to those of natural teeth.

Decisions for Class I and II Situations

The obvious situation in which a single implant can make a major contribution to the success of an RPD is in the distal extension partial denture. Patients have often been dissatisfied with our best efforts, whether with conventional or precision attachment partial dentures, because of chronic soreness under the distal extension base. This is especially true in those situations where the opposing arch contains a full complement of natural teeth or fixed partial dentures. Implants placed with the intent of providing a distal abutment, ideally in the area of the second molar, effectively change the Class I or II situation to that of the Class III.[1] If necessary, positioning the implant in the first molar area typically achieves the same goal. The implant need not provide retention, since adequate retention is most always available from other abutments.

There is no reason for the denture base, when supported by an implant, to extend to the traditional borders. In fact, once posterior support is available, the design of the denture base should be altered to make its contours as much like those of a fixed restoration as possible (Fig 13-30; see also Fig 13-26). This means that there is no advantage to extending into the floor of the mouth, or onto the external oblique ridge.

If the implant is distal to the first molar, it is not essential that a denture tooth be placed, especially if space is lacking. Occlusion through the first molar, when the base is well-supported posteriorly, will provide adequate mastication. If controlling the contact location or protecting the thin base is important, the limited space situation can be handled with metal overlays or copings as discussed. It is generally possible to cantilever one occlusal unit posterior to the area of implant abutment support. This is done when

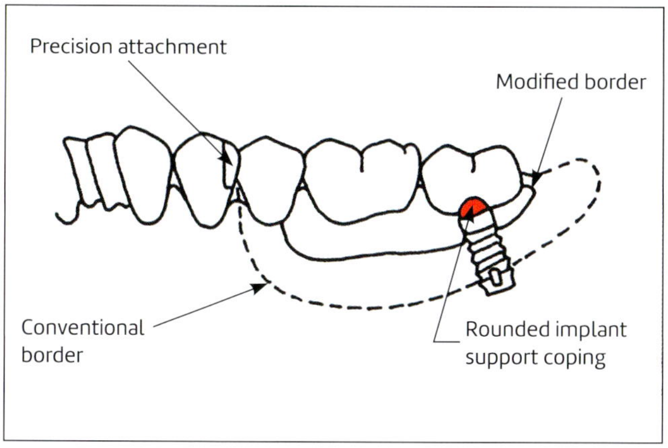

FIG 13-30 Modification of conventional denture borders with posterior implant support of Class I RPD.

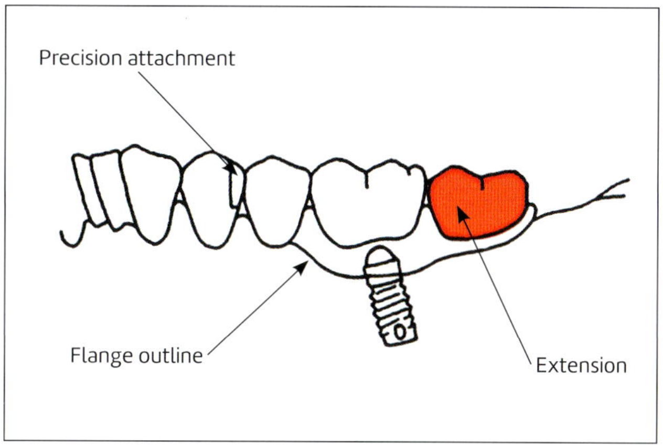

FIG 13-31 Posterior extension of one denture tooth beyond implant support.

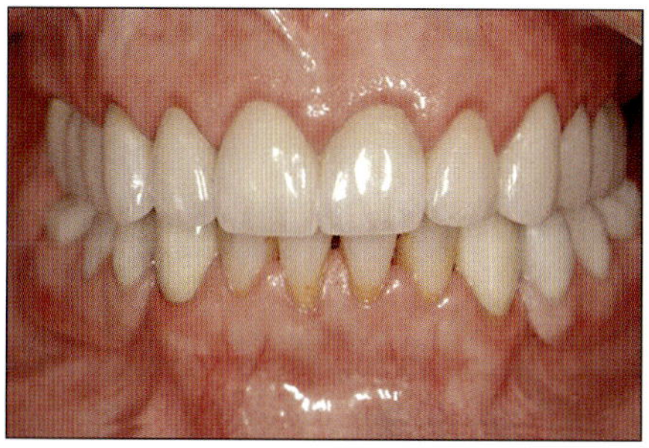

FIG 13-32 Posterior implants with OSO attachments facilitated the elimination of clasps.

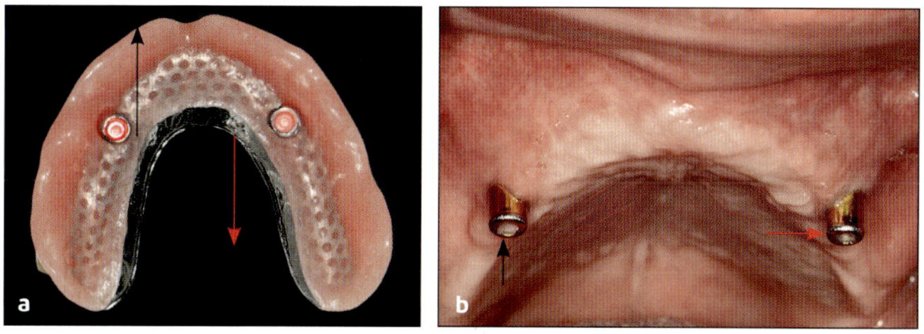

FIG 13-33 *(a)* Overdenture that rocks both anterior and posterior due to implant position. *(b)* Rocking of overdenture resulted in rapid wear of Locators at premolar sites.

a skeletal Class II malocclusion complete maxillary denture patient requires second molar contact yet the mandibular implant support is located at the first molar (Fig 13-31).

The next most commonly discussed position option for implants in a Class I arch is the premolar region, often the space adjacent to the canine.[6,7] The argument for placing the implant in this location is to eliminate anterior clasping. This again demonstrates the general hyperfocus on clasping rather than on support and stability. Placing an implant at a first premolar location does little to improve the situation and in fact can be detrimental to long-term outcomes. The statistics in favor of and clinical experience with Class III partial dentures is far superior to that of Class I partial dentures. The opportunity to make a case Class III should always be chosen over eliminating the anterior clasps. This is all the more obvious having seen the previous examples and knowing that the anterior clasping can be eliminated when the posterior implants are designed accordingly (Fig 13-32). Surgically, the placement of an implant just distal to the last remaining tooth is often as complicated as the second molar site. The risk of damage to the adjacent tooth or of having a significant discrepancy in gingival margin heights is real. The mental foramen, just apical to this general area, reduces the available fixture length and increases the risk of nerve damage in mandibular situations. Because the bone around the remaining canine must be preserved, the first premolar implant will often be placed as shallow as possible. This leaves less space for all of the necessary components, unless a full crown contour is planned. Then there is the postsurgical recession on the adjacent abutment tooth to be concerned about. Any root recession in the proximal area adds to an already heightened caries risk. This highlights once again the concern over continued disease and tooth loss. Despite the best efforts of patients and dentists, there are situations where disease will continue and the remaining teeth will be lost. If this occurs in a case that has had implants placed at the first premolar region, the result is a major complication for the now complete overdenture (Fig 13-33a). The inevitable anteroposterior rocking of the overdenture on the first premolar implants, positioned neither anterior nor posterior within the arch, often becomes a chronic problem solved only by burying the implants and losing retention, or adding additional implants (Fig 13-33b).

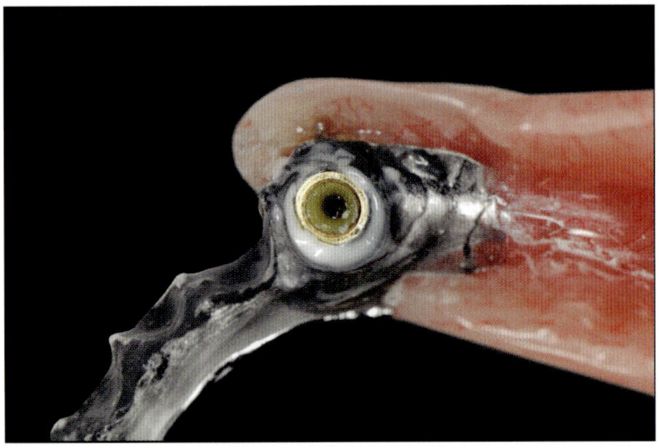

FIG 13-34 OSO attachment selected for terminal abutment canine.

If an implant is positioned as a terminal abutment for a Class I situation, it would make sense to consider stress relief to allow for soft tissue support (Fig 13-34). A properly integrated implant, by definition, will not move. Not incorporating stress relief leaves an extensive lever arm, the same as with any cantilever from a terminal implant. Due to the risk of damage to the implant or screw, it seems best to design and fit the partial denture with the same philosophies as if the abutment were a natural tooth. If a full contour implant crown is used as a terminal abutment, this means functional relief of the casting. If an attachment is used, the more resilient examples, along with the usual attention to base fit and long-term management, would achieve stress relief. In contrast to this, if implants are placed at the second molar locations to modify the arch to a Class III situation, the anterior retentive components no longer need to offer any stress relief. The case is no longer tissue supported and therefore will not torque the anterior abutments to a significant degree. This is why attachments or conventional clasping can be used effectively, if they are needed at all, in the now Class III situation (see Figs 13-3 and 13-4).

The clinical experiences described here have a growing base of scientific support. An early case series from the University of Washington demonstrated the benefits of these distal implants.[1] An excellent multicenter prospective evaluation of patient satisfaction with implant-supported Class I partial dentures showed significant benefits with the distal implant concept.[3,4] Whether healing abutments or ball attachments were used, patient satisfaction was higher than with conventional partial dentures in the same arch. This group also found a preference for the prefabricated attachment abutment, ball attachments, over the simpler healing abutment design.[4] This particular study made a point to use the ball attachments for support as well as retention. This fact may partly explain the improved patient response. Similar positive responses to these concepts have been found by other authors as well.[8,9] The standardization of the clinical situations in RPD research is critical to maintain validity as numerous but various classifications tend to be included to increase the sample size. This makes it difficult for clinicians to draw reliable or relevant information from much of the published research on this topic.[10–13]

Decisions for Class III and V Situations

In general, adding implants for Class III situations is contraindicated when an RPD is planned. If implants are feasible, a fixed prosthesis should generally be discussed. While it can be argued that the implants would facilitate elimination of the anterior clasping, this is possible even without the aid of implants or attachments, as has been discussed throughout this book. This makes the additional expense and risk a questionable investment.

There are, however, tooth-bound situations where strategic implants are of great value. Recall Applegate's suggestion of the Kennedy Class V as a Class III with a very weak anterior abutment tooth. The common clinical scenario is when a canine is lost in an otherwise Class III Mod 1 arch. Per Applegate, this would then be a Class V Mod 1 arch. The obvious area of most concern, and probable location of failure, is the weak incisor that would have to function as a primary abutment. An implant, strategically placed at the missing canine, per Rule 9, would convert this arch back to a Class III Mod 1 arch (Figs 13-35a and 13-35b). The improvement in force management and distribution would significantly improve the long-term prognosis of the arch (Fig 13-35c). This strategic use must be distinctly contrasted with the same placement location when there are no posterior teeth present. As mentioned in the introduction, replacement of a canine with an implant when the only other remaining teeth are the incisors and contralateral

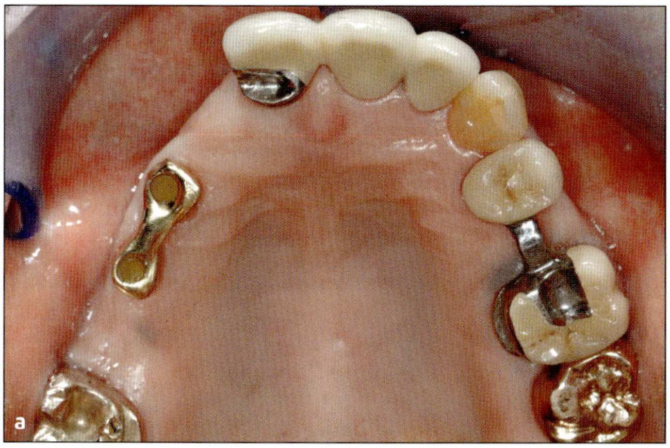
a

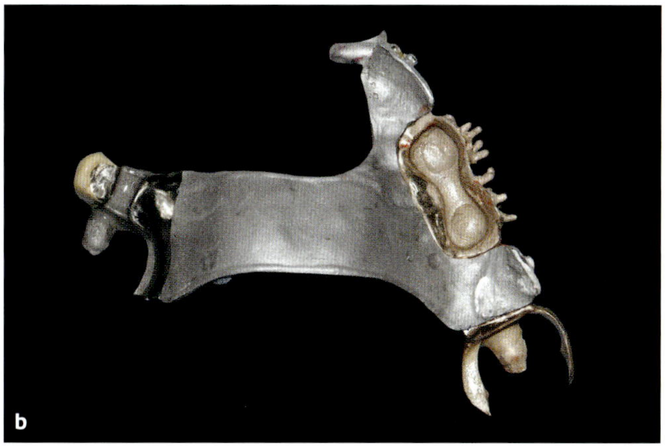
b

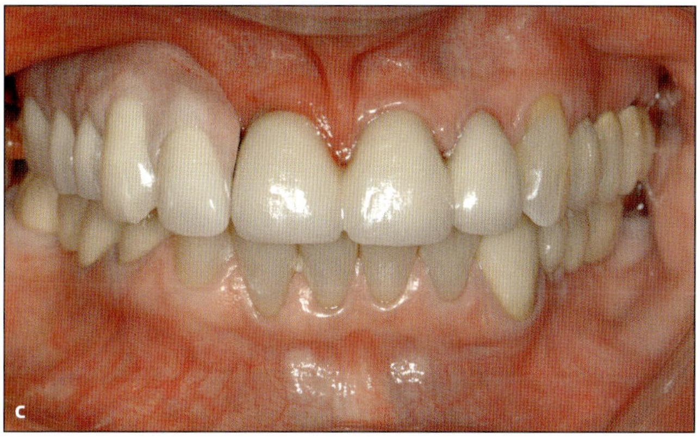
c

FIG 13-35 *(a)* Implants within the edentulous segment, per Rule 9, create a Class III arch. Note the splinted weak anterior abutment. *(b)* Custom overlay for maxillary left second premolar and custom housing for implant bar create maximum stability, reducing clasping. *(c)* Protecting the weak incisor and maximizing support are key to longevity with Class V arches opposing fixed dentitions.

canine does not seem to provide a significant improvement in long-term prognosis compared with a tissue-supported implant-retained overdenture. That being said, reports of implants in these situations have demonstrated positive outcomes,[11,13] at least in the majority of situations.

Decisions for Class IV and Extreme Situations

Class IV situations missing only the incisors generally do not allow enough space to consider implant support. Likewise, if implants are feasible, the fixed replacement of a fairly limited edentulous segment tends to be the preferred option. This explains the gradual reduction in prevalence of Class IV partial dentures as implants have become more common. When the fixed option is cost prohibitive, the rotational path partial denture, without implant support, is an excellent alternative. Adding implants would complicate the rotational placement design and would generally not be needed to support the small segment anyway.

That being said, when the Class IV defect becomes more significant in size and scope, implant support can be a vital means to maintain what remains of the residual ridge. If the Class IV situation involves missing posterior teeth, for example a patient with only molars remaining, the mechanics of the prosthesis are similar to that of a Class I, but in reverse. The edentulous span, exclusively in the anterior region, results in a lengthy cantilever. To make this situation worse, the edentulous segment is often opposed by mandibular anterior teeth (Fig 13-36a).

The strategic placement of an implant stop or multiple implants and a bar will protect the delicate anterior residual ridge during loading (Fig 13-36b). In addition, despite the use of ideal guiding planes, these larger defects will suffer from lack of stability and retention when the remaining abutments are far from the prosthetic anterior teeth (Fig 13-36c). Remember that without the implant support, some form of stress relief would otherwise be indicated to prevent overloading the remaining teeth holding the cantilever. While limited space is a contraindication with conventional Class IVs, the larger defects where implants are indicated tend to have significant interocclusal distance (Fig 13-36d). When vertical space is still an issue, it is best to use the prefabricated abutment as a support-only option.

The location of the implant or implants in these situations is often determined by the surgical limitations. This is especially true when the space is a cleft palate situation

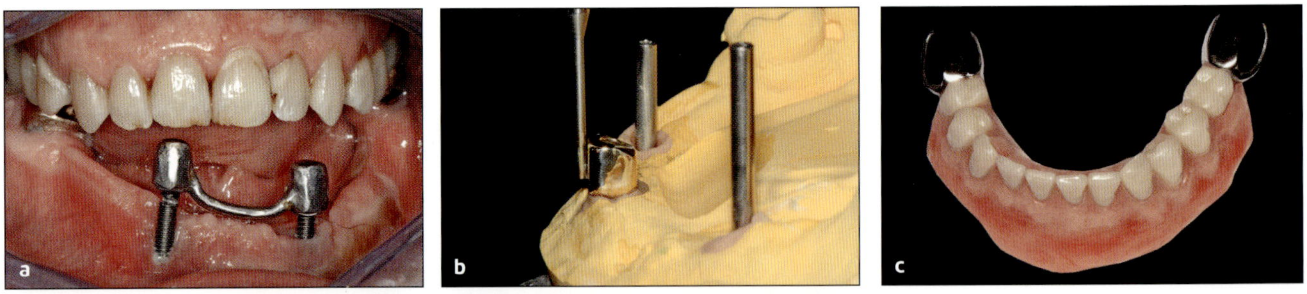
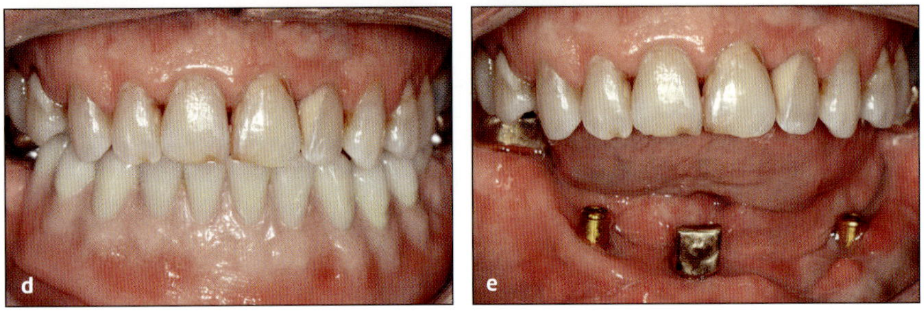

FIG 13-36 *(a)* Failing mandibular staple will leave a large anterior defect; healthy molars remain. Class I mechanics in reverse? *(b)* With only molars remaining, implants will support the anterior segment. *(c)* Without anterior implants, this RPD would lack adequate support. *(d)* Partial dentures can facilitate reconstruction of extensive defects. *(e)* Distribution of implants will allow conversion to a complete fixed or removable prosthesis should the teeth fail.

and the anterior maxilla was never fully formed or formed at all. When there is the opportunity to choose, it seems logical to place an implant as far to the end of the cantilever as possible, while still having the abutment design of choice fit within the planned dimensions of the prosthesis (Fig 13-36e). In a typical arch, this would mean the central incisor location. If a bar is planned, then the space between the implants must be considered. Remember, however, that if canine sites are selected, the bar often cannot connect the implants in a straight line. The curve of the arch form would cause a straight bar to cross over the anterior palate and disrupt normal contour and speech.

These large defects, and others like extreme Class II or unilateral situations, require thorough consideration before implants are placed. Even greater attention to the principles discussion in chapter 1 is required to avoid putting a patient through repeated reconstruction efforts. Consider that many of the already rare instances where maintaining a limited number of natural teeth is indicated are elderly patients with a limited life expectancy. These patients are normally high disease risks and poor surgical candidates. Add to this the maxillofacial segment of patients, some of whom have had radiation therapy, and another pool of potential situations is contraindicated for implants. The point of these facts is to once again reinforce the need to consider the cost-benefit analysis of implant placement for RPD therapy in comparison to the lower disease risk and very successful implant therapy available for the completely edentulous situation.

The number of implants in these situations is a critical question. In general, the larger the defect, the greater the necessity for multiple implants (Fig 13-37). A good basic planning philosophy is to consider that an arch has four corners, just as a Class III partial denture has four widely spaced abutment areas. In terms of specific teeth, if strong second molars and canines are present, the arch has quite a good amount of available support. When considering a large defect, ask how many corners are missing adequate support. If the arch is an extreme Class II arch (missing all teeth on one side), then the arch is missing two corners, so a minimum of two implants—properly spaced—are therefore required. Failure to restore support in all four corners leaves fulcrum lines and base extensions that will complicate force management (Fig 13-38). This is little more than using our ability to modify Kennedy's classification to our advantage.

Another major consideration in these limited abutment arches, more so than in others, is what would happen should any of the remaining natural teeth be lost. The implants being placed in these complicated situations absolutely must be placed with the knowledge that future edentulation is a real possibility (Fig 13-39a). The position must therefore allow adequate overdenture or fixed complete denture therapy in the future. If the abutments planned for use under the RPD could also serve under a future complete overdenture, a significant service and long-term cost savings has been provided to the patient (Fig 13-39b). While typically it is the teeth that are most at risk, some poorly controlled situations may contribute to the failure of the implants themselves (Fig 13-39c). When this occurs, it is tempting to wonder if the implants would have survived under different conditions.

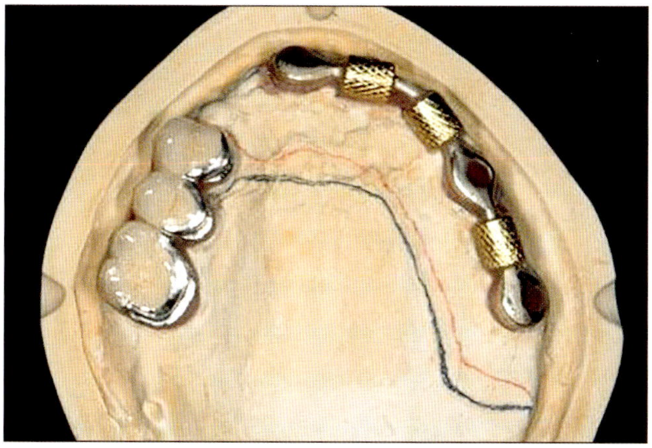

FIG 13-37 Extreme Class II modified with three implants and a bar to become fully supported.

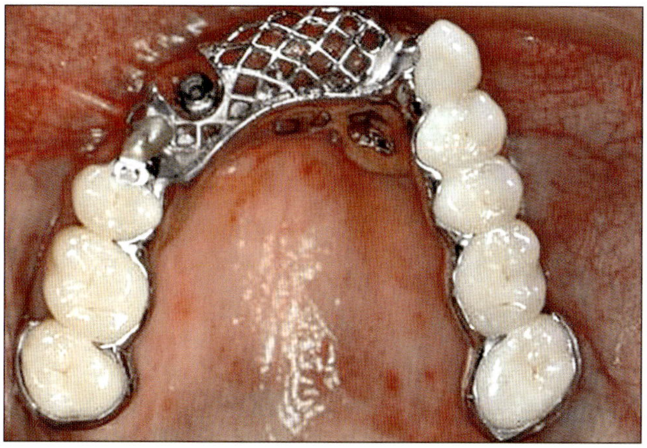

FIG 13-38 A single implant is placed to support the missing canine "corner."

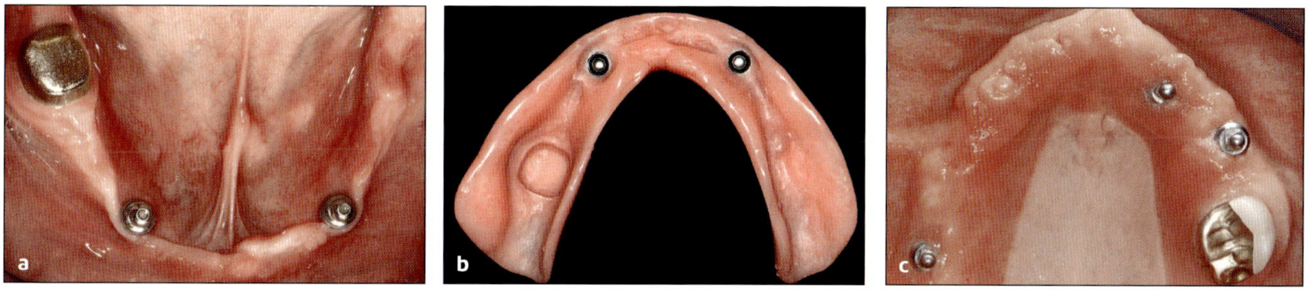

FIG 13-39 *(a)* Anterior implants placed 15 years prior in patient with ectodermal dysplasia. The mandibular left second molar was recently extracted. *(b)* Overdenture design, with teeth and implants, allows conversion when teeth are lost. OSO attachments are used for this reason. *(c)* Single molar complicates function on what was a total of five implants.

Surgical Considerations

In almost all cases, the implant will be placed at the beginning of treatment. After healing, the remaining natural tooth abutments are modified prior to implant abutment fabrication in order to maximize the implant position and angulation that was provided (Fig 13-40). There are situations where it is advisable to construct the definitive RPD first and then retrofit the implant under the prosthesis. The indication for this approach is when conditions preclude the construction of quality provisional prostheses or when continued use of an existing and ill-fitting prosthesis might compromise the surgical aspect of implant placement and integration. There are special design and construction implications for this approach in that the framework must allow enough space below the meshwork to insert the implant and its abutment under the completed partial denture. This decision is made by the clinician and surgeon before treatment begins, and the laboratory is instructed as to the relief, both vertical and horizontal, necessary to raise the mesh off the tissue enough for the planned implant abutment (Fig 13-41). Obviously, this approach is only feasible when there has been extensive resorption of the edentulous area and works best when a prefabricated abutment is being used as support only.

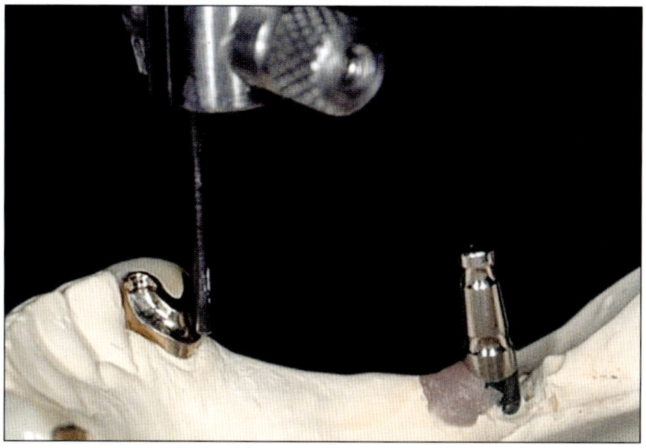

FIG 13-40 The surveyed crown is designed to be parallel with the distal implant.

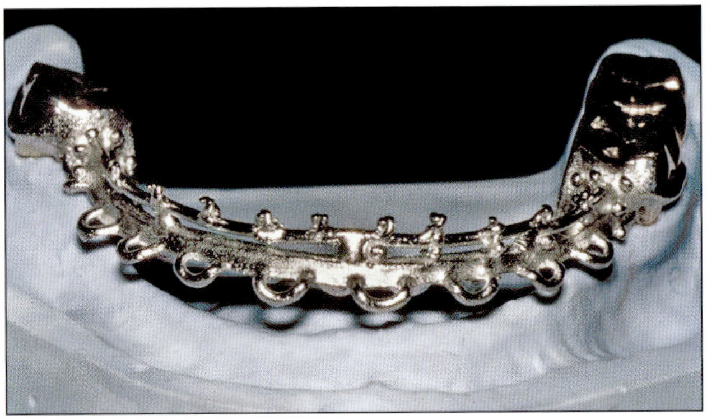

FIG 13-41 Raised mesh allows space for future implant support in the anterior region.

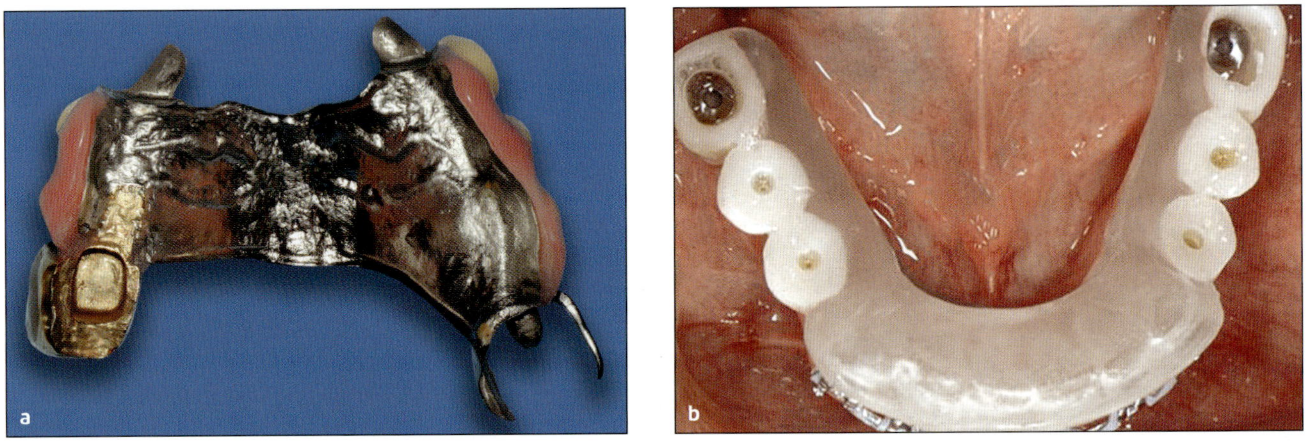

FIG 13-42 *(a)* An interproximally placed implant complicated this coping design. *(b)* A surgical guide facilitated accurate mesiodistal positioning. Future conversion to fixed partial dentures is made possible.

Failure to guide the surgical placement of the implant, at least in some fashion, can lead to major prosthetic complications. Despite having a denture base overlaying the area, the mesiodistal position of the implant is important. Placement in an interproximal area can limit the available space for coping and attachments that may be the preferred design (Fig 13-42a). Centering the implant according to an ideal tooth position will allow easier conversion to a fixed prosthesis should this become possible or preferred in the future (Fig 13-42b). The buccolingual positioning of the implant is considered important to keep the implant aligned with the expected direction of masticatory force. From a prosthetic perspective, an implant located far off-center to the buccal or lingual has the potential to alter the denture base or even tooth contour. The greater the degree of skeletal malocclusion, the greater the need for an accurate diagnostic arrangement to determine the relationship of the future prosthetic teeth to the available bone.

How the implant will be designed to connect to the partial will determine how critical the angulation will be. This will in turn determine how much effort is required to ensure accurate implant positioning. There are several surgical guide designs, digital or analog, that can assist the surgeon with accurate implant angulation (Fig 13-43). The topic of surgical procedures and guides is beyond the scope of this book. For the most part, as long as the implant abutment is not expected to carry an attachment component, the angulation of the implant relative to the remaining abutments is not critical. However, for those situations

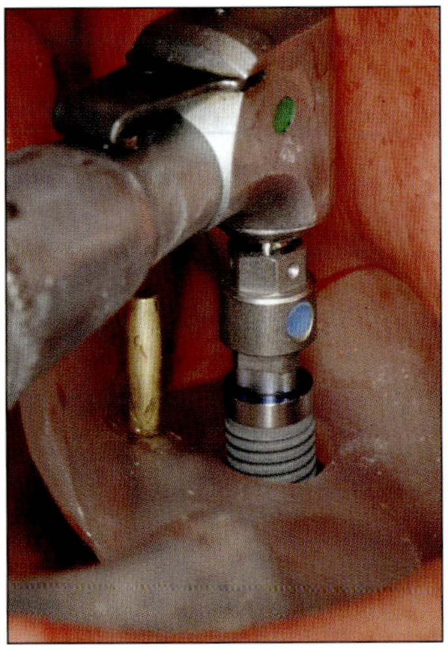

FIG 13-43 Surgical guide with angulation reference pin matching the planned path of insertion.

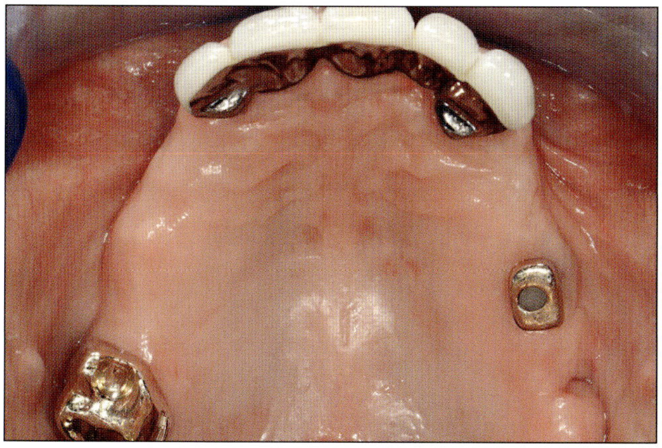

FIG 13-44 A pneumatized sinus and lack of bone were the reasons for first molar implant position. This is now a Class V arch.

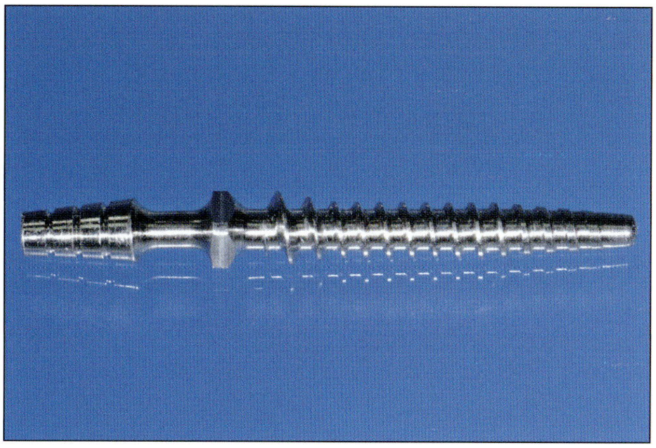

FIG 13-45 A 1.8-mm-diameter solid-body implant designed for provisional use. Many similar designs < 3 mm in diameter exist.

where a prefabricated attachment abutment is planned, the angulation is absolutely essential (see Figs 13-36 and 13-40). If the fixture is not placed in the long axis of the remaining abutments, parallel to the path of insertion, its attachment may not engage. Even if it does, it will suffer from rapid wear and degradation. Knowing this, the newest version of the Locator system, R-Tx (Zest Dental Solutions), claims to provide the ability to engage up to 30 degrees off-center for a total 60-degree convergence range. This is double the extended range inserts in its traditional design. Regardless of whether this attachment will reliably engage at these ranges, the wear of the insert and abutment will be increased. This complication is partially mitigated by placing the implant first, with an eye to matching the path of insertion, and then completing the mouth preparations to match the angulation of the implant (see Fig 13-40). Because it is technically very challenging, and often impossible, to ideally match the angulation of a second molar implant to existing abutments as far anterior as the canine, designs relying on prefabricated attachments with a limited range of function should be avoided.

Unfortunately, because of long-term ridge resorption, finding sufficient bone in the distal extension base area—where we often prefer to place the implant—becomes a major impediment. While extensive bone grafting is often possible, the additional cost and morbidity is often not indicated. Accommodations in implant position must be considered if the alternative is no implant at all (Fig 13-44). One way to help avoid compromised positioning, or to allow placement at all, is to use smaller implant dimensions.[14–16] Traditional studies with machined-surface, straight-bodied, external hex implants showed that implant loss is proportional to the length of the implants used, with special concern for the 7-mm and shorter implants. These studies have evaluated the implants for lateral stability and retention as well as vertical support. With improved surface design and chemistry, even shorter fixtures might now be used in some situations. The smallest of these are intended for extraoral maxillofacial use and measure 2.5 to 3.5 mm in length. These implants have been used for some time and have shown some potential for intraoral use.[14] While shorter, these types of implants are 3 to 5 mm in diameter and therefore still require significant width to the residual bone. Thin-ridge situations require narrow-diameter implants if more extreme grafting or ridge-splitting procedures are not advised. Research into these narrow designs is inconclusive at this point, and considering the extensive number of possible variables with RPD clinical care, ideal comparisons are not expected soon. One point of note on narrow-diameter fixtures is that diameters below the 3-mm threshold are almost always solid-body implants. This means there is no abutment screw channel. While some designs allow the replacement of a prefabricated attachment abutment, many platforms are simply solid abutments extending supragingivally (Fig 13-45). These designs are not only weaker, due to the narrow implant body, but they limit the prosthetic design flexibility. For these reasons, they are rarely considered for long-term applications. Advocates of these much smaller-diameter solid-body implants would point out the lower surgical risk involved as well as a greatly reduced surgical overhead cost that can be passed on to the patient. At the very least, the large variety of implant designs gives clinicians options. Certainly, if the fixtures are to be used for vertical support only, perhaps the shorter and narrower implants may suffice?

Preplanning implant position is clearly essential. However, experienced restorative dentists are realizing that the number of debilitated dentitions requiring reconstruction, in whom dental implants are already present, is growing. This means that preplanning implant position may not be

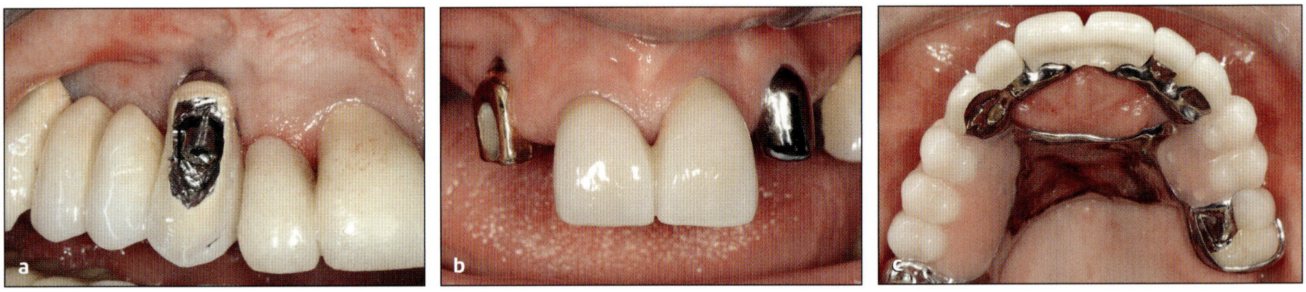

FIG 13-46 *(a)* Steep facial inclination of implant used for failed fixed reconstruction. *(b)* Reangulation of implant no. 6 to match path of insertion and coping on no. 11. *(c)* Failed fixed reconstruction converted to RPD with minimal surgical intervention. Overlay of root at no. 2, prefabricated Locator abutment on previous implant at no. 3, coping on previous implant at no. 6, splinted nos. 8 and 9, coping on no. 11, and surveyed crown on no. 14 all support a laser-welded RPD made with custom housings at nos. 6 and 7 as well as nos. 10 and 11. See also Figs 12-21, 12-28, and 12-29.

an option. Rather, the various customized designs discussed in this book will be more frequently necessary to manage difficult implant angulations and positions from failed previous treatments (Fig 13-46).

As this chapter explained, we have come to believe that the best use of a dental implant with an RPD is as a stop. This relatively simple modification helps manage what is perhaps the most challenging aspect of RPD therapy, the mechanical difference between soft and hard tissue support, seen most commonly with a distal extension base. The use of implants in conjunction with RPDs is no longer new or uncharted territory. Just as with the ever-changing collection of attachment systems, new implants, surgical techniques, and components will become available. However, the principles used to incorporate them into RPD therapy is not expected to change. As long as they are used in conjunction with thorough mouth preparation of soft and hard tissues, employ precisely fitting castings, and are cared for with regular recall and appropriate maintenance, we can be confident that they will improve the quality of RPD therapy. However, to expect them to be a solution for all our problems without this level of careful adherence to basic principles is foolhardy.

References

1. Mitrani R, Brudvik JS, Phillips KM. Posterior implants for distal extension removable prostheses: A retrospective study. Int J Periodontics Restorative Dent 2003;23:353–359.
2. Kaufmann R, Friedli M, Hug S, Mericske-Stern R. Removable dentures with implant support in strategic positions followed for up to 8 years. Int J Prosthodont 2009;22:233–242.
3. Payne AGT, Tawse-Smith A, Wismeijer D, De Silva RK, Ma S. Multicentre prospective evaluation of implant-assisted mandibular removable partial dentures: Surgical and prosthodontic outcomes. Clin Oral Implants Res 2017;28:116–125.
4. Wismeijer D, Tawse-Smith A, Payne AGT. Multicentre prospective evaluation of implant-assisted mandibular bilateral distal extension removable partial dentures: Patient satisfaction. Clin Oral Implants Res 2013;24:20–27.
5. French D, Naito M, Linke B. Interproximal contact loss in a retrospective cross-sectional study of 4325 implants: Distribution and incidence and the effect on bone loss and peri-implant soft tissue. J Prosthet Dent 2019;122:108–114.
6. Jensen C, Raghoebar GM, Kerdijk W, Meijer HJA, Cune MS. Implant-supported mandibular removable partial dentures: Patient-based outcome measures in relation to implant position. J Dent 2016;55:92–98.
7. Jensen C, Speksnijder CM, Raghoebar GM, Kerdijk W, Meijer HJA, Cune MS. Implant-supported mandibular removable partial dentures: Functional, clinical, and radiographical parameters in relation to implant position. Clin Implant Dent Res 2017;19:432–439.
8. Suzuki Y, Kono K, Shimpo H, Sato Y, Ohkubo C. Clinical evaluation of implant-supported removable partial dentures with a stress-breaking attachment. Implant Dent 2017;26:516–523.
9. Ohkubo C, Kobayashi M, Suzuki Y, Hosoi T. Effect of implant support on distal-extension removable partial dentures: In vivo assessment. Int J Oral Maxillofac Implants 2008;23:1095–1101.
10. Park JH, Lee JY, Shin SW, Kim HJ. Effect of conversion to implant-assisted removable partial denture in patients with mandibular Kennedy classification I: A systematic review and meta-analysis. Clin Oral Implants Res 2020;31:360–373.
11. Bortolini S, Natali A, Franchi M, Coggiola A, Consolo U. Implant-retained removable partial dentures: An 8-year retrospective study. J Prosthodont 2011;20:168–172.
12. Mekawy NHE, El-Negoly SAE, Grawish ME, El-Hawary YM. Intracoronal mandibular Kennedy Class I implant-tooth supported removable partial overdenture: A 2-year multicenter prospective study. Int J Oral Maxillofac Implants 2012;27:677–683.
13. Mijiritsky E, Lorean A, Mazor Z, Levin L. Implant tooth-supported removable partial denture with at least 15-year long-term follow-up. Clin Implant Dent Relat Res 2015;17:917–922.
14. Minoretti R, Triaca A, Saulacic N. The use of extraoral implants for distal-extension removable dentures: A clinical evaluation up to 8 years. Int J Oral Maxillofac Implants 2009;24:1129–1137.
15. Threeburuth W, Aunmeungtong W, Khongkhunthian P. Comparison of immediate-load mini dental implants and conventional-size dental implants to retain mandibular Kennedy Class I removable partial dentures: A randomized clinical trial. Clin Implant Dent Relat Res 2018;20:785–792.
16. Bellia E, Audenino G, Ceruti P, Bassi F. Clinical assessment of short implants retaining removable partial dentures: 4-year follow-up. Int J Oral Maxillofac Implants 2020;35:207–213.

FRAMEWORKS FOR IMPLANT OVERDENTURES

14

If we can make it, they can break it.

As Dr Jeffrey E. Rubenstein was apt to say to numerous uninitiated graduate prosthodontics residents, "If we can make it, they can break it." This piece of treatment planning advice is perhaps most applicable in removable prosthodontics where most prostheses are resin based. Unfortunately, fracture of denture bases is a common complication. It is even more common in overdentures due to the stress concentration areas created by the abutments.

While this is a textbook on RPDs, the modern techniques described within also apply to edentulous patients with dental implants. If we follow the modified Kennedy classification described in chapters 3 and 13, then an implant overdenture with fixtures at both mandibular canines, using individual stud attachments, would be classified as Class I Mod 1. There appears to be no reason why the functional movements of a removable device with shared hard and soft tissue support would be significantly different in these instances. Certainly, the management of the implants themselves is a lengthy conversation, but once determined, the design and use of the removable prosthesis itself becomes very much like an RPD.

Material Advantages

Co-Cr, Ni-Cr, titanium, and the other alloys used to cast an RPD framework may be used for overdenture frames as well. Obviously, their great advantage over the all-resin base is one of strength and thereby a reduction in thickness. Thin metal will tend to be more comfortable for the patient, as there will be less volume of material and thus a less objectionable contour. This ability to reduce thickness is critical to manage the lack of space caused by malpositioned dental implants or their many components. The fit of a metal casting is also considered more accurate due the inherent processing shrinkage with heat-polymerized, nonmilled acrylic resins. Traditional mucostatic techniques relied on metal castings for a more ideal tissue-base relationship. As will be discussed with bar and clip cases, this allows for an opportunity to manage the abutment-frame interface much the same way as the tooth-frame interface in conventional RPDs. Metal is also far more hygienic than traditional acrylic resin due to its lack of porosity. This results in less plaque retention and can be a critical factor in maintaining delicate peri-implant tissue health. This tissue tends to be more susceptible to inflammation when debilitated mouths lack the keratinized tissue present around teeth.

From the standpoint of practical clinical techniques, a major advantage of a metal base is that the retentive attachments, whatever they may be, can be joined to the base as soon as the fit of the base has been verified. This allows the base to have its final stability and retention while maxillomandibular relationship records are made and a trial evaluation completed. Not only will this provide

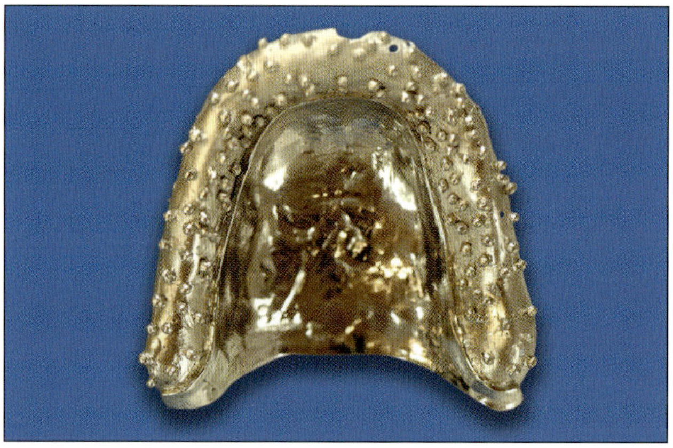

FIG 14-1 Typical metal base casting design.

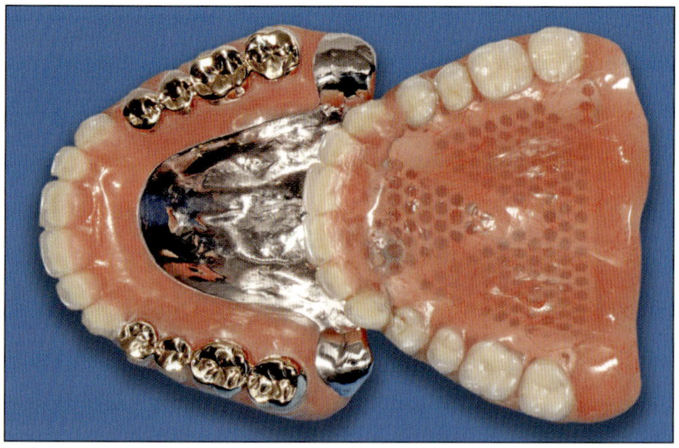

FIG 14-2 Metal base on the *left* and internal metal reinforcement on the *right*.

more accurate results, but the patients realize the benefits provided by the implants even before the prosthesis is completed. Experienced clinicians also realize significant chairside efficiencies as the aforementioned advantages occur. There is no doubt that these benefits and savings are worth the relatively minor additional cost.

Castings for Complete Dentures

Going back to the era of the swaged gold plate, metal bases for complete dentures have been a special but universal component of prosthodontics. Many alloys have been used in their construction; those mentioned earlier as well as aluminum are well documented in the literature. The form of the bases has changed over time, with metal coverage past the ridge crest, bead retention, and a lingual external finish line now considered routine (Fig 14-1). In this design, the base includes the posterior palatal seal, and it extends just to the point where buccal undercuts begin. Some feel that the posterior seal should be in resin so it can be relined if the final seal is inadequate. Others would say that if you can't capture that area accurately, you shouldn't be doing this level of prosthodontic care. For those concerned about being unable to reline this type of denture, it is obvious that the denture-bearing tissue must be mature before considering this option. While the denture cannot be relined, it certainly could be rebased. For designs not concerned with base thickness, castings composed of raised mesh that are for reinforcement only are possible, but even these tend to have the depth of the palate in metal only (Fig 14-2).

Details on specific impression techniques for these metal bases are plentiful in the complete denture literature. Because it relates to RPD castings, one point to be discussed here is the management of the external finishing line. In almost every instance, the placement of the external finish line is guided primarily by the position of the prosthetic teeth. If the finish line is too far coronal, the joint between metal and acrylic will be distorted. Specifically, it will either be an undercut in the resin contour, a forced narrowing of the denture tooth, or a situation in which the resin will overlay the polished metal surface. The first two are detrimental to the feel and function of the denture, and overlaying the metal will result in leakage and peeling of the resin after a short period of time.

To avoid this, a trial tooth arrangement should be completed prior to waxing of the framework pattern. In most instances, this does not require additional chairside procedures but will require careful laboratory transfers. The critical evaluation location will be the lingual contour of the prosthetic teeth in relation to the contour of the palatal ridge. To facilitate this evaluation, a matrix is made from light-cured composite in order to suspend the prosthetic teeth over the ridge after the trial base and wax has been removed.[1] This type of indexing was used by laboratory technicians in the 1990s to assist with the proper contouring of implant-supported fixed complete dentures. Used for several decades now at the University of Washington, this style of index is typically called a *spider* due to its distinctive appearance (Fig 14-3). Traditional buccal putty matrices tend to do a poor job of retaining the prosthetic teeth. The spider, as it is made out of rigid composite, is often more reliable and stable.

Because the trial evaluation included a final wax-up, there should not be deep undercuts around the teeth. This, combined with lubrication and careful placement of the occlusal/incisal bar of the spider, prevents complete locking of the denture teeth within the composite. This occlusal bar is generally laid on after several vertical extensions have been positioned. These vertical "feet" extend into grooves cut in the land area of the definitive cast. By placing the bar on last, the pressure to blend the material does not result in excessive composite overlaying and thus locking into

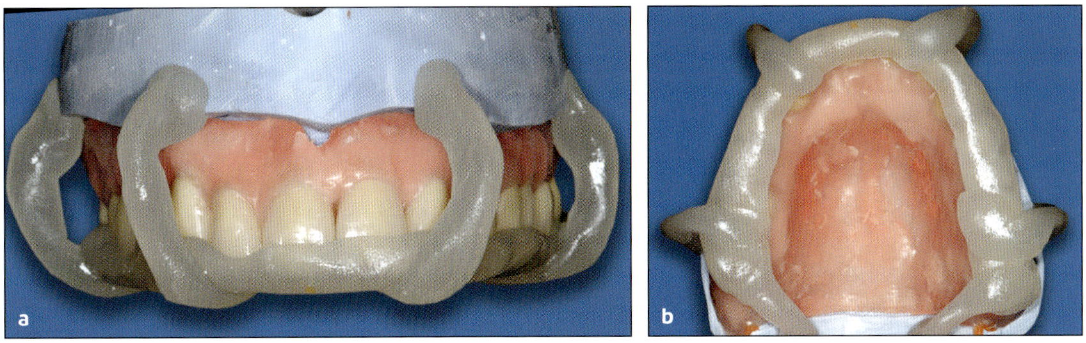

FIG 14-3 *(a and b)* Spider indexing.

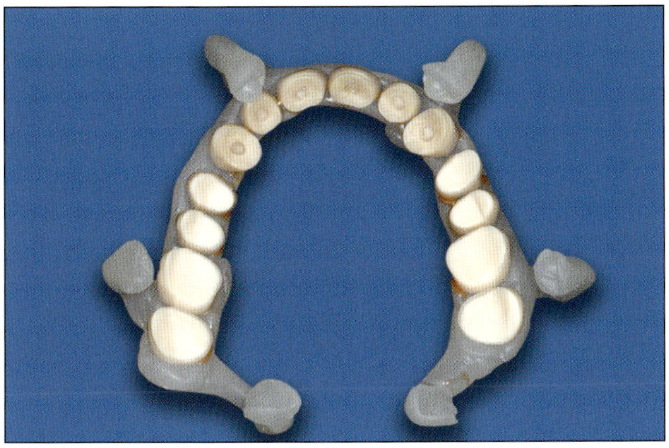

FIG 14-4 Spider after trial base removal.

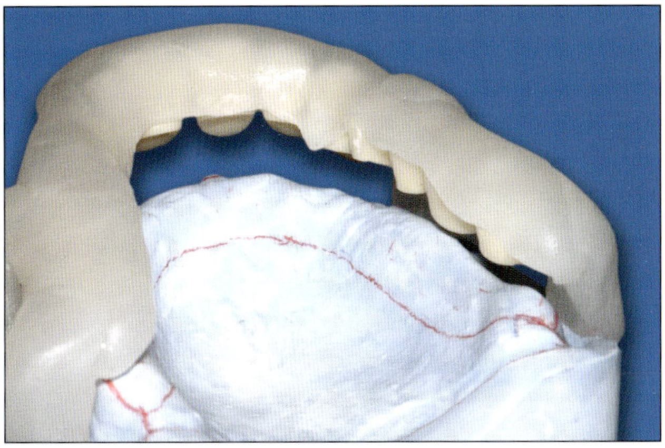

FIG 14-5 A spider back on the definitive cast to evaluate available space. The *red line* denotes the planned external finish line.

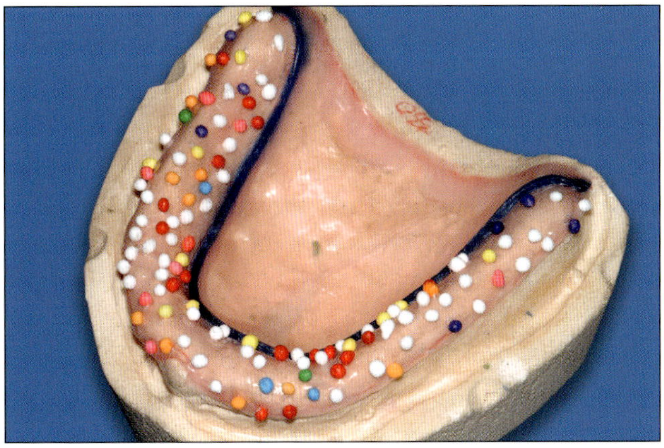

FIG 14-6 Base waxed on refractory, external finish line in *blue*. The indices are duplicated on the land area for the spider.

the heights of contour of teeth. After curing, the spider will typically lift off the cast and away from the wax on the trial base that was softened by the heat of the light. The prosthetic teeth, however, remain held within the occlusal/incisal overlay portion of the spider (Fig 14-4). After a bit of cleanup, the spider is placed back on the definitive cast without a trial base present. Any denture teeth that are loose can be retained more tightly with a small bit of sticky wax. The prosthetic tooth–edentulous anatomy relationship can now be visualized without interference (Fig 14-5). This technique is also valuable for implant space evaluations.

Positioning the external finishing line is now a matter of finding a point at which the lingual contour of the denture will flow smoothly from the denture teeth, apically to the depth of the palate. Because the acrylic requires some thickness and the goal for metal thickness is between 0.3 and 0.4 mm, the metal thickness at the point of the external finish line will increase (Fig 14-6). Ideally, this will occur at the same point at which the residual ridge begins to curve over the palatal crest. At this point, the increased thickness will not be noticed as a bump in contour but instead a smooth continuation once the resin is processed.

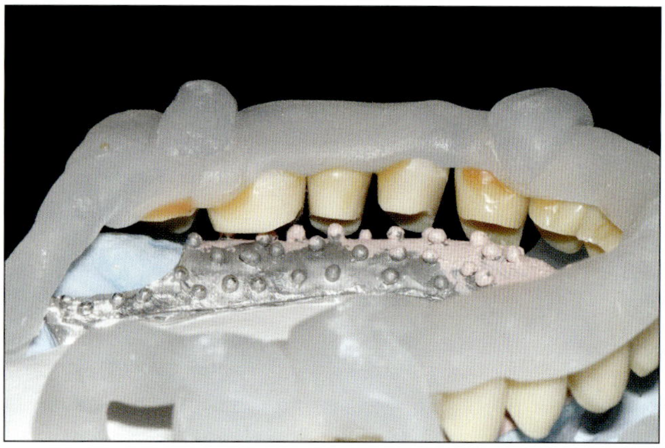

FIG 14-7 Confirmation of finish line prior to final waxing on metal base.

The exact dimensions and location of this transition are, as noted, dependent on the position of the teeth (Fig 14-7). In general, the more lingual the teeth are positioned, the more apical the external finish line will need to be, while the more buccal or facial the teeth are, the more coronal it should be. Situations where an excessive amount of residual ridge resorption has occurred will find a significant vertical distance from the prosthetic teeth to the palatal ridge crest. The metal finish line in these instances should not be brought as far coronal as it would be if the ridge were present, since the large increase in volume of metal will weigh down the denture and increase the negative effect of gravity on prosthesis retention.

The previous, now wax-free, trial base is placed back on the cast below the spider, and the planned location of the external finish line is drawn on it with a black marker. This should be enough for an experienced laboratory technician to accurately locate the finish line when the frame is waxed on the refractory cast. However, in challenging situations, it may be necessary to evaluate the finish line position on the refractory. The thickness of the waxed casting can also be evaluated if this is done. This is another advantage of the spider, as it can typically be positioned with a fair amount of accuracy on refractory casts when the land area, and therefore the indices, are properly duplicated. If necessary, the laboratory can easily trim away this land area after the wax-up and finish line position is confirmed.

Castings for Tissue-Supported Implant-Retained Overdentures

A consensus on effective and efficient terminology for implant prosthetics continues to be a challenge. The current definition of "implant-supported dentures" according to the *Glossary of Prosthodontic Terms*, 9th edition, is the following[2]:

> **Implant-supported denture:** Dental prosthesis, such as fixed complete denture, fixed partial denture, removable complete overdenture, removable partial overdenture, as well as maxillofacial prostheses, which can be supported and retained in part or whole by dental implants.

From the more advanced perspective of this textbook, this definition does not reflect the major differences in movement of various types of prostheses. Just as tooth-borne and tooth-tissue-borne RPDs are separated for design purposes, the clinician should separate implant prostheses the same way. The term *tissue-supported implant-retained overdenture* is therefore frequently used. For complete removable prostheses, this term immediately clarifies that the primary means of support will come from the soft tissue and that every attempt will be made to have the dental implants provide only retention. This idea, similar to that of Class I situations, is to limit the pressure applied to the small number of abutments present.

The risk of base fracture for implant overdentures cannot be understated (Fig 14-8). Between the limited amount of proprioception on the implants, the reduced thickness of overlying resin, and the stress concentration on a limited number of locations, the eventuality of overdenture base fracture must not be overlooked (Fig 14-9). Metal frameworks should be used in nearly all implant overdentures. The few situations where they may not be required are limited to frail edentulous patients who lack significant bite force and situations with dramatic interarch space resulting in a bulk of resin that provides the necessary strength. Even in these situations, a mandibular overdenture dropped on the bathroom floor by an elderly patient with poor dexterity is far more likely to survive when reinforced with a metal casting. Once an implant overdenture base fractures over or around one of the implants, it will never be the same. The

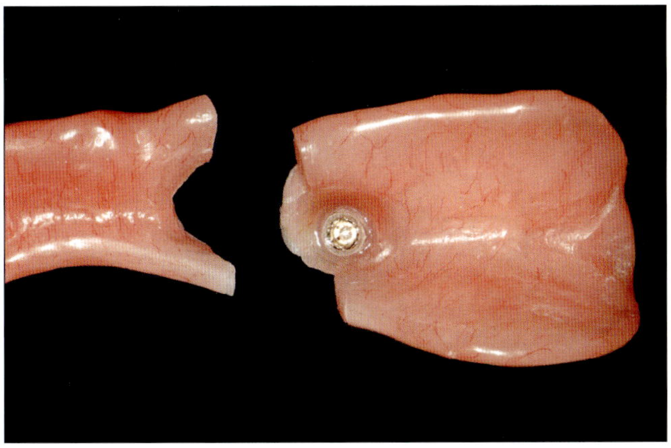

FIG 14-8 Base fracture through the thin area above a stud attachment. After repeated fractures, this overdenture was eventually remade with a reinforcing metal frame.

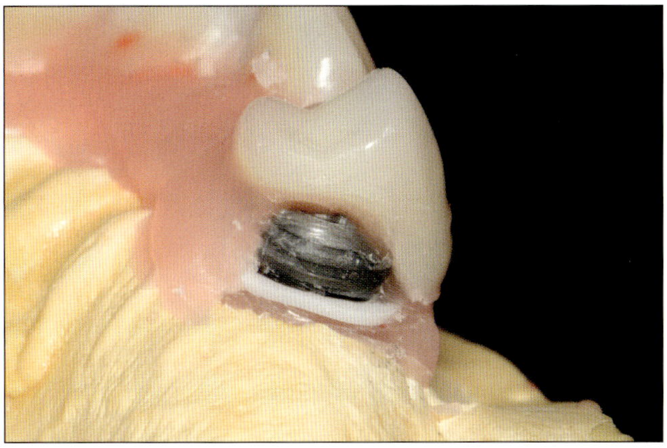

FIG 14-9 Demonstration of a limited space situation with spacer, housing, minimal wax, and denture tooth totaling 5 mm. This case requires a casting to prevent fracture and to protect the attachment housing.

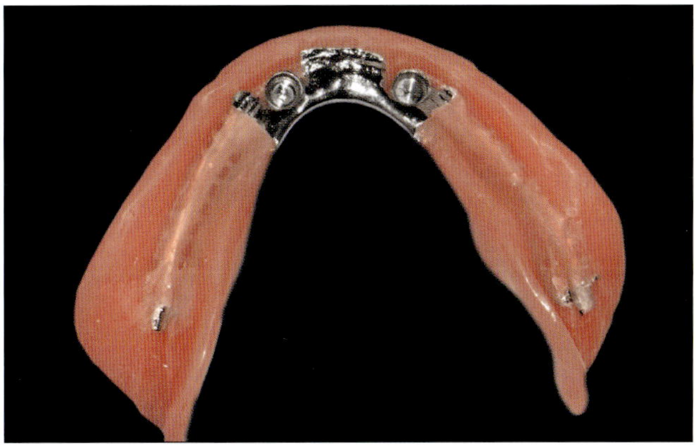

FIG 14-10 Intaglio view of a metal casting used to reinforce a mandibular tissue-supported implant-retained overdenture.

ability to accurately relate the pieces and maintain strength is limited. Considering the time, effort, and expense of the repairs, the best course of action in the long run is typically remaking the prosthesis with a metal casting, as should have been done in the first place.

Stud attachments

The decision to utilize stud attachments for tissue-supported implant-retained overdentures is most often one of convenience and cost. However, it is also defended as a means to incorporate some level of resiliency as described in chapter 11. With that in mind, the purpose of the casting in these situations is limited to providing strength, improved peri-implant tissue response, and a more effective means to pick up the attachment housings.

When designing this casting, a lingual bar shape is ideal for the limited space that often exists to the lingual of the mandibular anterior residual ridge. This design transitions easily with external finishing lines to the lingual and both distal extensions as the space opens into those areas. The surface area of exposed metal in this lingual bar area will help keep the invested framework in position after the wax is boiled out during processing. Bead retention with the metal base directly onto the anterior segment is, as noted, the most hygienic method. It also leaves the greatest amount of space available to set anterior teeth. The beads around the implant attachments can be raised slightly, if necessary, so that the vertical position of the housing is near the location of the actual union with resin. If the implant abutments have been selected correctly, this should not be more than a millimeter or two off the tissue. Once the metal base extends 3 mm distal to the implants, a transition is made to raised mesh retention in order to facilitate relining of the distal extensions just as with Class I situations (Fig 14-10).

Traditionally, implant overdenture cases were long-time edentulous patients who wanted to improve the function of their prostheses. In these situations, further significant residual ridge resorption was not likely for many years. As patients look to avoid the complete mandibular denture, it has become common to transition quickly from a few remaining anterior natural teeth to a mandibular

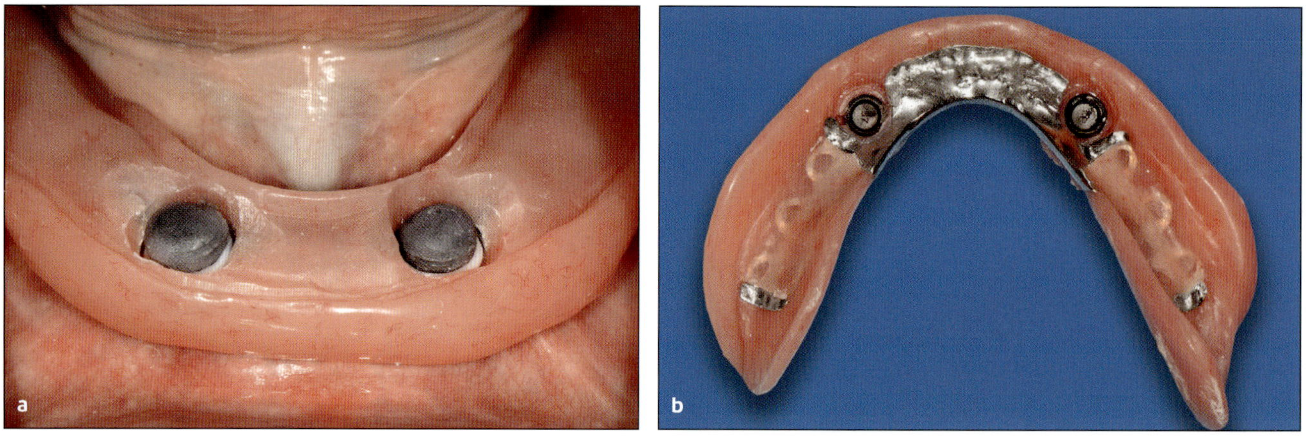

FIG 14-11 *(a)* Cameo view of processed base over casting. Pretreated Locator housings are placed over spacers and ready for pickup. *(b)* Intaglio of another processed base over casting. Note that the attachment housings have been picked up. Final records are now made.

overdenture using anterior implants. With this timing, extensive remodeling is to be expected, and the amount of metal base bead retention will need to be limited to a 2- to 3-mm horseshoe around the proximal and lingual surfaces of the implants. This will make the inevitable future reline or rebase less complicated, but will of course eventually result in acrylic around the implant abutments.

These frameworks are made after a definitive cast has been fabricated. The impression for this cast is made as if for a conventional denture. Either healing abutments or the definitive attachment abutments are in position for this impression with no need to record the implant-level connection. The general implant location and height are all that is necessary on the definitive cast. The metal casting is made first. This casting is fit to the definitive cast to make sure adequate distance exists around the implant abutments. Because the goal is tissue support, the metal of the casting must not contact the implant whatsoever. The only connection between the prosthesis and the implants will be through the resilient attachment or attachments. Once this is confirmed, the clinician can choose to add temporary denture bases for support so that records can be made. This would be a similar process to making records after an altered cast impression. However, this situation is ideal for the processed base technique. With the frame made and position confirmed, the laboratory can process the final resin base over and around the casting. The laboratory would therefore return a reinforced, completed overdenture base. This allows the clinician to make all further records and evaluations with an ideal tissue-base relationship and without any extra hassle of mobile trial bases or inaccurate tissue-base relationships during the pickup procedure. This processed base technique eliminates the need for any additional appointments because of the presence of the dental implants. The pickup of the attachment housings is made as described in chapter 11 with both metal-resin interfaces previously bonded under laboratory conditions (Fig 14-11). The gap for this final resin-to-resin pickup is managed simply the day of the records appointment by adjusting the resin to ensure that no base-abutment contact exists. The efficiency of this sequence should be obvious, as the need for a patient remount is often also eliminated. Further details on the processed base technique for complete dentures is available in the complete denture literature.

Bar and clip

When a bar-clip is used as the attachment for a tissue-supported implant-retained overdenture, there is an opportunity to manage lateral forces with the contact between the bar and the metal casting. Implants that are splinted by a bar are able to reliably withstand more force then individual implants. When compared with individual stud-type attachments, the components of the bar-clip tend to last significantly longer periods of time. This is partly due to the fact that the bar reduces off-angled dislodgement of the prosthesis, which tends to wear resilient components more rapidly.

Using the philosophies described throughout this text, there is an opportunity to create both support and stability on a specifically designed bar. First, the abutment portion of the bar is created somewhat more broadly so that an occlusal platform exists. Second, the lateral surfaces of the abutment portion of the bar are created as if they are guiding planes. The resulting form is that of a box. A typical bar complex is therefore two boxes connected by the bar of choice (Fig 14-12a). The coronal edges of the boxes are rounded slightly to allow easier duplication and fitting.

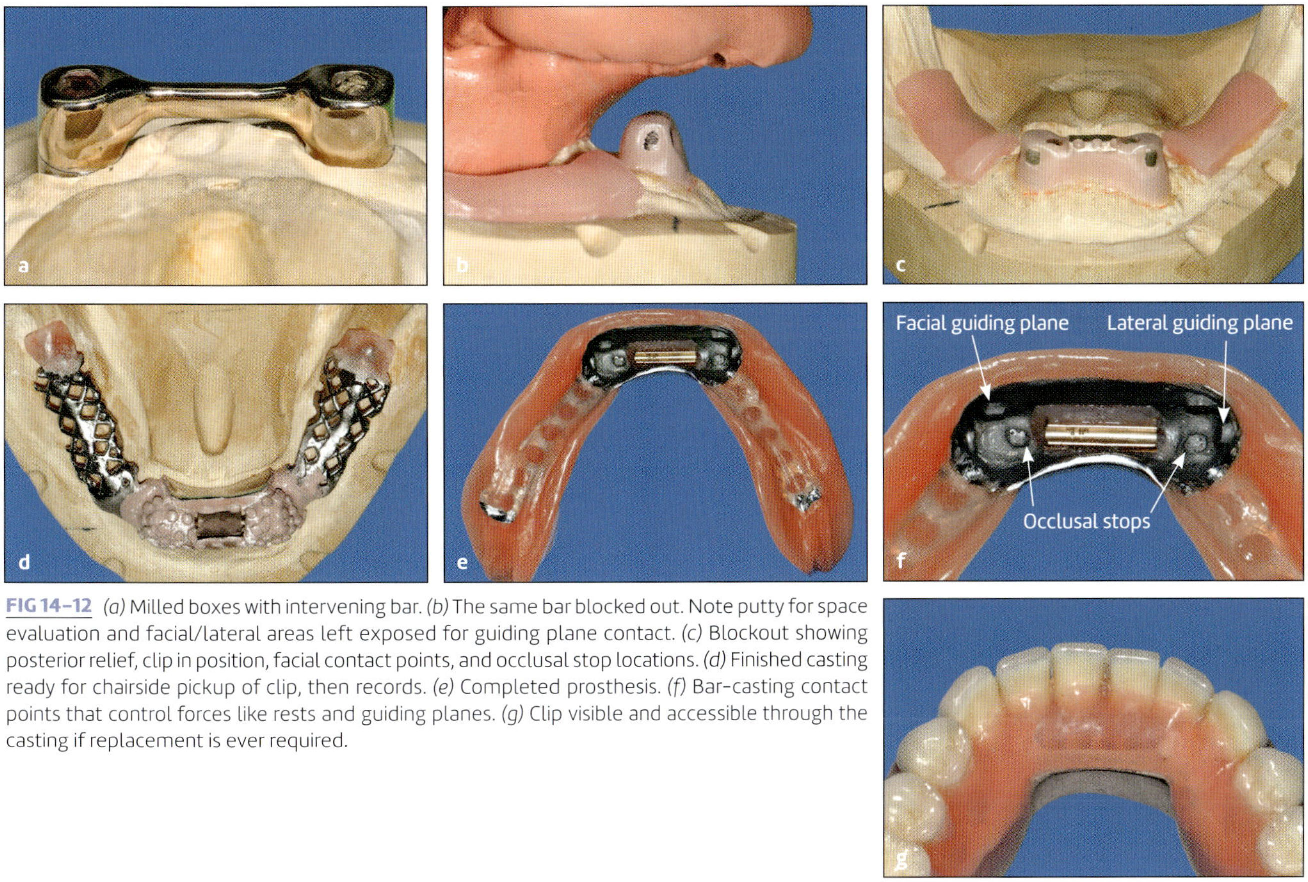

FIG 14-12 *(a)* Milled boxes with intervening bar. *(b)* The same bar blocked out. Note putty for space evaluation and facial/lateral areas left exposed for guiding plane contact. *(c)* Blockout showing posterior relief, clip in position, facial contact points, and occlusal stop locations. *(d)* Finished casting ready for chairside pickup of clip, then records. *(e)* Completed prosthesis. *(f)* Bar-casting contact points that control forces like rests and guiding planes. *(g)* Clip visible and accessible through the casting if replacement is ever required.

This shape allows support through vertical contact with the tops of the boxes and lateral stability through guiding plane contact on the opposing lateral surfaces (Fig 14-12b).

Just as described in chapter 11, the definitive cast is created to also have the actual implant bar present. The facial and distal portions of the two abutments are milled just as if they are guiding planes on surveyed crowns. The lingual surface is generally left slightly tapered to the gingival, and the mesial surfaces are tapered into the connection with the bar. The blockout of the cast allows for customization of the amount and exact location of the surface contact desired (Fig 14-12c). As demonstrated in Fig 11-17, when discussing semiprecision attachments, the goal is to allow rotation of the bilateral distal extension areas of the overdenture in the anteroposterior plane. This is allowed by only using the guiding plane contact on the lateral surfaces of the properly aligned and milled bar. The facial guiding plane contact is present to resist distal displacement of the prosthesis but will "lift" when the functional forces of mastication are placed on the posterior teeth. It is important to not contact the lingual surface of the bar, as this would lock and create a bilateral cantilever that would eventually harm the bar or implants. The gingival taper and blockout of the lingual area ensures that no binding will occur on the lingual of the abutments.

The casting, once made, is handled as if it is an RPD framework. Much the same as with a pickup cast, the frame is typically fit to the bar on the definitive cast (Fig 14-12d). Once the specific abutment-framework interface is established, the clip is picked up in the mouth and records completed. Processing follows as usual. The specific abutment-framework contact areas are visible and easy to verify due to the specific blockout (Figs 14-12e and 14-12f).

Using this design concept helps to differentiate the treatment planning choice between stud attachments and bar-clips when the typical two-anterior-implant situation exists. Studs are certainly more efficient and less expensive. However, they only work well when the implants are quite parallel and there is at least a reasonable amount of available keratinized tissue to support the prosthesis. The need for a bar-clip is evident when the implants are off-angled or when the need for reduced maintenance frequency is desired (Figs 14-12g and 14-13). Now, with the ability to control lateral forces more predictably than with stud attachments, bars are also indicated when the quality of remaining soft tissue support is poor. This is fairly common in patients

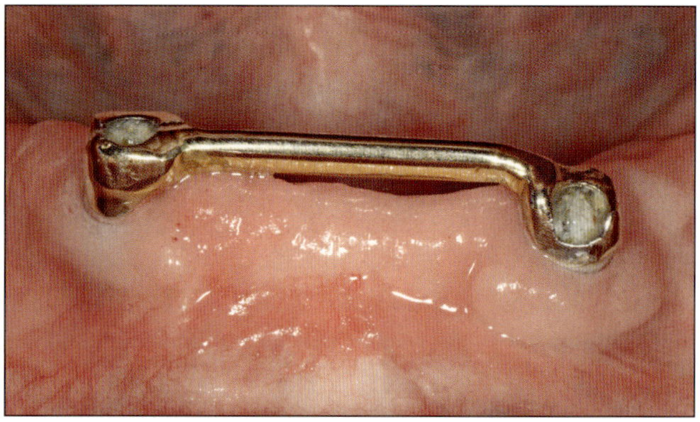

FIG 14-13 Bar on off-angled implants after 12 years of use. The same clip/denture is still in use. The box design allowed rest and guiding plane concepts to be used.

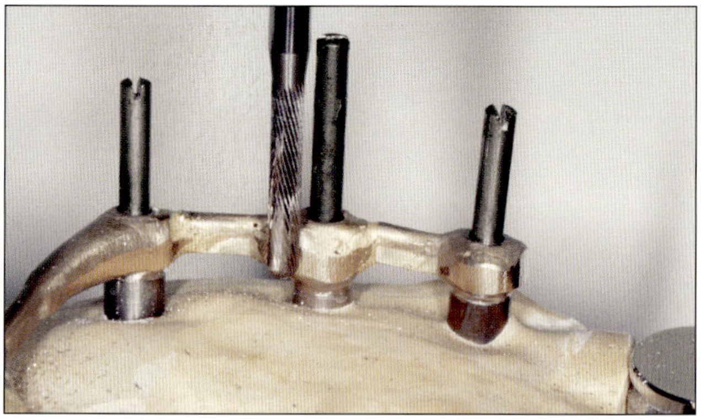

FIG 14-14 A cast bar being milled.[3] Note the Hader clip between the two distal implants.

with combination syndrome (sometimes referred to as *Kelly syndrome*) or those with extensive posterior residual ridge resorption that lose their remaining mandibular anterior teeth. A bar designed to function as a Class I RPD, with both vertical and lateral support, will reduce—although not eliminate—the reliance on soft tissue for support.

Castings for Implant-Supported Overdentures

When anterior and posterior implants are present bilaterally, as in a Class III situation, the term *implant-supported overdenture* is appropriate since the influence of soft tissue support is minimal. With this distribution, support (as previously defined) is provided entirely by the implants. The extensive effort and planning that is necessary for these types of cases requires that all efforts be taken to ensure longevity. Similar to the creation of custom housings for precision attachment partial dentures, castings for implant-supported overdentures are often required due to space. They can take many forms, but their primary purpose of strength remains.

While there are clinicians fabricating implant-supported maxillary overdentures on six or even sometimes four well-distributed stud attachments, the lack of truly reliable splinting of the implants may be a compromise. The best results for this type of prosthesis appear to come from implants joined by a bar. These full-arch bars provide an excellent means of support and stability where the lone-standing stud attachments cannot. There are many different types of attachments that will provide a means of retention. Whatever the exact attachment used, having this type of bar allows the creation of an extensive milled surface area that can in turn be used as a guiding plane surface against which a casting will function.[3]

When the overdenture casting contacts these surfaces, as described fully in earlier chapters, the stability is greatly increased along with the possibility for some frictional retention. Another very obvious advantage of the bar is that the path of insertion of the prosthesis is determined by the milled surfaces, not by the alignment of the implants. The specific shape of the bar depends on the position of the implants and the space available for the denture. The actual form must allow access for hygiene under the bar and around the implant fixtures as well as adequate space above for the cast base, the denture teeth, and sufficient resin to join these components. Great ingenuity is often required to comply with these restrictions (Fig 14-14).[1]

The milling is performed on the lingual side of the bar only. Early attempts with this design milled both sides, but it was found that the milled surfaces were so close together that the fitting of the framework was very difficult. Using guiding surfaces on the lingual only has proven to provide enough surface area to stabilize the completed prosthesis. The labial surface is therefore tapered to around 5 degrees, which also creates more space for the necks of the denture teeth. These bars are now typically milled using CAD/CAM technologies to assure ideal fit and strength. This will require more communication with the laboratory, as the implant-minded technicians designing the bar on the computer are almost always unaware of the concepts discussed here. They also tend to know less about denture contours, which directly relate to the design.

Laboratory processing inserts and housings are placed on the attachments with the bar on the definitive implant-level cast prior to blockout. The blockout is completed around these housings to create spaces in the resultant framework that will allow for the future pickup (Fig 14-15).[3] The fitting

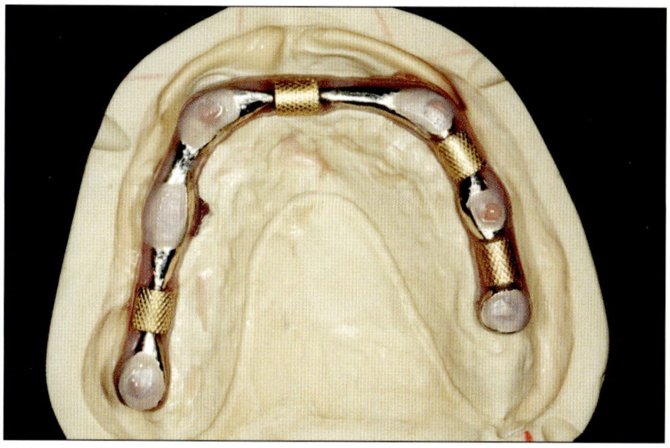

FIG 14-15 Blocked-out bar with housings in place ready for duplication.[3]

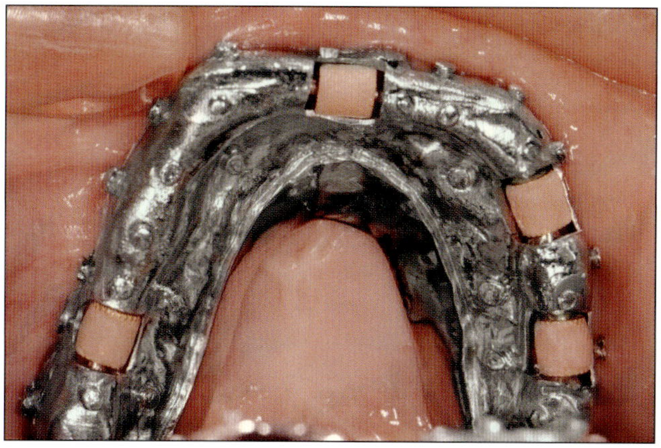

FIG 14-16 Finished casting fit to the mouth with clips on bar and ready for pickup with resin.[3]

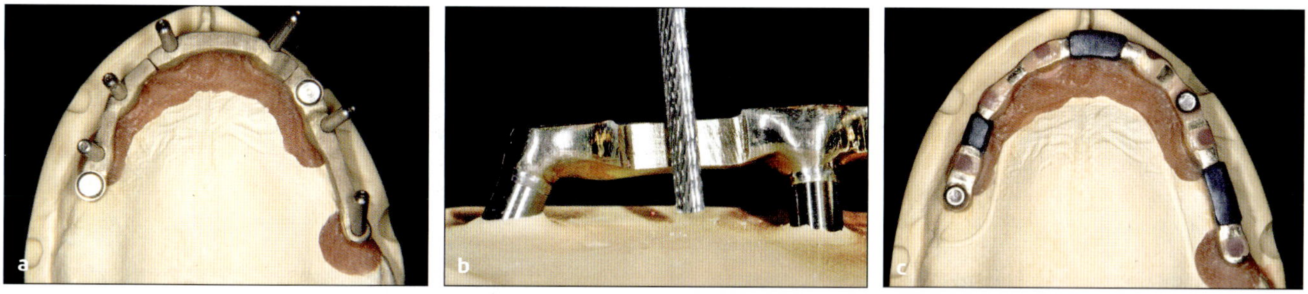

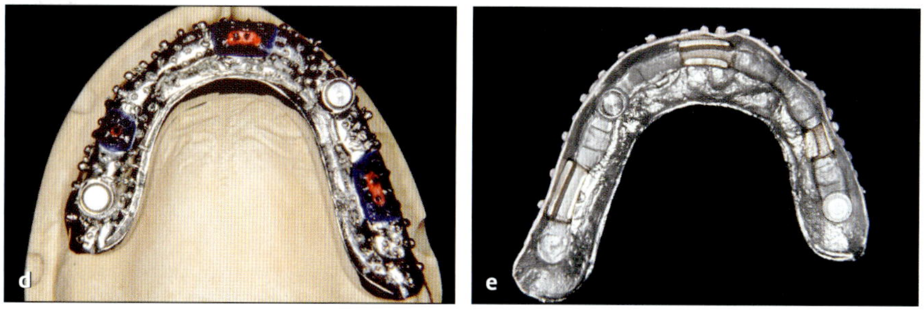

FIG 14-17 *(a)* A cast bar has the ability to reorient the path of insertion when flared implants are present. *(b)* The bar is milled to zero degrees at the lingual guiding plane areas. *(c)* The bar is lightly blocked out to ensure that contact will only occur on guiding plane clips once in position. *(d)* The framework is fit to the cast, showing the final occlusal waxing of guiding plane clips seen in part c. *(e)* The guiding plane clips are cast, fit, and laser welded into position. Note the laser-welded Locator housings.

of the casting can take place on the definitive cast since the only contact with the underlying tissue is through the contact areas adjacent to the clips. The process for fitting the framework is the same as for the RPD, but because of the multiple contact areas, it is most often a frustrating and time-consuming task. The pickup procedure is completed as described in chapter 11. This pickup will always take place in the mouth after the casting has been fitted to its underlying bar assembly (Fig 14-16).[3] It is critical that the pickup resin completely seal off the interface between clip and casting to keep the denture base material from entering the attachment area under the force of packing the resin.

It is typical to only utilize some of the attachments present on the bar. It is common that only two resilient attachments are enough to hold this guiding plane–stabilized prosthesis in position. Despite this, all available attachments should be picked up at the time of fabrication. If needed in the future, the housings are already present, making it a simple matter to add one of the vinyl clips or snaps when it is deemed necessary.

Because of the difficulties experienced in the fitting of the casting to the bar, the bar can be made with only isolated areas of parallelism. The reduced area of parallelism allows the milling to occur on both sides of the bar, which will be contacted by laser-welded gold clips. They will not be retentive attachments but precise guiding planes. These parallel surfaces will provide the highest level of stability and restriction of the path of removal (Fig 14-17). This demonstrates that one is able to design the bar surface with any combination of attachments or guiding planes. As the surface area and distribution of opposing guiding planes increases, the number of required retentive attachments will decrease. Castings stabilized by guiding plane surfaces are sometimes referred to as

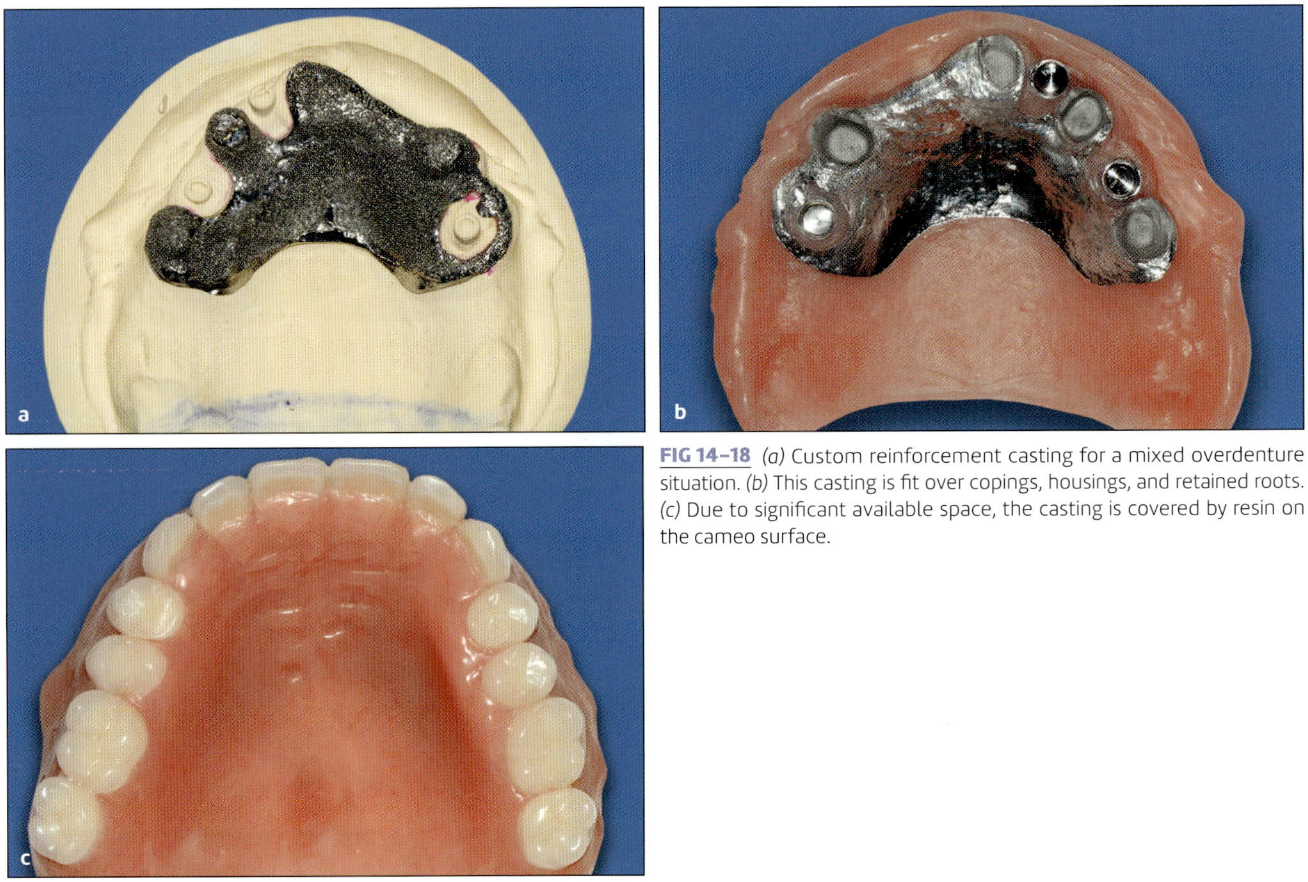

FIG 14-18 *(a)* Custom reinforcement casting for a mixed overdenture situation. *(b)* This casting is fit over copings, housings, and retained roots. *(c)* Due to significant available space, the casting is covered by resin on the cameo surface.

"poor-man's spark erosion" in homage to the more expensive spark-erosion prostheses that use the frictional fit concept.

The basic laboratory steps for blockout, waxing, and fitting of these overdenture castings are the same as described throughout this text. This design has proven to be most effective in that laboratory time has been reduced without loss of stability or frictional retention. The principles shown here should be adaptable to any of the implant overdenture situations that can be expected in the future.

Failed implant cases are an unfortunately common experience, especially for the prosthodontists tasked with the post-failure reconstruction effort. Conversion to some form of implant overdenture is a common management strategy. These cases will be in need of unique and specific castings (Fig 14-18). We have discussed the most common types of castings for edentulous situations. The principles are meant to be customized for the specific situations of unique patients. The various forms and designs are therefore potentially limitless.

References

1. Shor A, Chigurupati K, Goto Y. A denture tooth position index fabricated with light-polymerized acrylic resin. J Prosthet Dent 2003;89:515–527.
2. The Glossary of Prosthodontic Terms: Ninth Edition. J Prosthet Dent 2017;117(5S):e1–e105.
3. Brudvik JS, Chigurupati K. The milled implant bar: An alternative to spark erosion. J Can Dent Assoc 2002;68:485–488.

LESSONS FROM RPD EVOLUTION

15

High cost of alternative treatments, technical improvements, and significant demand have driven RPD innovation.

Note: This chapter is a summary of a previously published article on turning points in RPD history.[1]

Historical biases persist in RPD construction perhaps more than in any other aspect of prosthetic dentistry. Lack of understanding regarding dental disease etiology, absence of appropriate dental materials, and the complex and varied nature of RPD applications were all large obstacles to the logical or sequential development of RPD philosophy. Operator experience, rather than standardized clinical comparison, tended to drive changes in removable partial prosthodontics. In North America, where this textbook originated, the modern everyday result seems to be a design with little philosophical difference from the first one-piece castings described in the early 1920s. This is unfortunate considering that historical design concepts predate key design, material, and philosophical advances in RPDs. Ultimately, due to late discovery of the true etiologic factors for many of the clinical problems associated with partial dentures, well-intentioned design modifications addressed consequences rather than causes. The question exists if this was and continues to be due to the profession's overwhelming desire for efficient and productive treatment strategies or a lack of understanding regarding developments in RPD construction.

Early Developments: The Band, the Clasp, and Sectional Construction

Several excellent review papers describe the early development of RPDs in greater detail.[2–4] Some of the earliest partial prosthetic tooth replacements were carved ivory, stone, or detached tooth crowns that were ligated to adjoining teeth with gold bands or wire ligatures.[3,5,6] According to some, the first recorded description of an RPD was a block of bone carved to fit the mouth in 1711.[7] Terrell discusses similar examples and how early authors were focused primarily on the esthetic rather than functional improvements offered by these prostheses.[5]

Dentistry moved beyond this very crude "carved fit" stage with Fauchard's innovative RPD designs.[8] In 1728, he described and demonstrated the use of a connector. This connector joined the prosthetic teeth together to thereby create a single prosthesis. Fauchard used both a labial and lingual metal bar to achieve rigidity in the prosthesis.[2] Several reviews credit Mouton and Bourdet as the first to describe the use of retentive clasps or wires that would grab onto and hold an abutment tooth.[9,10] By 1810, Gardette of Philadelphia began using wide wrought metal bands wrapped around teeth in an attempt to improve prosthesis retention.[11] Much like current orthodontic bands, these bands completely encircled the tooth and often extended into the gingival sulcus (Fig 15-1). The commonly encountered destruction of marginal gingiva and teeth, due to constant vertical

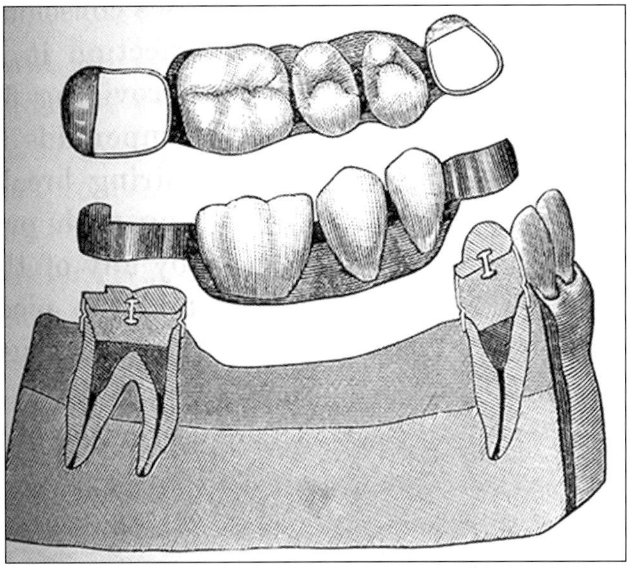

FIG 15-1 A later example of a band-clasp RPD, *Dental Cosmos* (1900).

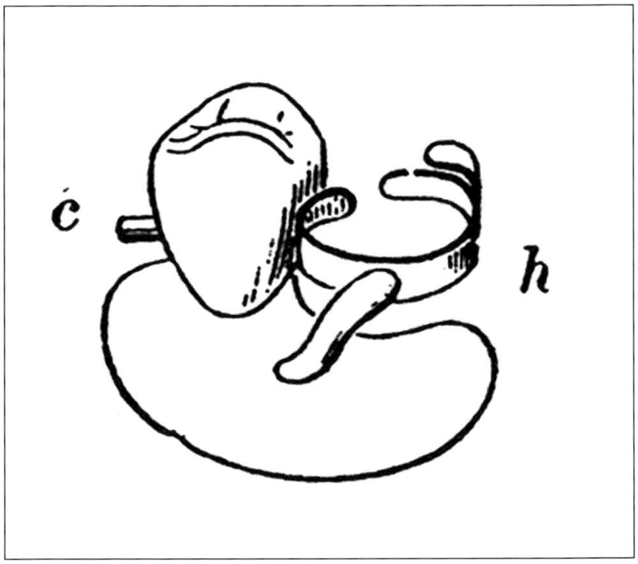

FIG 15-2 Bonwill's depiction of his new clasp design.[14]

movement of the prosthesis, led to the first description of an occlusal rest in 1817.[12] Delabarre described "little spurs" or horizontal extensions onto the occlusal surfaces of teeth. These spurs, now called *rests*, were meant for prevention of excessive vertical settling of the RPD and the resulting gingival or abrasion issues. By 1820, dentistry had already discovered three of the four primary RPD components: the connector, the clasp, and the rest.[2,4]

Little changed until the late 1890s, when Bonwill described the common consequences of RPD use at the time.[13,14] These included movement of the teeth, gross caries, wear of abutment teeth, and the clinician's inability to achieve a well-fitting prosthesis.[13] Bonwill attempted to manage RPD fit by fabricating in pieces prior to joining the parts with solder. An intraoral index or impression of the parts in close proximity to each other was used to relate the pieces. Today this would be called a *pickup impression*. This sectional construction method was dictated by the materials available at the time. The only available impression materials at the turn of the century that were stable enough for use in RPD creation were plaster or compound, both of which are very rigid once set.[15] This limited the clinician's ability to manage unusually shaped or malpositioned teeth. Imagine removing set plaster from someone's mouth as it engages around a lone-standing tooth.

Another obstacle was the inherent limitations of the available prosthetic materials. Acrylic resin would not be used regularly in prosthodontics for several more decades. The various gold, nickel, titanium, or chrome alloys used today did not exist. In fact, precision castings of any material were not available until William Taggart popularized the lost-wax casting technique for dentistry in 1907.[3] Instead, various gauges (diameters) and dimensions of gold wire or plate had to be bent, cut, and/or swaged to create the metal components.[16,17] Having a precise fit or rigid connector was a major challenge with this technique.[2]

Bonwill's main focus was his desire to move away from the use of bands for RPD retention (Fig 15-2).[13,14] The high incidence of gross caries due to food impaction between the imprecisely fit bands and teeth was of obvious concern. Bonwill therefore advocated a change to a retentive mechanism with much less vertical height. He suggested that an arm (soon to be called a *clasp*) be used instead of a large band. Such a dramatic reduction from a band to a clasp arm surface area was possible due to Bonwill's attention to fit, support, and stability of the prosthesis. Bonwill stated that occlusal rests and preparation of the tooth to accept them were absolute necessities.[14] Through clinical experience, Bonwill believed that much of the damage to the tooth and surrounding gingiva was prevented by using rest seats. This routine use of rest seats and attention to an accurate fit reduced the need for the clasp arm to provide support. This was an early example of how improving fit and maximizing tooth support benefited long-term clinical results. With the reduction in band size, Bonwill was able to discuss details regarding clasp flexibility. His statement regarding thickness and length as variables in clasp flexibility foreshadowed modern force management and clasp dimension strategies. Although the band design continued to be used for some time, their frequency faded quickly following the turn of the century.[16,18]

Hunter's Sepsis: A Force for Change

Increased attention brought major advances in RPD technology and construction at the turn of the century. The demand for RPDs was increasing because of major issues with the fixed partial dentures (FPDs) at the time. Turn-of-the-century FPDs suffered from the same material and method shortcomings as RPDs. Bonwill stated that "it requires no skill to whittle a natural crown to a point and slip over it a loose gold crown cap and cement it to fill up a bad fit."[14] The combination of poor retainer fit and weak water-soluble cements encouraged debonding and marginal leakage, followed quickly by decay. These consequences were often irreparable because the remaining retainers held the bridge in place, thus preventing diagnosis of the issue. Even if diagnosed, endodontic understanding and technology was still in its infancy despite the frequent use of posts (Fig 15-3).

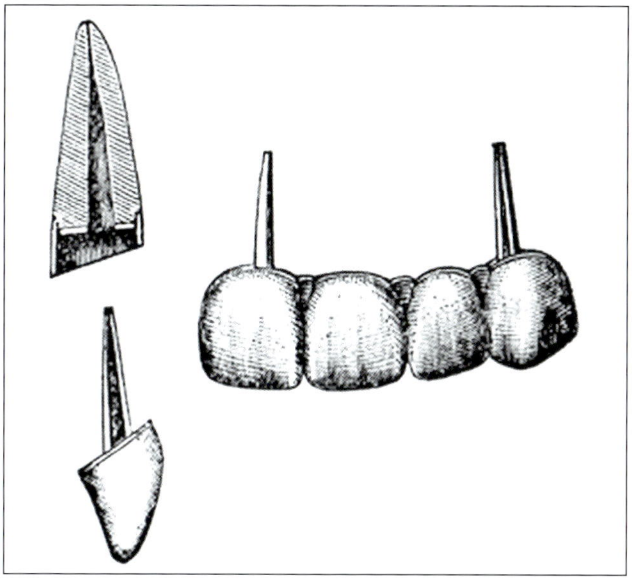

FIG 15-3 A typical prefabricated crown-post system, circa 1908, prior to reliable endodontics.

The inability to remove the FPD for cleaning was seen as the reason for all these problems. Consequences of this poor-quality care became so pervasive that a physician from Britain named William Hunter campaigned against dental practices of his time.[19] Beginning with his 1900 publication, Hunter proposed a causal connection between oral disease and systemic disease.[19] This connection was made after he repeatedly found multiple carious and abscessed teeth present in the mouths of patients with FPDs. His vivid descriptions are direct in their assessment of cause: "The worst cases of anemia, gastritis, colitis, obscure fever of unknown origin, or nervous disturbances of all kinds are those which owe their origin to, or are gravely complicated by, the oral sepsis produced in patients by these gold traps of sepsis."[20] The dental disease that he found was rightly attributed to the aforementioned FPDs, which he termed gold traps of sepsis, mausoleum of gold over a mass of sepsis, or septic dentistry.[20] He attacked the dental profession for its lack of attention to patient oral hygiene and prosthesis cleanability. These harsh attacks from the medical profession had a profound effect on prosthetic dentistry. Clinicians, afraid of being accused of causing "Hunter's sepsis," began focusing their attention on RPDs. The ability to remove and clean the partial denture was supposed to prevent the septic infections caused by FPDs. Indeed, the most prominent dental professionals at that time were strongly in favor of removable over fixed bridgework for this reason.[14,21–23]

The ultimate result of this RPD enthusiasm was significant advancement in its development. Clasp designs evolved quickly. Roach was a leader in infrabulge and wire designs,[21,24–28] while Nesbett was the first to publish on cast clasp arms in 1916.[22] It took a mere 20 years to move from the band clasp to the circumferential cast clasp still used frequently today. Hunter's sepsis was the primary driving force to reduce or minimize clasp size, since this would supposedly improve oral hygiene and reduce plaque retention. Some authors at this time took this idea even further: Several believed in minimal or no clasping.[16,29–31] To accomplish this, and still have a retentive RPD, these authors focused on stability and a precise fit. Using sectional construction, Woodworth believed clasps should merely aid in retention of the well-fitting RPD.[29] By 1915, Chayes was creating complex RPDs using attachments, sometimes referred to as *removable bridgework*.[31] Parallelism of the abutment surfaces and attachment devices were the hallmark of his RPDs. Prothero stated that by using frictional contact between teeth and the RPD, stability is maximized, thus reducing the need for clasps.[30] These authors proved that this design philosophy could improve esthetics, hygiene, and retention. While these designs did exist, they were for society's elite.[32] Very few dentists possessed the clinical or technical expertise to create such prostheses, and few patients could afford to pay the high cost to have one made. In addition, the complexities of these designs meant frequent adjustments, repairs, and often substantial tooth preparation.[33] For these reasons, most dentists in this time period continued to utilize conventional RPDs for their patients.

Because RPDs were being hand-made in sections, with limited material choices, the time and effort to achieve an accurate fit was substantial. Soon after William Taggart introduced the lost-wax technique to dentistry in 1907, this principle was applied to RPDs by Norman B. Nesbett (Fig 15-4).[22] In 1916, he described the technique for casting

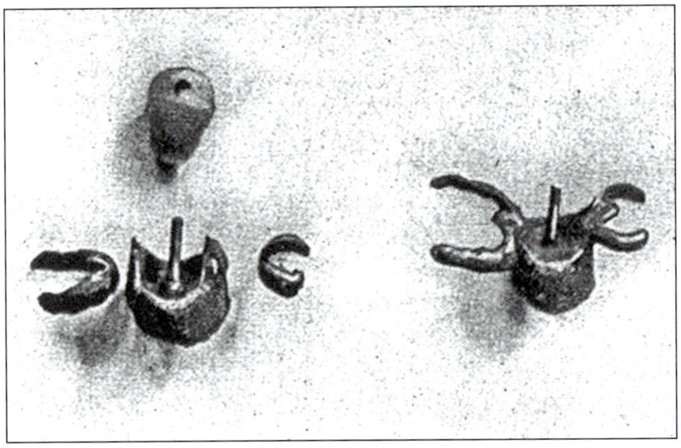

FIG 15-4 Nesbett was using lost wax to create custom-fitting sectionally constructed RPDs by 1916.[22]

clasp assemblies for RPDs. His refinement of the alloy and prosthetic tooth attachment allowed the successful creation of short-spanned well-fitting unilateral RPDs. Nesbett described the "inlay fit" of the clasp assemblies that was attained after assembling the separately cast components on a plaster cast. At that time, casting RPDs in one piece was not done. Nesbett says why: "Under no circumstances should the attempt be made to cast the two clasps and middle section in one piece, for while this can easily be done, no proper fit can be obtained. The warpage and shrinkage of such a large and irregular casting is uncontrollable."[22] This statement is very telling when one considers that it applies to small single-tooth RPD castings.

Rudd preferred to deal with the challenges of RPD fit in the laboratory.[34] To do this, he created a full-arch definitive cast. This was a major feat in the 1920s. Full-arch impressions with plaster were challenging to accurately make, let alone reassemble, after being removed in pieces to preserve the undercuts. In addition, the lack of refined dental stones required the creation of amalgam dies. However, if all went well, the benefit was a large reduction in the amount of chair time since the major fitting procedures occurred without the patient present.[34] The RPD was cast in pieces as normal, but each piece would then be fitted back to the definitive cast. Once fit, the pieces were soldered using an index from the cast rather than the mouth. After assembly, the RPD was again fitted back to the definitive cast. This basic technique sequence would continue to be used after RPD castings were made in one piece.

Access to Care: Akers' One-Piece Casting Technique

The leap into full-arch one-piece RPD castings was officially made by Akers when he published this technique in 1925.[35] The obvious allure was its efficiency. The time savings meant the possibility of offering RPD service to the general public. At the time, Akers was a strong proponent of improving access to quality dental care, and he stated that from an economic standpoint, RPDs made this way could be utilized by the person of average means.[35] Access to care was very much a hot-button issue for dentists in that era. Part of the "Hunter's sepsis" scare included Hunter's observations that those most affected by dental disease and low-quality care seemed to be those of lower socioeconomic status.[20] It is clear these attacks on the profession were taken to heart by many prominent dentists.[36] It appears that Akers' one-piece casting technique was not only a great contribution but a positive response to the issue.

Not everyone was as excited about the one-piece technique as Akers. Indeed, a heated debate as to the quality of these restorations began. As making RPDs in pieces was routine, to change this meant a major change in construction philosophy. In the discussion section following the Akers article, Roach responded by supporting the benefits of sectional construction.[35] Roach argued that full-arch impressions, which were still being made with plaster, were challenging. In addition, it was observed that the shrinkage of the large and often complex castings resulted in poor fit of the prosthesis just as Nesbett had discussed.[22] Three major reasons existed as to why the one-piece casting technique gained almost complete support within a decade. First, the admonishment of fixed bridgework by Hunter was still fresh in people's minds, resulting in great built-up demand for affordable RPDs.[20,36] Authors often encouraged this demand by citing supposed benefits of RPDs, such as positive effects upon underlying bone structure and cleanliness when compared with fixed bridgework.[37] Second, improvements in refractory materials and gold casting alloys continued.[38] This resulted in more reliable materials to manage the technical issues of the fabrication process. Third, the one-piece technique was much easier for the dentist. The many challenges

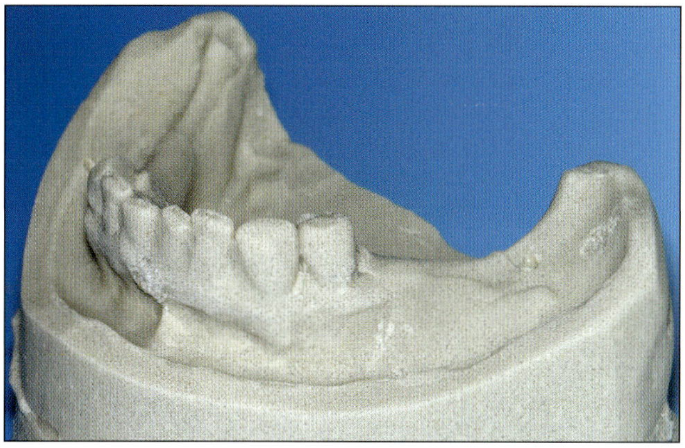

FIG 15-5 Being able to create a reliable, accurate, one-piece refractory cast was a major technologic advancement in the 1920s. Without it, the one-piece casting technique was not possible. Elastomeric impression materials make this process even more efficient than when it was first conceived.

of the sectional technique included multiple sectional impressions with rigid materials, pickup impressions, and soldering. These assembly procedures eventually gave way to the time-saving single impression and one-piece casting (Fig 15-5). Widespread acceptance was evident within a matter of years.[39,40] By 1930, a mere 5 years following the Akers article, even the former opponent Roach was using the one-piece casting technique.[25]

It is interesting to note that the unilateral tooth-bound RPD contributed greatly to the success of the one-piece casting. Schott in particular advocated how the unilateral RPD restoring a solitary bounded space could become practically a fixed bridge.[39] Roach preferred making separate rather than a single RPD when more than one tooth-bound space existed.[41] No doubt the reduced volume of metal resulted in better control over the casting shrinkage. With improved FPD treatment and passing of the Hunter's sepsis scare, the unilateral RPD would slowly lose favor. However, issues such as occasional swallowing of the prosthesis were also to blame.[42] The unilateral RPD restoring a bounded space eventually became an extremely rare treatment.[43] Of recent interest is the advertising by laboratories promoting polyamide materials to create these previously discouraged unilateral prostheses.

Early Standardization: Improved Evaluation of the Clinical Situation

Persistent use of old methodologies and lack of standardization complicated consistent and proper application of the many rapid developments.[23] In an attempt to address this issue, Cummer provided an excellent summary of the theory and practice of partial denture service.[44] In 1922, he discussed the design of RPDs as it related to the four basic components then being used. The terms used are now considered standard: saddle (base), connector, retainer, and occlusal rest.[44] Cummer promoted new force management strategies such as use of an indirect retainer (auxiliary rest), limiting clasps to one on either side of the fulcrum line, and rebasing of the saddle areas when appropriate. He also repeatedly commented on the major clinical challenge of RPD fit management. Of particular interest is his outline regarding the sequence of RPD service. A distinction is made between the four phases: design, construction, insertion, and maintenance. In essence, this article is a predecessor in thought and organization to the RPD textbooks that have followed since. This fact must be considered when evaluating the validity of the principles within these textbooks. For example, when reviewing the second edition of McCracken's textbook, you will find it nearly identical in thought to the 10th edition, despite the passage of nearly 50 years' time.[45] Likewise, if the philosophy from Cummer's 1922 article was the basis of these texts, one is reading and being taught a philosophy of RPDs from the 1920s. The principles typically considered foundational may no longer be valid, now nearly 100 years later, after several areas of significant philosophical and scientific change.

With the RPD having become a much more common treatment, it became apparent that the profession also still lacked a standardized classification system. Lack of agreement regarding what type of clinical situation was being discussed prevented agreement about the principles with which to approach each case. When discussing force management strategies (how an RPD would function when used), authors of the time rarely agreed because they were often promoting or debating strategies that applied to entirely different partially edentulous situations. While several classification systems had been introduced, none had proven simple and applicable on a consistent basis until Edward Kennedy presented his system.[29,44,46] The Kennedy classification system was simple, easy to use, and proved almost universally applicable. As was noted in chapter 3, its main differentiating factor is its ability to quickly and clearly

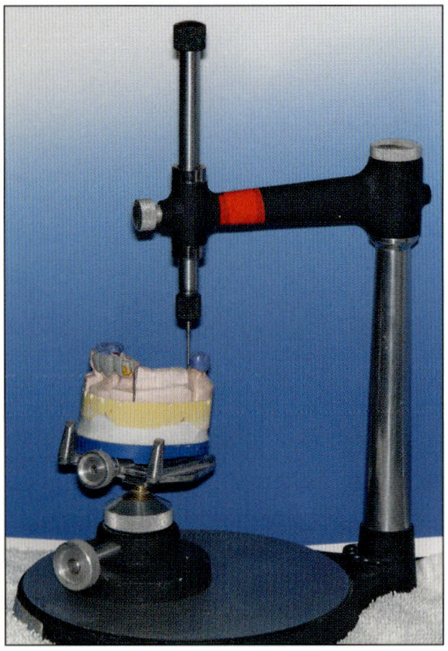

FIG 15-6 Dental surveyors led directly to the development of advanced RPD concepts such as guiding planes.

demonstrate the location of tooth support in relation to edentulous spaces. While not universally accepted for some time, strong established support for this system in both practice and education appeared by 1933.[47] Maintenance of this success is evident in that it is still the dominant partially edentulous classification system used by most popular RPD textbooks in the United States today.[45,48]

Another major advancement for RPDs in the 1920s occurred with the advent of the dental cast surveyor. A surveyor is a paralleling instrument used to locate and delineate the contours and relative positions of abutment teeth and associated structures. Chayes had developed a parallelometer to help guarantee parallel precision attachment alignment, both clinically and in the laboratory.[31] However, it is believed to be Fortunati who was first to demonstrate the advantages of using a mechanical device to map the contours of abutment teeth.[49] In 1921, Weinstein and Roth marketed the first commercially available surveyor.[49] However, its use was not routine until the advent of hydrocolloid impression materials in the 1930s. Dentacol hydrocolloid became available in 1926 and was among the first commercially available elastomeric impression materials. This allowed more accurate full-arch dental casts to be created. Prior to the use of elastic materials, the undercut areas of the teeth were often blocked out, relieved, or lost during impression procedures.[25,35,47] This tended to complicate framework fit due to the lack of control over the height of contour of the abutment tooth. However, by analyzing a dental cast that replicated the actual clinical situation, one is able to determine which area of an abutment tooth might require modification (Fig 15-6). Although descriptions of these line tracings on the teeth occurred prior to this time, the term *height of contour* is credited to Edward Kennedy.[49]

Willis was among the first to describe in writing the technique for dental model surveying.[50] He mentioned that blocking out of "undesirable undercut areas" was not new but that establishing a common vertical plane angle was. He appears to be the first to use the term *path of insertion* for RPDs in relation to a chosen plane. This term references the specific direction in which a prosthesis is placed. The process of surveying allows visualization and blockout of undercuts on the definitive cast prior to creating a refractory, a critical step leading to the RPD framework casting. Willis describes tripoding to record the path of insertion, and along with others, promotes the use of reversible hydrocolloid as the impression material of choice for RPDs.[47,50] This technique allows the dentist to improve two major aspects of treatment. First, the dentist is able to more accurately design the RPD and confirm mouth modifications. This was required for a more scientific debate regarding force management strategies and eventually led to the use of guiding planes as key features of RPDs.[1,31,51] Second, using a surveyor further incorporates the dental laboratory into the RPD construction process. After the dentist records the path of insertion and then designates a design, the remaining laboratory procedures may be delegated to the laboratory. The basic technique sequence described by Willis in 1935 continues to be used in almost identical fashion for the majority of RPDs made today. Soon after, most prominent authors were using surveyors from the diagnostic stages on.[52]

Consequences of Efficiency: Challenges with Framework Fit

With further refinement of the one-piece casting technique, demand for this method continued to grow.[40] Dental laboratories had quickly become a common and indispensable part of RPD therapy. Dentists, who due to the nature of the sectional construction technique had previously completed all framework fabrication steps in-office, now began delegating this step.[53] The difficulties in mastering the new and ever-developing process of creating a refractory cast, patterning a wax framework, investing, and casting was time-consuming for the average dentist.[34,54] The time savings of delegating this process allowed the dentist to treat greater numbers of patients, thus improving access to RPD treatment. In response to this, the number of dental laboratories began to increase. Unfortunately, in many cases the laboratory was soon given the task of designing the RPD without being aware of the clinical situation.[55,56] The resulting designs were not based upon biologically sound philosophies and often violated the few principles adopted by that time.[47]

Even with the addition of the surveyor, the fit of the framework continued to be a major issue due to the inherent shrinkage of the large castings.[22,44,57] Despite improvements in refractory materials and duplication techniques, the expansion and contraction of materials was not perfected.[38] To make matters worse, handling of the casting often compounded the misfit.[57,58] By accepting the task of framework creation, laboratories were often making decisions regarding elimination of undesirable undercuts on the cast by blockout. Blockout in this context was typically the application of wax to the cast so that the metal casting would not bind or be held up by areas that had been cast into an undercut. Extra blockout meant a greater likelihood of the framework easily seating to place in the mouth due to fewer tooth-frame contacts. However, it also meant reduced stabilization or tooth contact. The lack of knowledge most dentists had regarding the framework creation process and how this could handicap their ability to address fit issues was being mentioned as early as 1931.[56] Further control over framework fit was lost when laboratories polished all surfaces of the casting in order to maximize cleanliness.[40] Nesbett, the original author of cast clasps, recommended polishing of all metal surfaces.[22] This polishing altered the tooth-contacting surfaces more still.[58] Addressing this issue, Chappelle proposed fitting the casting as cast. He points out that laboratory-fabricated RPDs were "usually polished to the extreme," and to save time, they were ground with coarse-grit stones and polished with fast-cutting abrasives, further compromising accurate contact.[58]

The end result of these uncontrolled aspects of laboratory procedures was an RPD that did not necessarily fit as it was intended to. Authors such as McLean pointed out that "resilience of the Roach bars and the tolerance of the mucosa cloak the misfit of the average one-piece casting, but they do not eradicate it."[57] Cummer stated that the major clinical challenge in RPD construction was the maintenance of accuracy.[44] It is interesting then how the vast majority of authors in the 1930s, 1940s, and 1950s debate various methods of force transmission, stress distribution, and design, while the RPD frameworks in general use often lacked precise fit as discussed above.[28,41,59–63]

Even frameworks that did fit well had some concerns. By the 1930s, rigidity of the framework was an established principle.[29,58,59,64] However, rigidity of the major connectors was not universally achieved.[2,59] While the comparatively soft gold alloys used at the time did lend themselves to fitting procedures since they would show "facets" on prematurities, they were also known to flex or even permanently distort under enough force. The size of major connectors and continued use of stock wire bars for bar-type connectors was also to blame.[2,59] In these instances, RPD philosophies dependent upon rigidity could be questioned.

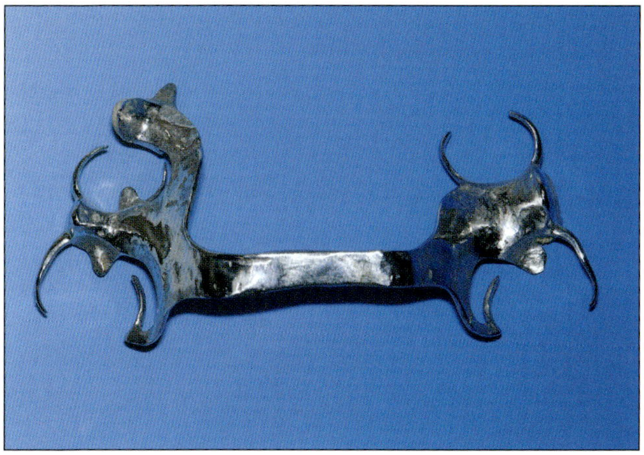

FIG 15-7 An example of a clasp-first mentality with all of its aforementioned negative effects.

Clasp-First Mentality: Complicating Design Philosophy

In an attempt to deal with these issues, clinicians tended to add multiple clasp arms to the RPD design (Fig 15-7). This generally was done under the premise of preventing abutment tooth drifting or to improve support, stability, or retention. The ill-fitting RPDs made at the time placed uncontrolled forces upon the abutment teeth, thus encouraging them to move away from the partial denture.[25,58] The band retainers that had been used at the turn of the century hid this consequence of misfit by encircling the clinical crown of the abutment tooth. With the advent of modern clasp arms, encirclement was no longer inherent to the design. The immediate solution to this tooth displacement problem was to encircle each abutment tooth with a second clasp arm on the opposite side of the tooth as the retentive arm in order to prevent its migration.[25,44,58] Roach, who is among the first to describe reciprocation, was aware that most retentive clasps were actively exerting force on the abutment teeth.[25,41] The need for encirclement is still more evident considering that some authors encouraged the placement of an active force upon the tooth by the clasp.[26,53,64] The profession seemed to persist in using retentive clasps with active pressure, believing that this kept the RPD in place. In 1935, Willis said the old idea of gripping a tooth with a clasp for retention has been so impressed on our minds that it is difficult to forget.[50]

In addition to reciprocation, it was believed that additional clasps and encirclement would improve the RPD's lateral stability in function.[2] According to Roach, these additional clasp arms also improved support for the RPD.[25] Of more obvious consequence to novice clinicians was the retentiveness of the prosthesis. To avoid patient complaints, or to achieve what they felt was the primary goal of the RPD, designs often included numerous retentive clasps. While the result was often a retentive partial denture, it was most likely not a well-fitting one. In fact, additional clasps only made RPD frameworks more complicated, which made them more difficult to fabricate and less likely to fit. Certainly, the numerous clasps added to the oral hygiene maintenance challenges that some associated with RPD components. Woodworth noted these trends and stated that clasps have been misused through expecting them to do too much, noting that they will hold the RPD in place when it really does not fit.[29]

By accepting the chronic poor fit of the RPD frameworks amidst the challenge of shared tooth and tissue support, dentists were constantly faced with what they felt were the consequences of RPD use in general. Dentists soon began blaming the RPD for destruction of the supporting periodontal tissues. With the major etiologic factors of dental disease still not clearly determined, a period of great debate raged about how to manage the forces placed upon abutment teeth. As demonstrated in this review, the heightened importance of laboratory science reinforced the belief that an engineering solution existed to this issue.[65] The ingenious use of stress breakers is one example of the profession's attempt to solve the clinical challenge of combined tooth and tissue support through engineering.[32–34,58,66,67] Unfortunately, few RPD authors focused on the etiology of the disease causing the dental destruction.[68] It was not until the 1950s with the advent of published research that some of these clinical debates were resolved with an evidence-based approach. By this time, poor clinical results and dramatic improvements in fixed prosthodontics combined to greatly reduce the level of respect for the RPD both by the public and within the profession.[69,70]

A Lost Battle for Respect: 1960s to Present

It is unfortunate that the negative attitude toward RPDs continues. This negative perception is felt from both dentists and patients. After tremendous amounts of extremely valuable evidence was published in the late 1960s through the 1980s, each passing decade seems to find less high-quality published research on RPDs. With time, it appears that the average practitioner understands less of the RPD framework creation process than previous generations.[56,71] A trend was noticed in U.S. dental school curricula in the 1980s, where time spent on removable prosthodontic education was reduced.[72] This trend continued into the 2000s and 2010s. Likewise, in continuing education, which is a good barometer of what clinical dentists are interested in, it is currently extremely rare to find independent evidence-based lecturers discussing RPDs. The effort and attention of the profession is clearly directed toward fixed prosthodontic efforts. While conventional fixed prosthodontics became Treatment Plan A by the 1960s, it is dental implantology that is now thought of as Treatment Plan A for an even larger number of clinical situations. One need only listen to advertising about dental implants or conduct an internet search on missing teeth to discover preferences of the public. The generalization of the concept that RPDs are inferior to other treatment alternatives is unfortunate since it blinds providers and patients to the numerous situations where RPDs can and should be the preferred treatment choice. It also tends to change how a provider approaches the treatment, often resulting in decisions meant to reduce time or money spent on care.[73–77] In the face of this pervasive negative perception, one should not be surprised that clinical analyses of noninstitutionalized treatment in the United States demonstrate a high frequency of defects. A past review of the National Health and National Examination Survey (NHANES III) evaluated 7,374 persons of whom 1,306 (18%) were using an RPD.[78,79] A mere 36% of RPDs were free of defects. Frank et al and colleagues from the University of Washington studied whether RPDs made in community practices met the standards of design and fabrication.[80] More than half (43/82) of the RPDs met four or fewer standards. Previous to this study, Frank et al conducted a survey of patients in the same dental plan and metropolitan area.[81] Only 40.3% of the patients were completely satisfied with their distal extension RPD.

The reality is that the demand for RPDs is likely to remain high for the foreseeable future. Over 90 years ago, Hillyer pointed out that as the edentulous conditions decrease, the partially edentulous will increase.[18] More recent investigations have analyzed trends in demand for prosthodontics in the United States and tend to support this idea.[82,83] Despite decreasing rates of tooth loss, the need for removable prosthodontic treatment remains high.[78,84,85] It appears that a consequence of the profession's improved preventive measures has been an increase in the number of patients who require partial prosthodontic treatment.[86] Likewise, an aging population retaining more teeth results in an increased number of teeth at risk for disease. Joshi et al and Manski et al have evaluated some of the aspects of the "more teeth more disease" hypothesis.[87,88] Fixed prosthodontic treatment modalities used to treat partial edentulism, such as dental implants, also happen to be the most expensive. This and other issues continue to limit their availability to middle and lower socioeconomic groups in whom the highest rates of tooth loss occur.[89–91] It should not be a surprise then that conventional removable prosthodontic treatment modalities continue to outnumber implant tooth replacements in general practice.[92] Further evidence in contrast to the negative attitude toward the RPD is the numerous studies revealing high rates of long-term success. As discussed throughout this text, modern RPD philosophy compares favorably with the much more expensive and often risk-involved procedures thought of as Treatment Plan A. Current and future dentists should therefore welcome this modern advanced approach. The etiology-based strategies will improve long-term outcomes, while the modern design philosophy will simplify the technical aspects, reducing the time spent to provide care to this debilitated patient group.

Conclusion

Key turning points in RPD philosophy included Bonwill's band-free RPD design, the Hunter's sepsis scare, Akers' one-piece casting technique, and the ramifications of the one-piece technique's application. The driving force behind these events appears to have been technologic improvements, high cost of alternative methods of tooth replacement, and high demand for RPDs. Unfortunately, other than material improvements or digitization, RPD framework fabrication and management within the United States remains basically the same as the mid 1930s. Due to these facts, it should not be surprising that modern RPD framework fit continues to be less than ideal.[93–98] Perhaps more importantly, RPD philosophy as practiced by the average dentist struggles to move beyond that which was established by the 1930s. The need for a modernized approach to RPD therapy is evident. Our hope as authors is that a modern presentation of what dentistry has learned about advanced RPDs over the past decades will increase the profession's attention to this neglected yet critical treatment modality.

References

1. Waliszewski MP. Turning points in removable partial denture philosophy. J Prosthodont 2010;19:571–579.
2. Giradot RL. History and development of partial denture design. J Am Dent Assoc 1941;28:1399–1408.
3. Tylman SD. Theory and Practice of Crown and Bridge Prosthodontics, ed 5. St Louis: Mosby, 1965:21–34.
4. Becker CM, Kaiser DA, Goldfogel MH. Evolution of removable partial denture design. J Prosthodont 1994;3:158–166.
5. Terrell WH. Use of partial dentures as an integral part of mouth reconstruction. J Am Dent Assoc 1933;21:240–248.
6. Kerr JG, Rogers LW. Chinese dentistry. Dent Cosmos 1877;19:385.
7. Altdorf (Heister description). De dentium dolore. Paris, France, 1718:618.
8. Fauchard P. Le Chirurgien Dentiste. Paris, France, 1728.
9. Mouton C. Essay d'odontotechnique, ou dissertation sur les dents artificielles. Paris, France, 1746:89.
10. Bourdet E. Recherches et observations sur toutes les parties de l'art du dentist, Vol 11. Paris, France, 1757.
11. Gardette J. New series. Am J Dent Sci 1850–51;1:375–382.
12. Delabarre CF. Discours d'ouverture d'un cours de medicine dentaire. Paris, France, 1817:390.
13. Bonwill WGA. New method of clasped plates versus movable or unmovable bridge-work. Int Dent J 1893;14:86–96.
14. Bonwill WGA. New methods of clasping artificial dentures to human teeth without injury versus immovable bridges. Dent Items Interest 1899;617–643.
15. Nichols IG. Prosthetic Dentistry: An Encyclopedia of Full and Partial Denture Prosthesis. St Louis: Mosby, 1930:567–575.
16. Southwell C. Removable bar fixture. Dental Cosmos 1904;46:542.
17. Pennington JA. Removable bridges with gold inlay abutments and saddle and vulcanite attachment. Dent Cosmos 1907;49:154–158.
18. Hillyer E. The retention of partial dentures. Dent Cosmos 1915;57:1019–1022.
19. Hunter W. Oral sepsis as a cause of disease. Br Med J 900;2:215–216.
20. Hunter W. The role of sepsis and antisepsis in medicine. Dent Brief 1911;16:850–862.
21. Roach FE. Double bow clasp. Dent Rev 1913;27:1007–1013.
22. Nesbett NB. Cast clasp in removable bridgework. Dent Items Interest 1916;38:581.
23. Beach JW. Removable hygienic bridge work and partial dentures. Dent Cosmos 1917;59:1225–1227.
24. Henrichsen SA. Ball clasps for partial dentures. Zahnaerztl Orthopaed U Prothese 1914. (Review in Dent Cosmos 1914;56:1194–1195.)
25. Roach FE. Principles and essentials of bar clasp partial dentures. J Am Dent Assoc 1930;17:124–138.
26. Stone ER. Tripping action of bar clasps. Dent Cosmos 1932;74:960.
27. DeVan MM. Embrasure saddle clasp—Principle and design. J Am Dent Assoc 1935;22:1352.
28. Stone ER. Tripping action of bar clasps. J Am Dent Assoc 1936;23:596–617.
29. Woodworth JG. Cast, continuous, lingual-clasp removable bridge work. Dent Cosmos 1922;64:290–300.
30. Prothero JH. Prosthetic Dentistry, ed 2. Chicago: Medico-Dental, 1916:247–250.
31. Chayes HES. A broad consideration of the principles involved in fixed and removable bridge work. Dent Cosmos 1915;57:783–790.
32. McLean DW. Stabilization of partial dentures. J Am Dent Assoc 1936;23:545–553.
33. Doskow S. The partial denture and its retention. Dent Cosmos 1923;65:242–247.
34. Rudd MB. Construction of partial dentures by an indirect method. Dent Cosmos 1923;65:1159–1169.
35. Akers PE. A new and simplified method of partial denture prosthesis. J Am Dent Assoc 1925;12:711–717.
36. Editorial. A renaissance in prosthodontia. Dent Items Interest 1916;38:864–867.
37. Weaver SM. Comparison of bone structure under movable and non-movable restorations. Dent Cosmos 1928;70:303–305.
38. Sweeney WT. Cristobalite for dental investment. J Am Dent Assoc 1933;21:108–119.
39. Schott CH. One piece cast removable appliances. J Am Dent Assoc 1928;15:1299–1310.
40. Bondy RM. Justification of the cast-clasp in partial denture restorations. Dent Cosmos 1928;70:310–313.
41. Roach FE. Mouth survey and design of partial dentures. J Am Dent Assoc 1934;21:1166–1176.
42. Hogan WJ. Swallowing of removable bridge: Report of case. Dent Digest 1935;41:301.
43. Owall BE, Taylor RL. A survey of dentitions and removable partial dentures constructed for patients in North America. J Prosthet Dent 1989;61:465–470.
44. Cummer WE. An outline of the theory and practice of partial denture service. J Am Dent Assoc 1922;9:735–754.
45. McGivney GP, Carr AB. McCracken's Removable Partial Prosthodontics, ed 10. St Louis: Mosby, 2000.
46. Kennedy E. Partial denture construction. Dent Items Interest 1928:2–8, 230–231.

47. Pasadena Prosthetic Study Club. A study in partial denture construction. J Am Dent Assoc 1933;20:598–614.
48. Phoenix RD, Cagna DR, DeFreest CF. Stewart's Clinical Removable Partial Prosthodontics, ed 4. Chicago: Quintessence, 2008:8–17.
49. Engelmeier RL. The history and development of the dental surveyor: Part I. J Prosthodont 2002;11:11–18.
50. Willis NG. Dental model surveying. Dent Digest 1935;41:222–228.
51. Tench RW. Fundamentals of partial denture design. J Am Dent Assoc 1936;23:1087–1092.
52. Applegate OC. Use of the paralleling surveyor in modern partial denture construction. J Am Dent Assoc 1940;27:1397–1407.
53. Sayre LD. Partial denture work. Dent Cosmos 1931;73:383–390.
54. Cummer WE. Supplementary notes on "impressions in partial denture service." Dent Cosmos 1929;71:58–66.
55. Roth GL. Tissue support in partial denture construction. Dent Cosmos 1929;71:25–27.
56. Van Minden F. Fitting, placing, and maintenance of cast partial dentures. J Am Dent Assoc 1931;18:442–449.
57. McLean DW. Factors of partial denture success or failure. Dent Cosmos 1935;77:256–263.
58. Chappelle W. Partial denture design. Dent Cosmos 1934;76:183–193.
59. Schuyler CH. Stress distribution as the prime requisite to the success of a partial denture. J Am Dent Assoc 1933;20:2148–2154.
60. Granger ER. Mechanical principles applied to partial denture construction. J Am Dent Assoc 1941;28:1943-1951.
61. Van Minden F. Ideal stressbreaking for partial dentures. J Am Dent Assoc 1943;30:657–669.
62. Neurohr FA. Health conservation of the periodontal tissues by a method of functional partial denture design. J Am Dent Assoc 1944;31:59–70.
63. Steffel VL. Simplified clasp partial dentures designed for maximum function. J Am Dent Assoc 1945;32:1093–1100.
64. Elliot FC. A method that simplifies the design of partial dentures. J Am Dent Assoc 1940;27:1263–1268.
65. Little AP. Partial denture construction from an engineering point of view, based upon the physiologic requirements. J Am Dent Assoc 1928:15:69–74.
66. McAfee SH. The essentials in avoiding trauma to clasped teeth with partial denture appliances, including a form of hand-made joint. J Am Dent Assoc 1928;15:127–133.
67. Neurohr FG. The spring lock dental restoration and the distal extension bridge designed upon this principle. J Am Dent Assoc 1933;21:788–803.
68. Wilson GW. Some common causes of failure in partial denture service. J Am Dent Assoc 1933;21:287–292.
69. Steffel VL. Fundamental principles involved in partial denture design. J Am Dent Assoc 1951;42:534–544.
70. Devan MM. The nature of the partial denture foundation: Suggestions for its preservation. J Prosthet Dent 1952;2:210–218.
71. Lynch CD, Allen PF. Why do dentists struggle with removable partial denture design? An assessment of financial and educational issues. Br Dent J 2006;200:277–281.
72. Taylor TD, Aquilino SA, Matthews AC, Logan NS. Prosthodontic survey. Part II: Removable prosthodontic curriculum survey. J Prosthet Dent 1984;52:747–749.
73. Radhi A, Lynch CD, Hanningan A. Quality of written communication and master impressions for fabrication of removable partial prostheses in the Kingdom of Bahrain. J Oral Rehabil 2007;34:153–7.
74. Schwarz W, Barsby M. A survey of the practice of partial denture prosthetics in the United Kingdom. J Dent 1980;8:95–101.
75. Taylor TD, Matthews AC, Aquilino SA, Logan NS. Prosthodontic survey. Part I: Removable prosthodontic laboratory survey. J Prosthet Dent 1984;52:598–601.
76. Cotmore JM, Mingledorf EB Pomerantz JM, et al. Removable partial denture survey: Clinical practice today. J Prosthet Dent 1983;49:321–327.
77. Hardy F, Stuart LM. A critique of materials submitted by dentists to dental laboratories for the fabrication of removable partial dentures. Quintessence Dent Technol 1983;7:93–95.
78. Redford M, Drury TF, Kingman A, et al. Denture use and the technical quality of dental prostheses among persons 18–74 years of age: United States, 1988–1991. J Dent Res 1996;75(Spec Iss):714–725.
79. Hummel SK, Wilson MA, Marker VA, Nunn ME. Quality of removable partial dentures worn by the adult U.S. population. J Prosthet Dent 2002;88:37–43
80. Frank RP, Brudvik JS, Leroux B, Milgrom P, Hawkins N. Relationship between the standards of removable partial denture construction, clinical acceptability, and patient satisfaction. J Prosthet Dent 2000;83:521–527.
81. Frank RP, Milgrom P, Leroux BG, Hawkins N. Treatment outcomes with mandibular removable partial dentures: A population-based study of patient satisfaction. J Prosthet Dent 1998;80:36–45.
82. Douglas CW, Watson AJ. Future needs for fixed and removable partial dentures in the United States. J Prosthet Dent 2002;87:9–14.
83. Marcus SE, Drury TF, Brown LJ, et al. Tooth retention and tooth loss in the permanent dentition of adults: United States, 1988–1991. J Dent Res 1996;75(Spec Iss):684–695.
84. Ettinger RL, Beck JD, Jakobsen J. Removable prosthodontic treatment needs: A survey. J Prosthet Dent 1984;51:419–427.
85. Hunt RJ, Srisilapanan P, Beck JD. Denture-related problems and prosthodontic treatment needs in the elderly. Gerodontics 1985;1:226–230.
86. Harvey WL, Hoffman WM. Ten-year study of trends in removable prosthodontic service. J Prosthet Dent 1989;62:644–666.
87. Joshi A, Douglas CW, Feldman H, et al. Consequences of success: Do more teeth translate into more disease and utilization? J Public Health Dent 1996;56:190–197.
88. Manski RJ, Moeller JF, Maas WR. Dental services: An analysis of utilization over 20 years. J Am Dent Assoc 2001;132:655–664.
89. Burt BA, Ismail AI, Morrison EC, et al. Risk factors for tooth loss over a 28-year period. J Dent Res 1990;69:1126–1130.
90. Eklund SA, Burt BA. Risk factors for total tooth loss in the United States; longitudinal analysis of national data. J Public Health Dent 1994;54:5–14.
91. Dolan TA, Gilbert GH, Duncan RP, et al. Risk indicators of edentulism, partial tooth loss, and prosthetic status among black and white middle-aged older adults. Comm Dent Oral Epidemiol 2001;29:329–340.
92. Janus CE, Hunt RJ, Unger JW. Survey of prosthodontic service provided by general dentists in Virginia. J Prosthet Dent 2007;97:287–291.
93. Stern MA, Brudvik JS, Frank RP. Clinical evaluation of removable partial denture rest seat adaptation. J Prosthet Dent 1985;53:658–662.
94. Dunham D, Brudvik JS, Morris WJ, et al. A clinical investigation of fit of removable partial dental prosthesis clasp assemblies. J Prosthet Dent 2006;95:323–326.
95. Frank RP, Brudvik JS, Leroux B, et al. Relationship between the standards of removable partial denture construction, clinical acceptability, and patient satisfaction. J Prosthet Dent 2000;83:521–527.
96. Firtell DN, Muncheryan AM, Green AJ. Laboratory accuracy in casting removable partial denture frameworks. J Prosthet Dent 1985;54:856–862.
97. Brudvik JS, Reimers D. The tooth-removable partial denture interface. J Prosthet Dent 1992;68:924–927.
98. Keltjens HM, Mulder J, Kayser AF, et al. Fit of direct retainers in removable partial dentures after 8 years of use. J Oral Rehabil 1997;24:138–142.

INDEX

Page numbers followed by "t" denote tables; "f" denote figures; and "b" denote boxes.